W0112659

Colposcopy

Practice and Atlas

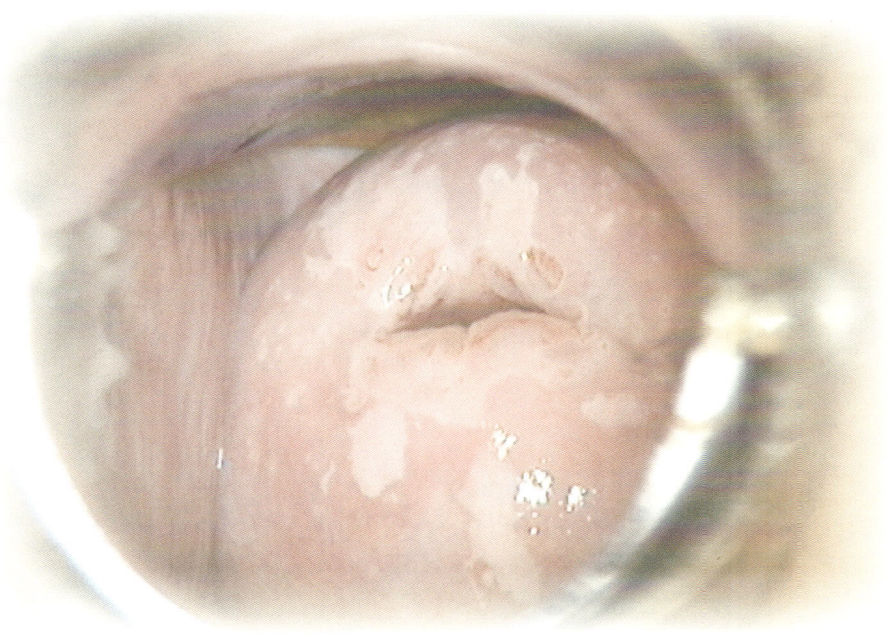

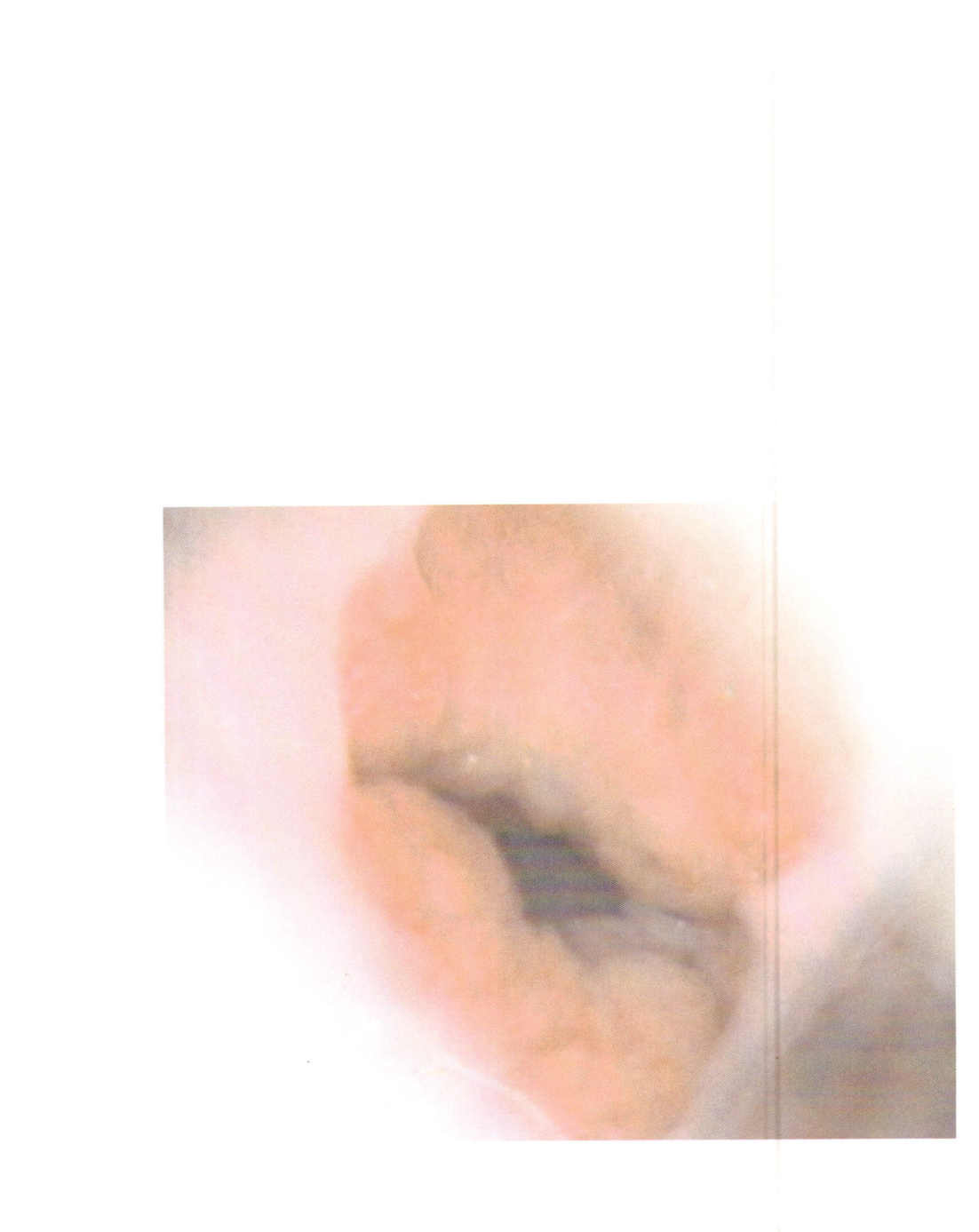

Colposcopy

Practice and Atlas

Aruna Batra

Consultant and Head
Department of Gynecology and Obstetrics
Vardhman Mahavir Medical College and
Safdarjung Hospital, New Delhi

Sudha Nigam

Consultant Gynecologist and Colposcopist
Lucknow Cancer Institute, Lucknow

S K Das

Consultant Gynecologic Oncologist
Action Cancer Institute, New Delhi

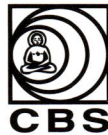

CBS

CBS Publishers & Distributors Pvt Ltd

New Delhi • Bengaluru • Chennai • Kochi • Mumbai • Pune
Hyderabad • Kolkata • Nagpur • Patna • Vijayawada

Disclaimer

Science and technology are constantly changing fields. New research and experience broaden the scope of information and knowledge. The authors have tried their best in giving information available to them while preparing the material for this book. Although all efforts have been made to ensure optimum accuracy of the material, yet it is quite possible some errors might have been left uncorrected. The publisher, the printer and the authors will not be held responsible for any inadvertent errors, omissions or inaccuracies.

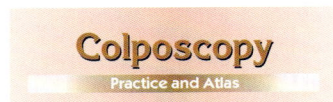

Colposcopy
Practice and Atlas

ISBN: 978-81-239-2403-8

Copyright © Authors and Publishers

First Edition: 2014

All rights reserved. No part of this book may be reproduced or transmitted in any form or by any means, electronic or mechanical, including photocopying, recording, or any information storage and retrieval system without permission, in writing, from the authors, and the publishers.

Published by Satish Kumar Jain for
CBS Publishers & Distributors Pvt Ltd
4819/XI Prahlad Street, 24 Ansari Road, Daryaganj, New Delhi 110 002, India.
Ph: 23289259, 23266861, 23266867   Fax: 011-23243014   Website: www.cbspd.com
                                                                                    e-mail: delhi@cbspd.com; cbspubs@airtelmail.in.
Corporate Office: 204 FIE, Industrial Area, Patparganj, Delhi 110 092
Ph: 4934 4934   Fax: 4934 4935   e-mail: publishing@cbspd.com; publicity@cbspd.com

Branches

- **Bengaluru:** Seema House 2975, 17th Cross, K.R. Road,
  Banasankari 2nd Stage, Bengaluru 560 070, Karnataka
  Ph: +91-80-26771678/79   Fax: +91-80-26771680   e-mail: bangalore@cbspd.com
- **Chennai:** 20, West Park Road, Shenoy Nagar, Chennai 600 030, Tamil Nadu
  Ph: +91-44-26260666, 26208620   Fax: +91-44-42032115   e-mail: chennai@cbspd.com
- **Kochi:** 36/14 Kalluvilakam, Lissie Hospital Road, Kochi 682 018, Kerala
  Ph: +91-484-4059061-65   Fax: +91-484-4059065   e-mail: kochi@cbspd.com
- **Mumbai:** 83-C, Dr E Moses Road, Worli, Mumbai-400018, Maharashtra
  Ph: +91-9833017933   e-mail: mumbai@cbspd.com
- **Pune:** Bhuruk Prestige, Sr. No. 52/12/2+1+3/2 Narhe, Haveli
  (Near Katraj-Dehu Road Bypass), Pune 411 041, Maharashtra
  Ph: +91-20-64704058, 64704059, 32392277 Fax: +91-20-24300160   e-mail: pune@cbspd.com

Representatives

- **Hyderabad**   0-9885175004   • **Kolkata**   0-9831437309, 0-9051152362
- **Nagpur**   0-9021734563   • **Patna**   0-9334159340   • **Vijayawada**   0-9000660880

Printed at Manipal Technologies Ltd., Manipal

to

---

the un-manifest supreme substratum of universe,
the conscient energy, without whose grace and blessings
it would not have been
possible to complete this work

Foreword

Every two minutes one woman dies from cervical cancer, the disease which can be prevented. Knowing this, it is our professional and human duty to do all we can to prevent cervical cancer. Increasing awareness and knowledge about cervical cancer among women and decision-making politicians is a very important part of this process. Equally important is to work on education of medical professionals. They have to be informed about recent advances in the field and to be able to apply them in the practice.

Colposcopy is an essential triage method for the management of women with abnormal cytology. It allows identification, localization and delineation of preinvasive lesions of the cervix and directs the biopsy site. It must be performed prior to any treatment of cervical pre-cancer because it helps planning the extent of the procedure and choosing the method that should be used.

Colposcopy requires long-term experience to acquire an expertize in colposcopic pattern recognition. It should never be forgotten that the primary goal of the colposcopist is to ensure that the invasive disease is not missed. This goal can be achieved only if colposcopy is performed by trained and experienced colposcopists, who audit their work and keep their colposcopic assessment and colposcopically directed treatment with internationally agreed standards.

The book *Colposcopy: Practice and Atlas* is a comprehensive and practical guide to colposcopic practice. This book covers all aspects of early detection of cervical cancer, from technique and equipment for colposcopy to very sophisticated discussion about the most challenging problems of modern lower genital system pathology.

The authors, Dr Aruna Batra, Dr Sudha Nigam and Dr SK Das, are brilliant professionals, who are not only well recognized experts in colposcopy but also sincerely dedicated to share their knowledge. Their long-term teaching practice in colposcopy is condensed in this book.

Good colposcopy requires the knowledge about histology and physiological changes of the cervix. This book is written in precise and clear style which enables understanding of colpscopic patterns and underlying pathological changes. It contains 16 chapters presented in 276 pages, 400 original photographs and 40 drawings. The text is easy-to-read and understand. It provides both basic information for the beginner colposcopist and practical guidelines for a more experienced colposcopist.

It is a privilege to write the Foreword to *Colposcopy: Practice and Atlas*, an exceptional book which, on the best way, continues the tradition of high quality education for colposcopy in India.

To be a good colposcopist one must love colposcopy. After this book, there is no other choice but to start loving it.

Kesic Vesna

Dr Vesna Kesic
President, European Society of Gynaecological Oncology
Medical Faculty, University of Belgrade
Institute of Obstetrics and Gynecology
Clinical Center of Serbia, Belgrade, Serbia
E-mail: vek1@open.telekom.rs

Foreword

It gives me immense pleasure in writing the Foreword to this book. Teaching and training in colposcopy and popularizing it has been the passion of Dr SK Das, Dr Aruna Batra and Dr Sudha Nigam. This book is one more milestone in this direction.

Colposcopy is a magnification system used to visualize the lower genital tract for evaluating abnormal Pap smear and visible epithelial abnormalities. A beginner can be master in colposcopic diagnosis and management of lower genital lesions with the help of this atlas.

Colposcopic pictures have been used to teach identification of squamocolumnar junction of the cervix, transformation zone, metaplasia, gland openings, abnormal vascularity, lesions suspicious of neoplasia and neoplastic lesions of lower genital tract and select the cases for directed biopsy of the lesion.

The authors have made colposcopy look simple by the relevant pictures. Illustrative cases have been discussed by clinical photographs to enable easy understanding and to sustain interest. Latest colposcopic terminology and using the different scoring systems for the cervix have been beautifully described. Problem-based management for different case scenarios is another highlight. Proper management depending upon the diagnosis is the key to reduce the burden of cervical cancer. An excellent effort has been made to compile different aspects of colposcopy. I wish them all success in their endeavor.

Dr. Swaraj Batra

Professor and Head
Department of Obstetrics and Gynecology
Hamdard Institute of Medical Sciences and Research
Ex-Director Professor and Head
Department of Obstetrics and Gynecology
Maulana Azad Medical College and Lok Nayak Hospital
New Delhi

Founder President
Indian Society of Colposcopy and Cervical Pathology
E-mail: drsbatra28@gmail.com

Contributors

Mithilesh Chandra MD, FICPath
Senior Consultant Pathologist and
Director, Tissue Path Lab
CEO, Digiscan (A house of digital images and e-modules)
B-6, Sector 27, Noida 201301, India
Ex-Deputy Director, National Institute of Pathology, ICMR, New Delhi
E-mail: docmchandra @yahoo.com

Amita Suneja MD, FICMCH, MAMS
Professor
Department of Obstetrics and Gynecology
University College of Medical Sciences and Guru Teg Bahadur Hospital
Delhi
E-mail: amita_suneja@yahoo.co.in

Preface

Cancer cervix is the second most common cancer globally as well as in India. Organized cancer screening programs along with well established colposcopy clinics in the developed countries have led to a marked reduction in cervical cancer incidence as well as mortality. Thus, there is a need for every gynecologist to know the fundamentals of colposcopy and master the skill so as to turn the dream of preventing an "easily preventable but not yet prevented" cancer into reality.

We had the opportunity to start the first 'dysplasia clinic' at Safdarjung Hospital, New Delhi, in 1985, followed by organization of a large number of colposcopy workshops all over the country. The vast experience gained over all these years has been compiled in this book, which is our second book in this field. The first book *Atlas of Colposcopy, Cytology and Histopathology of Lower Female Genital Tract* was published in 1995 and was appreciated greatly by the residents, postgraduates and practising gynecologists as well as cytopathologists. The current book focuses mainly on colposcopy.

Colposcopy practice continues to evolve. This book includes initial chapters on colposcopic equipment, technique, and histopathological basis of colposcopy along with the latest advancements in the field. Colposcopic nomenclature proposed by the International Federation of Cervical Pathology and Colposcopy (IFCPC) in 2011 has been explained in detail as the latest nomenclature attempts to bring greater clarity to terminology in diagnostic and therapeutic colposcopy practice. The atlas presents colposcopic pictures of normal cervix, vagina and vulva along with the abnormal findings of benign, preneoplastic and neoplastic lesions.

Recently updated practice guidelines (2012) of the screening and management of pre-invasive lesions of cervix are discussed along with the management of vulvovaginal lesions and the latest clinico/colposcopic terminology of vulva introduced by IFCPC which can be used by the gynecologists and the colposcopists for appropriate diagnosis and treatment as well as consistent reporting of vulvar lesions. The book also brings out the limitations of colposcopy and methods to minimize errors related to colposcopic practice. A chapter on problem-based management has been added to help in day-to-day practice. Also included is a chapter on cytology to highlight the practical aspects of sample collection, cytological techniques and interpretation for the gynecologists. We hope, this compilation of text and atlas would be beneficial in meeting our goals.

Aruna Batra
drarunabatra@gmail.com

Sudha Nigam
nigamsudha@gmail.com

SK Das
drskdas1315@gmail.com

Acknowledgments

We owe our expertize to the patients undergoing colposcopy by us overtime and whose colpophotographs have been included in this book, because of which compilation/formation of this book has become possible.

We also owe our knowledge to the participants of colposcopy workshops conducted by us over a span of many years, whose constant enquiries and curiosities encouraged us to enhance our skills in this field as well as keep our knowledge afresh. The constant encouragement and appreciation of all the gynecologists and colposcopists who had been the readers of our first book *An Atlas of Colposcopy, Cytology and Histopathology of Lower Female Genital Tract* resulted in the compilation of all our work in the form of this book. We are grateful to all these persons.

We are deeply grateful to Prof. Amita Suneja, Professor, Department of Gynecology and Obstetrics, University College of Medical Sciences and GTB Hospital, Delhi, for her critical appraisal of this manuscript and also giving useful advice from time-to-time. We also thank her for contributing the chapter on "Minimizing Colposcopy Errors". We are also very grateful to Dr Mithilesh Chandra, cytohistopathologist, for contributing the illustrative microphotographs and the chapter on "Cytology for Gynecologist".

We appreciate the great efforts put in by Dr. Madhu Nigam and thank her for contributing schematic diagrams in various chapters.

Finally, we are extremely thankful to the whole team of CBS Publishers & Distributors, Mr SK Jain, Chairman; Mr. YN Arjuna, Senior Director—Publishing; Ms Ritu Chawla, Production Manager; Mr Neeraj Prasad and Ms Preeti Khera, for their untiring support at every level of making of this book.

Contents

Abbreviations

AA	Acetic acid
AGC	Atypical glandular cells
AGUS	Atypical glandular cells of undetermind significance
AIS	Adenocarcinoma in situ
ASC–H	Atypical squamous cells—HSIL cannot be ruled out
ASCCP	American Society of Colposcopy and Cervical Pathology
ASC–US	Atypical squamous cells of undetermined significance
ATZ	Abnormal/atypical transformation zone
AW	Acetowhite
BCA	Bichloroacetic acid
Bx	Biopsy
CE	Columnar epithelium
CIN	Cervical intraepithelial neoplasia
CO_2	Carbon dioxide
Ct	*Chlamydia trachomatis*
DCC	Double crested capillaries
DES	Diethyl stilbesterol
DNA	Deoxyribonucleic acid
ECC	Endocervical curettage
Gr.	Grade
GO	Gland openings
HC 2	Hybrid capture 2
HPV	Human papillomavirus
HPV 2	HPV vaccine (bivalent)
HPV 4	HPV vaccine (quadrivalent)
HSIL	High-grade squamous epithelial lesion
IFCPC	International Federation of Cervical Pathology and Colposcopy
LBC	Liquid based cytology
LEEP	Loop electrosurgical excision procedure
LLETZ	Large loop excision of transformation zone
LSIL	Low grade squamous epithelial lesion
ME	Metaplastic epithelium
Mo	Mosaic
mRNA	messenger Ribonucleic acid
N:C	Nuclear: cytoplasmic
NETZ	Needle excision of transformation zone
NF	Nabothian follicle
N_2O	Nitrous oxide
OSCJ	Original squamocolumnar junction
Pap	Papanicolou
PCR	Polymerase chain reaction
Pn	Punctations
RCOG	Royal College of Obstetricians and Gynecologists
SCJ	Squamocolumnar junction
SE	Squamous epithelium
SPI	Subclinical papillomavirus infection
SSJ	Squamo-squamous junction
SWETZ	Straight wire excision of transformation zone
TCA	Trichloroacetic acid
TTZ	Typical transformation zone
TZ	Transformation zone
WHO	World Health Organization

Chapter

1

Introduction

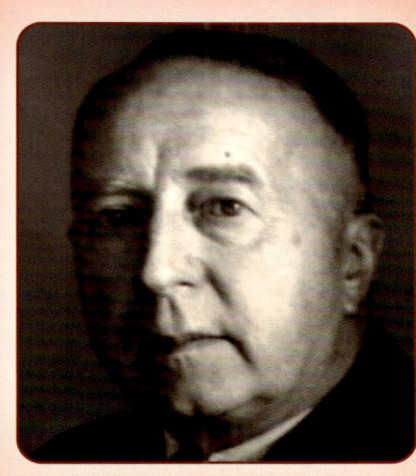

Hans Hinselmann
Father of Colposcopy

Chapter Outline

Literally translated, colposcopy (colpo: vagina and scope: to look) means to look into the vagina. Colposcopy is an optical method for visualizing lower female genital tract under bright illumination at a magnification between the naked eye examination and lower power of the microscope. It provides a study of the surface epithelium and the underlying connective tissue stroma along with its vascular network and is used as a diagnostic procedure for evaluating the lower genital tract in women with abnormal cervical cytology or clinically suspicious premalignant disease.

HISTORICAL ASPECTS

Colposcope was invented by Hans Hinselmann of Germany in 1925 as a screening tool for cervical cancer. Hinselmann hoped that by properly illuminating and magnifying cervix, precursor lesions might be identified early enough to allow effective treatment before invasive disease develops.

In the beginning, the technique of colposcopy was associated with difficulties due to short focal length of the lens, poor adjustment, and unsatisfactory diagnosis. With the help and technical cooperation of Reichert Co., it became possible to create a microscope with direct illumination which was able to evaluate different epithelial changes present on the surface after the application of some reagents, this machine was called colpomicroscope. In 1928, Schiller introduced the concept of placing iodine on the cervix to identify non-glycogen containing areas for biopsy.

Colposcopy remained confined to Germany initially because of lack of easily reproducible teaching material and resistance from the pathologists to accept Hinselmann's new terminology as atypical/abnormal epithelium and intraepithelial carcinoma. Later it got widely accepted in Europe as well, but it did not gain popularity in the United Kingdom primarily because of a cumbersome terminology that was difficult to translate into English.

In 1941, Papanicolaou and Traut published their report on the use of vaginal pool cytology for detecting cervical cancer. In 1949, Ayre developed the wooden cervical spatula, and it became possible to obtain abrasive cervical smears rather than exfoliative cytologic samples, which improved the detection of cervical neoplasia. The Pap smear, thus, became the accepted method of screening for cervical neoplasia.

In 1951, Kara-Eneff in Hamburg introduced electrical flash for production of satisfactory slides and photographs. A distinctive boom of colposcopy began in 1950s, with the advent of colpophotography, and the recognition of concept of carcinoma in situ by histopathologists. Colposcopy was essentially unknown in United States until the 1960s, when it was introduced in its current role as a confirmatory test for evaluation of women with abnormal cervical cytologic findings.

Cytology is an effective screening method, and colposcopy is the appropriate clinical diagnostic technique for evaluation of an abnormal Pap smear. Currently, it has near-universal acceptance as the most effective follow-up test for women suspected of having premalignant or malignant cervical lesions. The technique has become popular all over the world in the last four decades with the advances in the understanding of cervical carcinogenesis and development of appropriate colposcopic nomenclature reflective of the morphology.

INDICATIONS FOR COLPOSCOPY

Initially, colposcopy was used to identify asymptomatic early invasive disease, thereby improving patient survival. Subsequently, it helped in diagnosing pre-invasive lesions with resultant reduction in the incidence of cervical cancer and a significant drop in the number of diagnostic conizations. The ambulatory and conservative management of pre-neoplastic lesions was made possible only because of colposcopy, and now its role has been extended to the detection of sexually transmitted diseases, e.g. human papillomavirus, herpes simplex and Chlamydia infection.

Colposcopy is now routinely performed for the following indications (Table 1.1).

Table 1.1: Indications for colposcopy

1. Evaluation of women with abnormal Pap smear:
   - To localize the lesion
   - To map out the extent of the lesion
   - To select the biopsy site/s
2. Evaluation of women positive for high-risk HPV DNA
3. Evaluation of VIA positive women
4. Evaluation of suspicious cervix, and postcoital/postmenopausal bleeding, even if the Pap smear is normal
5. Unexplained abnormal lower genital tract bleeding
6. Persistent inflammatory/unsatisfactory cervical cytology despite appropriate treatment especially if high risk for carcinoma cervix
7. Evaluation of persistent abnormal vaginal discharge or pruritus vulvae
8. Identification and management of subclinical papillomavirus infection
9. History of inutero diethylstilbestrol (DES) exposure
10. Conservative management of intraepithelial neoplasia
11. Identification and management of vaginal extension of cervical neoplasia
12. Post-treatment follow-up
    - After treatment of intraepithelial and invasive carcinoma
    - Post-irradiation follow-up

The Colposcope and Ancillary Instruments

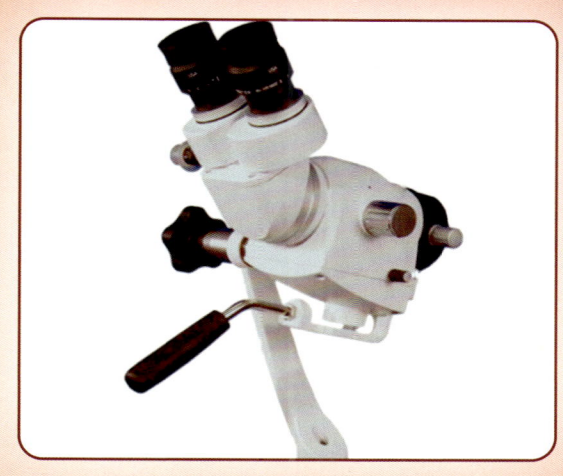

Chapter Outline

To make the best use of colposcope, one must be well familiar with the colposcope and the ancillary instruments required during colposcopy.

COLPOSCOPE

Colposcope is a low power, binocular microscope modified with the specific purpose for study of surface epithelium and underlying connective tissue stroma along with its vascular pattern.

Two varieties of colposcopes are available: Optical colposcope (Fig. 2.1A) and digital video colposcope (Fig. 2.2). Video monitor can be attached to optical colposcope also (Fig. 2.1B). Optical colposcope offers the advantage of stereoscopic or three-dimensional vision.

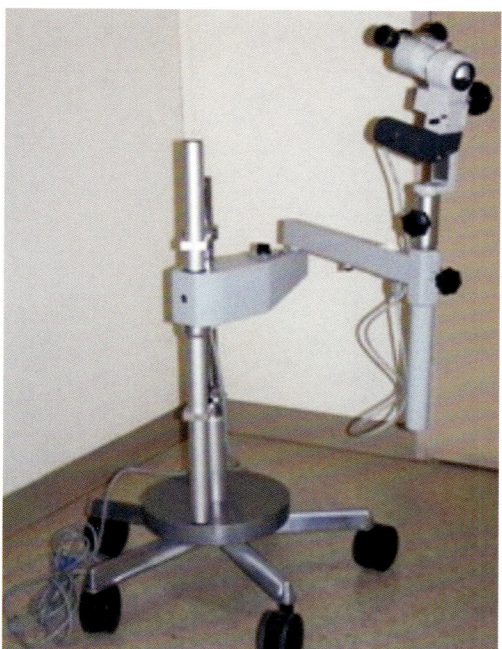

Fig. 2.1A: Optical colposcope

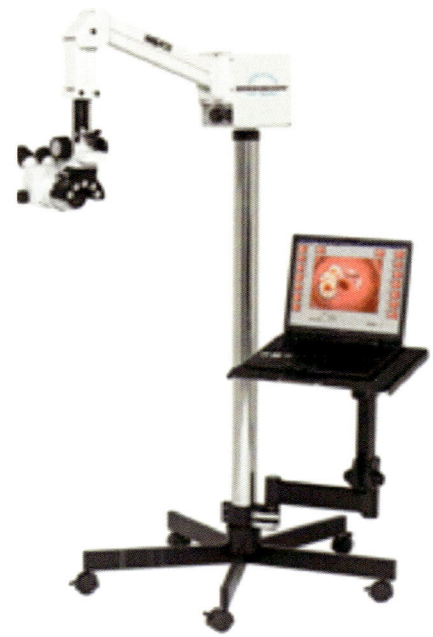

Fig. 2.1B: Optical colposcope with video monitor

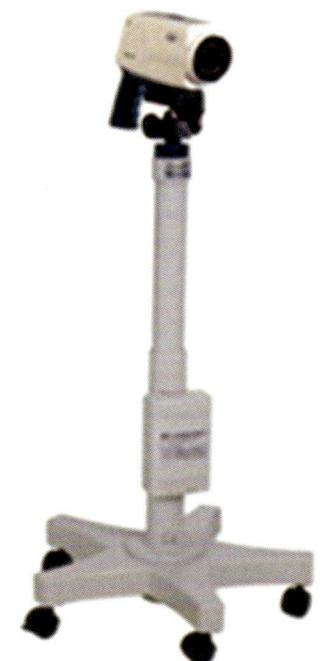

Fig. 2.2A: Digital video colposcope

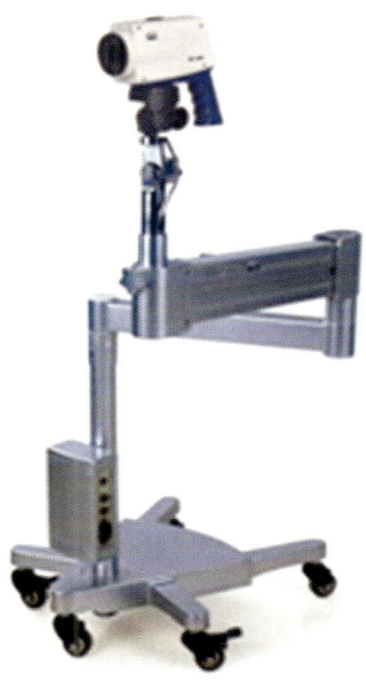

Fig. 2.2B: Digital video colposcope with spring arms

Optical Colposcope

Basic components of an optical colposcope (Fig. 2.3) include:

- Main objective lens
- Magnification changer
- Eyepieces
- Green filter
- Beam splitter
- Light source
- Stand

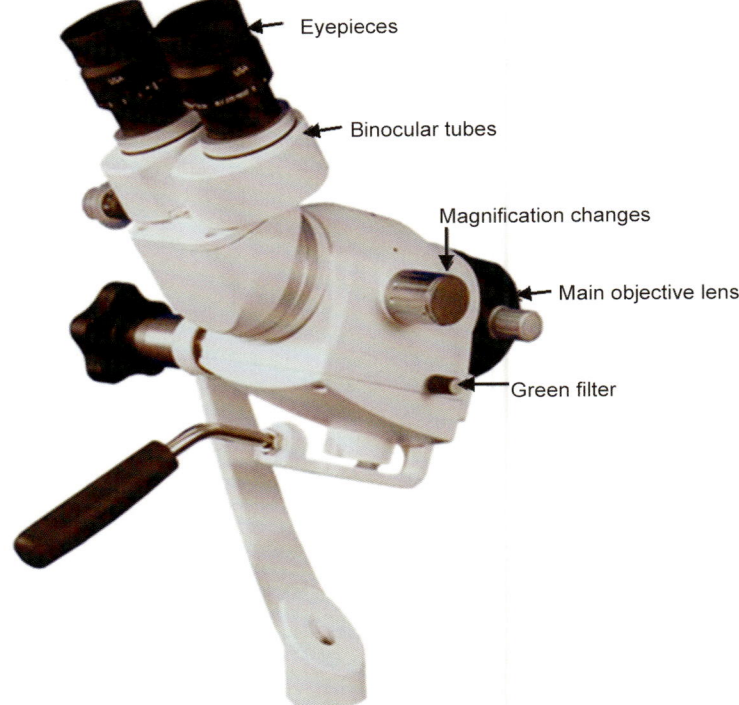

Eyepieces

Binocular tubes

Magnification changes

Main objective lens

Green filter

Fig. 2.3: Basic components of colposcope

Main Objective Lens (Fig. 2.4)

It gathers light from the object and produces an image, the brightness of which depends upon diameter and focal length of the lens. Larger the diameter, and lesser the focal length, brighter is the image. Main objective lens is available with different powers and it can be changed to alter the magnification and working distance of the colposcope.

Focal length determines the working distance between the lens and the target tissue. Most colposcopes have focal lengths of 250–300 mm. If focal length is too short, there will be limited space to maneuver the instruments in front of the lens. If too long, colposcopist will be placed too far to comfortably perform the examination and procedures. Focusing is obtained by either moving the colposcope itself or using the focus knobs on the instrument.

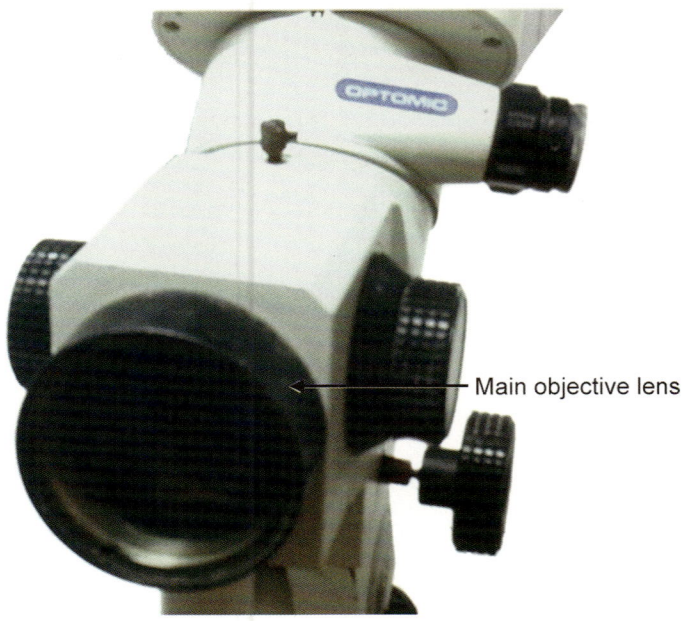

Main objective lens

Fig. 2.4: Colposcope (close up) showing main objective lens

Magnification Changer (Fig. 2.5)

All colposcopes follow similar principles. Most modern colposcopes have capability of variable magnification either by zooming through different magnification levels, or through separate discrete steps with the help of a magnification changer, in which multiple lens pairs are contained in a drum which can be rotated in either direction with an outside knob marked 0.4, 0.6, 1.0, 1.6, 2.5 to provide magnification ranging from 4× to 25×.

Low and medium magnifications are used for initial assessment. Low power (4× to 6×) is typically used for examination of vulva and male genitalia and for therapeutic purposes like LASER or LEEP so that entire transformation zone can be visualized in one field. Magnification up to 10× is sufficient for routine examination of cervix and vagina. Higher magnification (15× to 25×) is especially helpful for study of the finer details of vascular pattern. However, it decreases the field of vision and depth of field in focus.

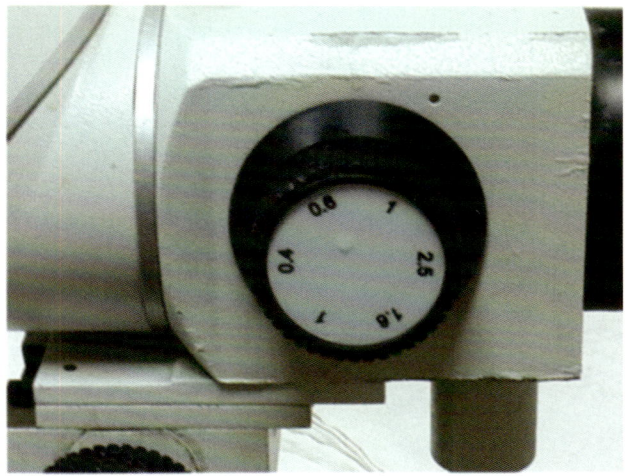

Fig. 2.5: Magnification changer

Filter

A green or blue filter is interposed between the light source and main objective lens, which absorbs red color from the light spectrum making red vessels appear blacker, standing out in sharp contrast against the surrounding epithelium. It helps in the study of vascular architecture.

Beam Splitter

For teaching purpose and photography, some colposcopes have a beam splitter in the form of semitransparent mirror interposed at 45° angle between the eyepiece and the binocular objective, so that some of the light rays go to the eye piece and some to the co-observer tube or the photographic attachment.

The co-observer tube does not provide stereoscopic, true three-dimensional view seen by the examiner.

Optical Pathway of the Colposcope

Light rays after passing through the main objective lens pass through the magnification changer and then through the optical system of the binocular tubes, i.e. binocular objective (converging optical system forming an intermediate real image) and then through glass-angled prisms. Prisms make the inverted image upright and allow the lateral parallel shift required for the adjustment of eyepieces to provide stereoscopic (3-dimensional) vision. Eyepieces further enlarge the intermediate real image and the enlarged parallel rays from the eyepieces are focused by the eye lens of the observer on the retina and this is how one gets the magnified view of an object (Fig. 2.6).

Total magnification of the colposcope depends upon the main objective lens, magnification factor of the magnification changer, binocular objective lens and eyepiece lens.

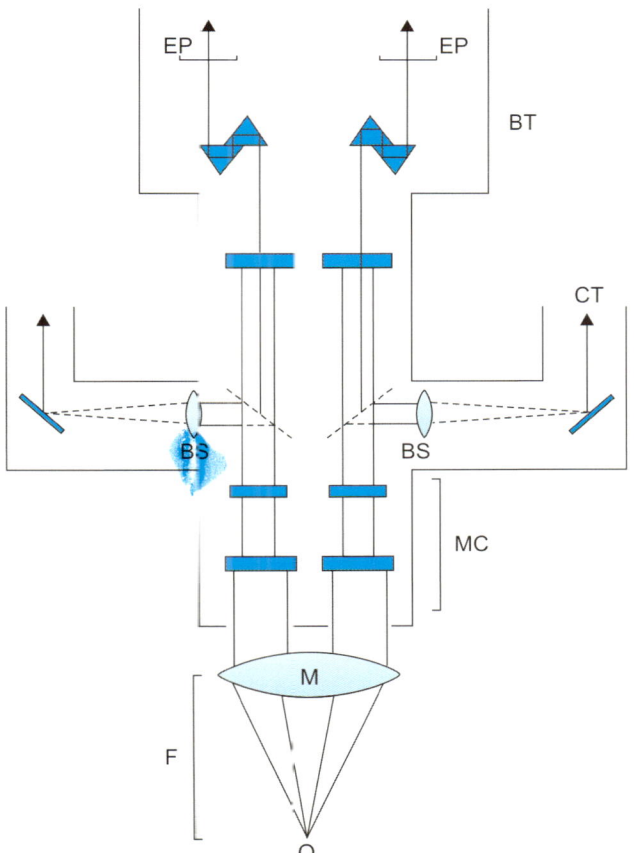

Fig. 2.6: Optical pathway of colposcope
EP Eyepieces; BT Binocular tubes; BS Beam splitter; MC Magnification changer; M Main objective lens; O Object; F Focal length of main objective lens; CT Co-observer tube

Eyepieces (Fig. 2.7)

The eyepieces can be moved away from or towards each other, to match the interpupillary distance of the colposcopist. This adjustment is essential as the viewer's pupils should be in line with the exit pupils of the colposcope. Otherwise images of both the eyes do not fuse and stereoscopic vision is not obtained. Interchangeable eyepieces with various levels of magnification are available for most colposcopes. Changing the magnification of the eyepieces alters the magnification levels achieved by the colposcope.

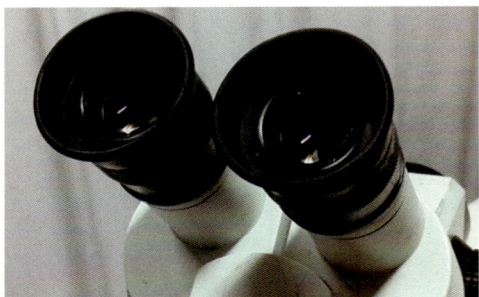

Fig. 2.7: Eyepieces

While viewing through the colposcope, eyes should be kept as near as possible to the eyepieces, as the distance decreases the brightness of the image. Eyepieces are provided with diopter adjustment also and colposcope can be used without spectacles. Eyepieces have marks '0', '+', '-'. '0' diopter is set for emmetropics and contact lens users, '+' for hypermetropics, and '-' for myopics, according to individual refractive error. Astigmatic person has to wear eye glasses.

Rubber cups are provided on eyepieces which protect the unguarded eye from the intense light and help in locating the exit point of the light rays. Persons who wear eye glasses should fold back these rubber cups to decrease the distance between the eye and the eyepiece.

Light Source

Coupled to the microscope is a halogen or xenon light source of high intensity. Remote light source with fiber-optic light does not give heat to the patient as well as the colposcopist. Light intensity should be at least 30000 lux. A rheostat is used to adjust the intensity of light. Newer colposcopes have LED (light emitting diode) light source which provides a higher luminous efficiency and improved contrast than halogen lamp and have a much longer lifespan in hours.

Stand

A good colposcope should be easily adjustable in both vertical and horizontal directions.

Colposcope may be mounted on a stand (Fig. 2.1) or may be affixed to the side of examination table (Fig. 2.8A) or even to the ceiling (Fig. 2.8B) or to the wall (Fig. 2.8C) according to the individual preference. Usually, colposcope is mounted on a mobile roller base. Base is heavy and wheels have a locking mechanism so that it does not move after it has been focused. A weighted or wide colposcope base prevents inadvertent tripping of the scope and damage to the head or to the optics.

Modern colposcopes are easily adjusted up or down by arms balanced with springs or hydraulic system.

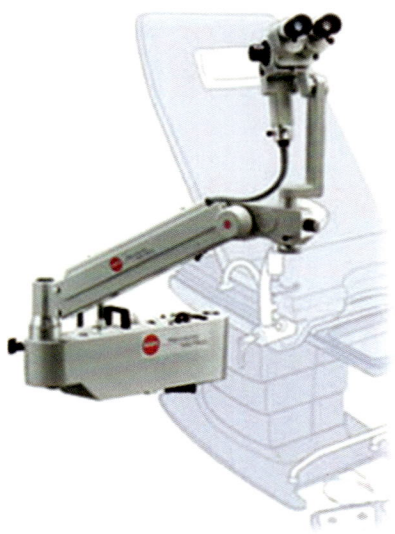

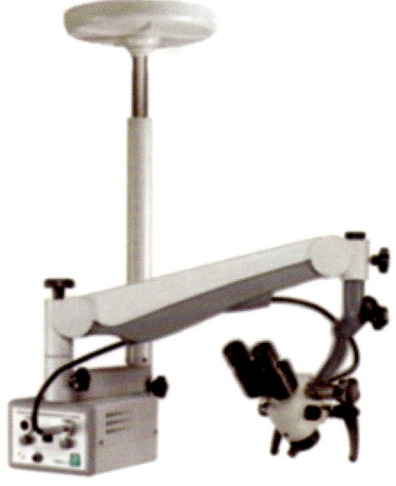

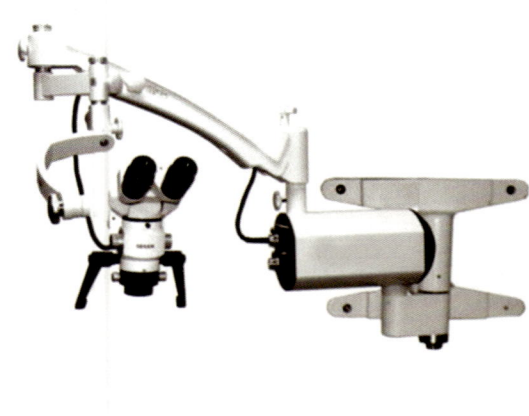

Fig. 2.8A: Table mount colposcope   **Fig. 2.8B:** Ceiling mount colposcope   **Fig. 2.8C:** Wall mount colposcope

Digital Video Colposcope

Video colposcope (Figs 2.9A and B) has a new method of providing magnification and illumination with the help of an inbuilt camera and strong light source (LED). Binocular eyepieces are not required and the colposcopic image is viewed on a high resolution video monitor. It has several advantages such as easy manipulation, co-visualization of image simultaneously by several viewers including trainees as well as the patient. It obtains permanent record of the findings in the form of replica of the image being seen by the examiner.

Recent innovation is linking a digital camera and a computer to the colposcope. The image and report are stored in the memory of computer and can be recalled later. With the advent of modern CCD cameras, electrical signals can be captured by computer and it became possible to create high-resolution digital images of the cervix that could be displayed real-time, printed, or manipulated by a computer. The image captured can be reviewed and recaptured. Images also can be stored and retrieved for comparison at future visits or for consultation with expert colpscopists. Digitised images can be transmitted to remote locations so that distant colposcopists can directly consult expert colposcopists via telemedicine. It provides a more quantitative method in the assessment of progression or regression of dysplastic lesions over time.

One of the main criticisms of video colposcope is that it gives a two-dimensional image rather than three-dimensional making assessment of the contour and density of lesion more difficult. Also it takes some time for colposcopist to adjust to the video colposcope to allow for development of psychomotor skills specially taking biopsy, etc. Others, however, feel there is no difference between optical colposcope and video colposcope in assessing the lesion. We, however, feel that the examination of endocervical canal is always better with the optical colposcope. Many colposcopes have both optical and video viewing and recording systems.

Examination Table

As the colposcopic examination takes a long time, comfort to the patient as well as to the colposcopist is a necessity. A height-adjustable stool should be used to allow proper back posture for the colposcopist. A height and tilt adjustable gynecologic table (Fig. 2.10A) with

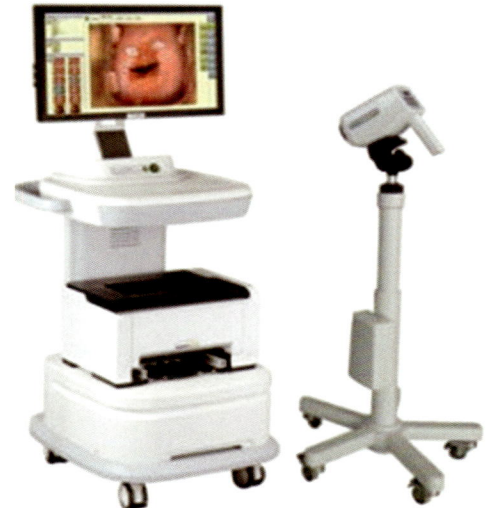

Fig. 2.9A: Digital video colposcope

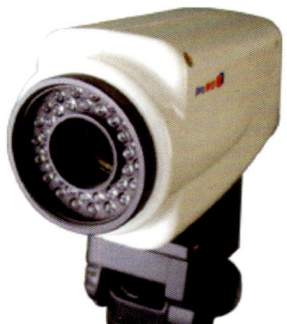

Lens and LED lights of
video colposcope

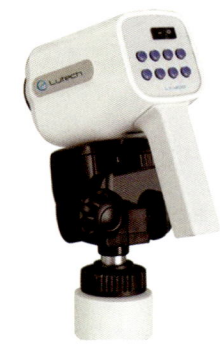

Function keys or buttons
on the head

Fig. 2.9B: Digital video colposcope

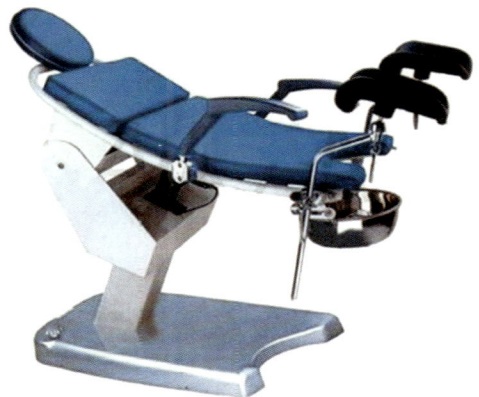

Fig. 2.10A: Hydraulic colposcopic table

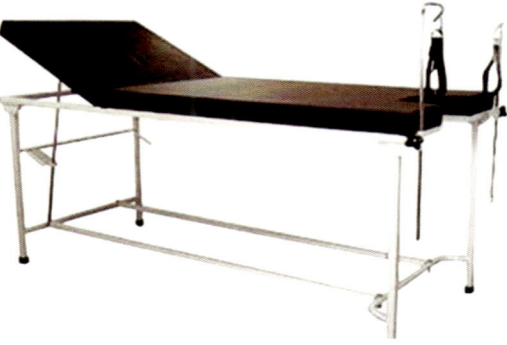

Fig. 2.10B: Ordinary gynecology examination table

special knee and calf supports should be used, so that the patient is comfortable and cooperative (Fig. 2.10A). It should have automatic foot control to adjust the height of the table so as to avoid the neck and back strain to the observer. In the absence of such a table, ordinary gynecologic table can be used which can be raised to desired height with the help of wooden blocks (Fig. 2.10B). There should be a basin for collection of blood or discharge and bleach solution for used instruments near the examination table.

ANCILLARY EQUIPMENT

Accessory equipment and reagents required for colposcopic procedure are listed below (Table 2.1).

All the accessory instruments and reagents are kept ready on a tray (Fig. 2.11) near the colposcopist's seat.

INSTRUMENTS

Speculum

Bivalve Cusco's or Pederson speculum should be used so that one hand remains free to carry out any manipulation or procedure, if required. Speculums should be available in various sizes to suit individual width and depth of vagina in multiparous, nulliparous or postmenopausal patient (Fig. 2.12). Insulated speculum with smoke evacuator should be available for LEEP, if required.

Vaginal Wall Retractor (Fig. 2.13A)

Vaginal side wall retraction may be required in multipara patients, if vaginal walls are lax and redundant and hamper the visualization of cervix. Vaginal wall retractor is specially designed to fit along-side a speculum and open with a ratchet mechanism.

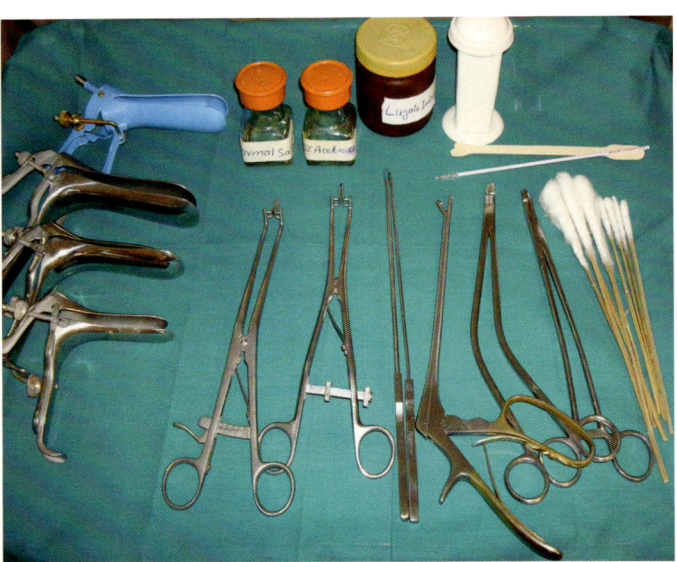

Fig. 2.11: Colposcopic tray containing, Cusco's speculum in various sizes, endocervical speculum, endocervical curette, cervical hook, biopsy forceps, ring forceps, small and large cotton-tipped applicators, normal saline, acetic acid, Lugol's iodine, Pap smear supplies

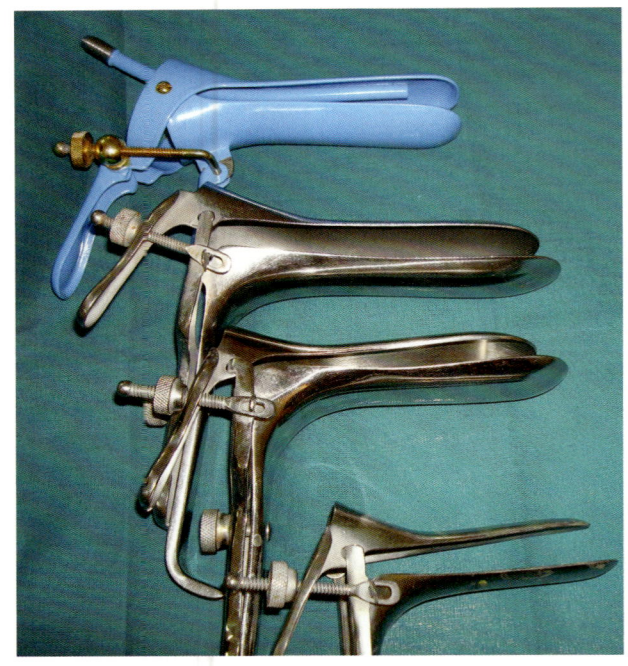

Fig. 2.12: Vaginal speculum in various sizes

Table 2.1: Ancillary equipment	
Instruments	**Electrosurgical unit** (for LEEP) with loops
• Bivalve speculum (different sizes)	**Cryocautery equipment**
Cusco's/Pederson	**Reagents**
• Endocervical speculum	• Normal saline
• Endocervical curette	• Acetic acid 1%, 3%, 5%
• Iris hook	• Lugol's iodine 50% aqueous solution
• Punch biopsy forceps	• Toluidine blue 1% aqueous solution
• Electrosurgical loops (different sizes)	• Ferric subsulfate (Monsel's) paste
• Small tissue forceps to pick up the biopsied material	**For Cytology**
• Needle holder for stitch whenever required	• Ayre's spatula, endocervical brush
	• Slides and glass marking pencil
	• Fixative: 95% alcohol and ether in equal proportion/cytospray

Complete opening may be hindered by hinges of speculum.

If a retractor is not available, a bivalve speculum covered with condom (Fig. 2.13B) can be used with its tip cut to achieve vaginal wall retraction.

Endocervical Speculum (Figs 2.14A and B)

Endocervical Speculum is required for examination of endocervix especially in unsatisfactory colposcopy to visualize the squamocolumnar junction or lesions extending into the endocervical canal. The head is placed into the external os and opened gently. It is available in different sizes of tips (length and width) to suit the cervices according to parity and stenotic cervices.

Punch Biopsy Forceps (Figs 2.15A and B)

Many varieties of punch biopsy forceps are available. Each obtains slightly different shaped but the tissue removed by all is small around 3.5 mm diameter. All have a long handle, shank and a head or tip whose jaws have an anchoring device and a mobile cutting edge. The cutting part is fenestrated so as not to crush the tissue, and the anchoring part has a grid to prevent the loss of specimen. Some shanks can be rotated 360° so that entire instrument does not have to be rotated. More important than design of biopsy forceps is that the cutting edge of the instrument is sharp as it reduces the pain perceived by the patient and the tissue is removed without distortion.

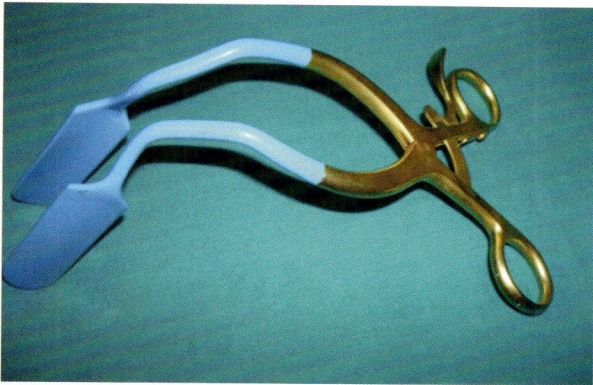

Fig. 2.13A: Vaginal wall retractor

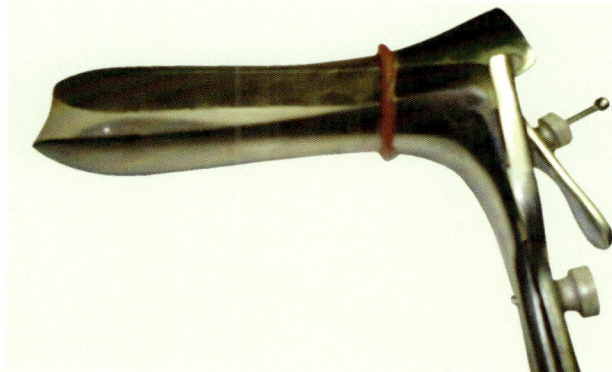

Fig. 2.13B: Speculum covered with condom

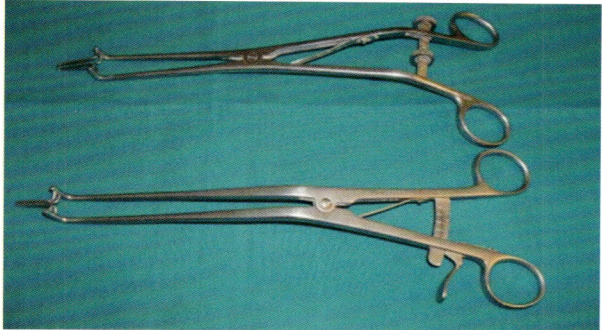

Fig. 2.14A: Endocervical speculum—different sizes

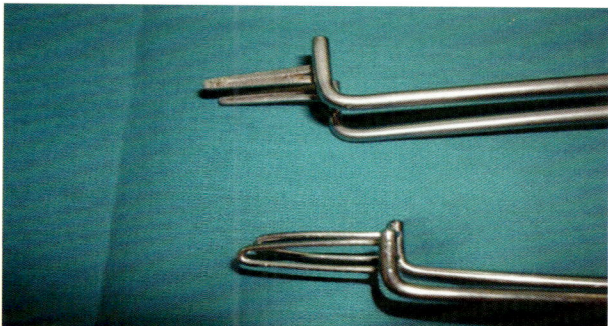

Fig. 2.14B: Head of endocervical speculum

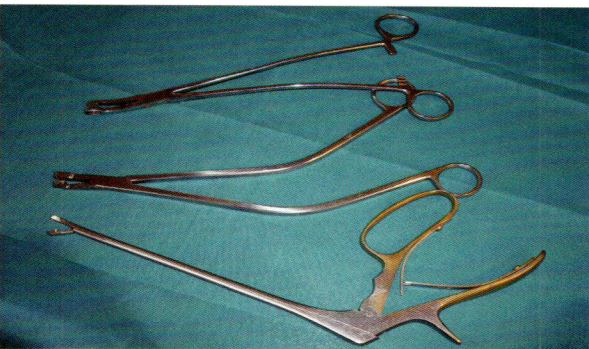

Fig. 2.15A: Punch biopsy forceps

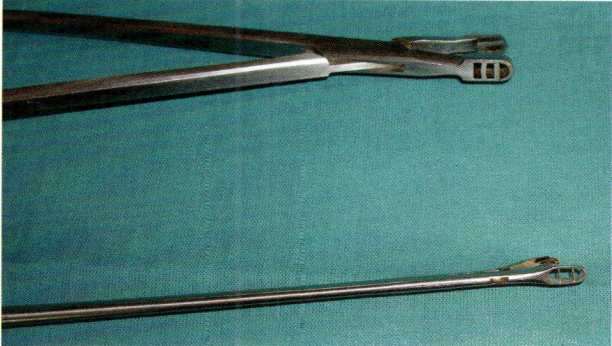

Fig. 2.15B: Heads of Kevorkian and Tischler forceps

Endocervical Curette (Fig. 2.16)

It is used for endocervical curettage, if a lesion is extending up into the canal or if colposcopy is unsatisfactory.

Iris Hook

Iris hook (Fig. 2.17) may be used to retract the cervical lips in cases of unsatisfactory colposcopy and also to stabilize the cervix while taking a cervical biopsy.

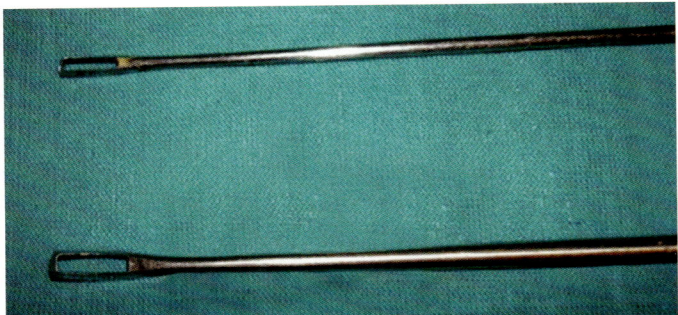

Fig. 2.16: Endocervical curettes

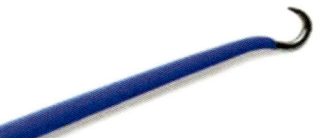

Fig. 2.17: Iris hook

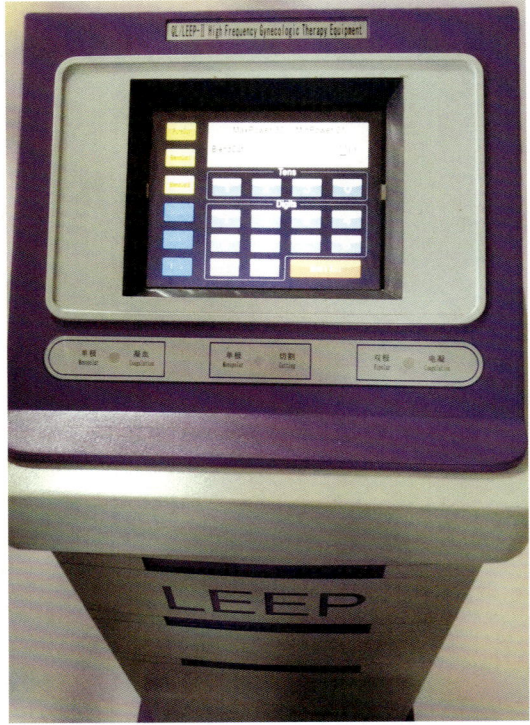

Fig. 2.18A: LEEP unit

LEEP (Loop Electrosurgical Excision Procedure) Equipment

Electrosurgical Unit

Monopolar electrosurgical unit (Figs 2.18A and B) having provision of cut, blend, and coagulation current should be available. It should be able to maintain a voltage of over 200 V through the procedure.

Electrosurgical Loop and Ball Electrode (Fig. 2.19)

Electrosurgical loops are used for excision of entire transformation zone. Small size loops can also be used as an alternative to punch biopsy forcep for taking colposcopy directed biopsies. Various sizes of loop are available. The tungsten wire loops have greater control

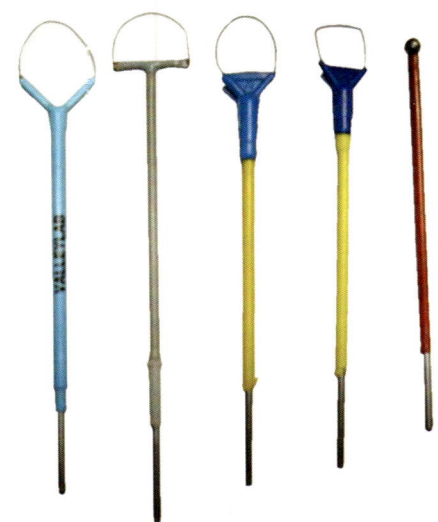

Fig. 2.19: Electrosurgical loops in various shapes, size and ball electrode

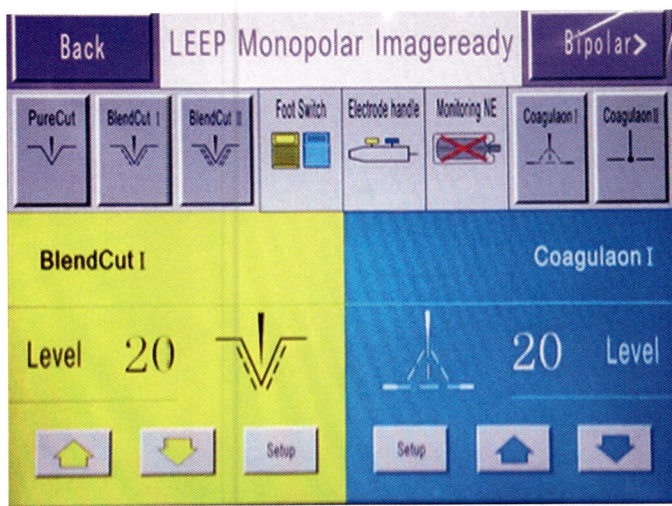

Fig. 2.18B: Front panel of electrosurgical unit

against bending and resist breakage even at higher power levels as compared to stainless steel loops.

Insulated Bivalve Self-retaining Speculum

Insulated bivalve self-retaining speculum with an attachment for smoke evacuation (Fig. 2.20) is useful for performing LEEP procedure.

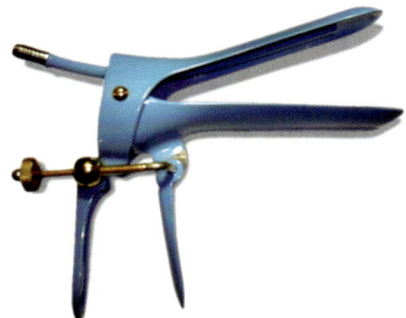

Fig.2.20: Speculum with attachment for smoke evacuation

Cryotherapy Apparatus

Cryotherapy apparatus consists of a handheld cryogun with probe and a cylinder containing carbon dioxide/nitrous oxide as refrigerant with a gauge for measuring the tank pressure (Fig. 2.21). Probes are available in various size and shape for use according to the size and location of different lesions (Fig. 2.22).

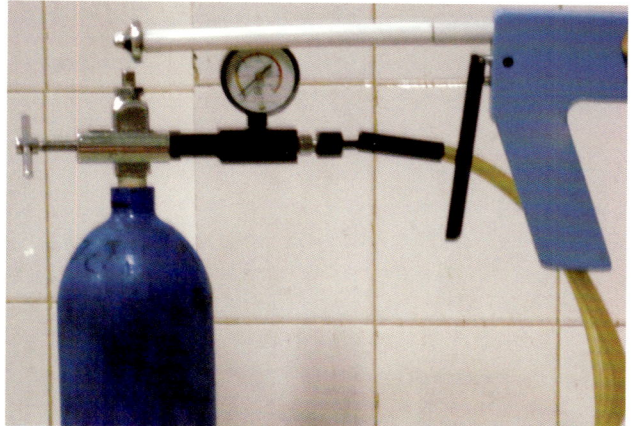

Fig. 2.21: Cryo gun with coolant cylinder

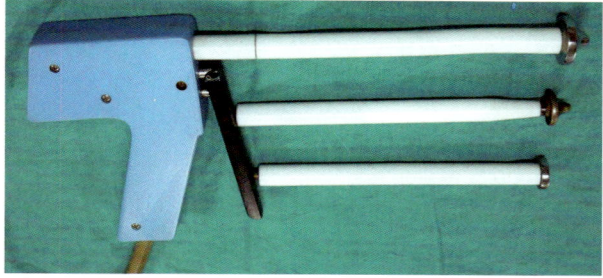

Fig 2.22: Cryo probes

Keye's Dermal Biopsy Forcep

Keye's dermal biopsy forcep (Fig. 2.23) is used for obtaining vulval biopsies. It has a cylindrical tip with cutting edge so that the tissue obtained is deep enough for appropriate histopathological evaluation.

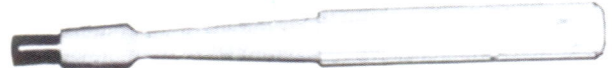

Fig. 2.23: Keye's vulval biopsy forceps

RECENT INNOVATIONS

Constant efforts are made to improve the quality of images and enhance the accuracy of colposcopic diagnosis. Newer technologies are based on digital image recognition or the physical properties of the underlying epithelium.

Digital Imaging Colposcopy

Advancements are being made in the digital image recognition of the features of abnormal transformation zone for prediction of underlying histopathology. Image processing techniques are used to enlarge, enhance and measure the abnormal lesions. The response of underlying epithelium to acetic acid is assessed by automated processing of digital outputs. Hence the grading of lesion becomes less subjective. One such system that allows objective quantitative assessment of the acetowhitening effect is the *dynamic spectral imaging system* (DySIS) which can be used by novice colposcopists for improved accuracy in diagnosis.

Biophysical Devices

Physical properties of the underlying epithelium are being explored to detect the changes associated with cervical intraepithelial neoplasia. These devices can be used as an adjunct to colposcopy to enhance its sensitivity in women with abnormal cervical cytology to discriminate between high- and low-grade intra-epithelial lesions or normal tissues so as to reduce the rates of under-treatment and over-treatment and unnecessary biopsies.

Electric impedance spectroscopy uses the electrical impedance of the biological tissues to detect the cytological changes in the cervical epithelium cells as they transform into CIN resulting in marked alteration in the cervical tissue's impedance spectra. This spectrum is measured at multiple points by a pencil probe incorporating electrodes. It is an objective technique and has been shown to be a potentially promising real-time screening tool for CIN with similar sensitivity and specificity to currently used screening tests.

LUMA cervical imaging system is an FDA approved optical detection system based on the properties of fluorescence, reflectance and spectroscopy intrinsic to in vivo tissues. The system shines a light on the cervix and produces a color map based on the response of different areas of the cervix to this light. The colors and patterns on the map help to differentiate between normal and abnormal tissues and take directed biopsies.

Truescreen or polar-probe is a real-time optoelectronic automated device that measures the response to optical and electrical stimulation of the cervix. It has a pen-shaped probe that delivers low level electrical pulses and optical signals to the cervical tissue and scans the whole cervix. The response is compared to the database stored in the computer-based system connected to the probe. The results are obtained immediately as normal, low- or high-grade abnormality, without the need of an expert physician.

Optical coherence tomography (OCT) is a non-invasive high resolution real-time imaging technique that can characterize microarchitectural features of subsurfaces up to 2 mm in depth. It is highly sensitive in identifying pre-invasive and invasive cancer of the uterine cervix and highly specific when used with computer-aided diagnosis (CADx).

Digital High Definition Video Exocolposcopy

VITOM® is a novel high-definition (HD) video exoscope based system consisting of a laparoscope, full HD camera system, high-quality optics, full HD monitor, a xenon light source and AIDA HD documentation system. The system supports a 25 to 60 cm working distance providing a comfortable workspace.

VITOM® (video telescopic operating microscope) is a safe and reliable system that has additional advantage over conventional colposcopy as it provides a full HD video documentation of colposcopic examination and allows its storage and reanalysis for teaching research.

Exocolposcopy with the VITOM® system is accurate and shows a good correlation with histological findings in high-grade cervical disease. It can be used in the operating theatre for conization procedures and LEEP as majority of operating theatres do not have colposcopes, but have a laparoscopic surgical unit available to which VITOM® system can be easily attached and most of the gynaecologists who perform conizations are also experienced in laparoscopy.

The use of laparoscopic equipment for conization procedures could improve the quality of conizations with a reduction in the volume of healthy cervical tissue removed unnecessarily in young women with CIN II-III.

REAGENTS

Normal Saline

Normal saline makes the surface epithelium transparent and gives a good view of the color, contour and underlying vascular pattern.

Acetic Acid

Acetic acid causes the sharpest contrast between the normal and abnormal epithelium. 3% concentration is preferred for application on the cervix, as 5% may cause irritation. 5% acetic acid is used for examination of vulva. 1% is used to wash away the toludine blue in collin's test during vulval examination.

5% acetic acid is prepared by adding 5 mL glacial acetic acid into 95 mL saline or distilled water. Bottle of glacial acetic acid should be closed airtight to prevent dilution by absorption of humidity from atmosphere. Acetic acid solution should be freshly prepared daily and unused acetic acid should be discarded at the end of the day.

Lugol's Iodine

Lugol's iodine is prepared by dissolving 10 g potassium iodide in 100 mL water, when completely dissolved, 5 g iodine is added. Solution is stirred well till iodine flakes are completely dissolved, filtered and stored in a dark brown bottle. Shelf-life is 3–6 months. Alcohol-based iodine solution should not be used as it could affect the epithelium and interfere with histological interpretation in case lesion needs to be biopsied.

Monsel's Solution (Ferric Subsulfate)

Monsel's solution (ferric subsulfate) is most common agent used to achieve hemostasis after biopsy or excision. It is available as readymade solution or can be prepared also (appendix 2).

It performs best when it has a thick, toothpaste consistency. It can be bought this way or produced by allowing the stock solution to sit exposed to the air in a small open container. This allows evaporation and thickening of the agent, a process that can be enhanced by placing the open container in a warm place. The resulting paste texture can be maintained by keeping the paste in a closed container.

Chapter

3

Technique of
Colposcopy

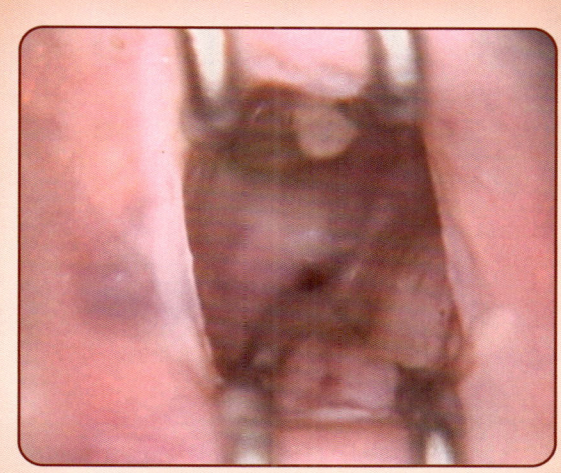

Chapter Outline

COLPOSCOPY OF CERVIX

Colposcopic findings should always be evaluated in conjunction with the history and clinical examination findings. A detail history and clinical examination is required before taking up the patient for colposcopy.

A written informed consent is to be obtained and patient identification data carefully recorded on the proforma to avoid any mix-up.

Timing of Colposcopy

Colposcopy should ideally be performed between 8th and 12th day of the menstrual cycle. At this time the external os is wide open and cervical mucus is abundant (Fig. 3.1) which acts as a refractory medium helping in visualization of endocervix. It should be avoided for a few days just after periods as menstrual blood causes maceration reducing the thickness of epithelium, hence minute lesions may be missed. This examination should also not follow any such procedures which may cause damage to the cervix such as hysterosalpingography, dilatation and curettage, cervical biopsy, etc. Findings may be misleading in such situations, as even minor trauma can cause inflammation and regenerative changes affecting the colposcopic appearance.

Ideally, colposcopy should be carried out in the presence of Pap smear report, as in the case of an abnormal smear, a thorough search has to be made to find the abnormality. Pelvic examination and Pap smear are to be avoided immediately before colposcopy as it may result in bleeding, scraping off dysplastic cells, and an erroneous interpretation.

Performing Pap smear following colposcopy may also give erroneous results as the abnormal cells can get desquamated following the application of reagents. But in case it has not been done earlier, it may be obtained gently at this time. If required specimen for culture or HPV DNA can also be taken simultaneously.

In case bleeding is too much, interfering with the view, colposcopic examination should be deferred. Sufficient time should be devoted to this examination. It should be carried out systematically.

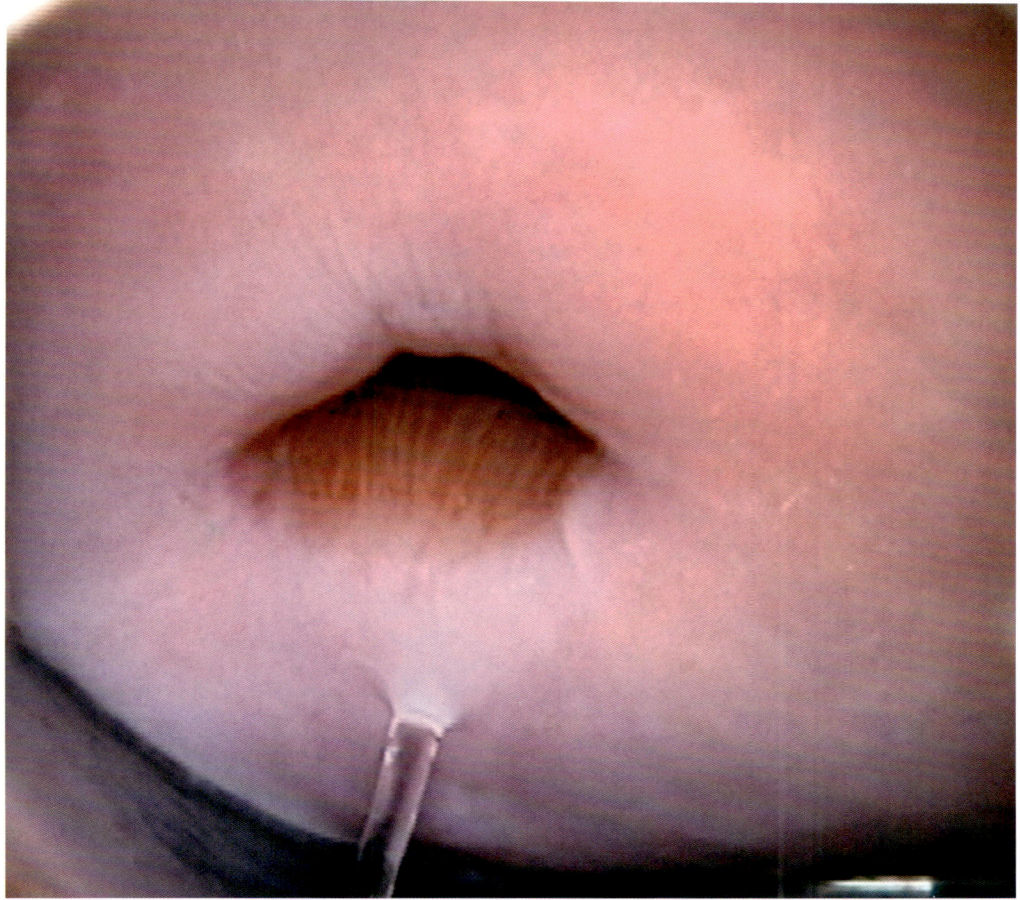

Fig. 3.1: Abundant clear mucus with open os in mid-menstrual cycle

Steps of Examination

Before starting the colposcopic examination, all the instruments and reagents should be available on a trolley nearby on the right side.

Patient is made to lie down comfortably in lithotomy position. Bivalve self-retaining speculum should be used so that one hand remains free for any manipulation required.

Vaginal speculum suitable for the individual patient is selected and inserted gently into the vagina parallel to the vaginal slit. After inserting it for a while, the blades are partially opened and rotated horizontally and as soon as the cervix is visible both the valves of speculum are opened.

Care should be taken not to traumatize the cervix as it may initiate bleeding hampering the colposcopic examination. With one hand the vaginal speculum is manipulated, while with the other hand the colposcope is brought forward and focused on the cervix.

Colposcopy is performed in a stepwise manner (Table 3.1).

Preliminary Inspection and Examination after Saline Application

First the cervix is visualized in natural state under low power magnification to note the amount and

Table 3.1: Steps of colposcopic examination
1. Inspection of cervix and vagina in natural state
2. Examination after normal saline application
3. Examination through green filter
4. Examination after 3% acetic acid application
5. Examination of vagina and vulva
6. Examination after Lugol' iodine application
7. Endocervical sampling and directed biopsy, if required
8. Documentation

nature of any discharge along with the gross findings (Fig. 3.2).

This is followed by examination after removing the mucus and discharge from the cervix with the help of a cotton swab soaked in normal saline (Fig. 3.3). Dry swab should not be used as it may initiate bleeding.

Normal saline makes the surface epithelium transparent and gives a good view of the color, contour and underlying vascular pattern (Fig. 3.4).

At this stage any gross lesion, opacity of epithelium and vascular details can be easily made out (Fig. 3.5).

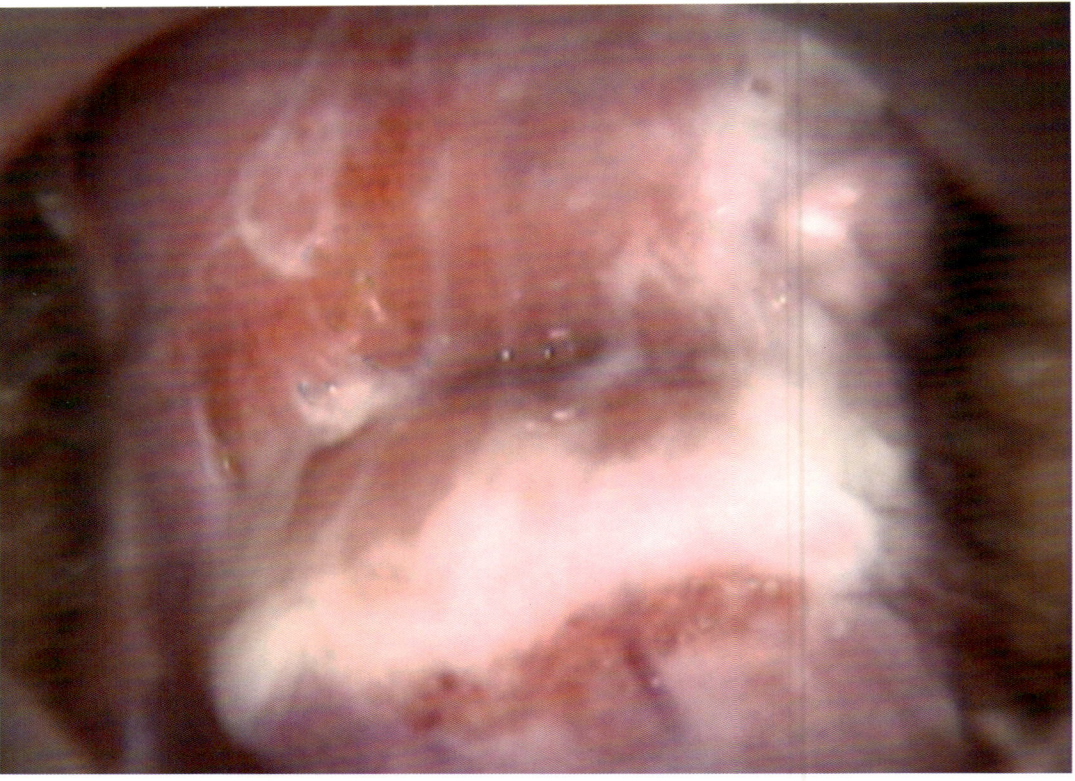

Fig. 3.2: Cervix in natural state: Copious discharge covering most of ectocervix

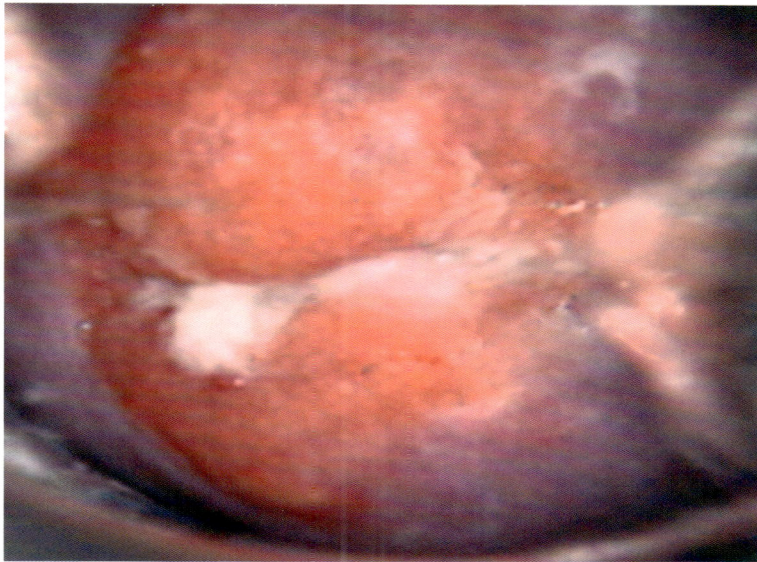

Fig. 3.3: Cervix after normal saline:Red velvety columnar epithelium with pink squamous epithelium at periphery

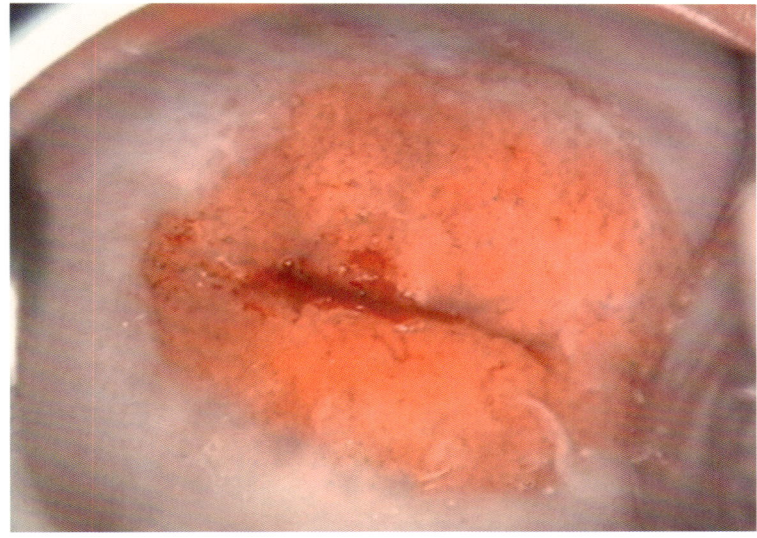

Fig. 3.4: Ectopy after saline application

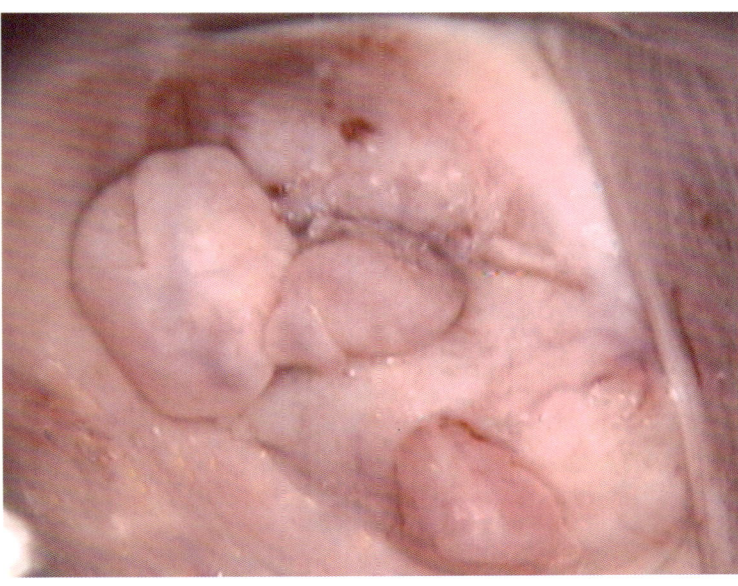

Fig. 3.5: Multiple polyps

Examination through Green Filter

Vascular pattern is studied in detail under higher magnification (20-fold plus). It is further highlighted by examination through green filter and vessels stand out as black streaks against background of translucent epithelium (Figs 3.6 and 3.7).

Abnormal epithelium may also at times be distinguished from normal epithelium through green filter. Study of angioarchitecture can be made in vivo using optical micrometer or by photography.

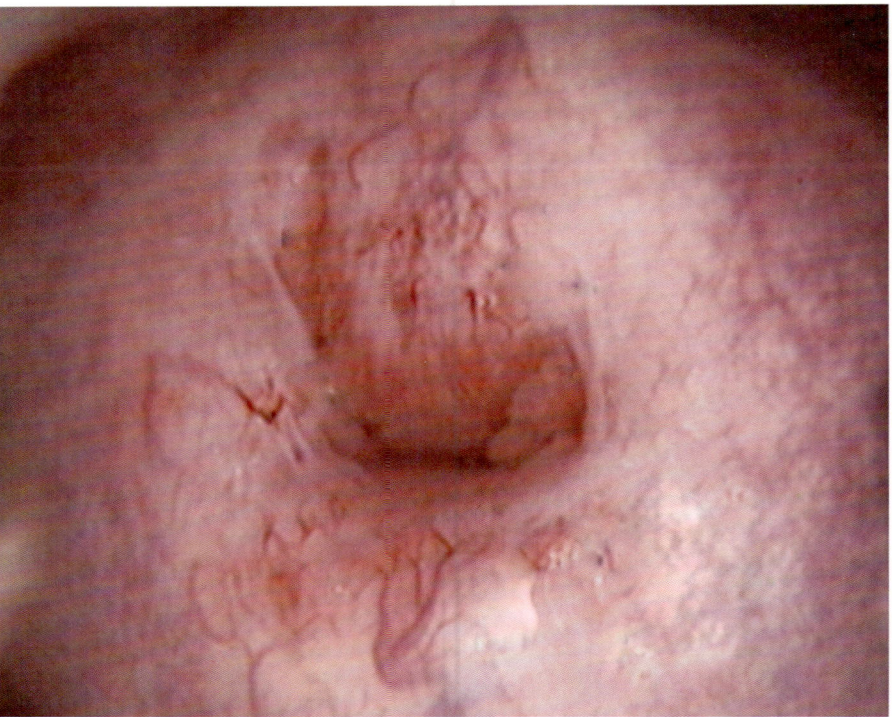

Fig. 3.6: Vascular pattern: After saline application

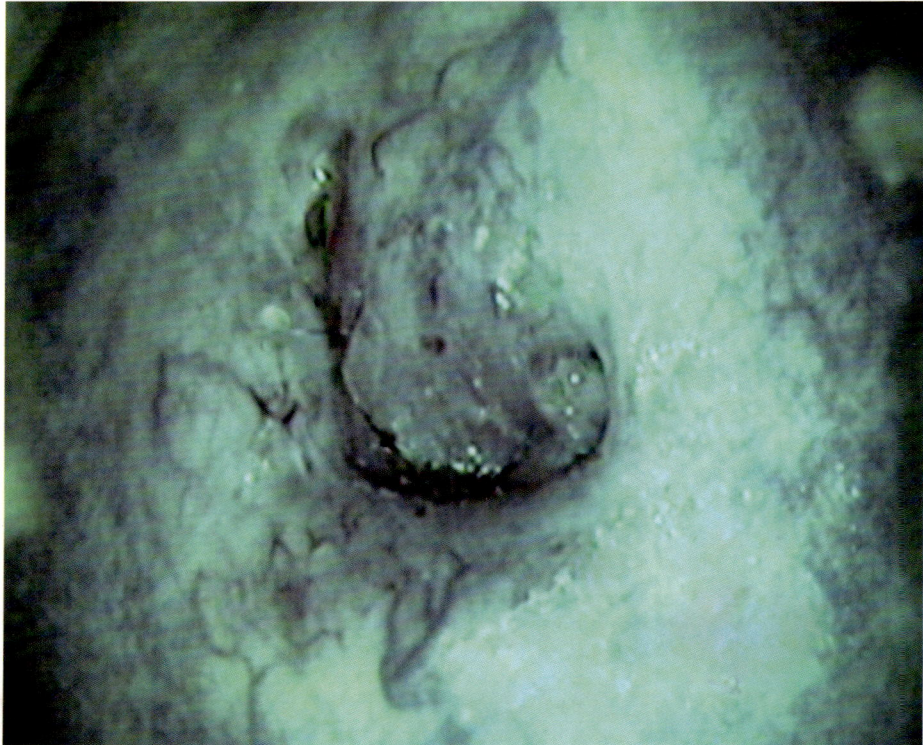

Fig. 3.7: Under green filter: Vessels seen as black streaks

Number of vessels, their caliber, tortuosity, shape, and the intercapillary distance are noted. Number of vessels is estimated by the abundance or scarcity of vessels in comparison to that in normal tissue. Regularity or irregularity of caliber is observed. Vascular pattern is noted whether typical (Fig. 3.8) or atypical (Fig. 3.9) in the form of mosaic, punctation, or abnormal vessels.

Intercapillary distance refers to the space between corresponding parts of 2 adjacent vessels or the diameter of fields delineated by network or network like, mosaic or mosaic like vessels.

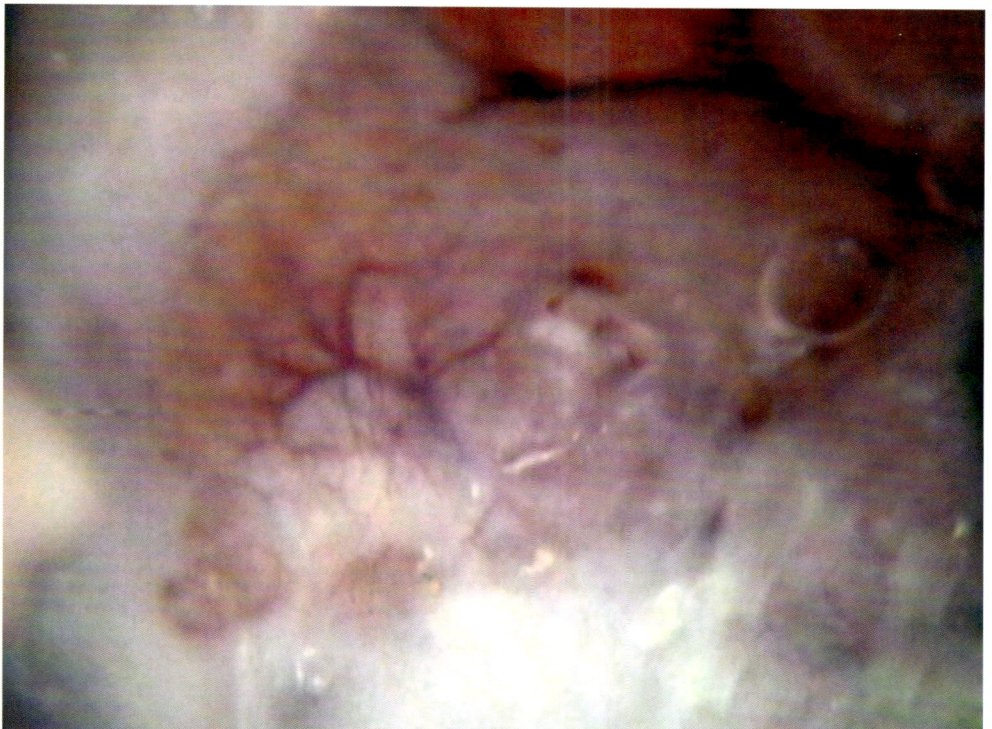

Fig. 3.8: Typical vessels with regular, dichotomous branching

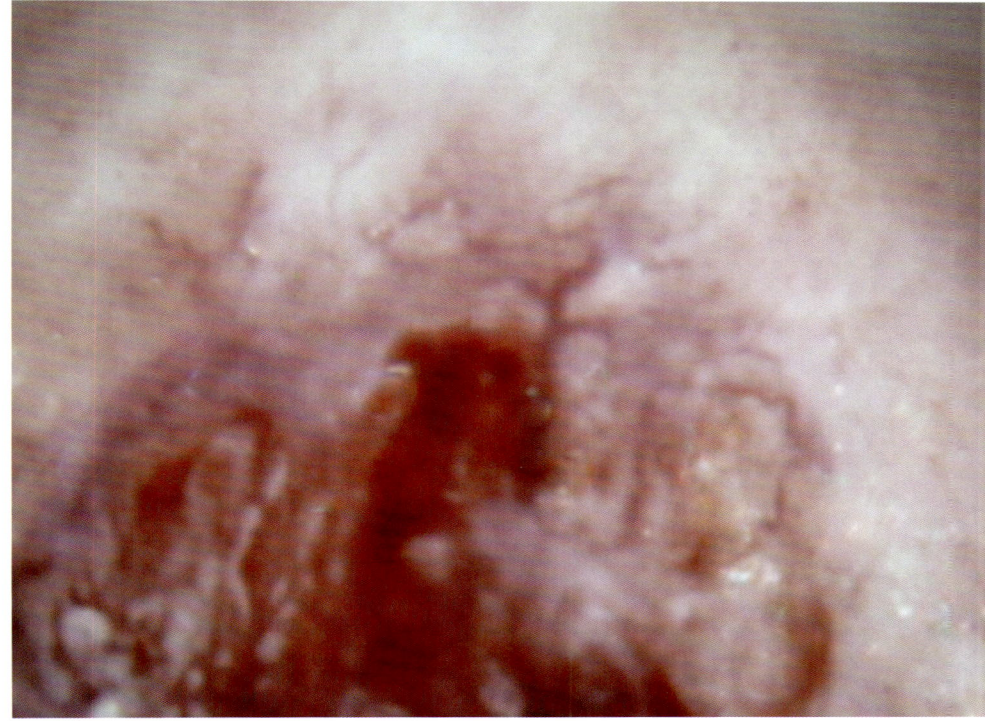

Fig. 3.9: Atypical vessels with irregular caliber and branching

Examination after Acetic Acid Application

This is the most important step in colposcopic examination. Acetic acid causes the sharpest contrast between normal and abnormal epithelium. It is used in 3–5% concentration. 3% concentration is preferred for mucosa of cervix and vagina and 5% for vulva. With 5% strength over mucosa, patient may complain of irritation while with weaker strength lesions take a long time to appear. Acetic acid is applied copiously with gauze/cotton, tipped swabs or spray bottle. Solution must be left in contact with tissue for about 1 minute. Excessive rubbing should be avoided as it may initiate bleeding.

After application of acetic acid, the columnar epithelium assumes grape-like appearance because of swelling of individual villi (Figs 3.10A and B) whereas metaplastic and dysplastic epithelia appear white (Figs 3.11 and 3.12).

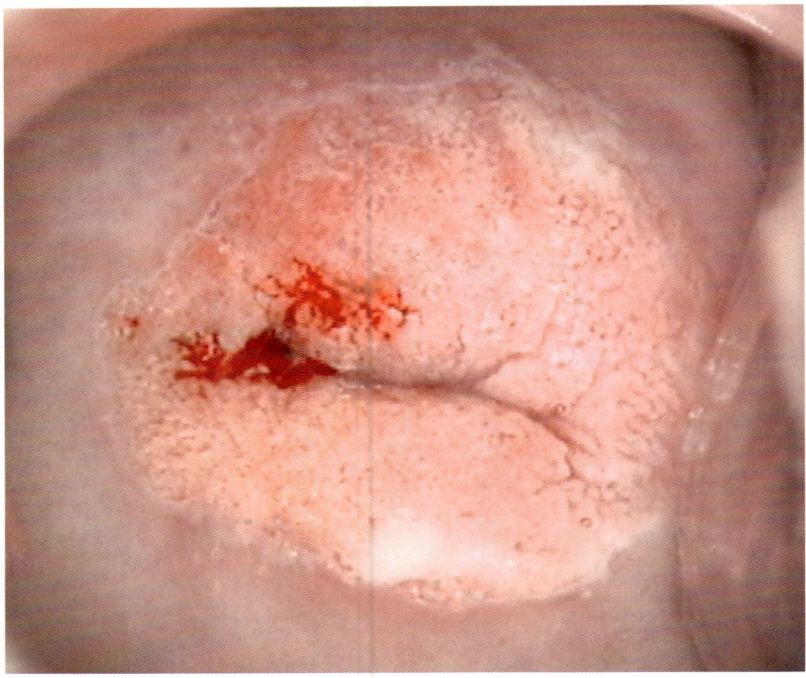

Fig. 3.10A: After acetic acid: Grape-like columnar epithelium

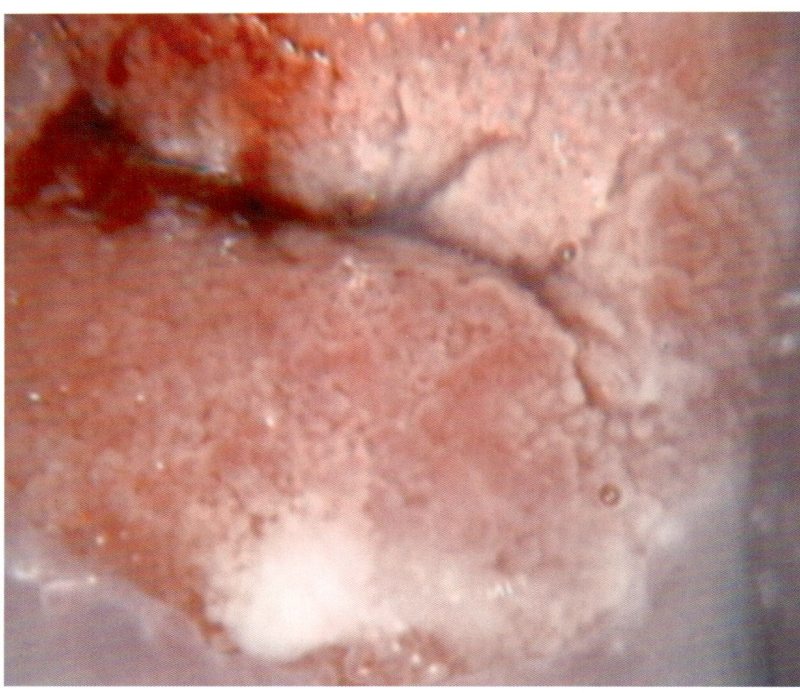

Fig. 3.10B: Same cervix under higher magnification: Grape-like columnar epithelium

The OSE, the CE, and the TZ are identified, and any lesion, if present is delineated. The lesion is assessed for the intensity of whiteness, speed of appearance, duration of stay, and speed of disappearance.

After 3% acetic acid, observable changes usually appear within 1 minute and remain for 2–3 minutes. This change is transient but reappears after reapplication of acetic acid. Repeated applications of acetic acid may be required.

After delineating the lesion, its limits have to be identified. Caudal limit of the lesion can be seen by manipulating the speculum. Sometime help of cotton wool pledget has to be taken to examine the whole lesion (Fig. 3.13).

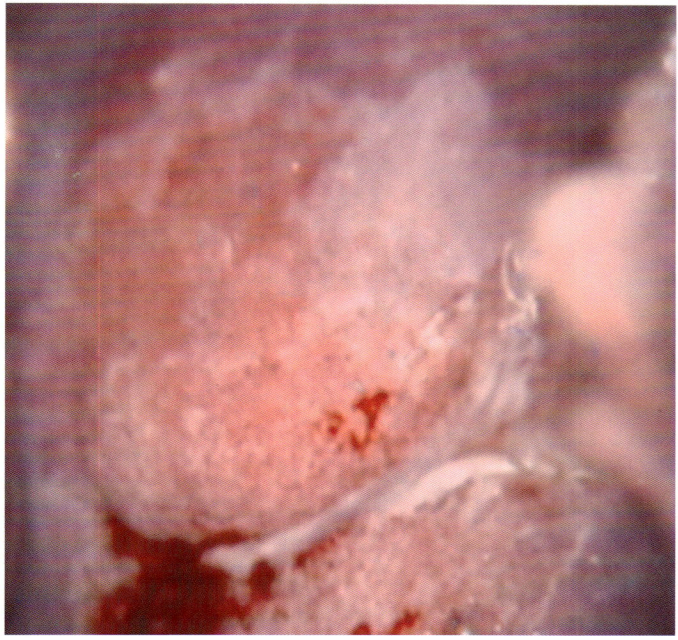

Fig. 3.11: After acetic acid application: AW epithelium over anterior lip at 1 O' clock

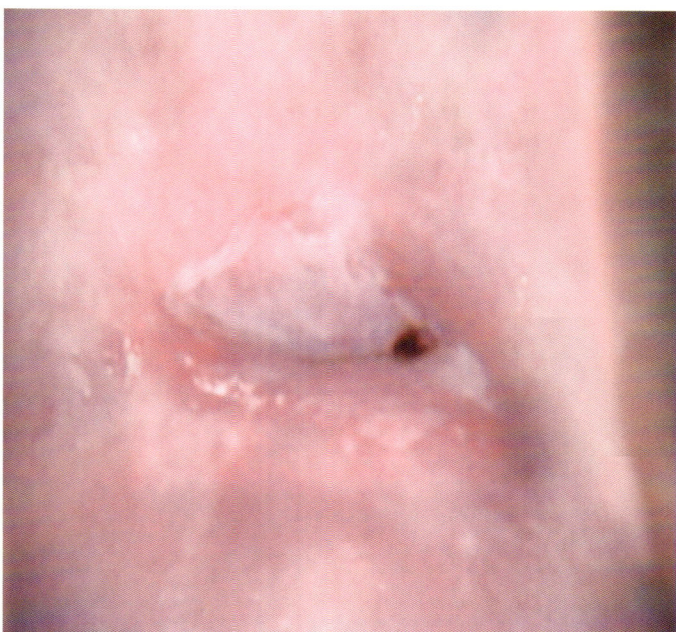

Fig. 3.12: After acetic acid application: Sharply demarcated AW epithelium reaching inside endocervix

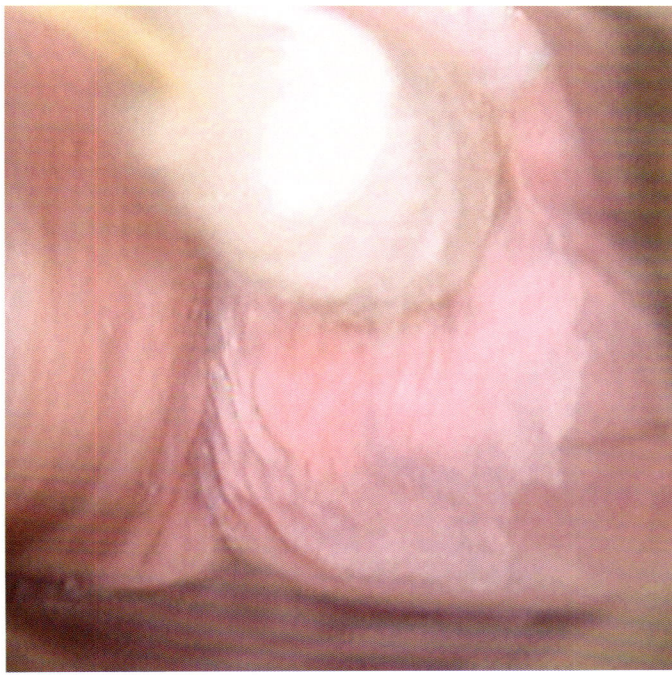

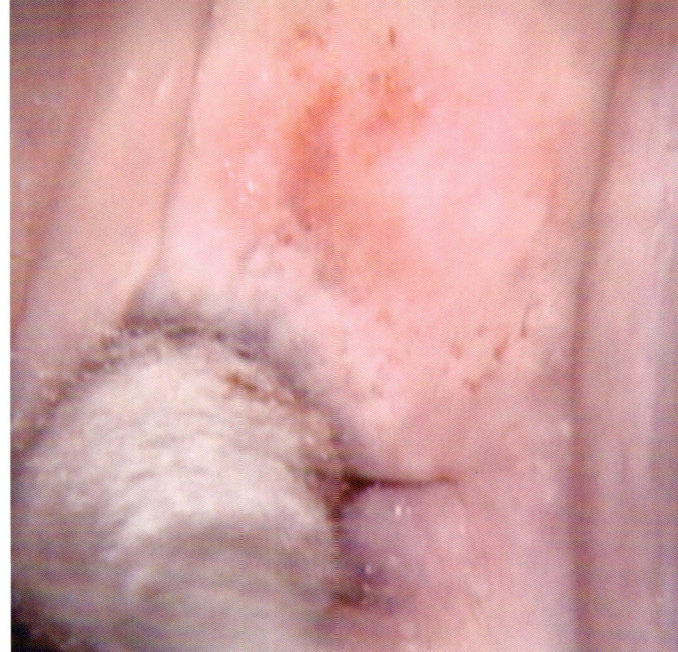

Fig. 3.13: Manipulation of cervix with cotton wool pledget to see whole lesion

Cranial limit of the lesion has to be identified along with evaluation of endocervical canal. Acetic acid is applied inside the endocervical canal with the help of a small cotton wool pledget.

Lower portion of the canal is usually seen easily in reproductive age group just by widely opening the valves of the vaginal speculum, but in about 10% cases, the colposcopist may need to apply pressure near the os with the cotton wool applicator (Fig. 3.14) in order to open the canal or the help of iris hook may be required. If this is not adequate for visualization, an endocervical speculum may be used.

Upper portion of ECC can be seen by using endocervical speculum, whereby at least 1.5 cm of endocervix can be observed in most of the patients (Fig. 3.15) and in multipara even entire length can be seen during reproductive age (Fig. 3.16).

If SCJ or the cranial limit of lesion cannot be seen, colposcopic examination is labeled as unsatisfactory.

As the acetowhitening starts fading, vascular patterns become more distinct. Normal and abnormal epithelium and vessel pattern should be mapped for documentation.

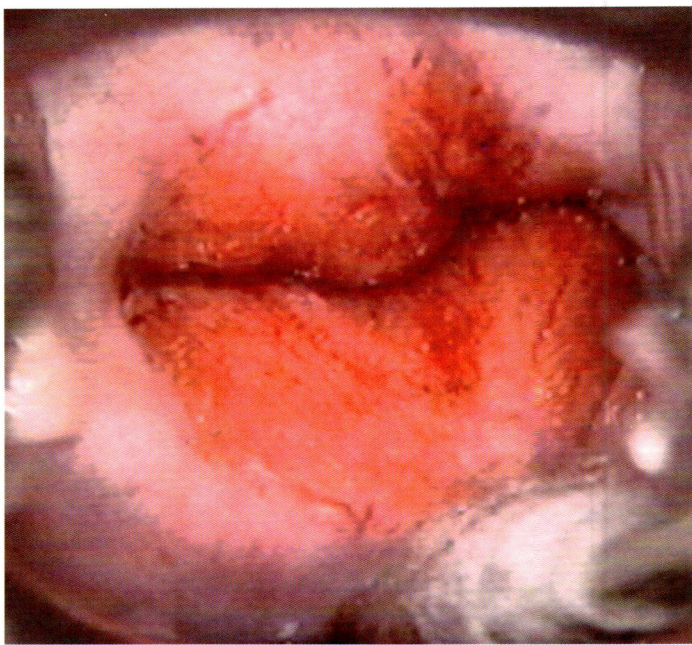

Fig. 3.14: Lower portion of endocervix seen with the help of cotton wool stick

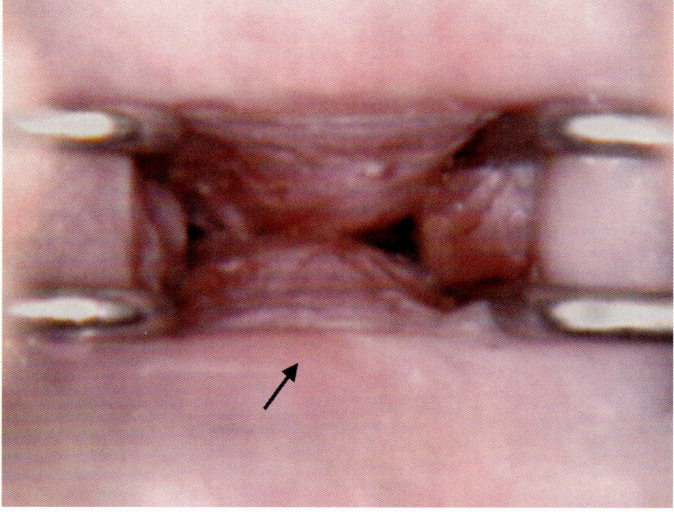

Fig. 3.15: Examination of endocervix through endocervical speculum

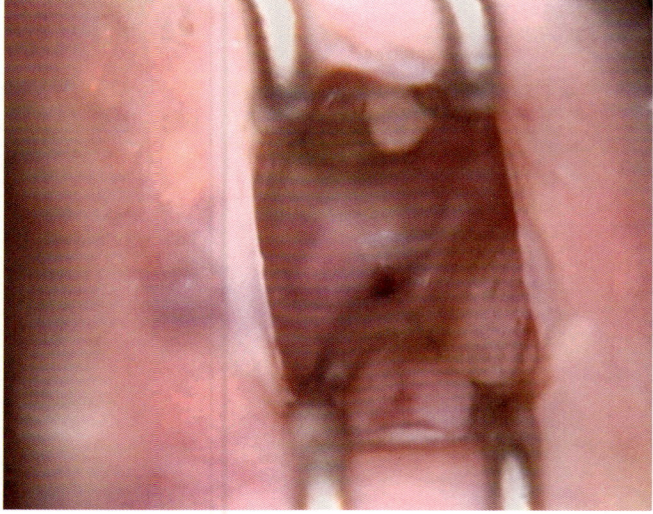

Fig. 3.16: Almost entire length of endocervical canal seen through endocervical speculum

Examination after Lugol's Iodine Application

Iodine staining concludes the colposcopic examination. After application of Lugol's iodine, mature squamous epithelium stains mahogany brown because of its glycogen content. Epithelium deficient in glycogen, such as columnar epithelium (Fig. 3.17) or abnormal epithelium (Fig. 3.18), does not take up stain and is termed as iodine negative.

Iodine staining is useful in distinguishing HPV lesions from significant dysplastic lesions and also in the evaluation of all the vaginal folds. It is also very useful for a novice colposcopist as it points out abnormal areas and confirms the colposcopic examination results. Iodine staining is a must before performing LEEP/conization or hysterectomy for preneoplastic and neoplastic lesions to ensure free margins of the healthy mucosa.

Some colposcopists have stopped using iodine staining because it is a non-specific test and both benign and malignant lesions may give positive reaction. Also it does not add much to evaluation, rather it might obscure very minute vascular details and may make it difficult to localize most abnormal area requiring directed biopsy.

If iodine staining is to be used, it should be done after examination of vagina is complete, by reinserting the speculum and liberally painting the cervix and vagina with iodine.

Iodine may produce intense allergy in some patients. Therefore history of previous allergies should be asked before iodine application.

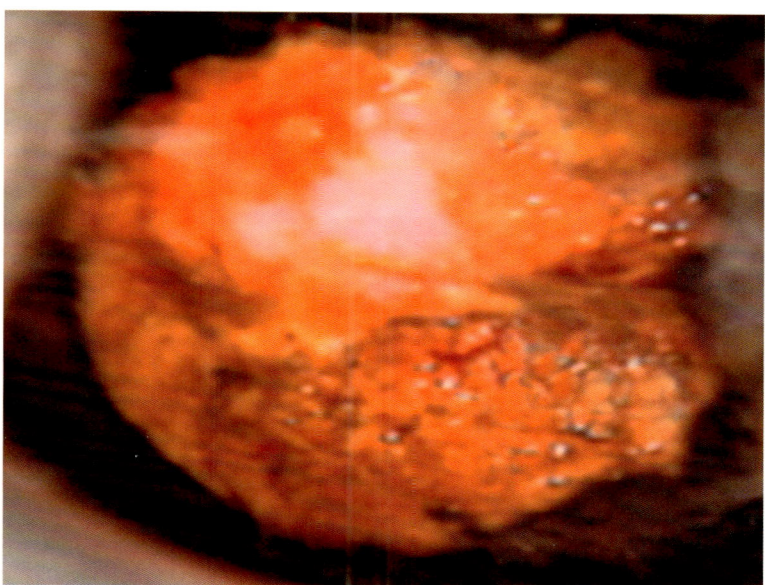

Fig. 3.17: After Lugol's iodine application: Mahogany brown squamous epithelium and Iodine negative columnar epithelium

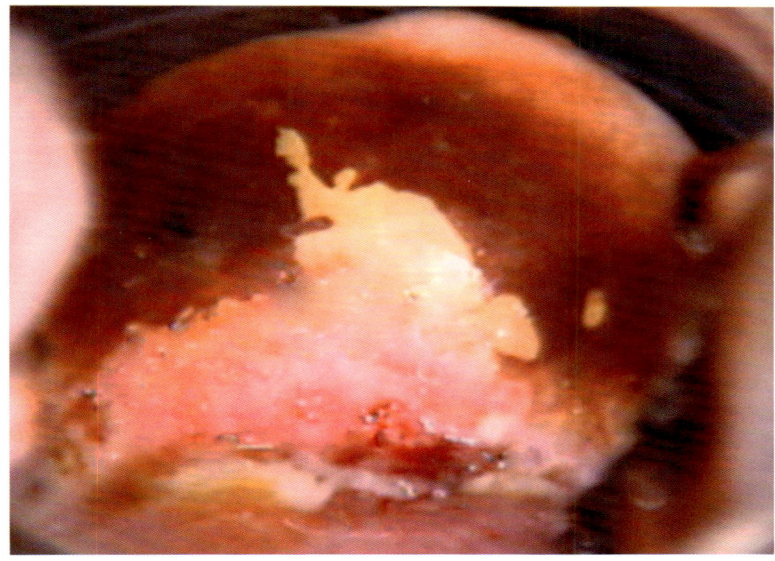

Fig. 3.18: After Lugol's iodine application: Abnormal epithelium as iodine negative area over anterior lip

Grading of Colposcopy Findings

After completing the examination of cervix and noting the details such as the site of new SCJ, limits of TZ, type of TZ, the colposcopy findings should be graded according to the classification/scoring system (Coppleson/Reid/Swede/IFCPC) with which the colposcopist is familiar. If any abnormal areas are identified, directed biopsies have to be taken after completing the examination of vagina and vulva.

Directed Biopsy

Following colposcopy, all lesions that appear to be abnormal should be biopsied. Biopsy should be taken under colposcopic guidance from a point within the most abnormal area. After taking biopsy, the sampled area should be visualized again through colposcope to ensure that biopsy has been taken from the right area only (Figs 3.19A to C).

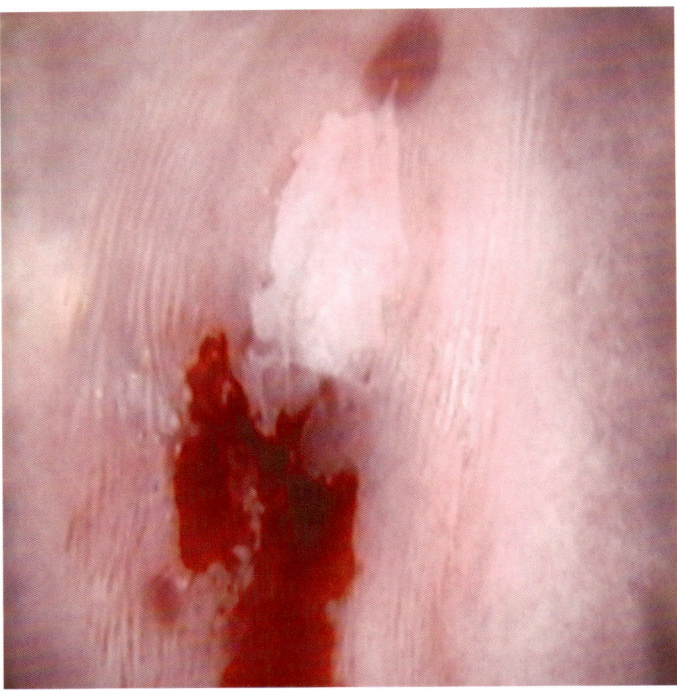

Fig. 3.19A: Lesion over anterior lip requiring biopsy

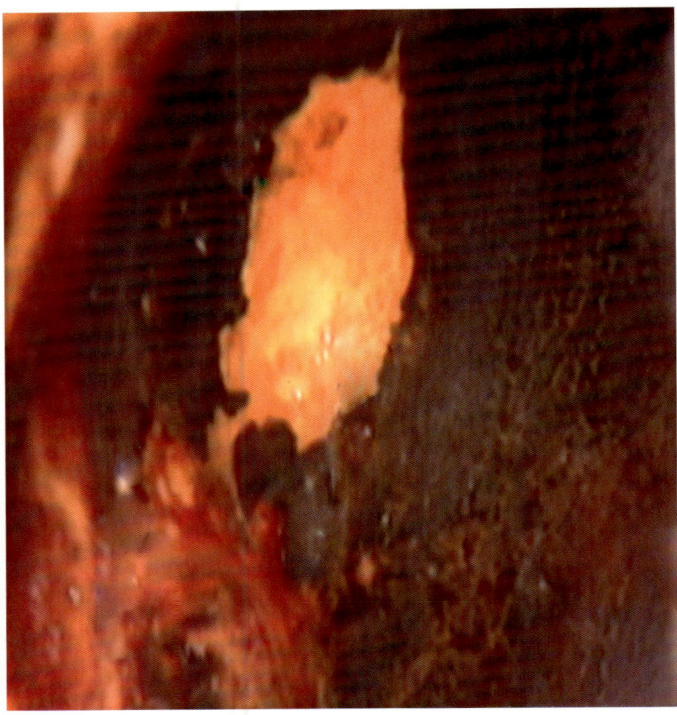

Fig. 3.19B: Same lesion after Lugol's iodine application

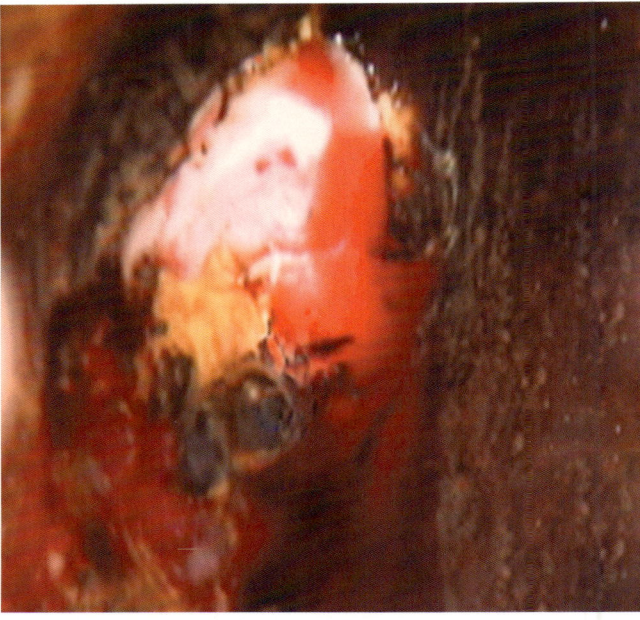

Fig. 3.19C: Checking biopsy site after taking biopsy which has been taken from within the lesion

If the lesion is large or there is more than one lesion, multiple biopsies should be taken for correlating the colposcopic findings with the histopathology result.

One can also perform electrosurgical excision of entire transformation zone (LLETZ) in such cases. If the lesion is going into the endocervical canal, taking a punch biopsy from the ectocervical portion of lesion may miss a lesion higher up in the canal. In such cases, one should resort to conization.

Biopsy can be taken using punch biopsy forceps, electrosurgical loop or as wedge biopsy using knife. Biopsy should be sufficiently deep to include adequate stroma to rule out invasion.

Punch biopsy: It does not require any anesthesia. Although not proven to reduce the pain, many colposcopists use topical anesthetic agent before taking biopsy. Biopsy forceps should be sharp enough to give a clean cut and should be able to take sufficient depth of stroma for accurate diagnosis to be made.

Compression of tissue should be avoided as crushing of the epithelium distorts the tissue architecture which may make correct histopathology interpretation difficult. Also tissue compression may lead to fragments of squamous epithelium getting buried within the connective tissue that may appear as a pseudo-invasive lesion, if the patient requires a cone biopsy or hysterectomy at a later stage.

Epithelium must be cut at right angle to the surface (Fig. 3.20). When multiple biopsies are required, biopsy from posterior lip should be taken prior to that from lateral or anterior lip of cervix as bleeding from the anterior lip may obscure the abnormal area over the posterior lip. Sometimes biopsy forceps slips on ectocervix. In such a case, tissue can be tented into the biopsy forceps with the help of iris hook so that biopsy can be taken easily.

Wedge biopsy: At times punch biopsy is not possible or may not provide sufficient stroma especially in postmenopausal and post-irradiation cases when the cervix is totally flushed with vagina.

Wedge biopsy can be taken with the help of small conical knife (Fig. 3.21) under local anesthesia. Hemostasis can be obtained with a stitch of catgut.

Electrosurgical loop biopsy: Thin wire loop 0.5 cm diameter size is used with blend current (Fig. 3.21). A deeper and wider chunk of tissue can be easily obtained under local anesthesia. Bleeding is minimal with this method.

Hemostasis after biopsy can be achieved simply by packing the vagina with gauze. Alternatively, Monsel's paste (ferric subsulfate) or silver nitrate stick can be applied at the biopsy site.

Such hemostatic agents should be applied only after taking all the biopsies as it may interfere with subsequent colposcopic evaluation. Extra Monsel's paste should be wiped out carefully before withdrawing vaginal speculum. Patient should be warned about having a charcoal-like tarry vaginal discharge for few days.

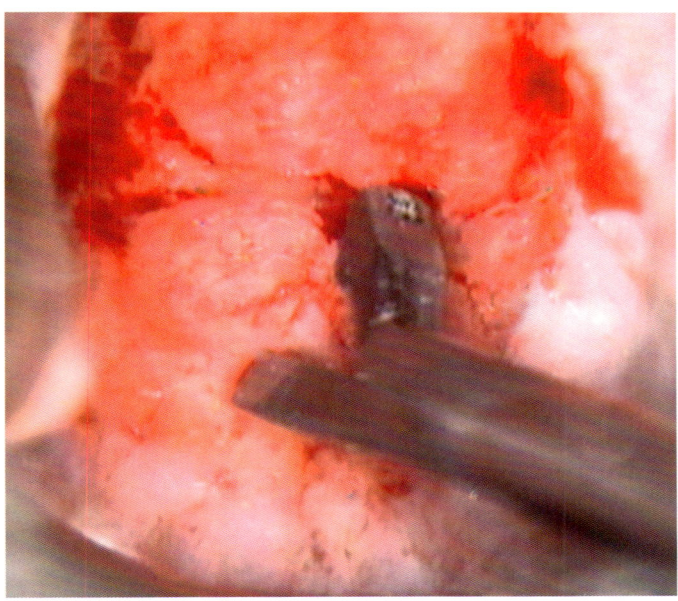

Fig. 3.20: Taking punch biopsy

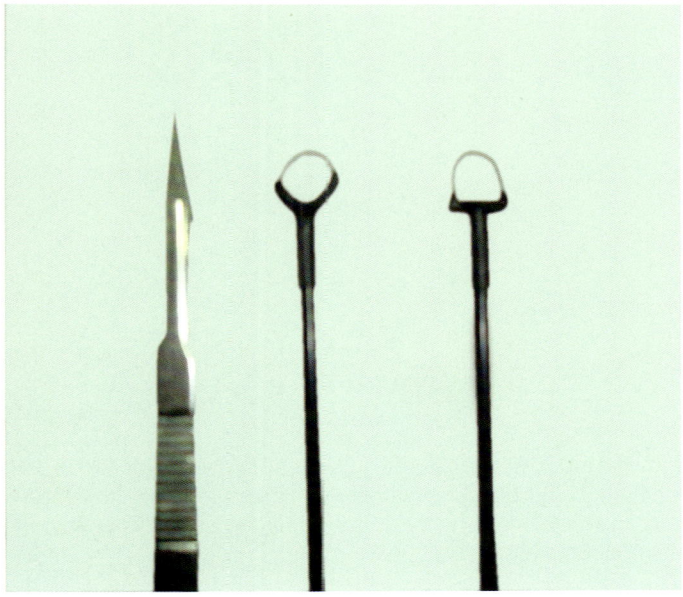

Fig. 3.21: Knife for wedge biopsy and small loops for biopsy

Endocervical Curettage

Endocervical curettage (ECC) aims to detect an endocervical glandular or squamous lesion that cannot be reached by a colposcopically directed biopsy. It cannot confirm the presence or absence of an invasive lesion because the specimen is often superficial, and the distinction between adenocarcinoma in situ and invasive adenocarcinoma is often compromised.

ECC is often carried out in conjunction with cervical biopsy in USA, but is used less frequently in Europe, where a diagnostic conization is often preferred when an endocervical lesion has to be excluded.

We believe that the endocervical curettage must be done, if the colposcopy is unsatisfactory (SC junction not visible) or if an abnormal lesion is extending up into the canal. The role of ECC in cases of satisfactory colposcopy/abnormal lesion visible completely on the ectocervix is controversial. In such case, one could do ECC, if the lesion is high grade or is large so as to avoid a false negative diagnosis.

The endocervical curettage is performed using an endocervical curette which is held like a pencil and introduced into the endocervical canal. With gentle strokes all around, tissue fragments of endocervical epithelium are curetted and transferred to formalin. Care is taken not to withdraw the curette on to the ectocervix as sample may get contaminated with the strip of abnormal epithelium from ectocervix and may give false positive results. Endocervical sampling using an endocervical brush is equally good and shows a lower false-negative rate than ECC.

Endocervical curettage should not be performed during pregnancy.

The biopsy samples should be carefully preserved in 10% formalin and labeled accurately before sending to the laboratory along with detailed proforma of patient identification, clinical and colposcopic findings.

Documentation of Findings

Serial documentation of colposcopic findings is very important to analyze progression or regression of the disease process. Documentation can be done by photography or by hand drawings. Modern digital videocolposcope is very helpful for keeping serial photographic records.

In absence of facility for photography, simple, clear, elaborate and explanatory hand drawings should always be made soon after colposcopic examination. Cervical findings along with location of SCJ are marked at the specific site. Both normal as well as abnormal findings are marked and specified with abbreviations like AW (acetowhite area), TTZ (typical transformation zone), PN (punctation), MO (mosaic), etc.

Many graphs have been devised to record the findings. Odell's diagram (Fig. 3.22A) is the simplest. Another is Hammond's graph (Fig. 3.22B) which has twelve sections divided by concentric circles to mark the findings at a more precise site. Biopsy sites should also be marked. Records should include demographic information, clinical findings and recommendations for follow-up and treatment.

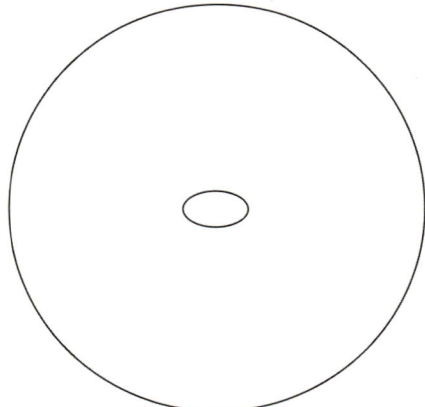

Fig. 3.22A: Odell's diagram. Cervical findings along with the location of squamocolumnar jucntion are marked at the specific site and the lesion can be specified by the side of the diagram using abbreviations

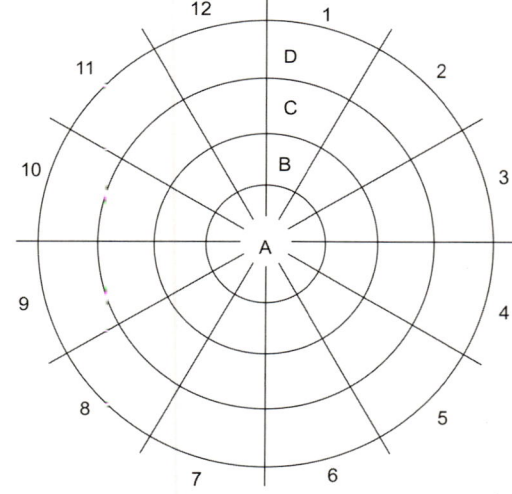

Fig. 3.22B: Hammond's graph. It has twelve sections divided by concentric circles to mark the findings at a more precise site. Lesions can be specified using the abbreviations

Abbreviations: EC Ectopy; TTZ Typical transformation zone; NF Nabothian follicle; GO Gland opening; ATZ Atypical transformation zone; PN Punctation; MO Mosaic; AW Acetowhite lesion

COLPOSCOPY OF VAGINA

Vagina is examined after the examination of cervix. Colposcopy of vagina is more tedious and difficult and technically challenging because of large surface area and vaginal rugosity.

Ideally vagina must always be examined after examination of cervix but it is especially indicated if cervix shows no abnormality in a case of abnormal Pap smear, after treatment of CIN, after hysterectomy for CIN or invasive disease, after radiotherapy, HPV associated disease, history of maternal DES exposure or any gross lesion on inspection or palpation.

Examination of vagina takes much longer time than cervix and is uncomfortable to the patient. Vaginal fornices can be examined along with the cervix, while the lateral, anterior and posterior walls along rest of the vagina, are examined by slowly and simultaneously withdrawing as well as rotating the vaginal speculum (Figs 3.23A and B)

All the folds of vagina are examined as they roll over the speculum blades during withdrawal. Appropriate size speculum with long blades should be used deep enough to examine uppermost vagina and can be easily rotated also.

To minimize discomfort to the patient, diluted 1–4% xylocaine solution can be applied to vagina beforehand.

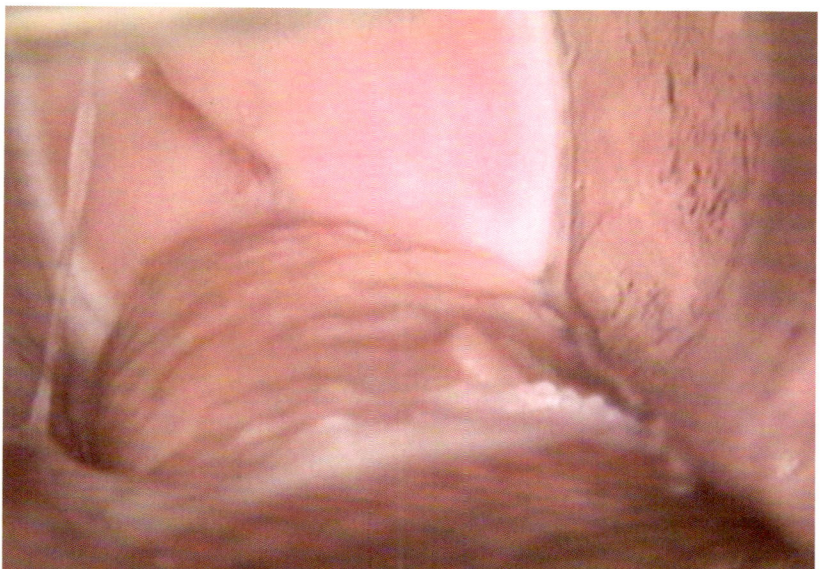

Fig. 3.23A: Examination of posterior vaginal wall

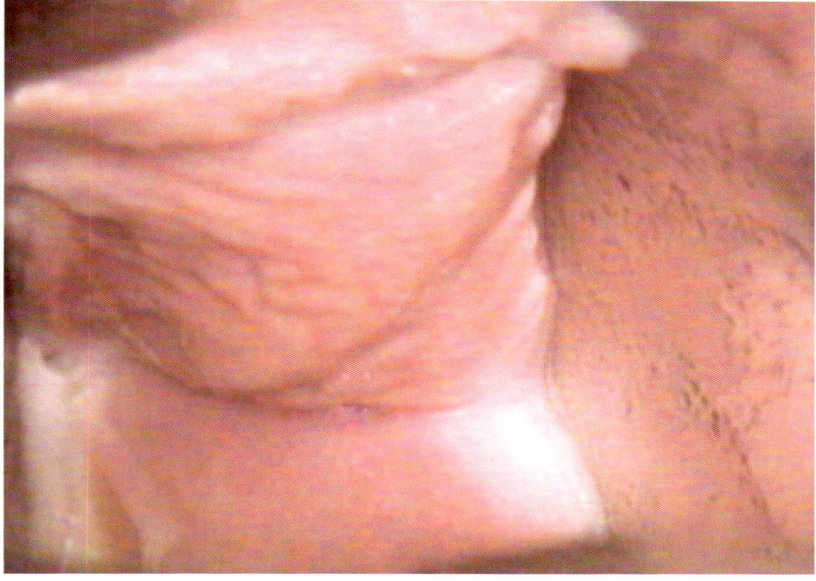

Fig. 3.23B: Examination of anterior vaginal wall

Instead of 3%, 5% acetic acid can be used for vagina so that even the subtle lesions may appear rapidly decreasing examination time. It should be liberally applied over the entire vaginal epithelium (Fig. 3.24A). A hook may have to be used to evaluate all the folds and angles of the vagina by stretching the mucosa and flattening the rugae.

Unlike other sites, application of Lugol's iodine is a must for vagina (Fig. 3.24B). It aids in detection of even the minutest lesion, which may otherwise be overlooked because of large surface area and multifocal lesions in vagina.

Vaginal biopsy site should be selected during colposcopy. Multiple biopsies may be required. Cervical punch biopsy forceps is used and biopsy is taken after elevating epithelium of biopsy site with the help of iris hook.

One should be careful because vaginal epithelium is not very thick. Superficial biopsy may not include the full thickness while deeper biopsy may injure deeper tissues. Hemostasis after biopsy can be easily obtained by local pressure or Monsel's solution. Rarely stitch may be required.

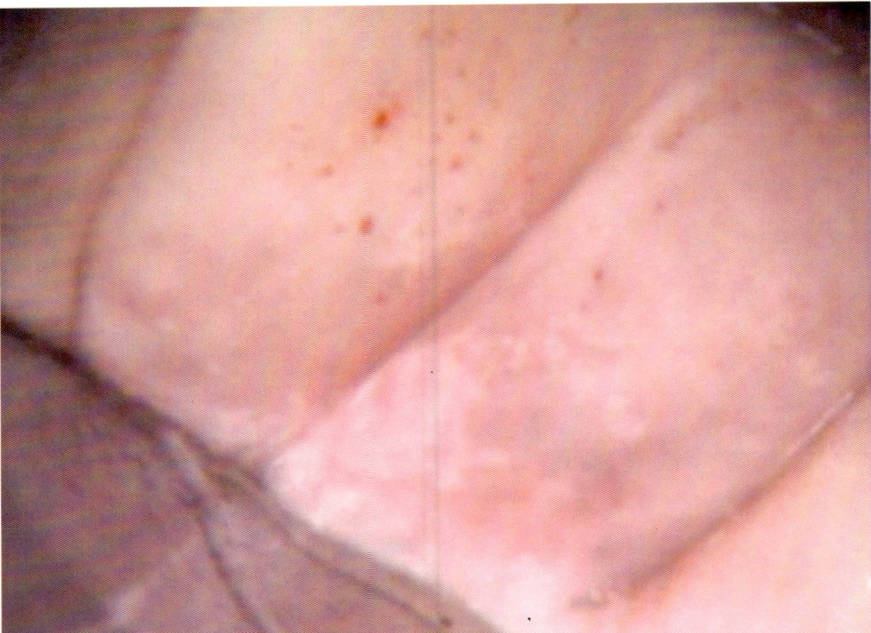

Fig. 3.24A: Vagina after acetic acid application

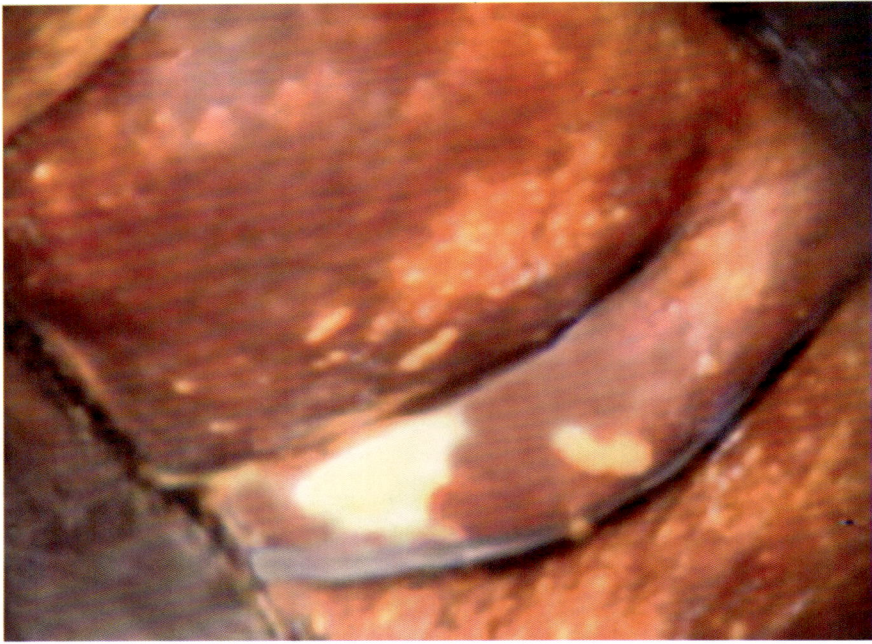

Fig. 3.24B: Vagina after Lugol's iodine application

COLPOSCOPY OF VULVA—VULVOSCOPY

Vulva is the part of the female genital tract located between the genitocrural folds laterally, the mons pubis anteriorly, and the anus posteriorly. Embryologically, it is the result of the junction of the cloacal endoderm, urogenital ectoderm, and paramesonephric mesodermal layers.

Epithelium of vulva is predominantly dry, hyperkeratotic and opaque which does not provide a clear view of the underlying vascular pattern. Therefore, in the past, colposcope was not considered suitable for evaluation of vulval lesions.

With the recognition of subclinical forms of HPV lesions of vulva, especially in young females with its multifocal pattern, colposcope has emerged as being a more accurate diagnostic technique. It helps in detection of acetowhite lesions or other less macroscopic lesions which may otherwise be missed by evaluation of the vulva by gross inspection only. Magnification provided by colposcopy aids in better appreciation of color changes and surface anatomy even of minute lesions. It also helps in identifying the multifocal lesions for directed biopsy as well as the treatment.

Vulva is divided into hairy and non-hairy areas. Non-hairy areas are clitoris, labia minora, inner surface of labia majora, vestibule, posterior fourchette and immediate perianal mucosa (Fig. 3.25).

Different epithelia, from keratinized squamous epithelium to squamous mucosa, cover the vulva. At the introitus, well-differentiated, glycogenated squamous epithelium of vagina terminates and vulval epithelium takes over which is a highly specialized, keratinized, non-glycogenated stratified squamous epithelium.

Central portion (non-hairy) of vulva is less keratinized and gradually becomes more keratinized towards periphery. It contains all the skin appendages like sebaceous and eccrine glands and a rich network of apocrine glands but has few sweat glands and no hair follicles. Epithelium of the vestibule is neither pigmented nor keratinized and contains eccrine glands and mucus secreting glands as well.

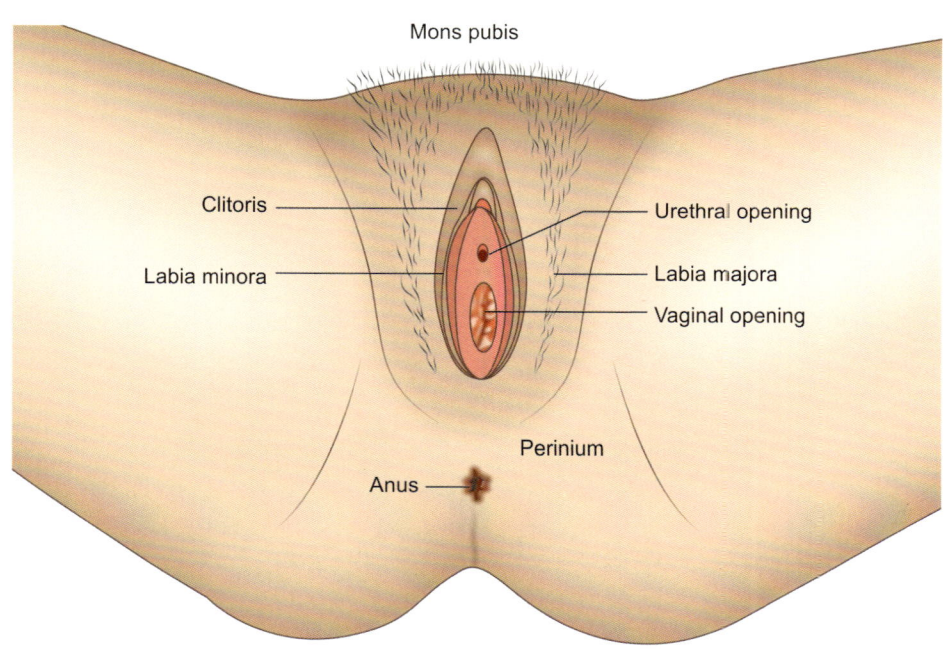

Fig. 3.25: Normal vulval anatomy

Technique

Vulval examination follows that of the cervix and vagina. Vulva is also examined in a stepwise fashion.

All the areas of vulva should be systematically examined, viz. vestibule, urethral meatus, labia minora, clitoris, prepuce and interlabial sulcus, perineal and perianal area including anus till its mucocutaneous junction.

Examination of Unprepared Vulva

It is done first by naked eye and then under low power magnification. Any leukoplakic patch pigmented or depigmented area and papule is noted; surface contour of the lesion is also noted, whether smooth, flat or papillary; any growth, ulcer or condyloma can also be made out (Figs 3.26 and 3.27).

Examination after Application of Normal Saline/Water Soluble Jelly

It decreases the keratinizing effect to a certain extent and assists in visualization of abnormal vessels.

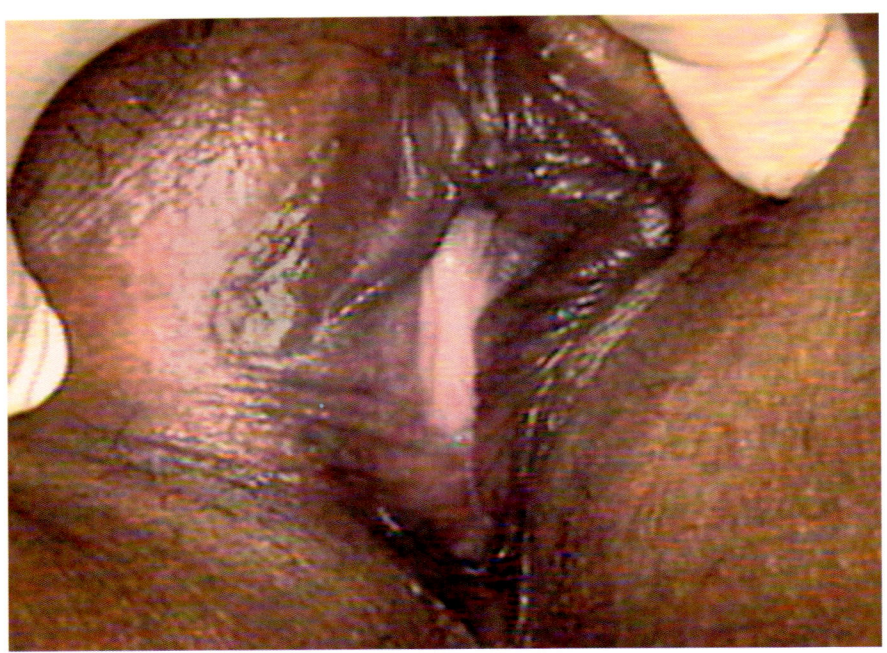

Fig. 3.26: Examination of vulva—naked eye

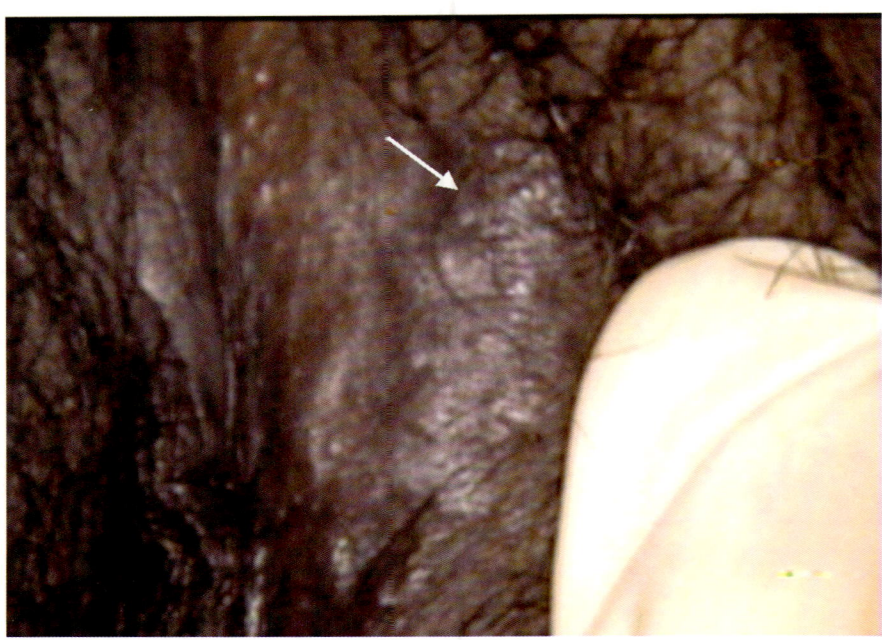

Fig. 3.27: Papules at labia majora

Examination after Acetic Acid Application

To be effective on vulval skin, acetic acid is used in more concentrated (5%) form, with the help of a swab. Vulva is soaked for about three minutes with large amount of acetic acid. Only this way, the lesions and underlying vascular aberration may become visible. Systematic observation is made under higher magnification (Figs 3.28A and B).

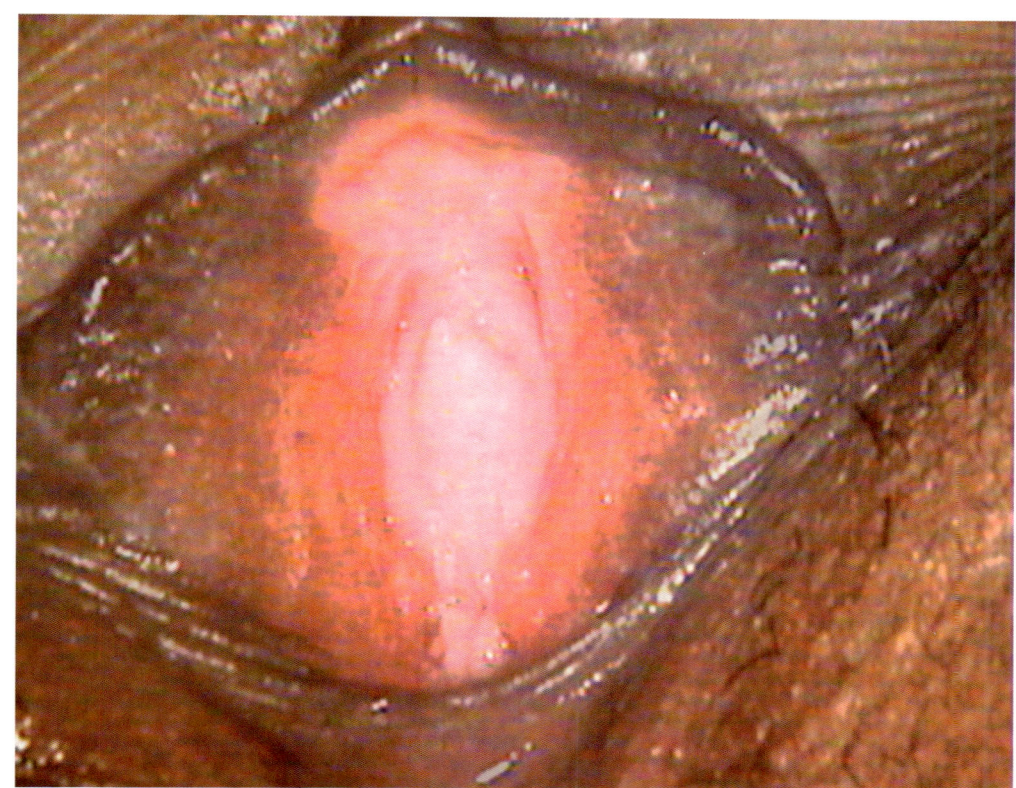

Fig. 3.28A: Examination of vulva after 5% acetic acid application

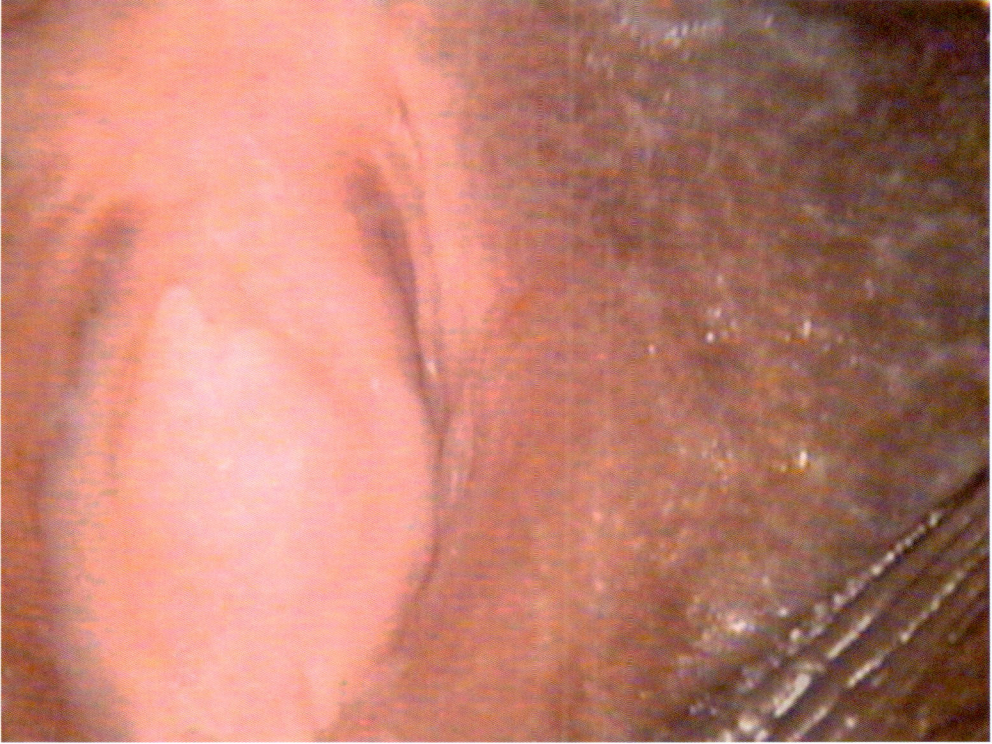

Fig. 3.28B: Examination of vulva after acetic acid application—magnified view

Examination after Toluidine Blue (Collin's test)

Toluidine blue is a nuclear stain. Normal keratinized anucleate cells of vulva do not take up this stain. 1% or 2% of toluidine blue is applied over the vulva and is left there for two minutes. Thereafter, it is washed away with 1% acetic acid.

Any condition that results in nucleated cells on the surface retains this dye as fine punctate blue dots which are easily recognized through the colposcope (Figs 3.29 and 3.30).

Nucleated cells in vulva may be due to immature squamous cells or parakeratosis. Both may be the result of variety of benign and neoplastic conditions.

Thus a positive test delineates a focus of abnormal squamous maturation and site for biopsy. This test is non-specific as the dye is retained by any erosion or ulceration also. Therefore, many people do not use this test.

Vulval Biopsy

Benign tumors of the vulva are relatively uncommon and may show non-specific clinical features. Therefore, a biopsy is often needed to exclude malignancy and to initiate proper treatment. It has to be done under local anesthesia. It can be easily taken with the dermatological punch biopsy forceps.

Alternatively, excision biopsy can be taken with knife. Bleeding is usually not much after punch biopsy; otherwise one stitch with plain catgut ensures hemostasis. The following points should be noted on vulval colposcopy:

1. *Surface contour:* Flat, raised, papular, micropapillary or condylomatous
2. *Color change:* Normal, white, red, brown, or other pigmentation.
3. *Blood vessels:* Absent, punctation, mosaic, atypical vessels. Punctations are seen occasionally in non-hairy portion. Mosaic is a rare finding in vulva.
4. *Location:* Unifocal or multifocal.

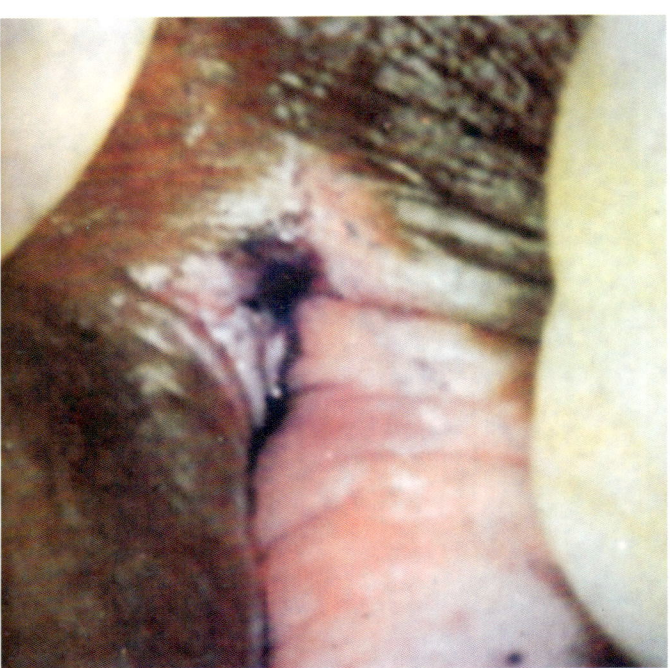

Fig. 3.29: Toluidine positive lesion pointing to abnormal area

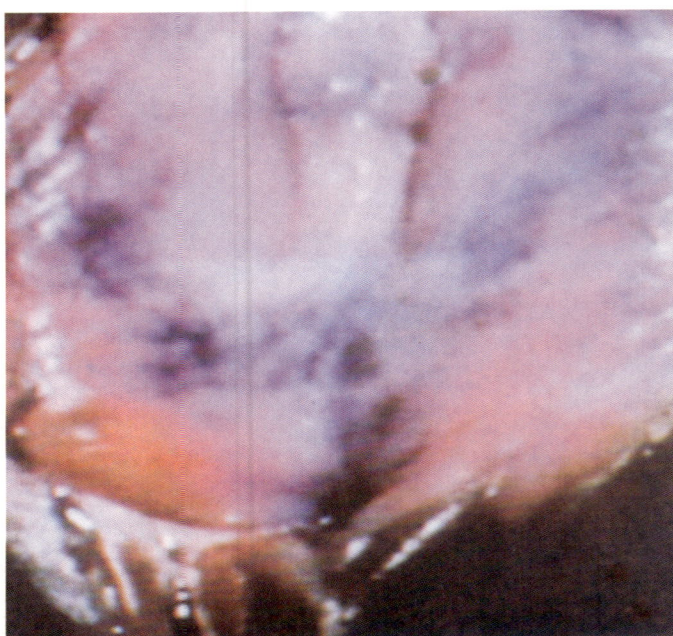

Fig. 3.30: Vulva after Collin's test — retention of blue dye seen as punctate blue dots

Chapter

4

Colposcopic Nomenclature

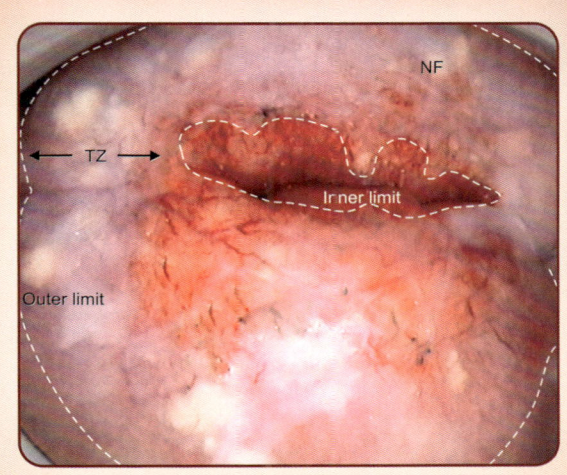

Chapter Outline

Original Hinselmann's nomenclature was purely descriptive and not related to histological characteristics. With the world over popularization of colposcopy, a need for universal colposcopic nomenclature was felt to describe and interpret the colposcopic findings.

Basic colposcopic terminology was approved in 1975 at the second world congress for cervical pathology and colposcopy, but this was applicable to cervix only.

In 1990, at seventh world congress, International Federation of Cervical Pathology and Colposcopy (IFCPC) approved a modified version which was applicable to the entire lower female genital tract (Table 4.1).

This was further modified in 2002 and 2008 after reviewing publications that critically analyzed each colposcopic sign, aiming to create an evidence-based terminology.

At the World Congress of Cervical Pathology and Colposcopy 2011, a new IFCPC nomenclature has been formulated to describe the colposcopic features to help identify significant disease, plan management in a rational way, and facilitate research collaboration. This includes terminology related to the cervix (Table 4.2), the vagina, and added an addendum to terminology of the cervix.

IFCPC recommends that the 2011 terminology should replace all other terminologies and be implemented for diagnosis, treatment and research.

Table 4.1: International (IFCPC) colposcopic terminology–1990

Normal colposcopic findings
- Original squamous epithelium
- Original columnar epithelium
- Transformation zone

Abnormal colposcopic findings
(Inside/outside transformation zone)
- Acetowhite epithelium (flat/micropapillary)
- Punctation (fine/coarse)
- Mosaic (fine/coarse)
- Leukoplakia (fine/coarse)
- Iodine negative epithelium
- Atypical vessels
- Colposcopically suspect invasive carcinoma

Unsatisfactory colposcopy
- Squamocolumnar junction not visible
- Severe inflammation or atrophy
- Cervix not visible

Miscellaneous findings
- Nonacetowhite micropapillary surface
- Exophytic condyloma
- Inflammation, atrophy, ulcer, and others

Table 4.2: International (IFCPC) colposcopic terminology–2011

General assessment		• **Adequate/inadequate for the reason…** (i.e. cervix obscured by inflammation, bleeding, scar) • **Squamocolumnar junction visibility** completely visible, partially visible, not visible • **Transformation zone types 1, 2, 3**	
Normal colposcopic findings		– Original squamous epithelium – Mature – Atrophic – Columnar epithelium – Ectopy – Metaplastic squamous epithelium – Nabothian cyst – Crypt (gland) openings – Deciduosis in pregnancy	
Abnormal colposcopic findings	**General principles**	**Location of the lesion:** Inside or outside the T-zone, location of the lesion by clock position **Size of the lesion:** Number of cervical quadrants the lesion covers; size of the lesion in percentage of cervix	
	Grade 1 (Minor)	– Thin acetowhite epithelium – Irregular, geographic border	– Fine mosaic – Fine punctation
	Grade 2 (Major)	– Dense acetowhite epithelium – Rapid appearance of acetowhitening – Cuffed crypt (gland) opening	– Coarse mosaic – Coarse punctation – Sharp border – Inner border sign – Ridge sign
	Non-specific	– Leukoplakia (keratosis, hyperkeratosis), erosion – Lugol's staining (Schiller's test): Stained/non-stained	
Suspicious for invasion		o Atypical vessels o **Additional signs:** Fragile vessels, irregular surface, exophytic lesion, necrosis, ulceration, tumor/gross neoplasm	
Miscellaneous findings		– Congenital transformation zone – Polyp (ecto/endocervical) – Congenital anomaly – Post-treatment consequence	– Condyloma – Stenosis – Inflammation – Endometriosis
Addendum to terminology of cervix			
Excision treatment types		**Excision types** 1, 2, 3	
Excision specimen dimensions		**Length:** The distance from the distal/external margin to the proximal/internal margin **Thickness:** The distance from the stromal margin to the surface of the excised specimen **Circumference (optional):** The perimeter of the excised specimen	

GENERAL ASSESSMENT

The popular terms "satisfactory colposcopy" and "unsatisfactory colposcopy" have been abolished in the new nomenclature. The opening statement of every colposcopic examination should be on **adequacy/ inadequacy of colposcopy** and the **visibility of SCJ**. The terms "adequacy" and "squamocolumnar junction visibility" are not mutually exclusive.

Adequacy/Inadequacy of Colposcopy

The term 'adequacy' is used to comment on the visualization of the cervix. If examination is inadequate, reasoning for inadequacy, such as cervix is obscured by inflammation, bleeding, or scarring, etc. should be mentioned (Figs 4.1 to 4.3).

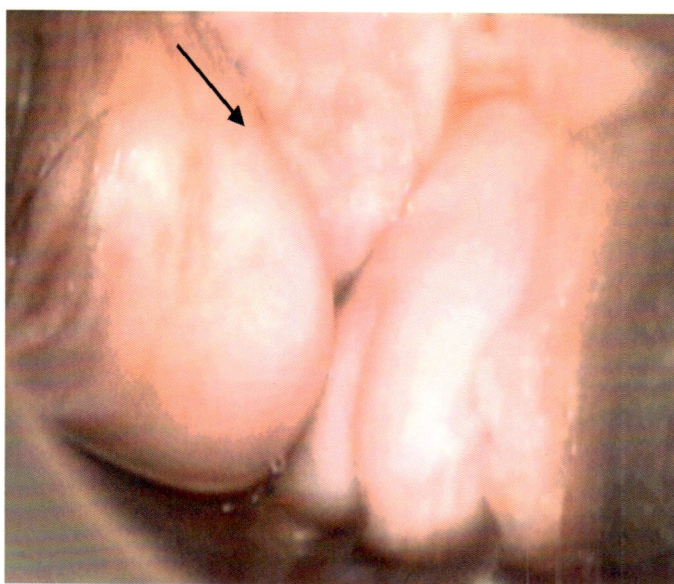

Fig. 4.1: Inadequate colposcopy—cervix obscured by vaginal cysts

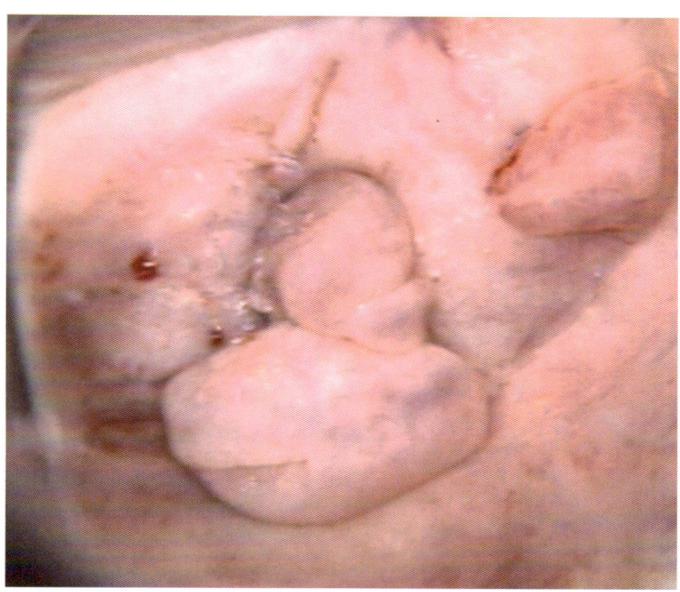

Fig. 4.2: Multiple polyps obscuring cervix

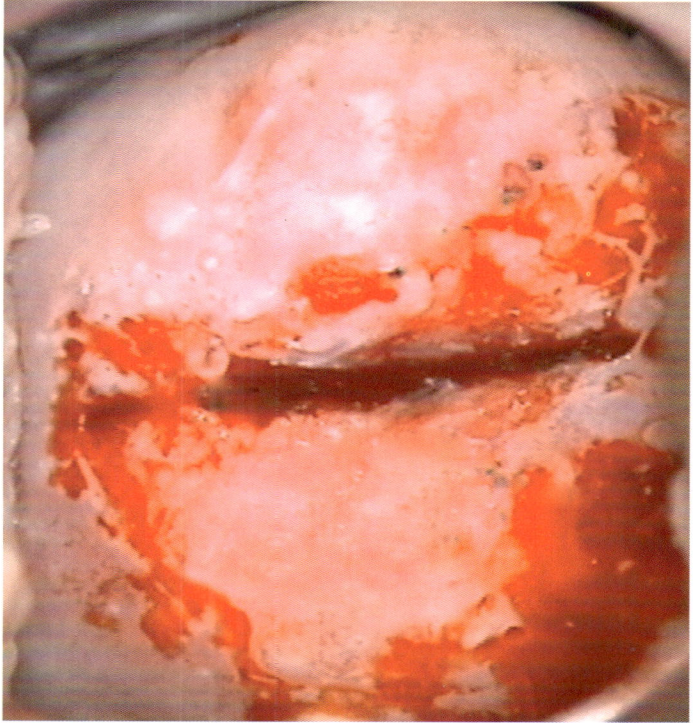

Fig. 4.3: Inadequate colposcopy due to bleeding

SCJ Visibility

The squamocolumnar junction is described as "completely visible" when 360° of the SCJ is seen (Fig. 4.4), and "not visible" when all or most of the SCJ cannot be seen because it is in the endocervical canal (Fig. 4.5). It is described as "partially visible" when most of the SCJ is visible but a section of it is inside the endocervical canal (Fig. 4.6) or when a lesion covers the SCJ with its inner border in the endocervical canal.

The squamocolumnar junction may be partially visible because a portion of its inner margin is located high in the endocervical canal, whereas the colposcopic examination is still considered adequate because the cervix itself is not obscured by blood or inflammation.

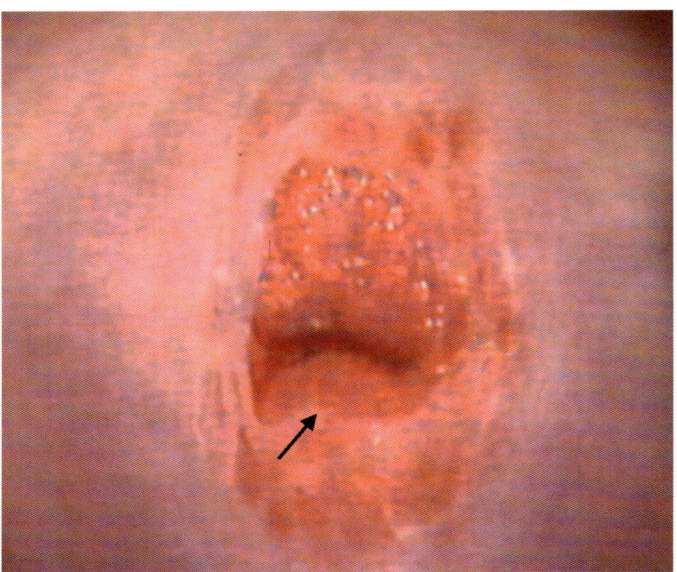

Fig. 4.4: Colposcopy adequate with SCJ completely visible

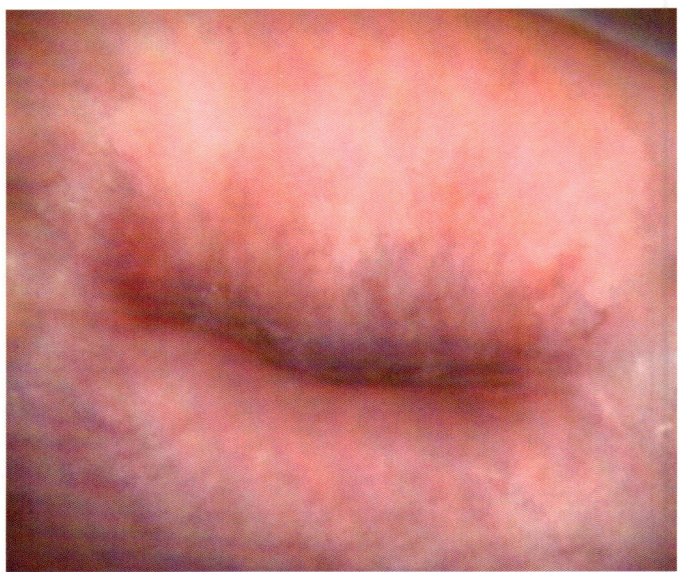

Fig. 4.5: Colposcopy adequate with SCJ not visible (inside endocervix)

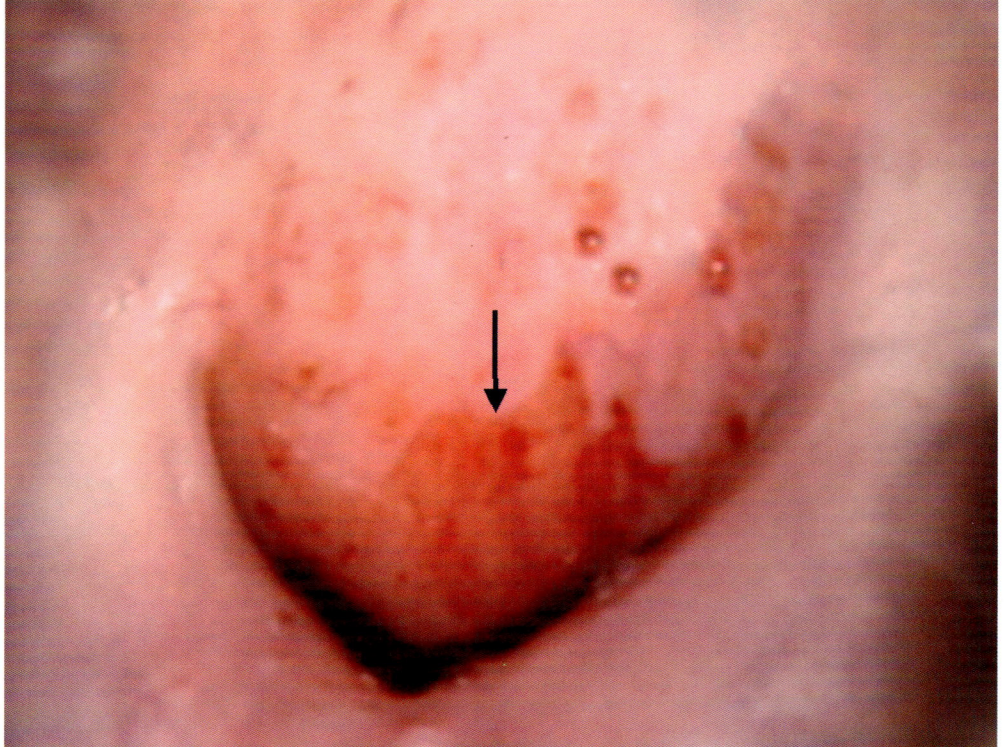

Fig. 4.6: Colposcopy adequate with incompletely visible SCJ (visible over anterior lip and not visible posteriorly)

Transformation Zone Types

The third parameter in general assessment involves assigning a transformation zone (TZ) type.

Type 1 TZ

TZ is completely ectocervical and fully visible and may be small or large (Fig. 4.7A).

Type 2 TZ

TZ has an endocervical component, is fully visible, and may have an ectocervical component that may be small or large (Fig. 4.7B).

Type 3 TZ

TZ has an endocervical component that is not fully visible, and may have an ectocervical component that may be small or large (Fig. 4.7C).

"TZ type" overlaps with the "visibility of the squamo-columnar junction" to some degree, but not completely. The TZ and the SCJ is not the same thing. The SCJ is the "inner" margin of the transformation zone.

Both types 1 and 2 TZ are "completely visible". The differentiation between two is important, mainly for planning treatment.

A fully visible and small TZ is easy to assess and simple to treat by ablation or excision, whereas a large type 3 TZ is not possible to completely assess colposcopically and also difficult to treat with increased risk of long-term morbidity and residual disease.

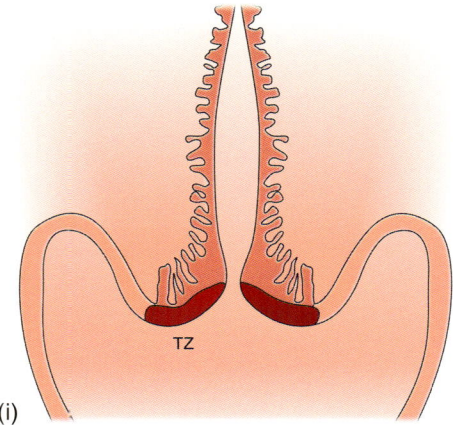

(i)

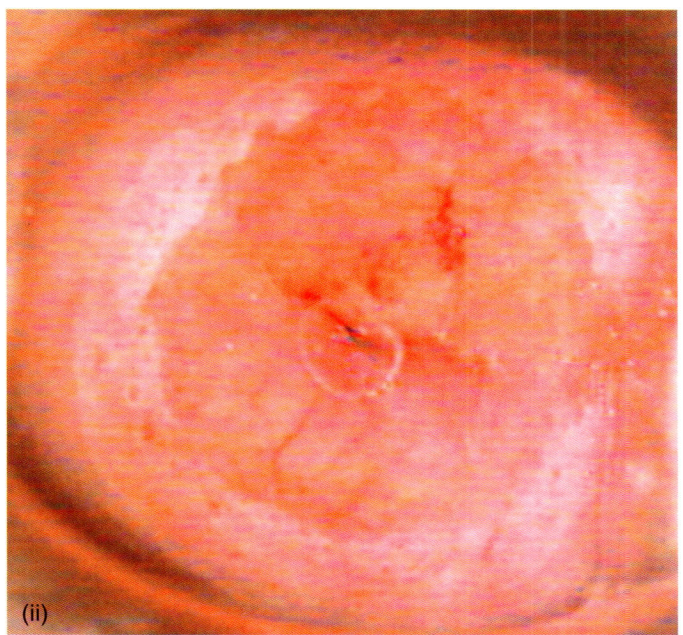

(ii)

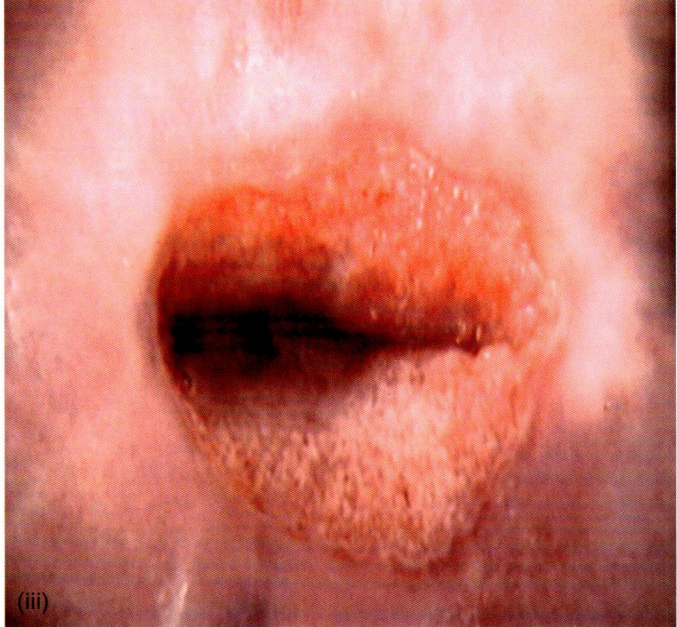

(iii)

Fig. 4.7A (i, ii and iii): Type 1 TZ

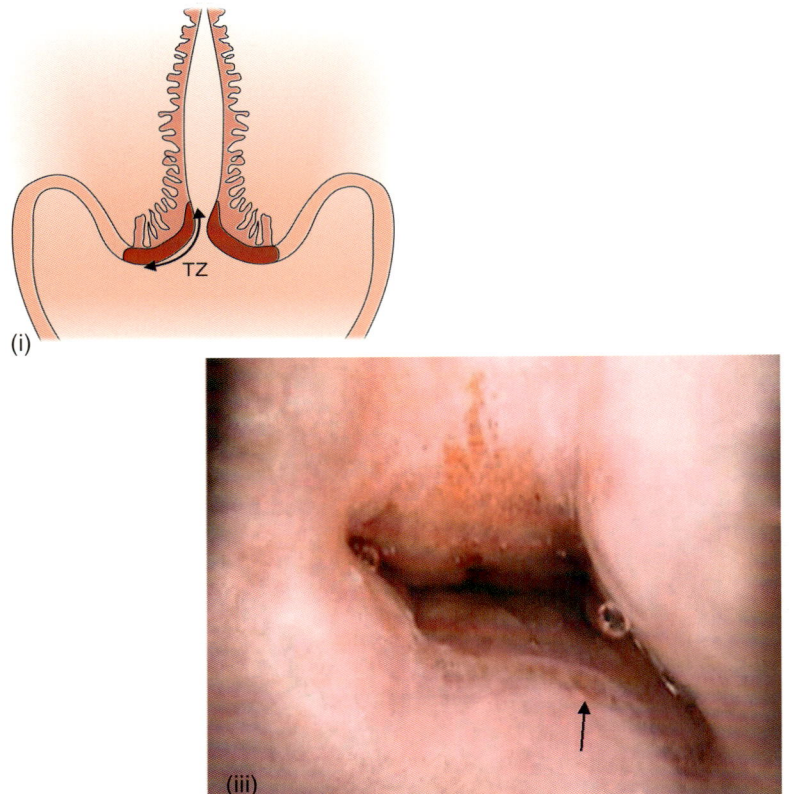

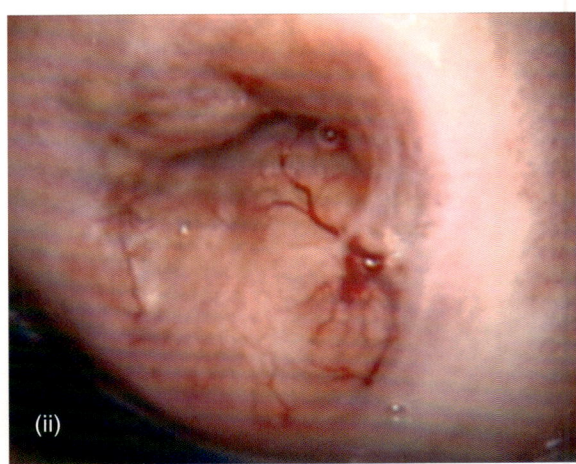

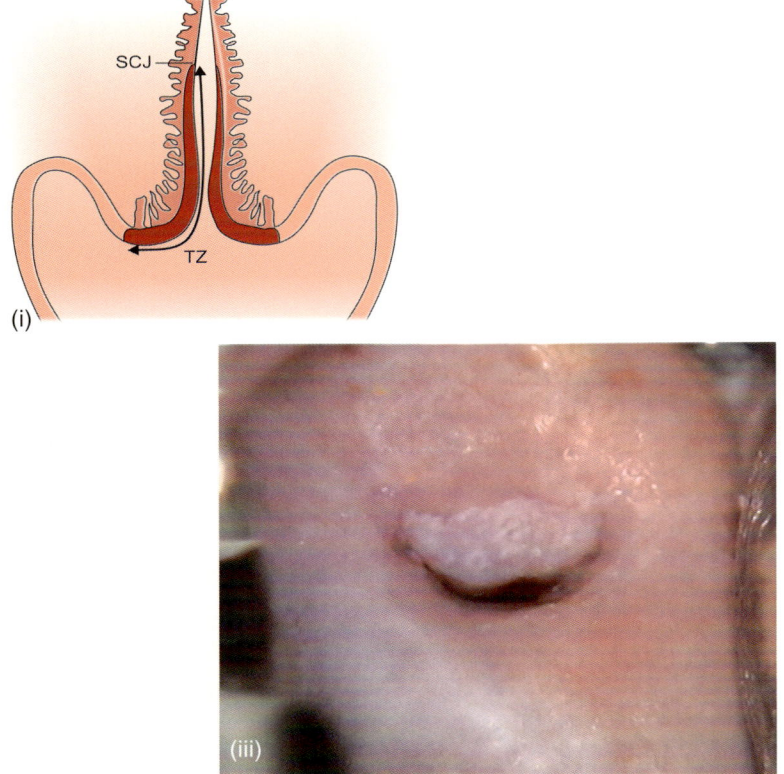

Fig. 4.7B (i, ii and iii): Type 2 TZ

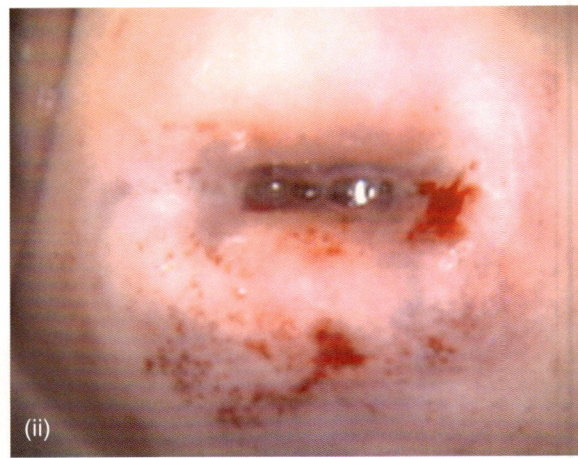

Fig. 4.7C (i, ii and iii): Type 3 TZ

NORMAL COLPOSCOPIC FINDINGS

Original Squamous Epithelium (OSE)

OSE is the epithelium in the region of ectocervix beyond the outer limit of the transformation zone. OSE looks translucent, flat, homogeneous, and uniformly pink in color, during the reproductive years (Fig. 4.8), whereas atrophic epithelium of the postmenopausal cervix appears pale and thin (Fig. 4.9).

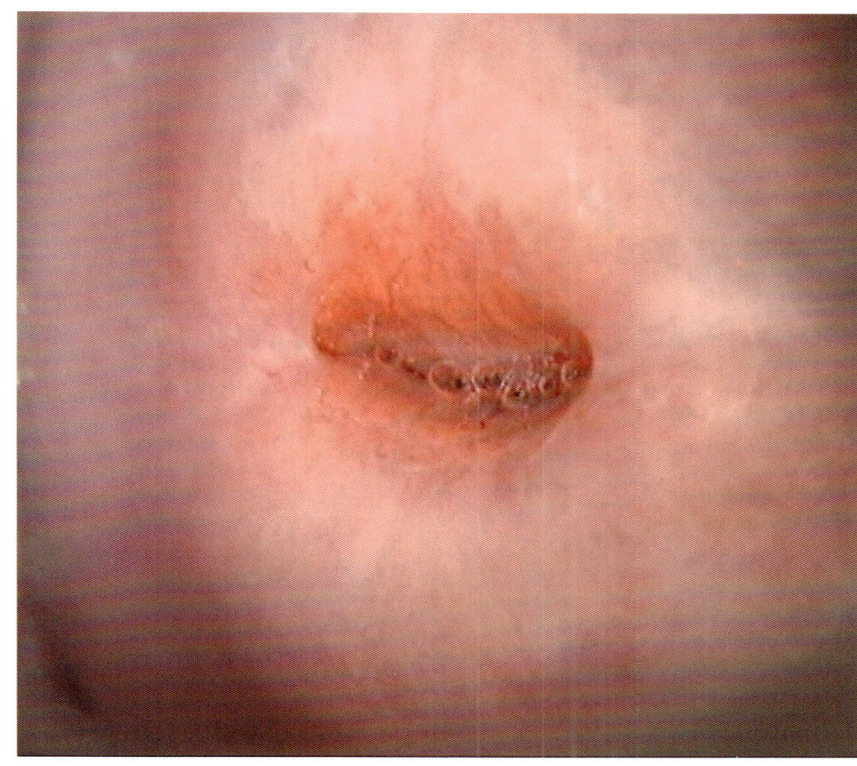

Fig. 4.8: Original squamous epithelium—during reproductive life seen as translucent, flat, homogeneous and uniformely pink surface

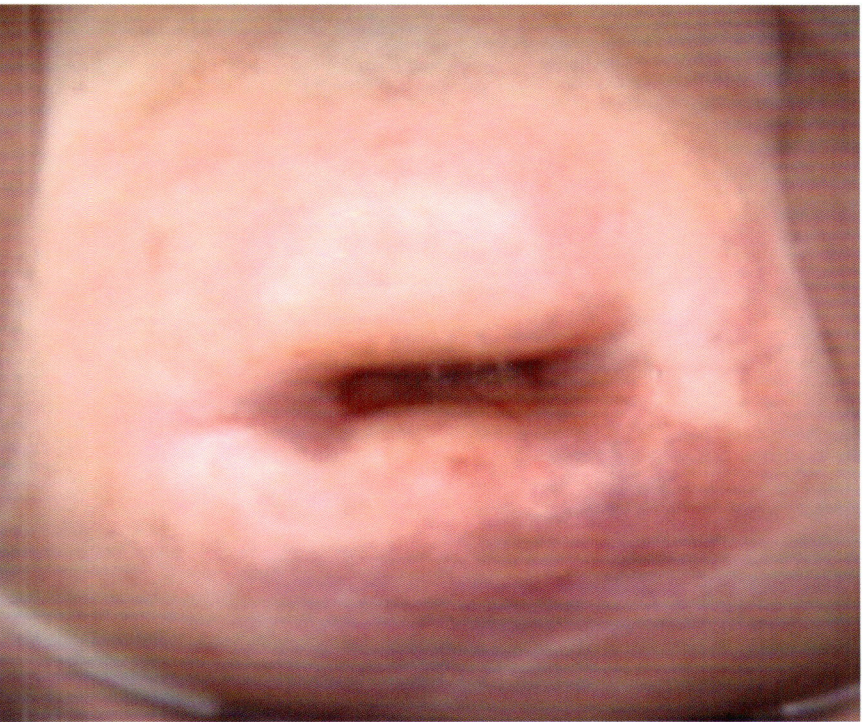

Fig. 4.9: Thin and pale, atrophic squamous epithelium in postmenopausal age

Columnar Epithelium

It is the epithelium lining the endocervical canal. When the columnar epithelium comes onto the ectocervix it is called *ectopy* (Figs 4.10 and 4.11). It has a red, velvety appearance (Fig. 4.10) which changes into grape-like structures after the application of acetic acid (Fig. 4.11).

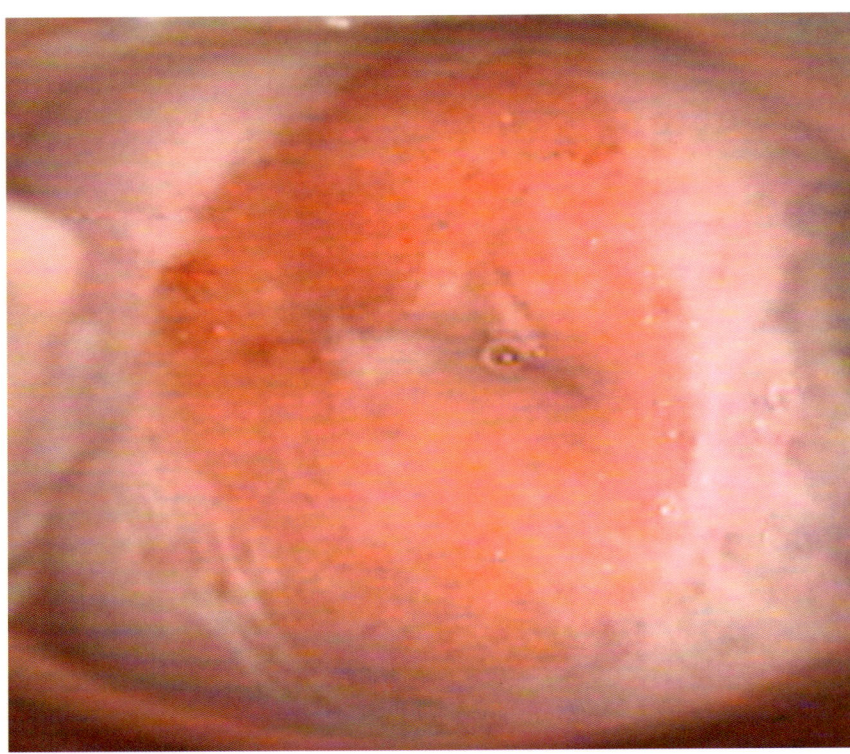

Fig. 4.10: Columnar epithelium as red velvety surface—ectopy

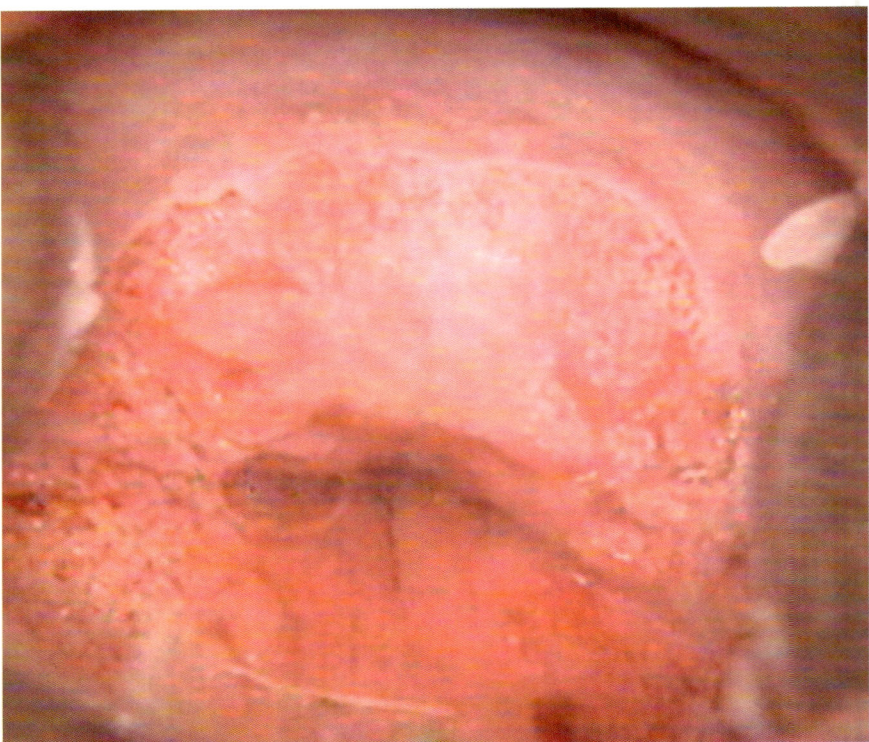

Fig. 4.11: After acetic acid application: Ectopy with grape-like columnar epithelium

Metaplastic Squamous Epithelium

The metaplastic squamous epithelium lies between the OSE and CE in the area of transformation zone. The metaplastic epithelium may be in different stages of maturation. Its inner boundary is the new SCJ and outer limit is the SSJ (old SCJ) and is marked by the presence of GOs and NFs (Figs 4.12 and 4.13).

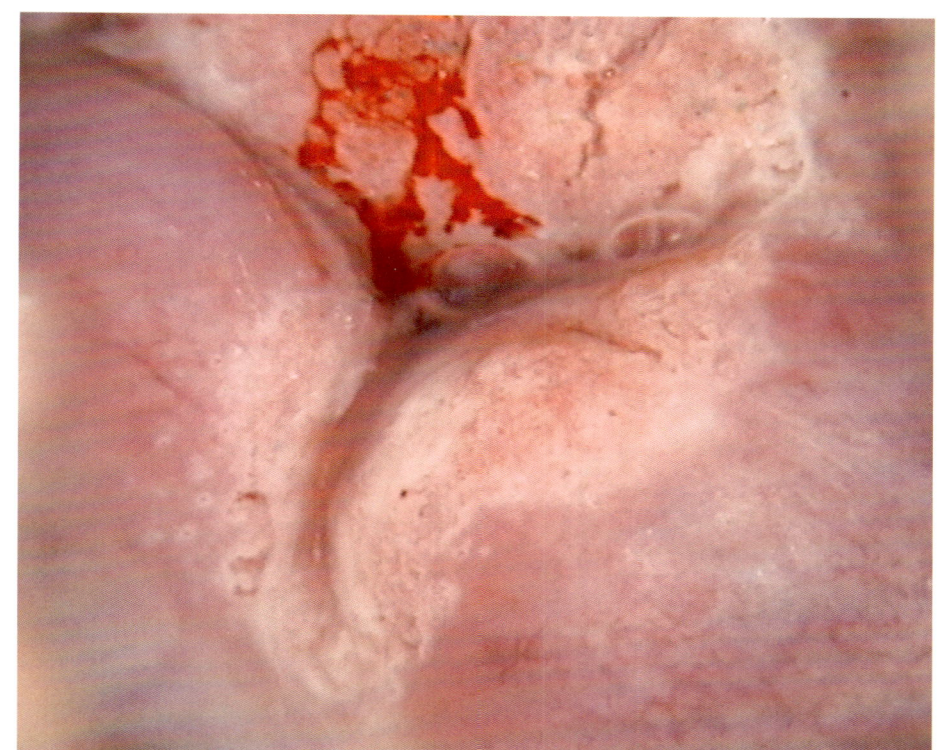

Fig. 4.12: After acetic acid application—mature metaplastic epithelium with multiple gland openings

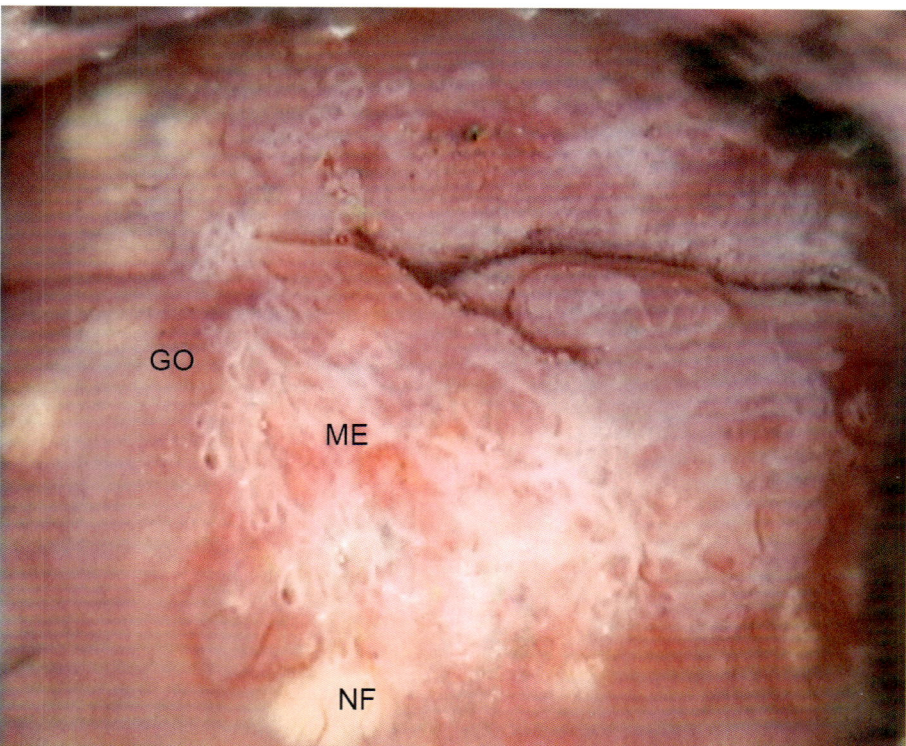

Fig. 4.13: Transformation zone with various stages of metaplasia, gland openings and nabothian follicles

ABNORMAL COLPOSCOPIC FINDINGS

General Principles

Location of the Lesion

Location of the lesion in relation to the transformation zone was part of the 1990 IFCPC colposcopic terminology, but not the 2002 terminology. However, a lesion within the transformation zone (Fig. 4.14), as opposed to one outside (Fig. 4.15), has been shown to be an independent predictor of a high-grade lesion or carcinoma. Hence it has been added again in the 2011 terminology. "Inside" location means within the boundaries of TZ. Location of the lesion should also be described by the clock position(s) (Figs 4.14 and 4.15).

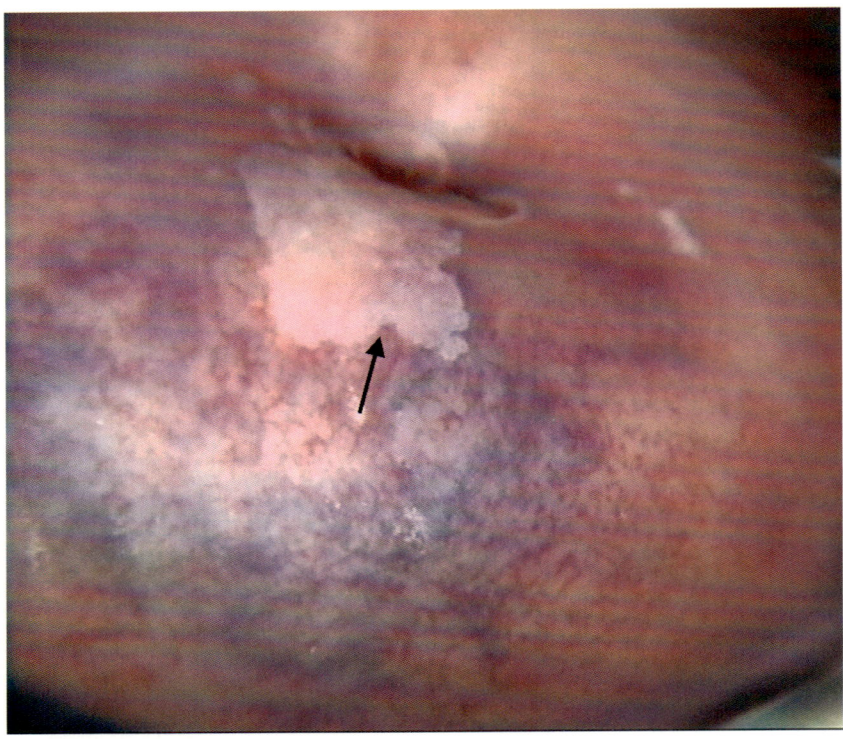

Fig. 4.14: Small grade 2 AW lesion seen inside TZ at 6–7 O' clock, occupying one quadrant only

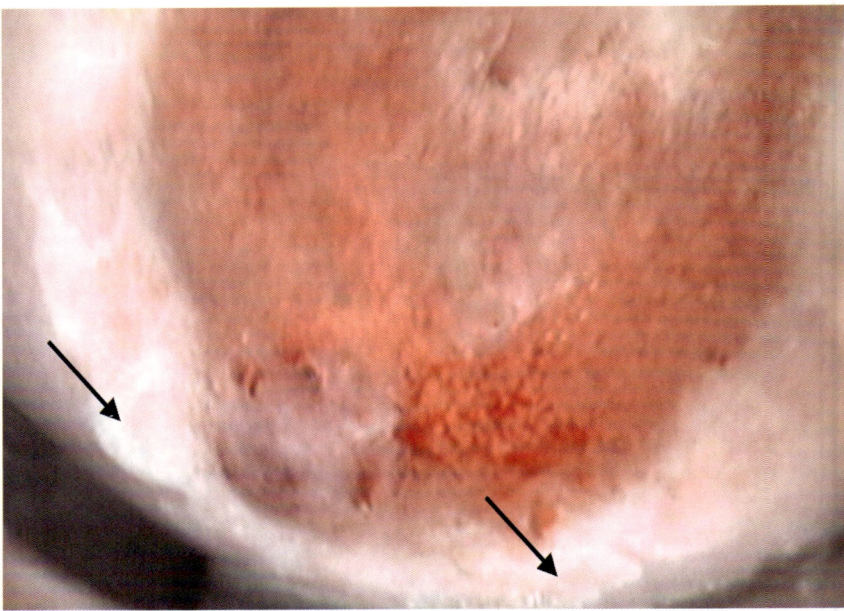

Fig. 4.15: Grade 2 AW lesion outside TZ from 5–8 O' clock, occupying 2 quadrants

Size of the Lesion

Number of cervical quadrants the lesion covers; and the size of the lesion in percentage of cervix has been added in the latest terminology, because the size of the cervical lesion has been found to have a predictive value for a high histologic grade. Both the size and location by quadrants have been added as these two parameters do not overlap; for example, a lesion can occupy three quadrants but be composed of a thin layer of abnormal epithelium that occupies only 10% of cervix (Figs 4.16 and 4.17).

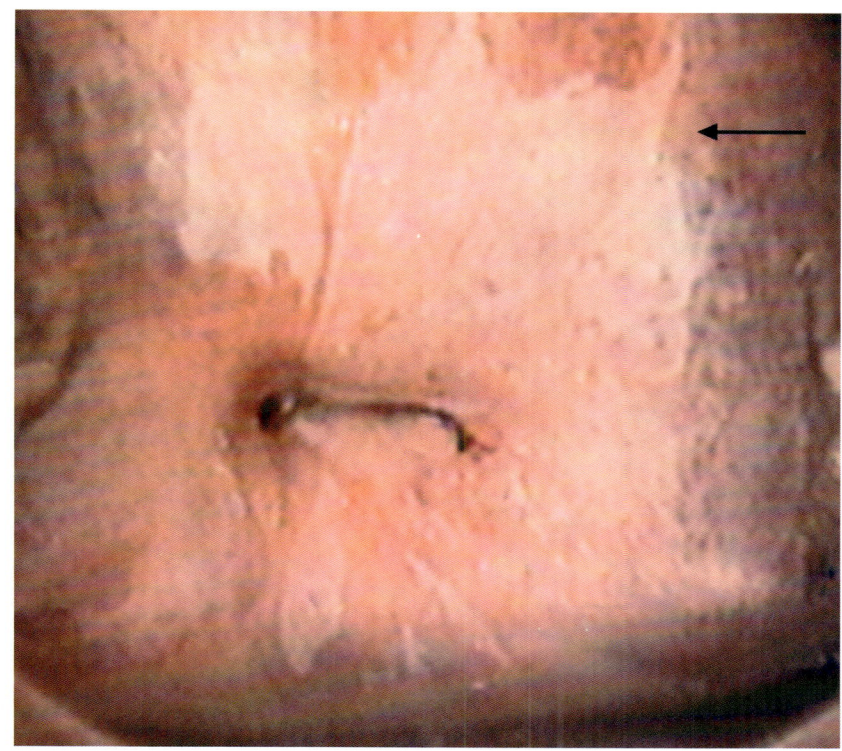

Fig. 4.16: AW lesion occupying 3 quadrants of cervix and 60–70% of the cervix

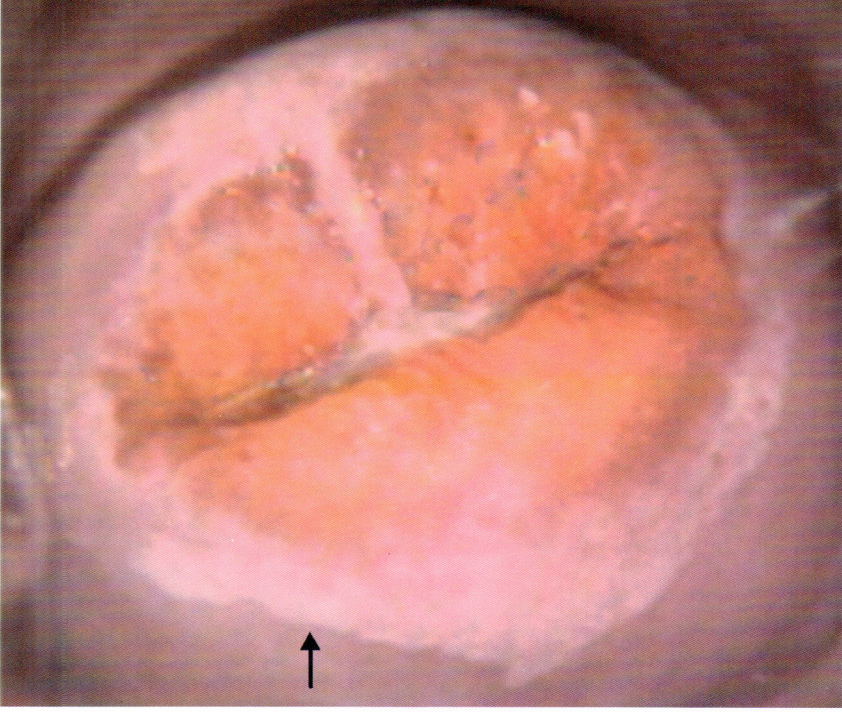

Fig. 4.17: Thin rim of AW lesion occupying 3 quadrants, but only about 10% of cervix

Grading of Abnormal Colposcopic Findings

Abnormal colposcopic findings are graded as minor, major, and non-specific.

Grade 1 (Minor)

1. Thin acetowhite epithelium (Figs 4.18 and 4.19)
2. Irregular, geographic border (Figs 4.18 and 4.19)
3. Fine mosaic (Fig. 4.18)
4. Fine punctation (Fig. 4.19)

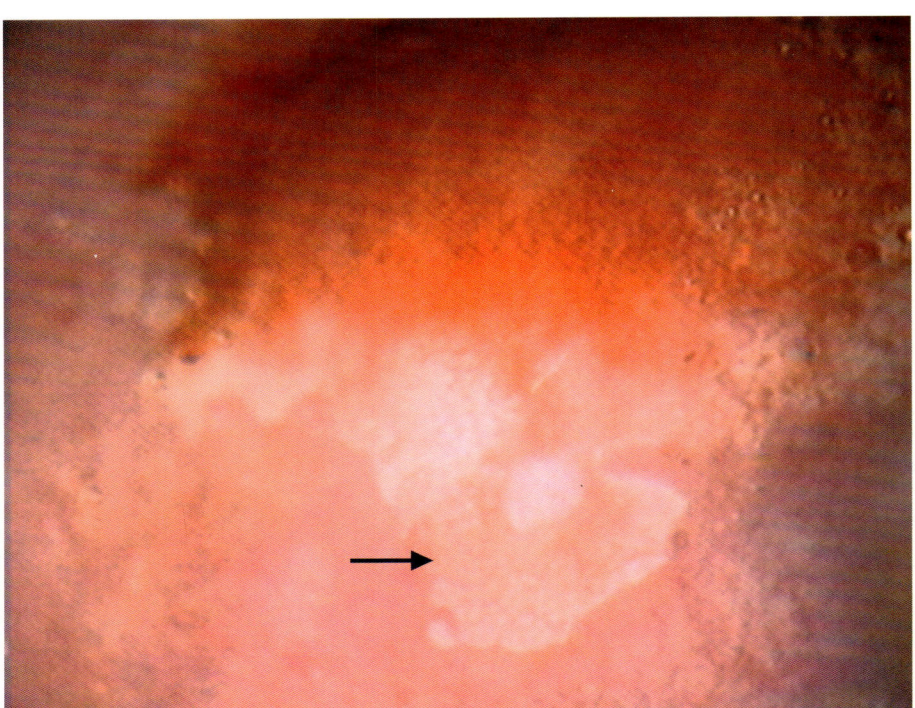

Fig. 4.18: Thin AW epithelium with geographical border and fine mosaic

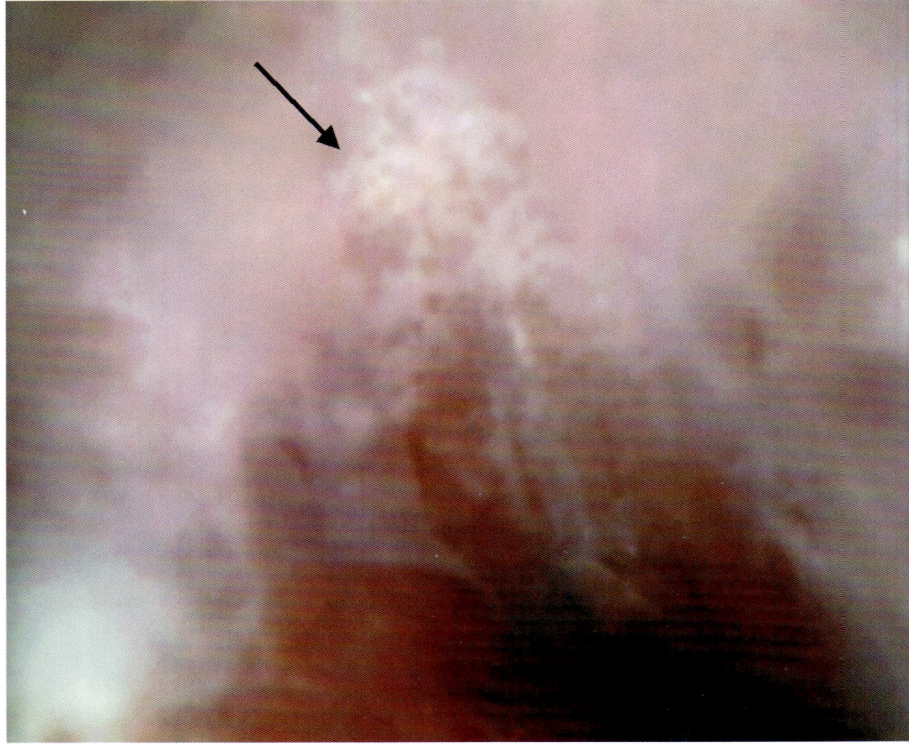

Fig. 4.19: Thin AW epithelium with geographical border and fine punctations

Grade 2 (Major)

1. Dense acetowhite epithelium (Fig. 4.20)
2. Rapid appearance of acetowhitening (Fig. 4.25)
3. Cuffed crypt (gland) opening (Fig. 4.21)
4. Coarse mosaic (Fig. 4.20)
5. Coarse punctation (Fig. 4.22)
6. Sharp border (Fig. 4.21)
7. Inner border sign (Fig. 4.23)
8. Ridge sign (Fig. 4.24)

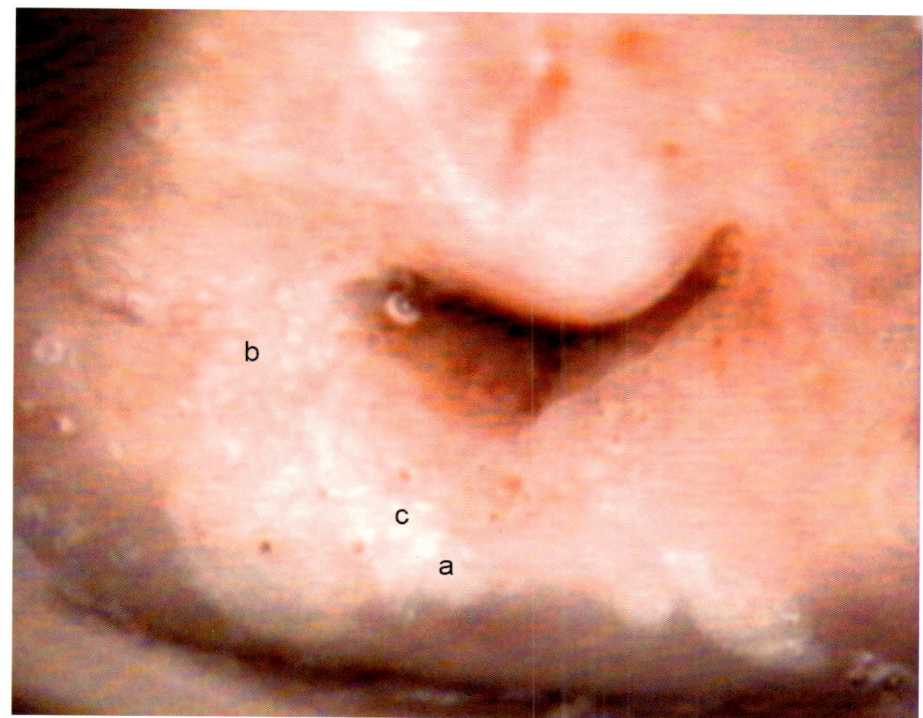

Fig. 4.20: Dense AW lesion (a), with coarse mosaic (b), and cuffed gland openings (c)

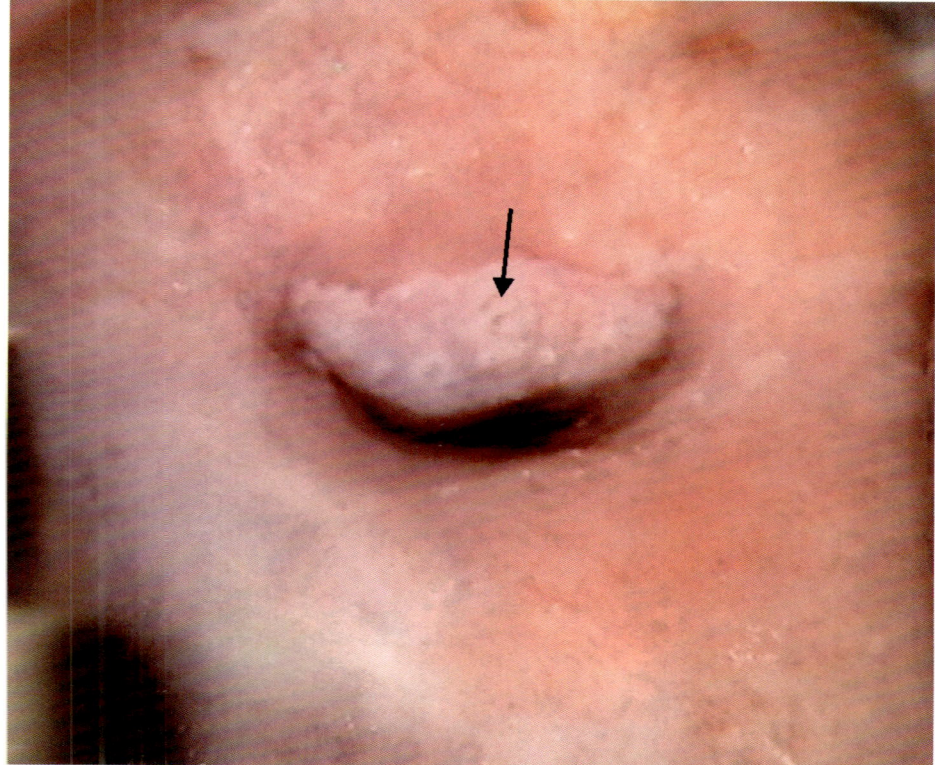

Fig. 4.21: Dense AW lesion with sharp border and cuffed gland openings

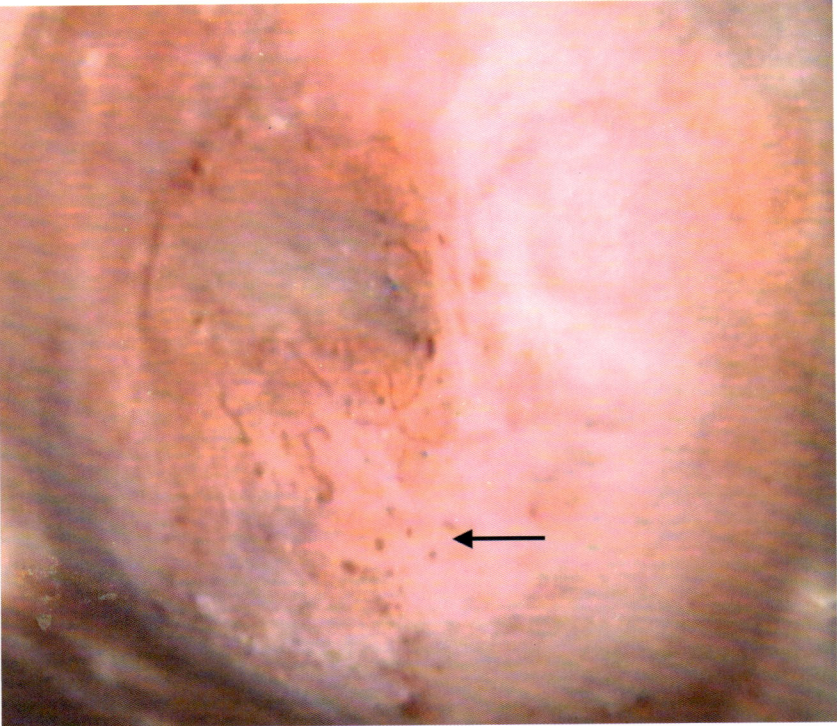

Fig. 4.22: Coarse punctations

The major signs are associated with a more severe lesion. Sharp border means a straight edge of an acetowhite cervical lesion. The inner border sign is a sharp demarcation between thin and dense aceto- white areas within the same lesion (Fig. 4.23). The ridge sign is an opaque protuberance at the area of a white epithelium within the transformation zone (Fig. 4.24).

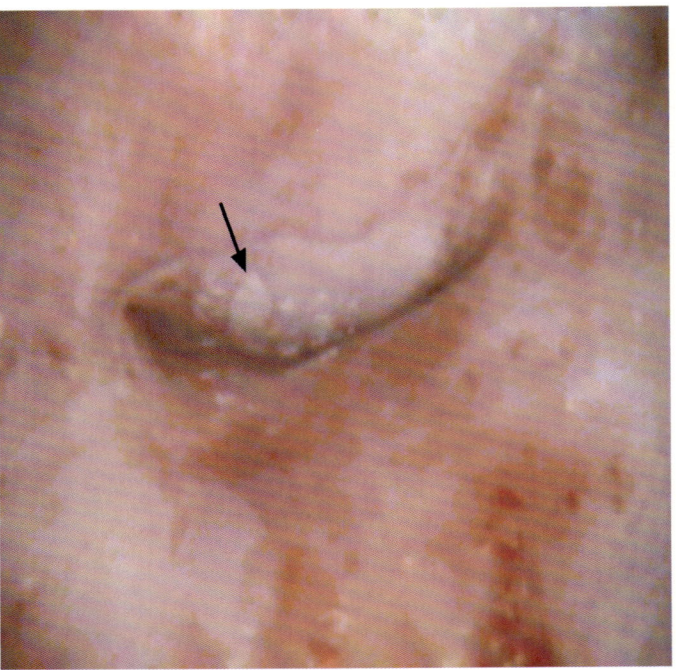

Fig. 4.23: Inner border sign: Dense AW epithelium with sharp border at 11 O' clock within a large thin AW epithelium

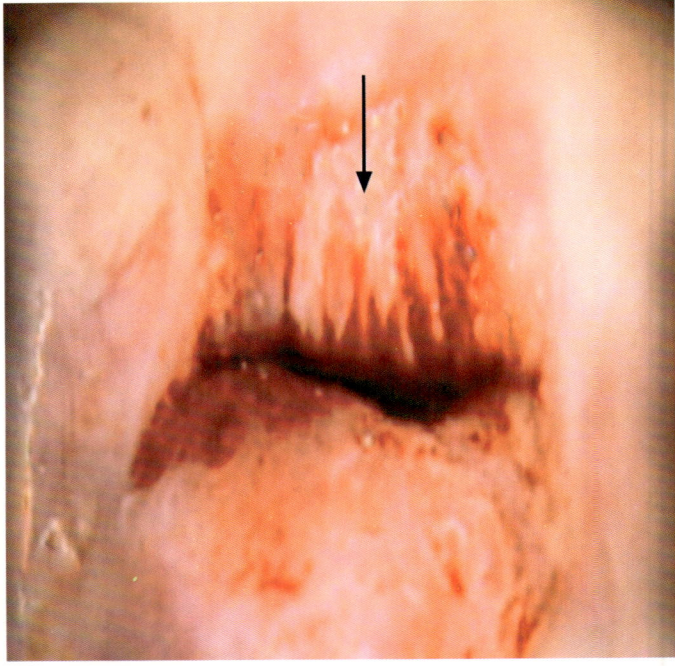

Fig. 4.24: Ridge sign: Thick opaque protuberance of AW epithelium with sharp border near SCJ

Another criterion associated with high grade CIN is rag sign (Fig. 4.26), which is an iatrogenic small erosion/sloughing of atypical squamous epithelium in a rag, caused by mechanical trauma of cervix during sampling of cervix for cytology/HPV DNA or while applying of acetic acid/Lugol's iodine. Part of epithelium is sloughed off and underlying erosion or detached epithelium resembling a rag is visible. Its presence alone or in combination of inner border or ridge sign is strongly associated with high grade CIN.

The ridge sign (Fig. 4.24), inner border sign (Figs 4.23 and 4.25) and rag sign (Fig. 4.26) are pathognomonic as they are objective, effective and are significantly associated with high grade CIN. They differ from the other existing criteria in that they are present or absent. They are to be dichotomously reported, and not graduated.

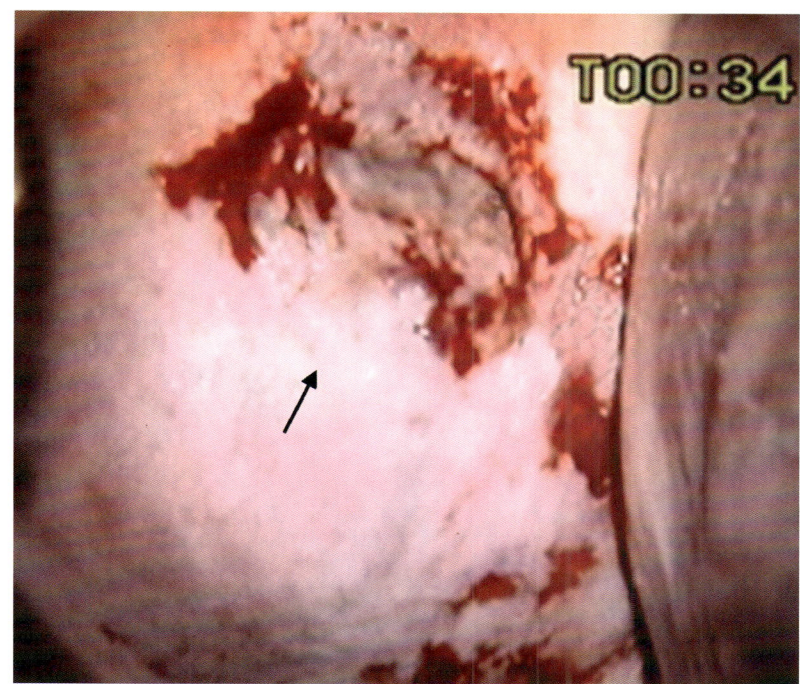

Fig. 4.25: Rapid appearance of acetowhitening: Dense AW epithelium with inner border and rag sign seen after thirty seconds only

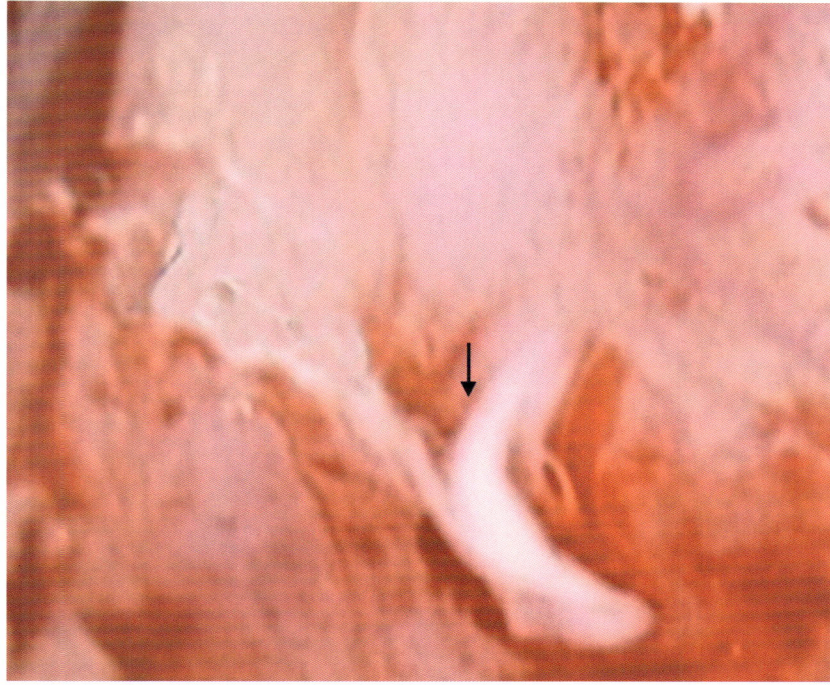

Fig. 4.26: Rag sign: Dense detached AW epithelium hanging from cervix like a rag after applying acetic acid

Non-specific

The term leukoplakia (Fig. 4.27) or keratosis was considered a major lesion in the first and second IFCPC terminologies but was reclassified in 2002 in the third IFCPC under "miscellaneous findings," to diminish its significance.

However, because leukoplakia or keratosis was shown to have a 25% independent predictive value of containing high-grade or invasive neoplasia, it has been returned to the abnormal colposcopic finding section, but to the non-specific category, because it may represent either a benign or a severe intraepithelial lesion.

Moving the test of Lugol's staining (Schiller's test) from the "minor grade" category to the "non-specific" category of the "abnormal colposcopic findings" section is because several studies such as those associated with the ASC-US-LSIL Triage Study showed poor reliability of Lugol's staining (Fig. 4.28).

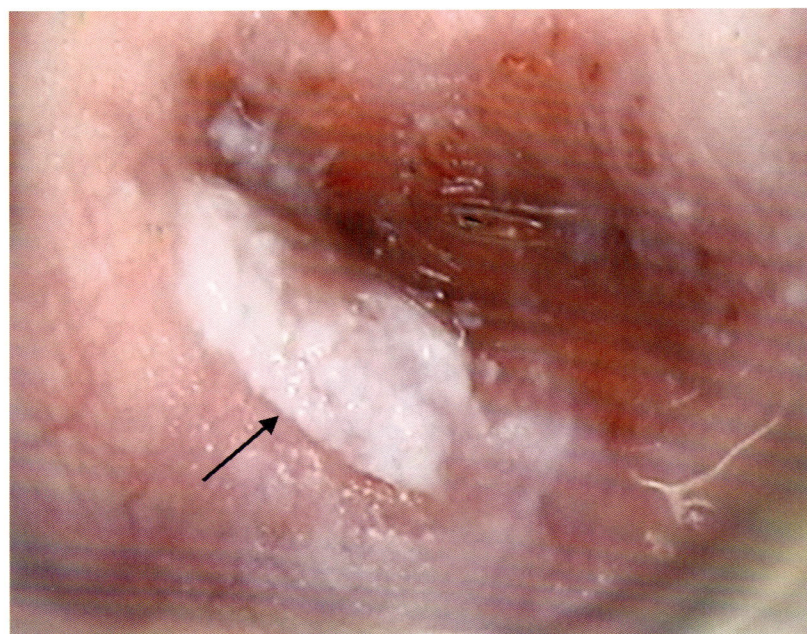

Fig. 4.27: Raised white leukoplakic lesion seen before acetic acid application

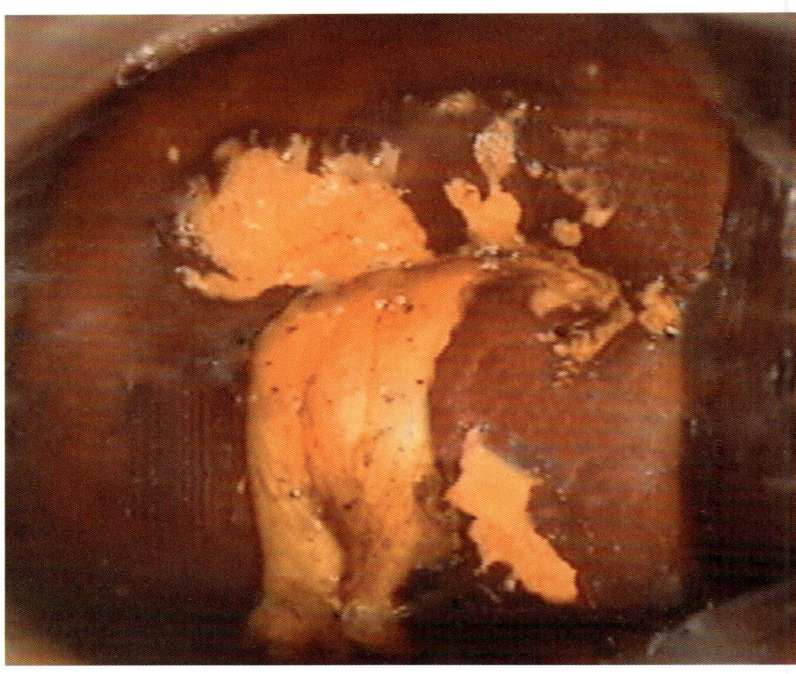

Fig. 4.28: After Lugol's iodine application: Abnormal lesion as iodine negative area

SUSPICIOUS FOR INVASION

1. Atypical Vessels

Atypical vessels are strikingly irregular in size, calibre, shape, course and mutual arrangement. They do not have dichotomous branching, instead may run parallel to the surface, with sharp irregular bends, may show constrictions and dilatations and may appear or disappear bluntly (Fig. 4.29).

2. Additional Signs

Fragile vessels, irregular surface, exophytic lesion, necrosis, ulceration (necrotic), tumor or gross neoplasm (Fig. 4.30).

MISCELLANEOUS FINDINGS

A cervical polyp is a common finding including its origin as being ectocervical or endocervical.

Post-treatment effect may or may not be an adverse feature, e.g. stenosis, deformation or distortion, scarring, thickening or increased fragility of the mucosa, cervical endometriosis.

Endocervical polyps are generally benign lesions resulting from focal hyperplastic growth of endocervical epithelium and stroma, often showing increased vascularity, inflammation and squamous metaplasia on the surface of the polyp. However, they must be biopsied and sent for histopathology as they might be arising from the endometrium and might be malignant.

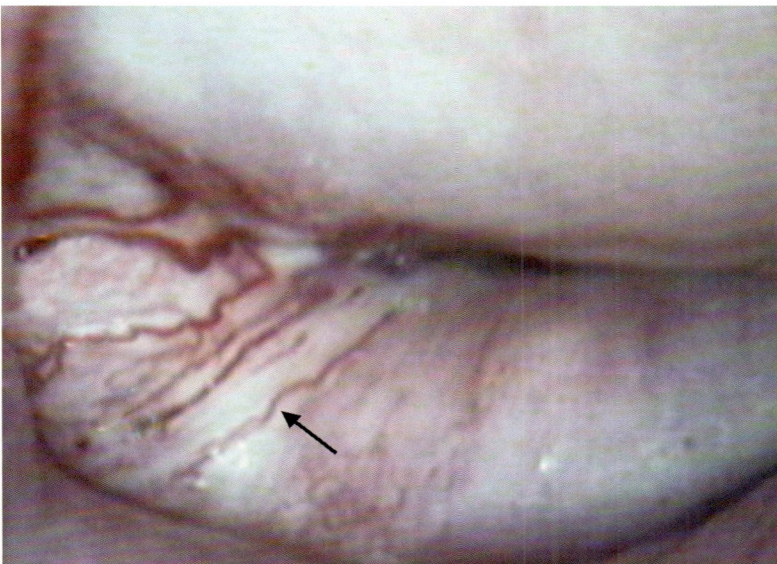

Fig. 4.29: Atypical vessels

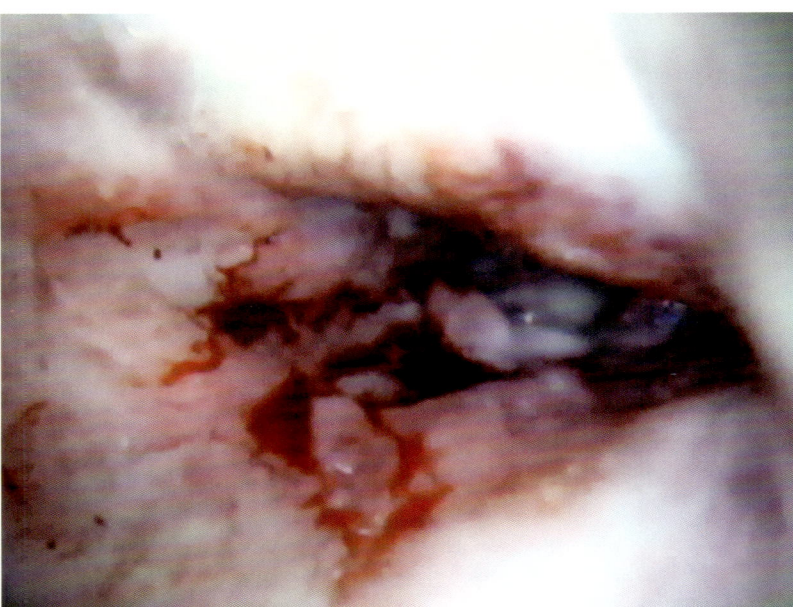

Fig. 4.30: Exophytic lesion with irregular surface and fragile atypical vessels under green filter

SCORING SYSTEMS

In order to predict the severity of the underlying histopathology, some scoring systems have been developed to grade the colposcopic lesion in a systematic way. Most of the systems (Tables 4.3 to 4.5) are based on a subjective evaluation of the colposcopic features.

Table 4.3: Reid's combined colposcopic index (1985)			
Colposcopic sign	*Zero points*	*One point*	*Two points*
Margin	– Condylomatous/micropapillary contour – Indistinct acetowhitening – Flocculated/feathered margins – Angular, jagged lesions – Satellite lesions and acetowhitening that extend beyond TZ	– Regular lesions with smooth straight white lines	– Rolled peeling edges – Internal demarcations between areas of differing appearances
Color	– Shiny, snow white color – Indistinct acetowhitening	– Intermediate shade (shiny gray)	– Dull oyster white
Vessels	– Fine caliber vessels – Poorly formed patterns – Condylomatous/micropapillary lesions	– Absent vessels	– Definite punctation and mosaic
Iodine	– Positive iodine staining	– Partial iodine uptake	– Negative staining of significant lesion

Score   0-2 predictive of minor lesion (SPI or CIN 1)
3–5 indicate middle grade lesion (CIN 1–2)
6–8 indicate significant lesion (CIN 2–3)

Table 4.4: Modified Reid index (2010)			
Feature	*Zero points*	*One point*	*Two points*
Margin and surface contour of AW lesion	– Feathered margins – Angular, jagged lesions – Flat lesions with indistinct margins – Microcondylomatous or micropapillary contour	– Regular lesions with smooth straight white lines	– Rolled peeling edges – Internal demarcations (a central area of high grade change and peripheral area of low-grade change)
Color of acetowhite (AW) area	– Low intensity acetowhitening – Snow-white shiny AW – Indistinct AW – AW beyond TZ.	– Gray white AW with shiny surface	Dull oyster-white, gray AW
Vessels	– Fine/uniform vessels – Poorly formed patterns or fine punctations and/or mosaic – Vessels beyond TZ margins – Fine vessels within microcondylomatous or micropapillary lesions	– Absent vessels	– Well-defined coarse punctation and mosaic
Iodine staining	– Positive iodine uptake giving mahogany brown color – Negative uptake of lesions scoring ≤ 3 points on above three categories.	– Partial iodine uptake by a lesion scoring ≥ 4 points on above three categories—variegated, speckled appearance	Negative iodine uptake by a lesion scoring ≥ 4 points on above three categories

Score   0–2 likely to be CIN 1
3–4 indicate overlapping lesion likely to be CIN 1–2
5–8 indicate significant lesion likely to be CIN 2–3.

A new scoring system was introduced by *Strander et al 2005*, at the Department of Obstetrics and Gynecology, Göteborg, Sweden, and subsequently validated at the Royal Free. It was the first scoring system to incorporate lesion *size* as a variable to evaluate a scoring system for high grade lesions as the size of lesion has been shown to be associated with increasing severity of CIN.

The Shafi-Nazeer scoring system is a clinico-colposcopic index (Table 4.6) that considers the age of the patient along with her smoking status and the index cytology report in addition to colposcopic features for prediction of histological grade. It is practical to use within a clinical setting. A maximum score of 10 can be obtained for each patient, the higher the score, the more significant the lesion.

Following one of these grading systems would help in analyzing the subjective findings in a systematic manner and enhance the diagnostic accuracy of colposcopy in differentiating between low- and high-grade disease.

Table 4.5: Strander's Swede Score (2005)

	Score 0	1	2
Aceto uptake	Zero or transparent	Shady, milky Neither transparent nor opaque	Distinct, opaque white
Margins and surface	Diffuse	Sharp but irregular, jagged, geographical satellites	Sharp and even, difference in surface level including 'cutting'
Vessels	Fine, regular	Absent	Coarse or atypical vessels
Lesion size	< 5 mm	5–15 mm or 2 quadrants	> 15 mm or 3–4 quadrants or endocervically undefined
Iodine staining	Brown	Faintly or patchy yellow	Distinct yellow

Total score = 10

Score   < 5 points— predicted to be benign— do not require biopsy

5–7 points – require biopsy for diagnosis

≥ 8 points clearly high grade lesions may be directly treated with 'see and treat' approach

Table 4.6: Shafi-Nazeer scoring system (Clinico-colposcopic index)

Variable	Zero points	One point	Two points
Index cytology	Low grade	–	High grade
Smoking status	No	–	Yes
Age (years)	≤ 30	> 30	–
Acetowhitening	Slight	Marked	–
Surface area of lesion	≤ 1 cm²	> 1 cm²	–
Intercapillary distance	≤ 350 μ — fine/no mosaic/punctation	> 350 μ — coarse mosaic/punctation	–
Focality of lesion	Unifocal/multifocal	Annular	–
Surface pattern	Smooth	Irregular	–

Score   0–2: Insignificant lesions

3–5: Mixed histological pattern, often CIN I or II

6–10: Generally high grade disease

Comparison of Scoring Systems

Figures 4.31 to 4.33 depict the scoring of lesions by different based on colposcopic features. However, the interpretation by all the three systems (Table 4.7 to 4.9) appears to the same. Therefore, one can use any system that one is familiar with.

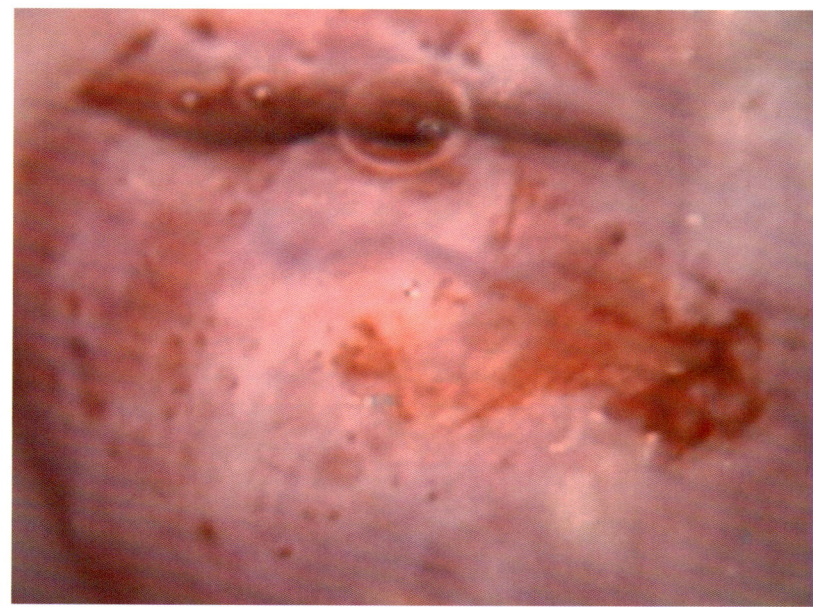

Figs 4.31A: After acetic acid

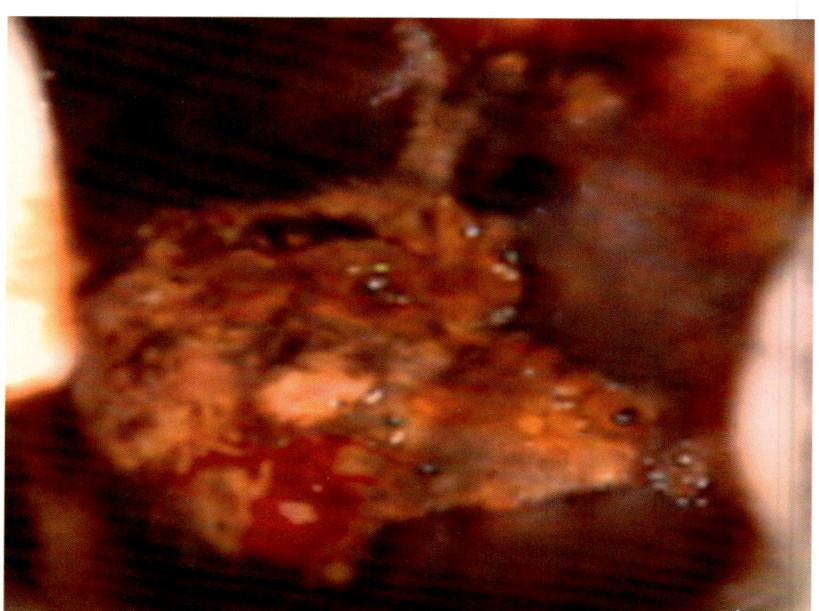

Fig. 4.31B: Same cervix after iodine staining

Table 4.7: Scoring of lesion in Figs 4.31A and B			
	Reid's	*Modified Reid's*	*Strander's*
Color/aceto uptake	0	0	0
Margin and surface	0	0	0
Vessels	1	1	1
Iodine staining	1	0	1
Size	–	–	1
Total score	2	1	3
Interpretation	**Benign/minor lesion**		

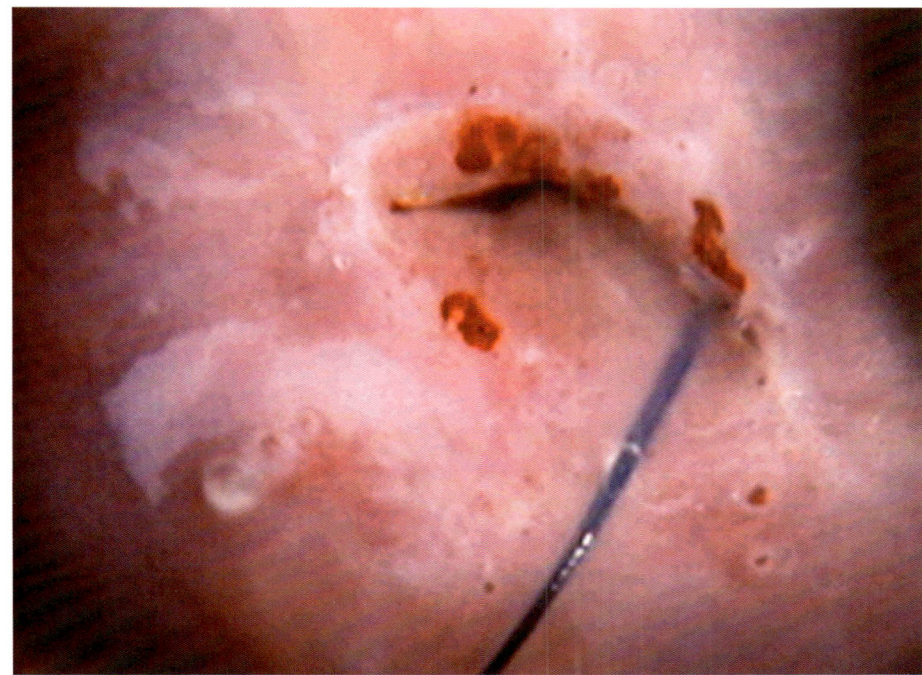

Fig. 4.32A: After acetic acid

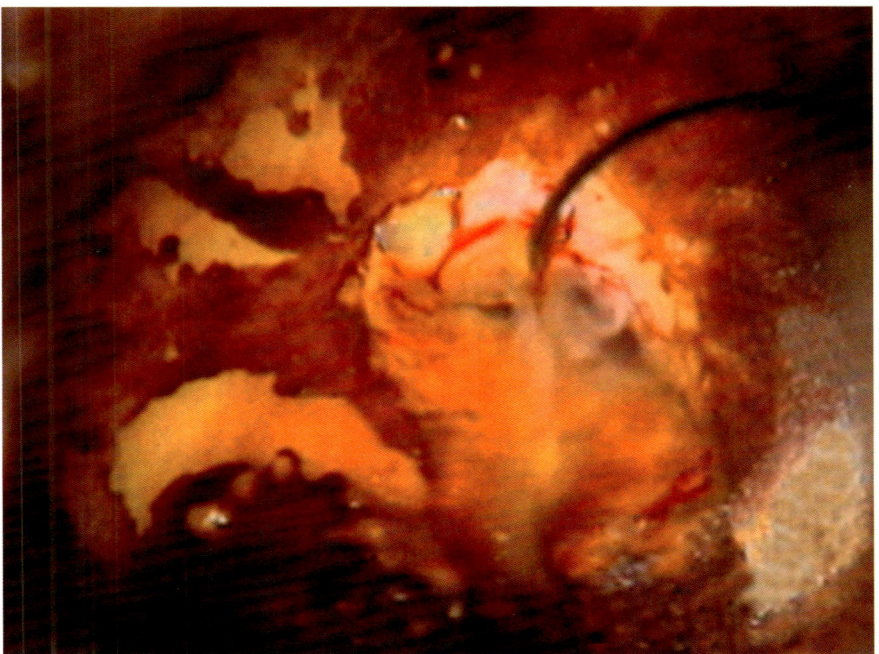

Fig. 4.32B: Same cervix after iodine staining

Table 4.8: Scoring of lesion in Figs 4.32A and B			
	Reid's	*Modified Reid's*	*Strander's*
Color/aceto uptake	1	1	1
Margin and surface	1	1	1
Vessels	1	1	1
Iodine staining	2	0	2
Size	–	–	1
Total score	5	3	6
Interpretation	**Middle grade lesion requiring biopsy**		

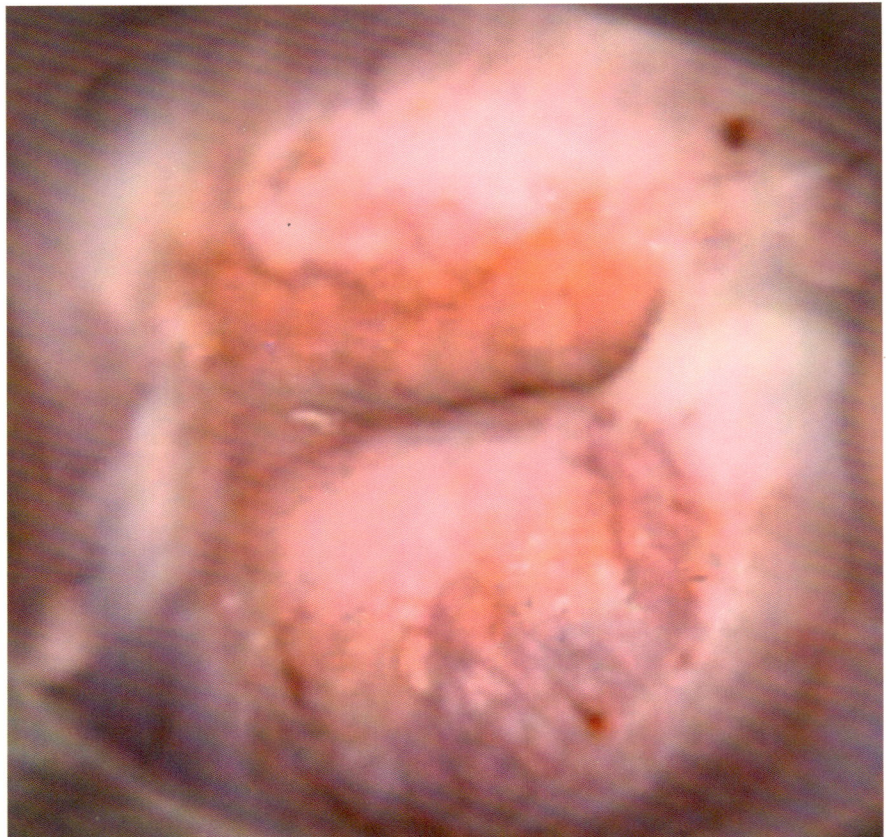

Fig. 4.33A: After saline: Local hyperemia and mosaic-like vasculature

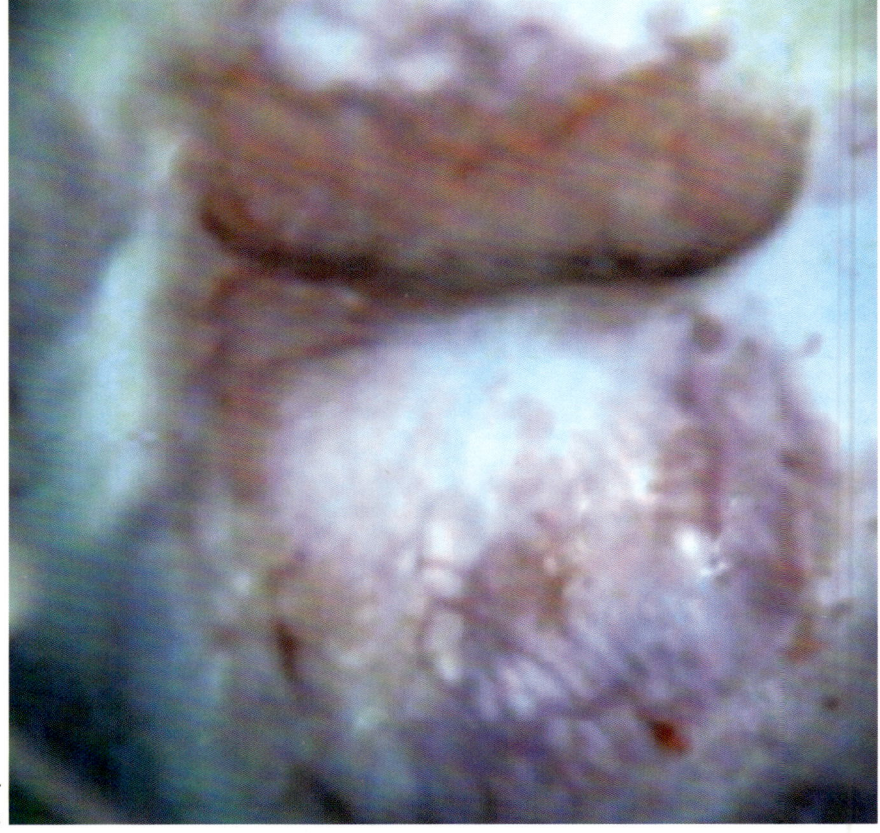

Fig. 4.33B: Same cervix under green filter with mosaic-like vessels

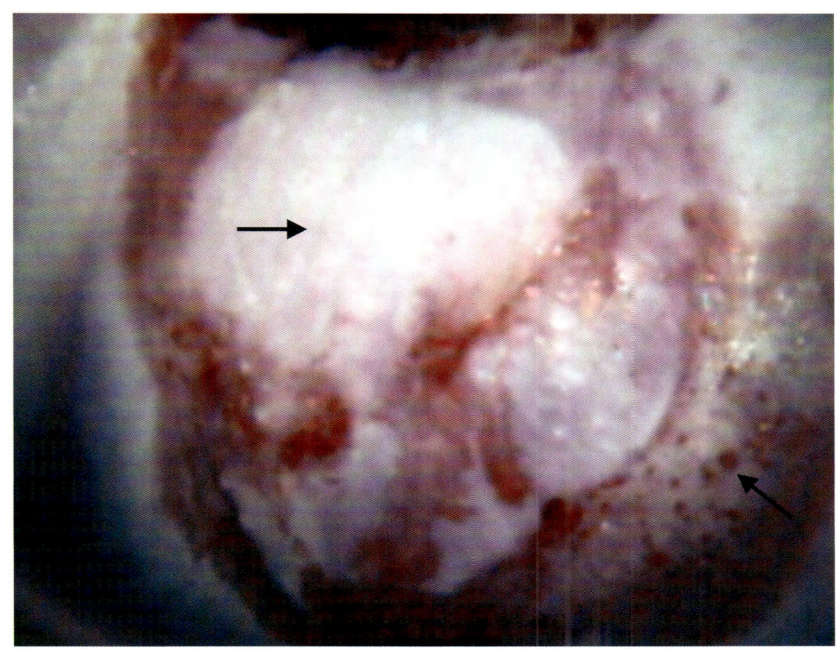

Fig. 4.33C: Same cervix after acetic acid application: Thick raised acetowhite epithelium with sharp internal borders and coarse punctations

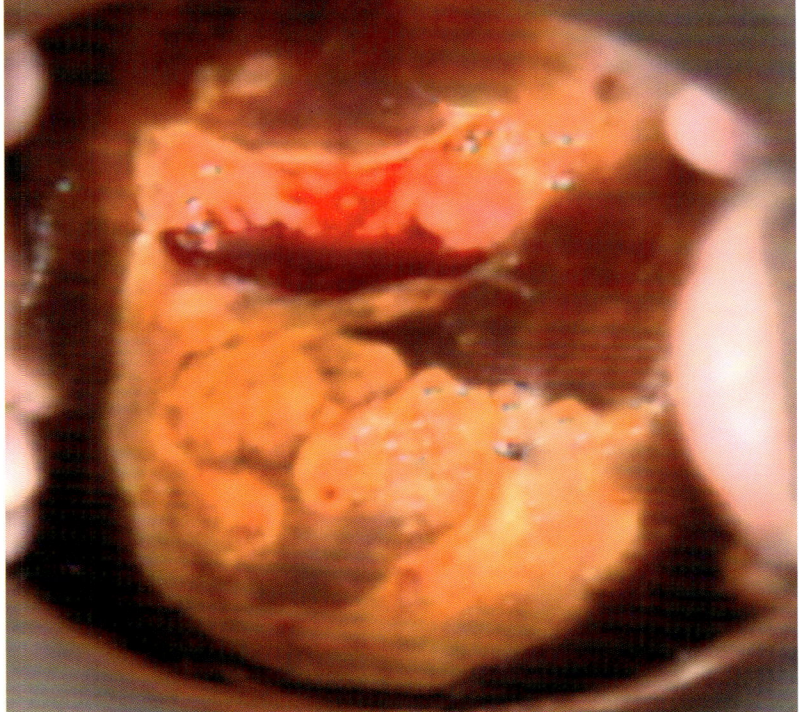

Fig. 4.33D: Same cervix after iodine staining

Table 4.9: Scoring of lesion in Figs 4.32A to D			
	Reid's	*Modified Reid's*	*Strander's*
Color/aceto uptake	2	2	2
Margin and surface	2	2	2
Vessels	2	2	2
Iodine staining	2	2	2
Size	–	–	1
Total score	8	8	9
Interpretation	**Severe grade lesion requiring biopsy**		

EXCISION TYPES

Type 1 excision (Fig. 4.34A) resects a completely ectocervical or type 1 TZ.

Type 2 excision (Fig. 4.34B) resects a type 2 transformation zone. It will resect a small amount of endocervical epithelium that is visible with a colposcope.

For a small TZ, a loop of 2 ×1.5 cm can be used for type 1 TZ and 2 × 2 cm for type 2 TZ, whereas for larger TZ, a wider loop or a combination of loops may be chosen.

Type 3 excision (Fig. 4.34C) resects a type 3 transformation zone. It resects a longer and larger amount of tissue than type 1 or type 2 excision and will include a significant amount of endocervical epithelium.

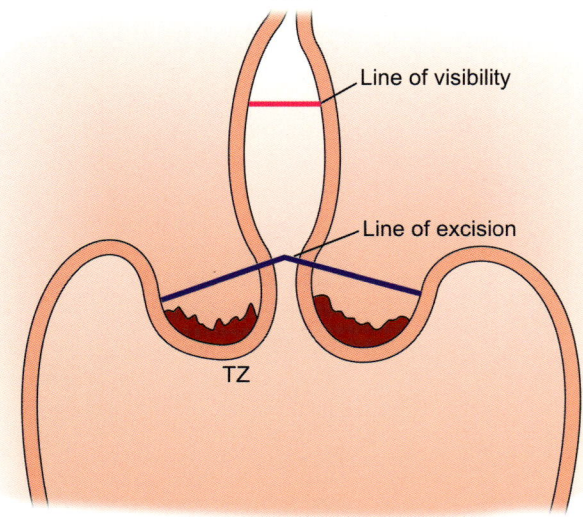

Fig. 4.34A: Type 1 TZ and type 1 excision

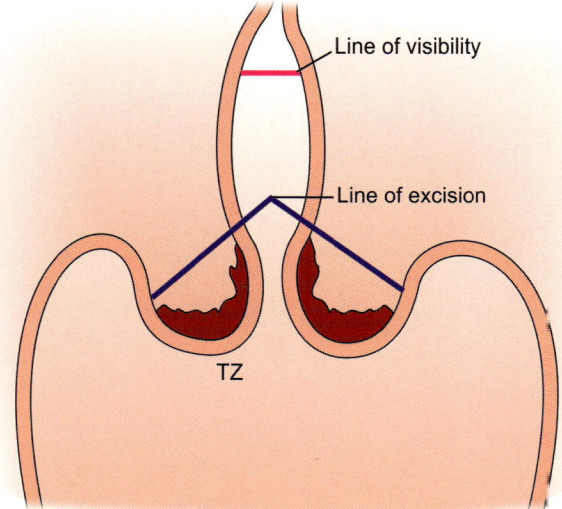

Fig. 4.34B: Type 2 TZ and type 2 excision

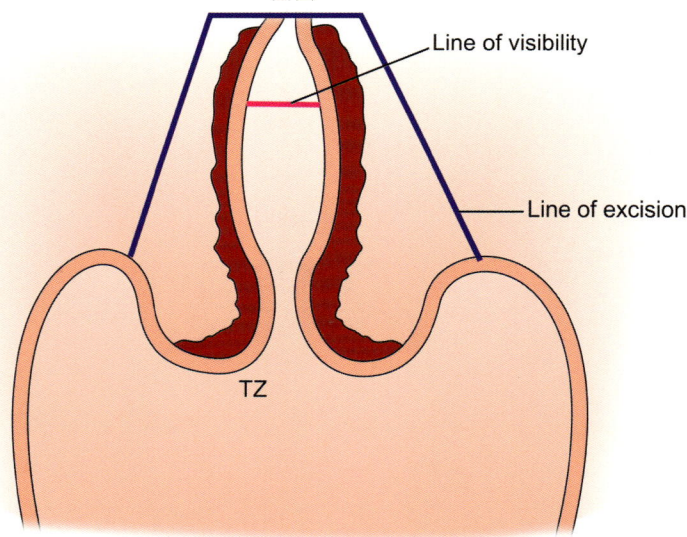

Fig. 4.34C: Type 3 TZ and type 3 excision

Histopathological Basis of Colposcopic Findings

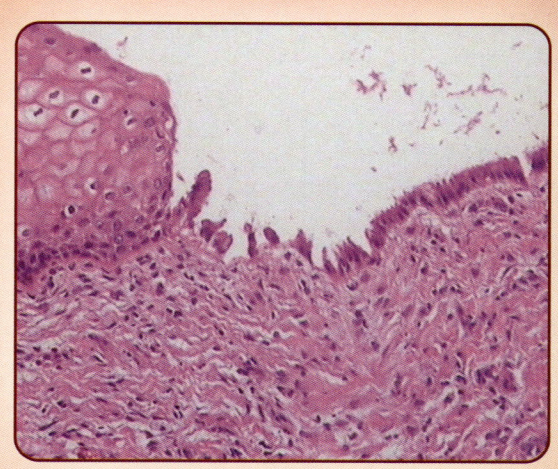

Chapter Outline

Colposcope is basically optical equipment with low power magnification. The light reflected from the cervix not only indicates changes in the covering epithelium but also of the underlying stroma and vascular bed. Any changes in any of these three components affect the colposcopic appearances.

Histopathological changes in the epithelium affecting the colposcopic image include thickness of epithelium, maturation of cell cytoplasm, and alteration in nuclear cytoplasmic ratio. When the incident light from colposcope falls on the surface epithelium, it may pass through the cell layers impinging on the underlying stroma and vasculature (Fig. 5.1A) or it may be reflected back by cells with large dense nuclei or by keratin deposition (Fig. 5.1B).

Thus the colposcopic image is determined by the ratio of reflected and absorbed light depending upon epithelial cell numbers, their organization, and morphology, as well as compactness of underlying stroma, the caliber of stromal vasculature with their branching pattern.

Therefore, it is of paramount importance to have a thorough knowledge of the tissue basis of colposcopic findings.

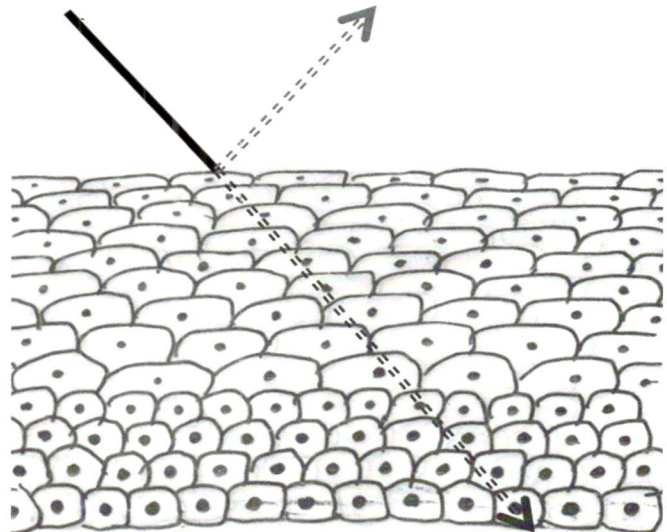

Fig. 5.1A: Light rays passing through normal squamous epithelium

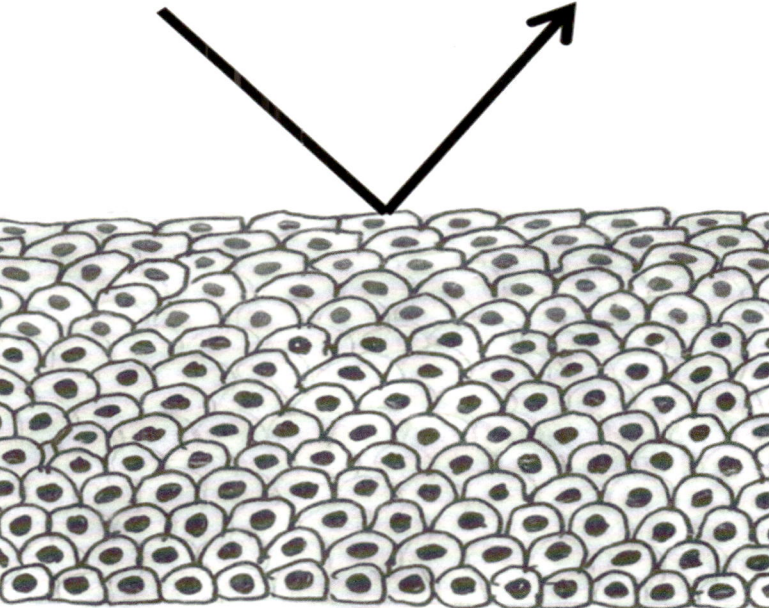

Fig. 5.1B: Light rays reflecting back from abnormal epithelium

NORMAL COLPOSCOPIC FINDINGS

Original Squamous Epithelium (OSE)

The epithelium originally laid down on the ectocervix and vagina during embryological development is called original squamous epithelium. It is stratified non-keratinizing multilayered epithelium resting on a thin undulating reticular basal lamina (Fig. 5.2). The underlying connective tissue stroma has a rich vascular network. Light passing uniformly through this multi-layered epithelium and impinging upon the vascular bed gives a pink appearance to the epithelium (Fig. 5.3).

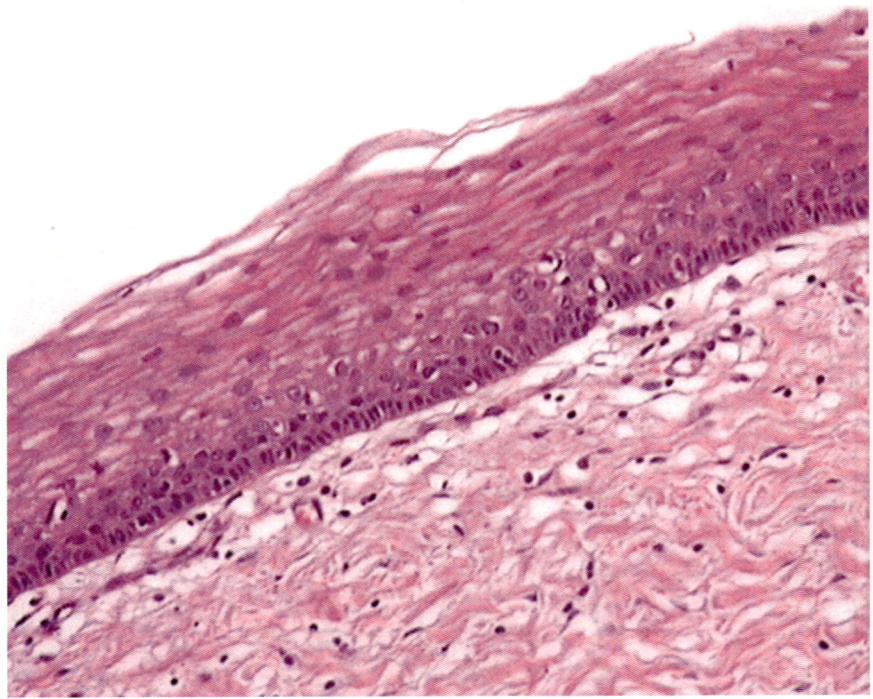

Fig. 5.2: Microphotograph showing original squamous lining of cervix, made up of multilayered epithelium resting on fibrous vascular stroma

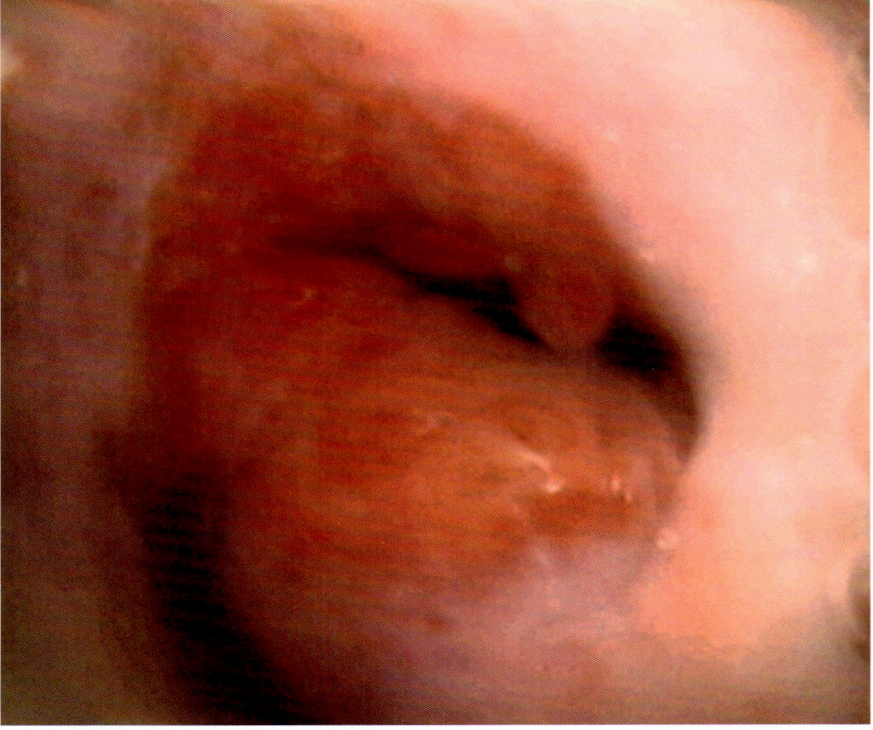

Fig. 5.3: Normal cervix during reproductive life: Squamous epithelium seen as flat, translucent, uniformely pink surface, and columnar epithelium as red velvety area surrounding external os

Columnar Epithelium

Normal columnar epithelium is a single layer of tall, mucus secreting, columnar cells lining the endocervical canal which may also extend on to the ectocervix during reproductive life. This epithelium is thrown into numerous villi and clefts, which appear on cut section as glands, hence erroneously called endocervical glands. Each villus has a core of connective tissue stroma containing a single vessel (Fig. 5.4).

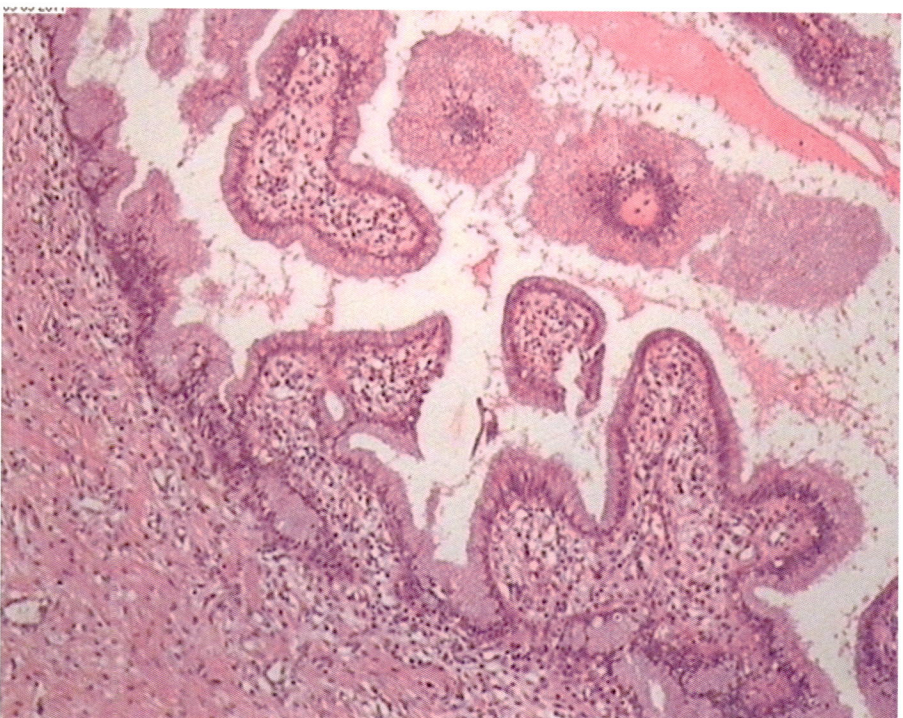

Fig. 5.4: Microphotograph showing endocervical lining thrown into villi, lined by mucin secreting columnar epithelium

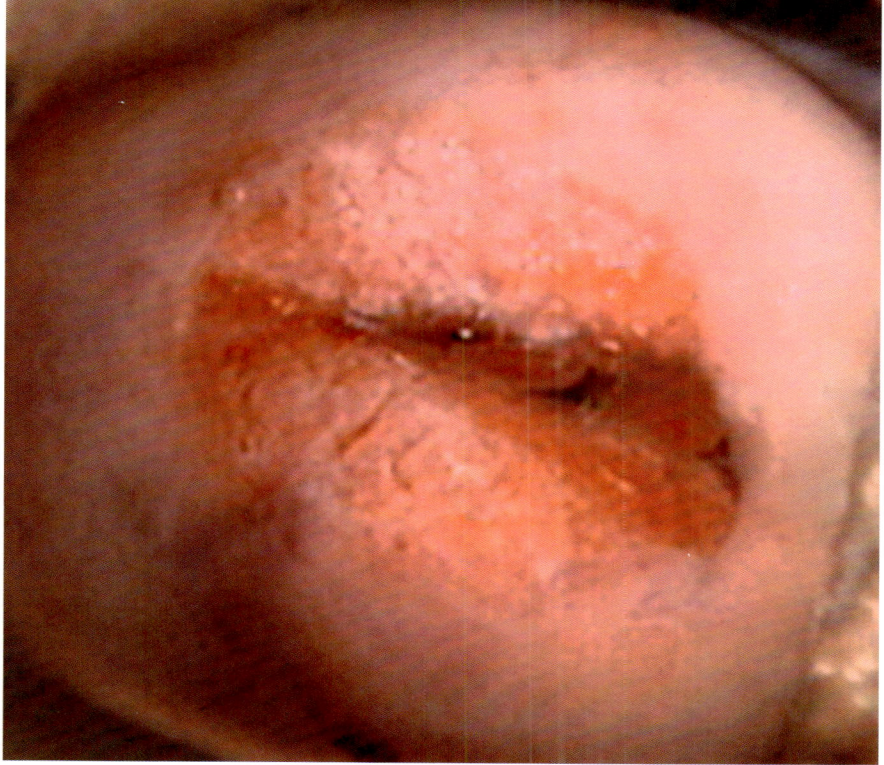

Fig. 5.5: Columnar epithelium after acetic acid application seen as granular surface (at low magnification)

Colposcopically this thin folded epithelium with close proximity to the underlying vasculature gives red, velvety appearance (Fig. 5.3) which changes into grape-like structures after the application of acetic acid (Figs 5.5 to 5.7).

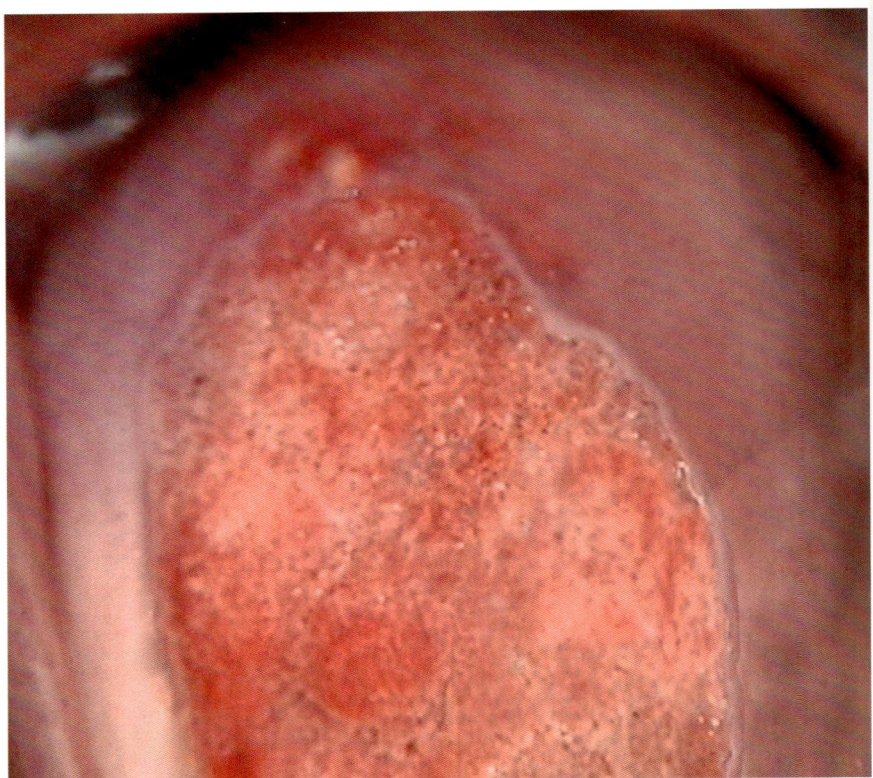

Fig. 5.6: Columnar epithelium after acetic acid application showing grape-like villi (higher magnification)

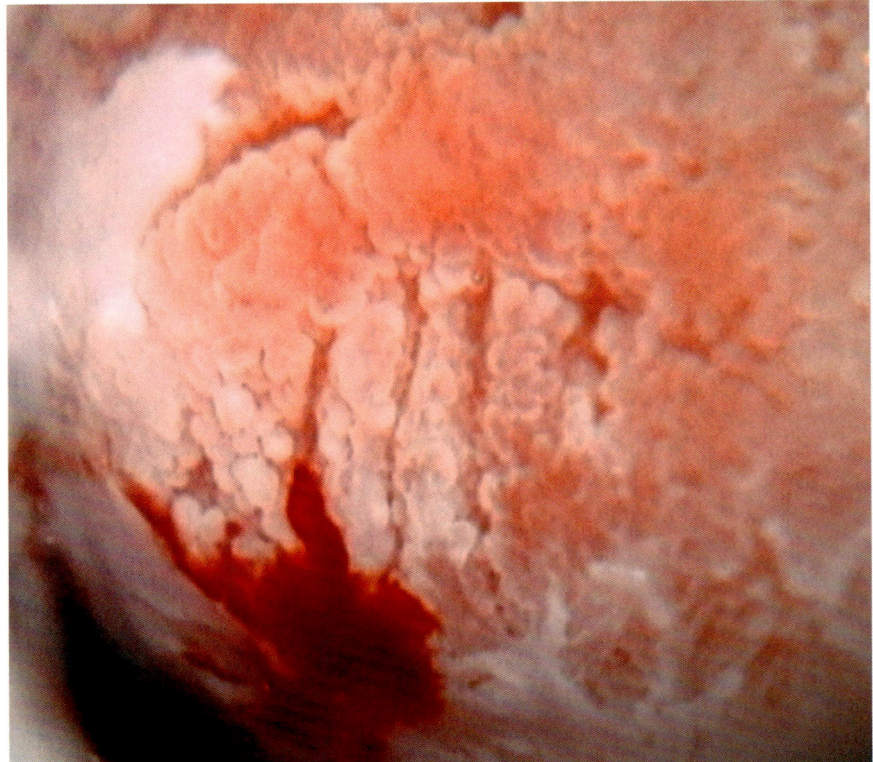

Fig. 5.7: Grape-like columnar epithelium under higher magnification

Squamocolumnar Junction (SCJ)

In the newborn female, the vagina and most of ectocervix are covered by original or native squamous epithelium, whereas endocervix is lined by columnar epithelium. The junction of these 2 epithelia called OSCJ (Fig. 5.8) usually coincides with anatomic external os (Fig. 5.9A), but its location is not static and changes in different phases of life, depending on the hormonal status.

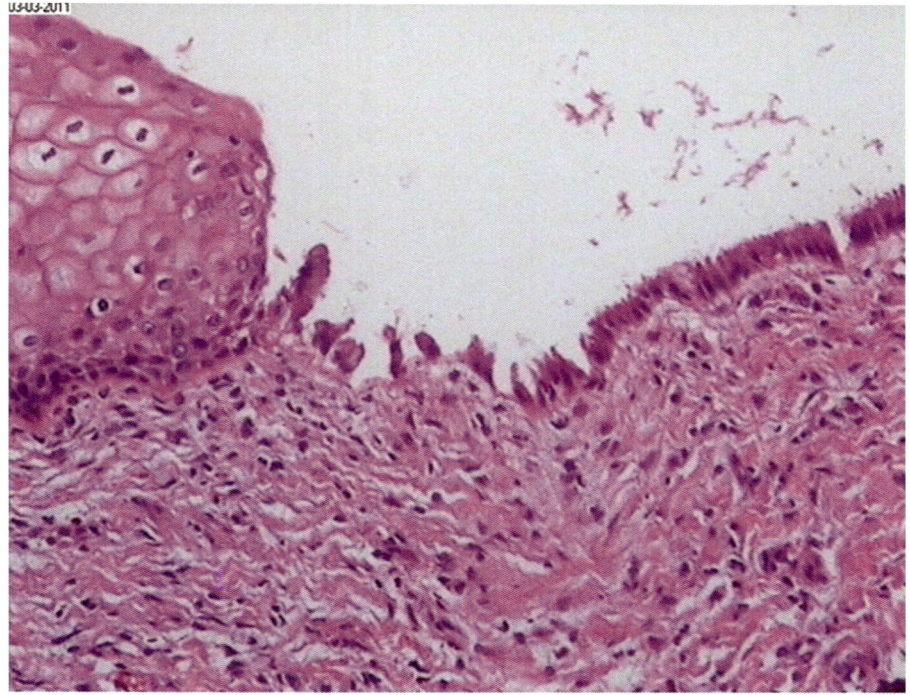

Fig. 5.8: Microphotograph—original squamocolumnar junction showing abrupt transition from squamous cell lining to columnar cells

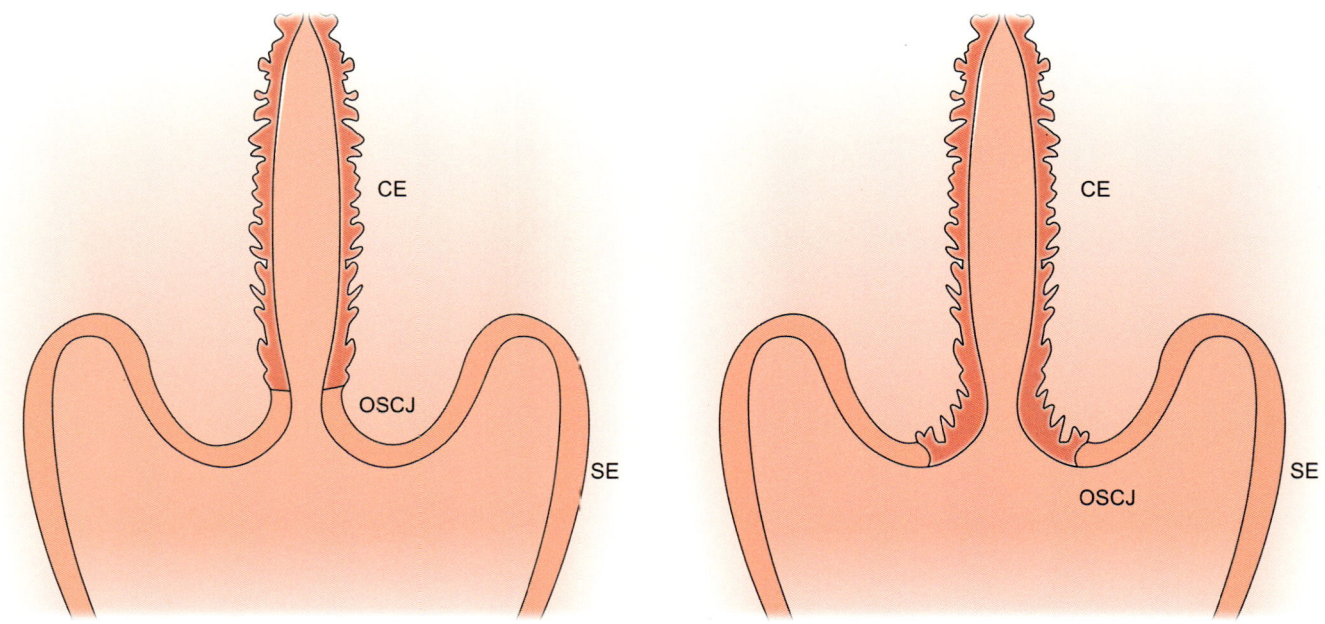

Fig. 5.9A: SCJ coinciding with anatomic external os   **Fig. 5.9B:** SCJ seen over ectocervix

OSCJ Original squamocolumnar junction; SE Squamous epithelium; CE Columnar epithelium

During menarche and 1st pregnancy, it comes onto the cervical portio, where it stays throughout a woman's menstruating life (Figs 5.9B, 5.10A). This deceptive movement is caused by the high estrogen level, which increases the mass of mesenchymal elements in the stroma, resulting in eversion of endocervix.

With the withdrawal of estrogens in the postmenopausal state, the SCJ recedes into the endocervical canal and may not be visible on the ectocervix (Fig. 5.10B).

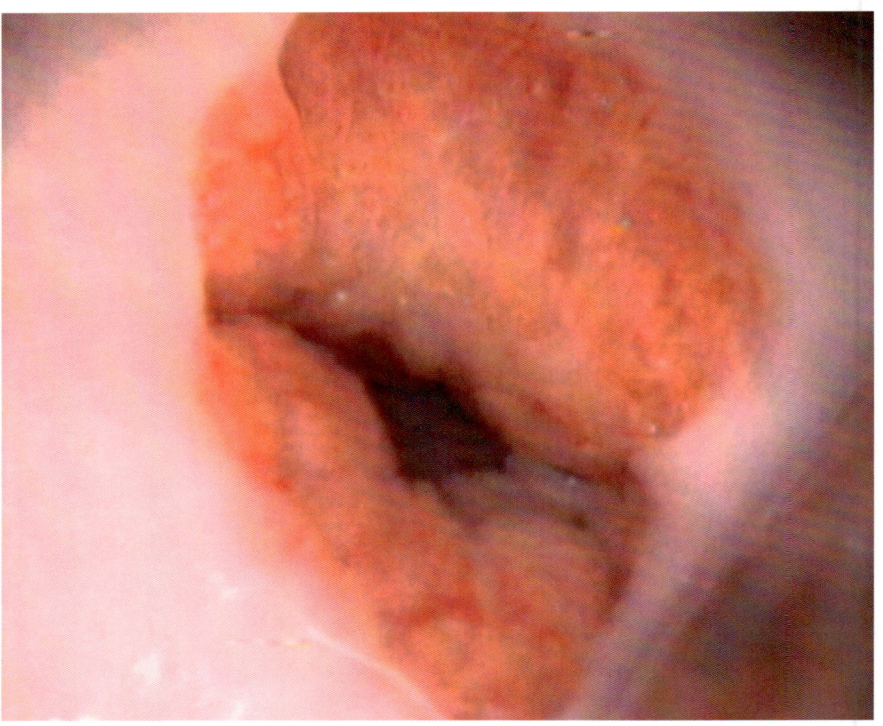

Fig. 5.10A: Cervix during reproductive age with SCJ on the ectocervix

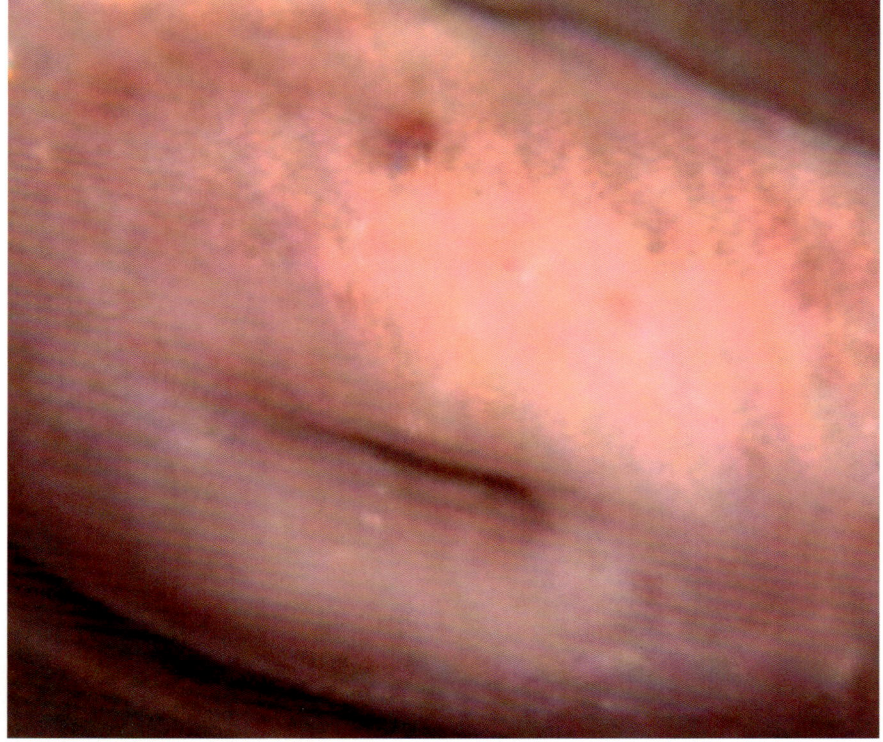

Fig. 5.10B: Postmenopausal cervix with SCJ receded in endocervix—not visible

Normal Metaplastic Process and Typical Transformation Zone (TTZ)

During the reproductive age, the exposed columnar epithelium under the influence of acidic milieu of vagina undergoes a gradual change into squamous epithelium.

This process of transition from columnar epithelium to squamous epithelium is called metaplasia and the dynamic area of physiologic metaplastic change is known as the normal or typical transformation zone (Fig. 5.11).

Transition from columnar epithelium to squamous epithelium is thought to begin with production of a new cell called reserve cell just beneath the basement membrane of the columnar epithelium. These reserve cells undergo hyperplasia (Fig. 5.12), lifting off the original columnar epithelium, replacing it with multilayered immature undifferentiated epithelium which ultimately undergoes differentiation and acquires glycogen and transforms into mature squamous epithelium.

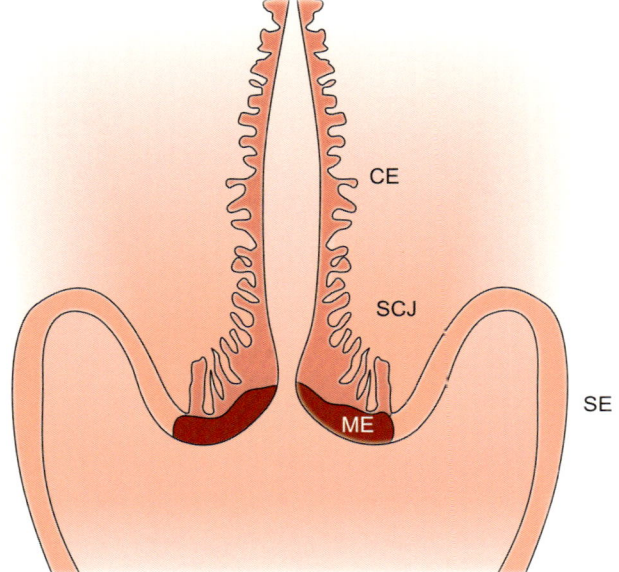

Fig. 5.11: Metaplastic epithelium and TZ
SCJ Squamocolumnar junction; ME Metaplastic epithelium; SE Squamous epithelium; CE Columnar epithelium

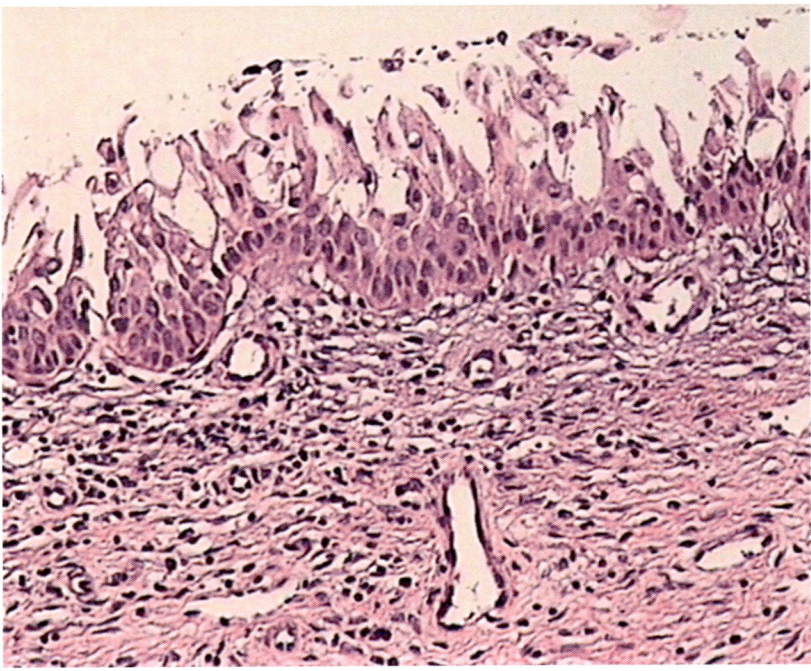

Fig. 5.12: Microphotograph showing reserve cell hyperplasia with columnar cells on the surface

Earliest Metaplastic Change

The metaplastic process begins at the tips of the villi (Figs 5.13A and B). This early metaplsia is seen colposcopically as loss of translucency at the tips of villi which stand out as small opaque areas against red background after application of acetic acid (Fig. 5.14).

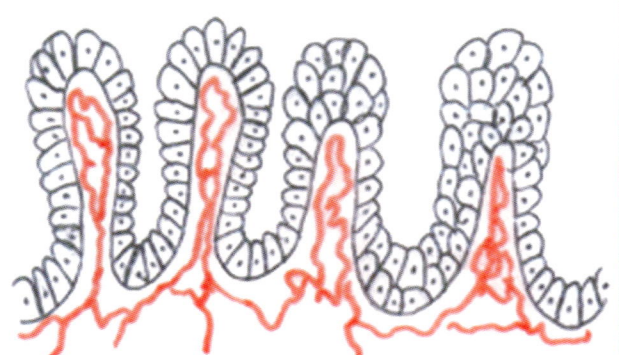

Fig. 5.13A: Metaplastic process beginning at tips of villi

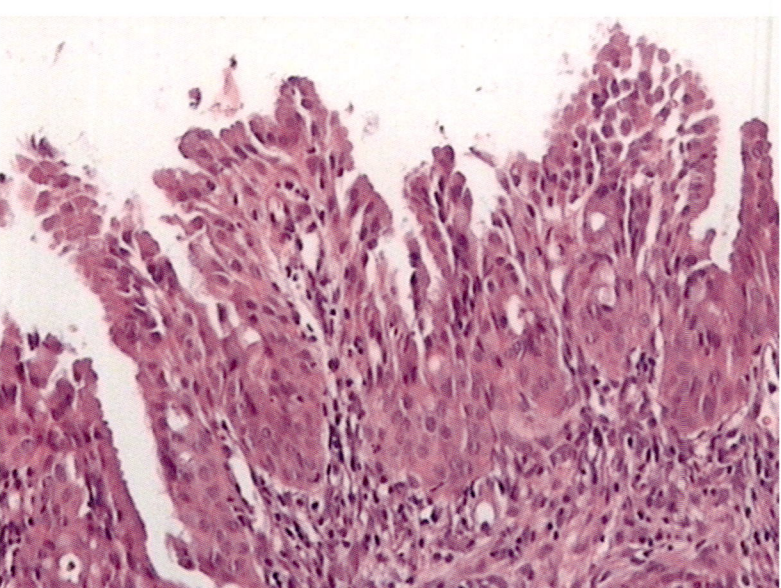

Fig. 5.13B: Microphotograph showing earliest metaplastic change seen as squamous transformation of columnar cells at the tips of villi. Some columnar cells are retained

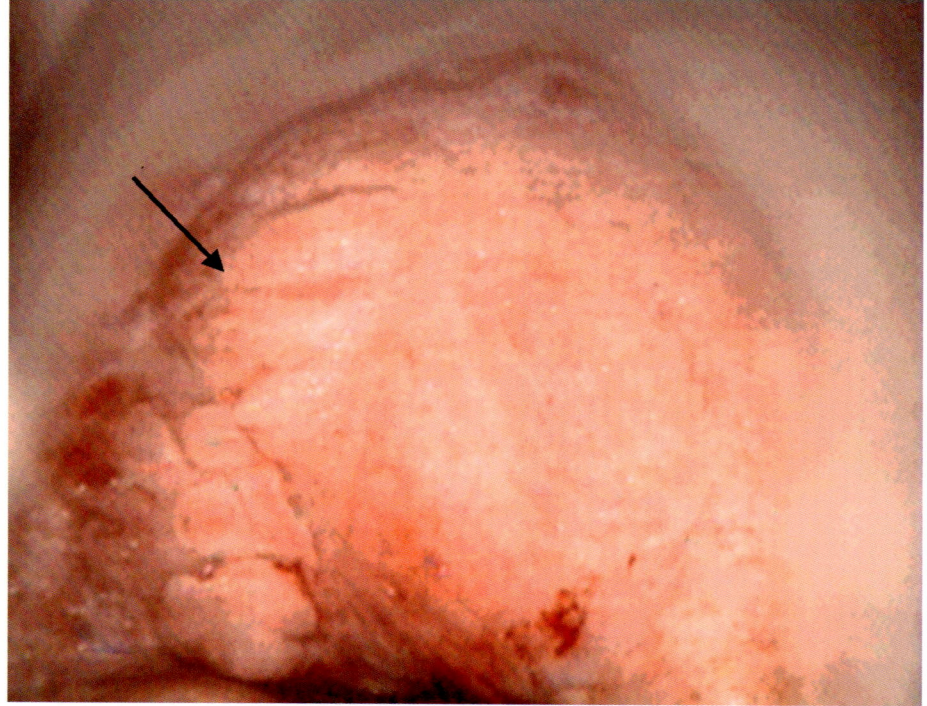

Fig. 5.14: Cervix after acetic acid application. Showing early metaplasia. Small opaque dots can be seen against red background representing metaplasia at the tips of villi

Early Metaplasia

With further proliferation of cells, opposing surfaces and tips of villi fuse with each other, pushing down the vessels of connective tissue papillae (Figs 5.15A and B). Colposcopically opaque villi appear fused but minute protuberances representing the tips of old villi may be seen (Fig. 5.16).

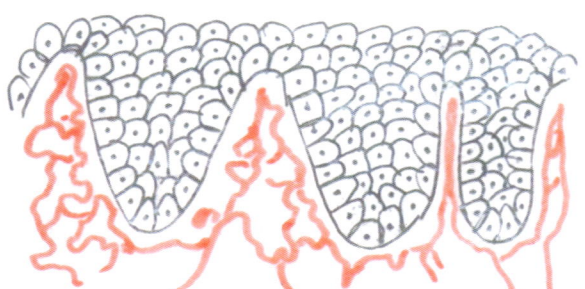

Fig. 5.15A: Immature metaplastic epithelium—vessels being pushed by metaplastic cells

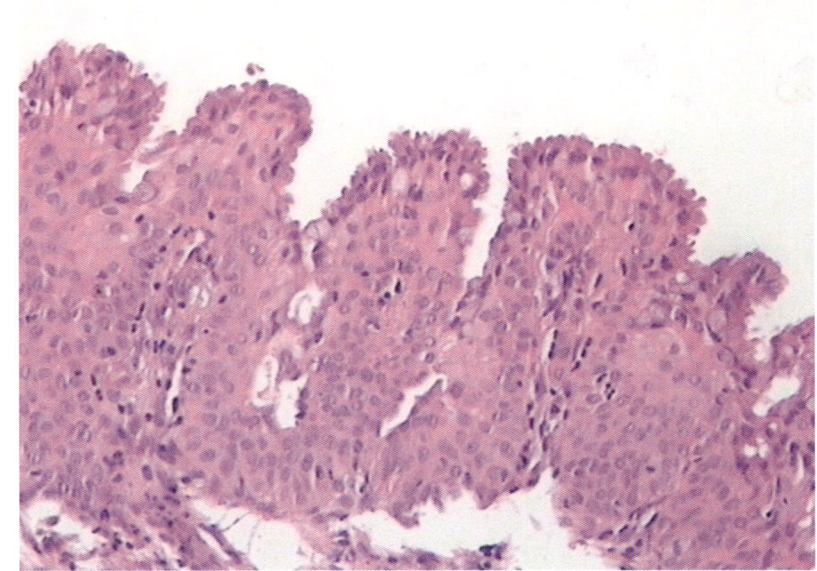

Fig. 5.15B: Microphotograph showing more marked proliferation of immature squamous cells in early metaplasia still retaining villous architecture

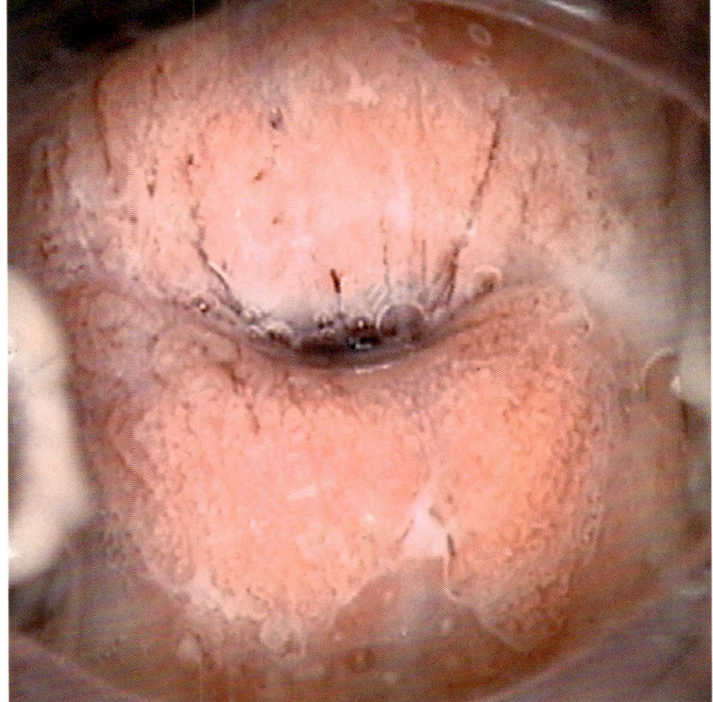

Fig. 5.16: Cervix after acetic acid application. Showing more advanced metaplasia seen in between columnar papillae. In peripheral zone, metaplasia is more advanced forming fairly smooth-layered metaplastic epithelium along with gland openings and nabothian follicles

Immature Metaplasia

With further maturation, a multilayered epithelium is formed but identity of individual cells is retained (Figs 5.17A and B). Colposcopically, a smooth surface is produced appearing as tongues of flat acetowhite epithelium (Fig. 5.18). The acetowhiteness of metaplastic squamous epithelium is because of immature cells having increased N:C ratio. As these cells lack glycogen, they appear iodine negative.

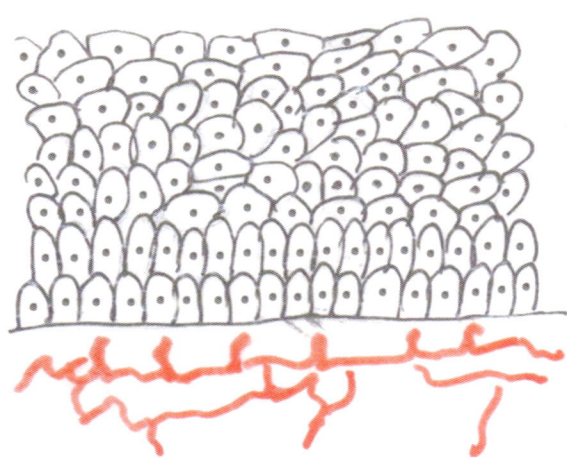

Fig. 5.17A: Immature metaplastic epithelium with undifferentiated cells

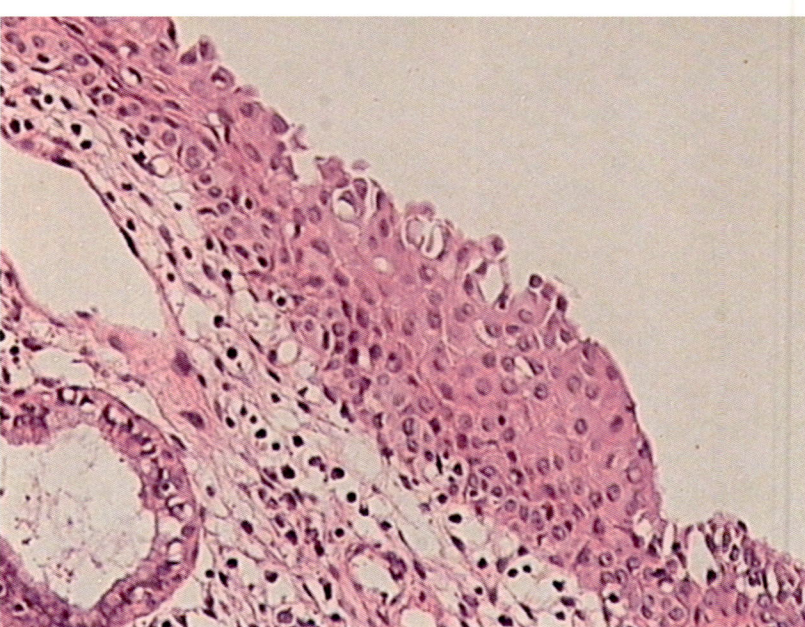

Fig. 5.17B: Microphotograph: Immature squamous metaplasia showing transformation of reserve cells into squamous cells. Some columnar cells can still be seen

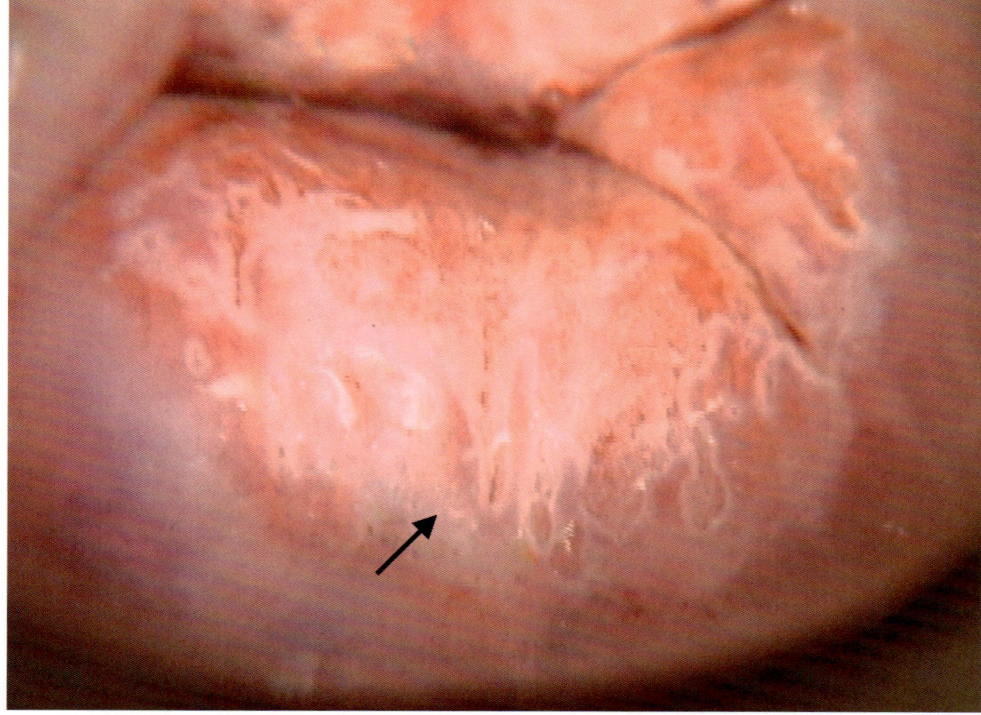

Fig. 5.18: Immature metaplasia seen as flat, smooth acetowhite epithelium

The metaplastic process usually begins in the distal zone adjacent to OSE and progresses to more proximal zones (Fig. 5.19), but it may be multifocal developing as discrete islands within the columnar tissue which gradually widen, coalesce and eventually join the peripheral components (Figs 5.20 and 5.21).

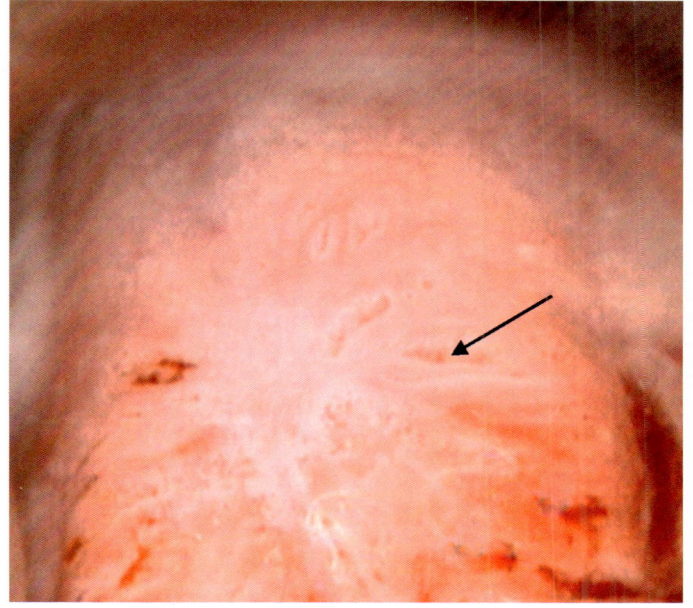

Fig. 5.19: More advanced metaplasia seen as tongues of flat, smooth acetowhite epithelium progressing from distal to more proximal zones

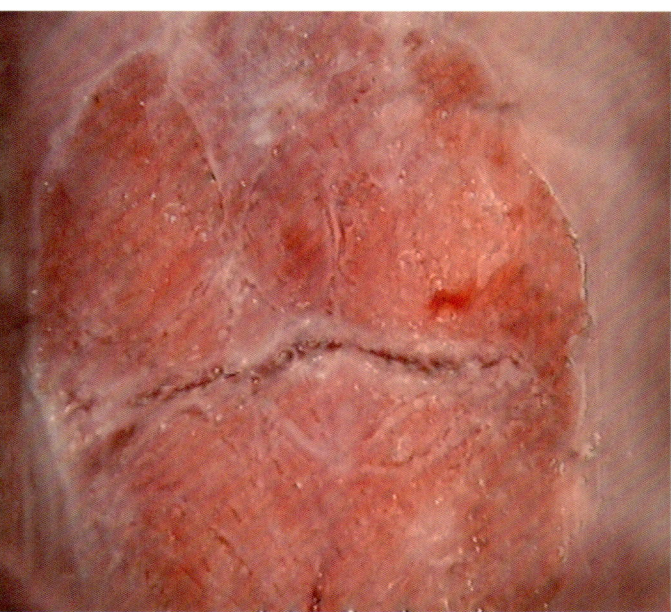

Fig. 5.20: Multifocal metaplastic epithelium in between columnar epithelium

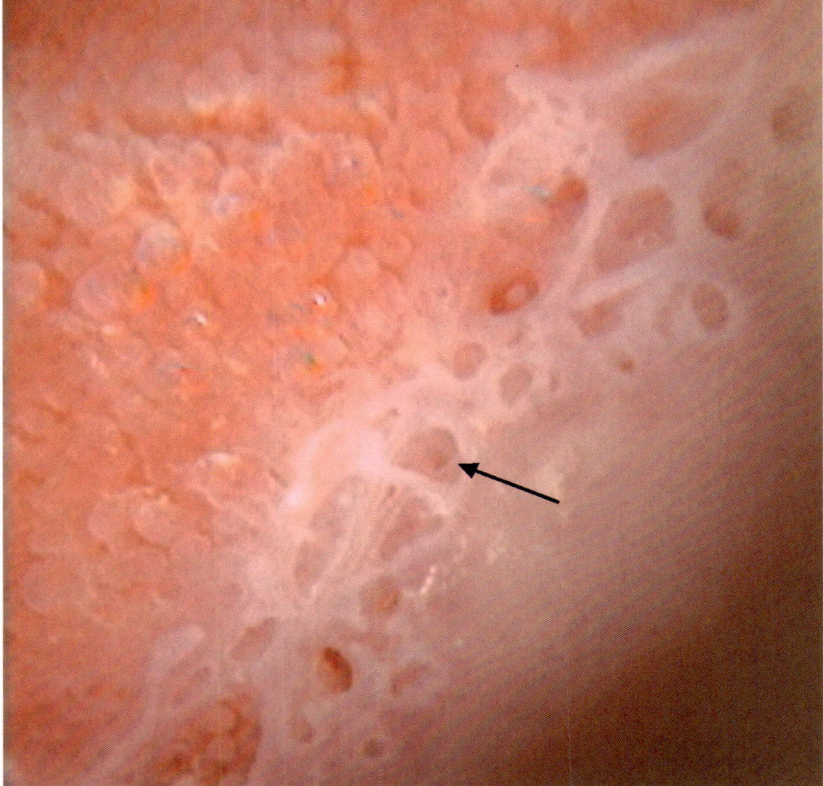

Fig. 5.21: Advanced metaplastic epithelium with windows showing columnar epithelium in between

Mature Metaplasia

Over a period of years, metaplastic epithelium differen-tiates further and becomes glycogenated, and fully mature forming a smooth well-differentiated epithelium having the same features as original squamous epithelium except that it may have remnants of columnar epithelium in the form of residual clefts without metaplasia seen as gland openings (Figs 5.22 and 5.23) or as nabothian cysts (Figs 5.24 and 5.25) which are formed, if the superficial portion of the endocervical cleft is occluded by squamous metaplastic tissue and columnar epithelium deep within the cleft continues to produce mucin.

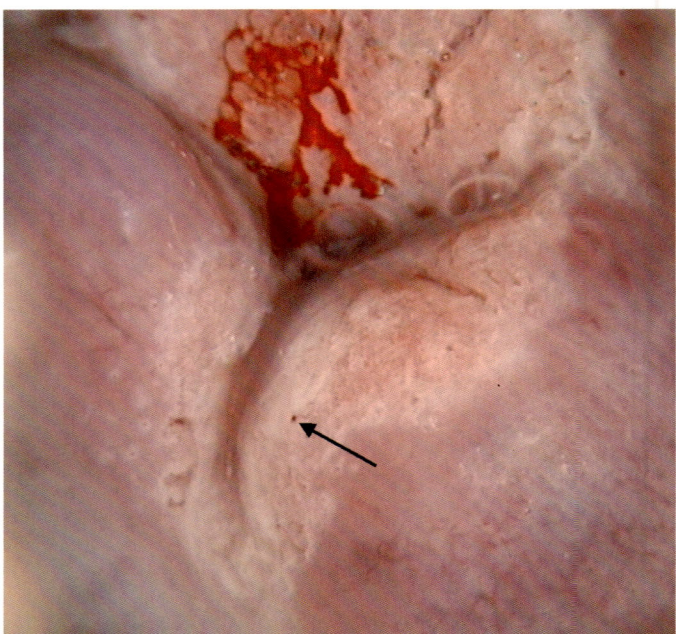

Fig. 5.22: Microphotograph showing mature metaplastic epithelium with normal looking squamous epithelium and residual cleft of columnar epithelium

Fig. 5.23: Cervix after acetic acid application showing mature metaplastic epithelium with multiple gland openings

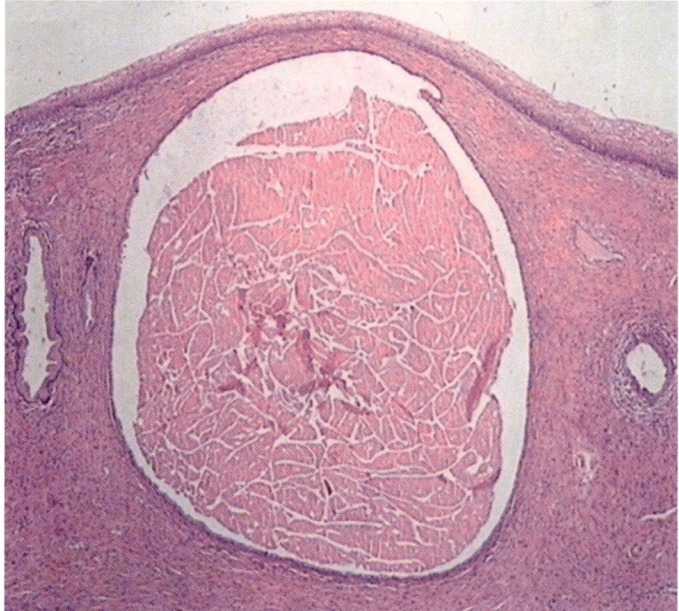

Fig. 5.24: Microphotograph showing metaplastic epithelium covering dilated crypt filled with mucin

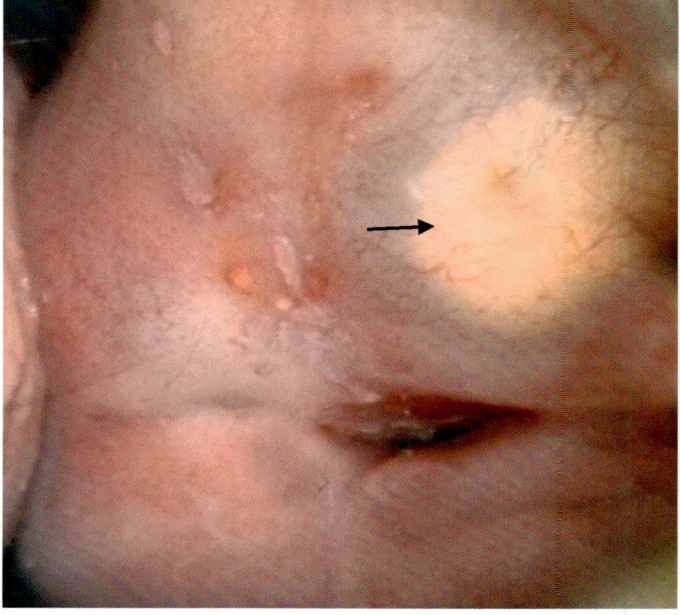

Fig. 5.25: Mature metaplastic epithelium with big nabothian follicle along with overlying normal arborizing vessels

Thus columnar epithelium gets eventually replaced by fully mature metaplastic epithelium. Original SCJ becomes the SSJ (squamo-squamous junction between the OSE and metaplastic squamous epithelium) and a new SCJ is formed between the metaplastic squamous epithelium and the original columnar epithelium.

The area between SSJ (caudal end) and new SCJ (cephalic end) is a dynamic area of physiologic metaplastic change and is called the normal or typical transformation zone (Fig. 5.26).

The normal or typical transformation zone (TTZ) is recognized colposcopically by the presence of metaplastic epithelium in different stages, GOs, NFs and normal dichotomously branching vessels (Figs 5.27 and 5.28). It is the area of maximum colposcopic interest as all pre-neoplastic and neoplastic changes are believed to originate in this region.

Mature metaplasia is a permanent change. It is the immature metaplastic change when epithelium may attain neoplastic potential and become atypical.

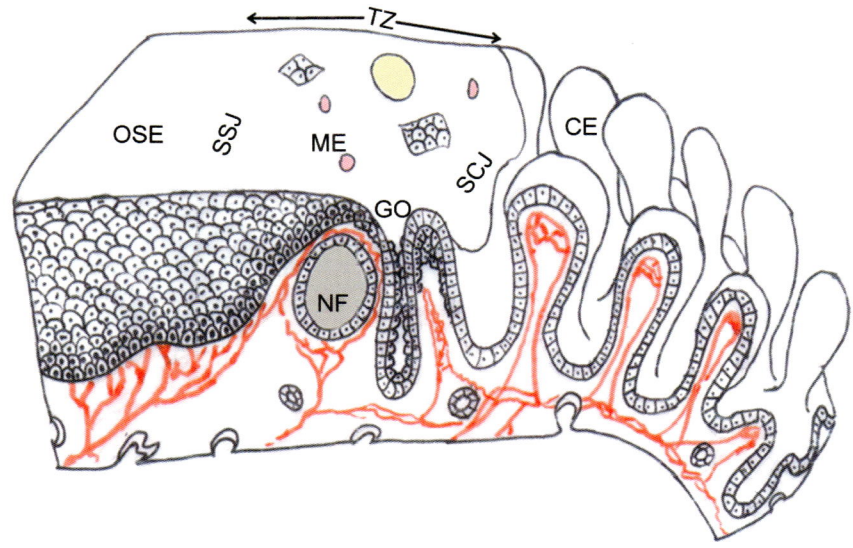

Fig. 5.26: Normal transformation zone ((diagrammatic representation)

OSE Original squamous epithelium; SSJ Squamo-sqamous junction; SCJ Squamo-columnar junction; ME Metaplastic epithelium; GO Gland opening; NF Nabothian follicle; CE Columnar epithelium

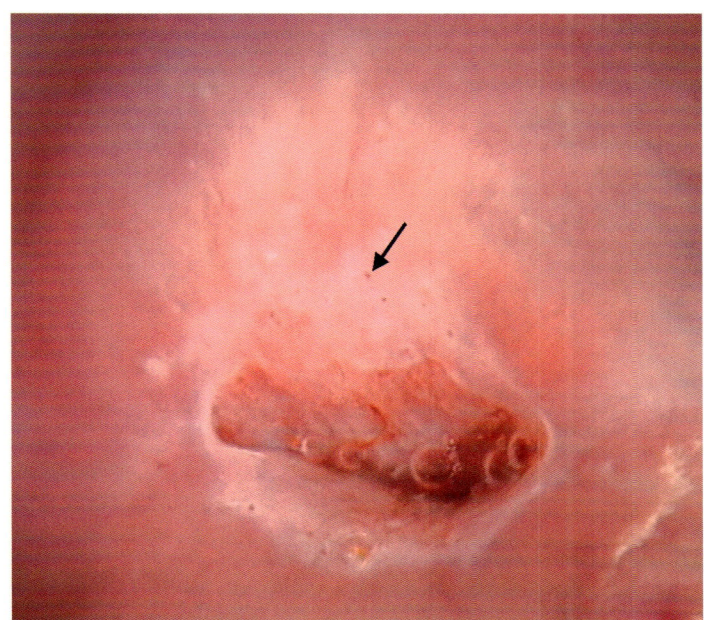

Fig. 5.27: TTZ with gr 1–2 gland openings

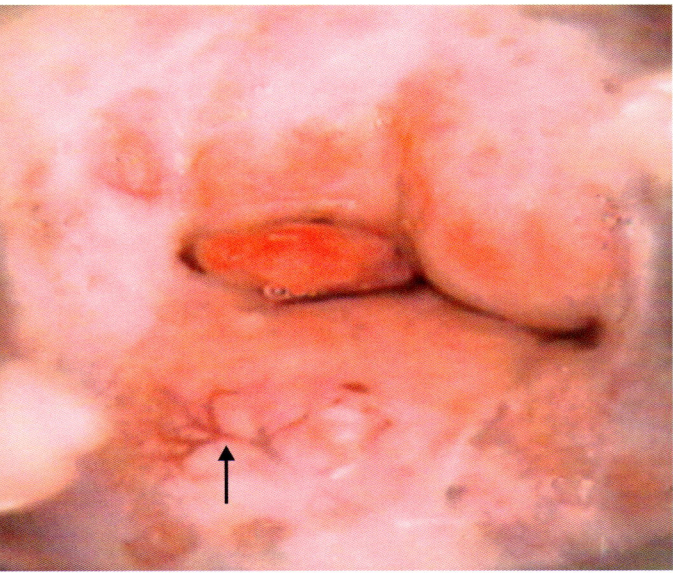

Fig. 5.28: Transformation zone showing metaplastic epithelium, multiple nabothian follicles and normal dichotomously branching vessels

ATYPICAL METAPLASIA AND ATYPICAL TRANSFORMATION ZONE

During the physiological process of metaplasia, if the environment contains some oncogenic factors such as human papillomavirus DNA, the metaplasing cells incorporate the oncogenic factor into its nucleus and take on a neoplastic potential. Instead of dividing and maturing into normal squamous epithelium, they divide into atypical cells giving rise to atypical transformation zone.

In the process of atypical metaplasia, there is increased proliferative activity. The atypical metaplastic squamous cells divide into blocks of tissue, invading and filling the surrounding clefts and folds, causing a

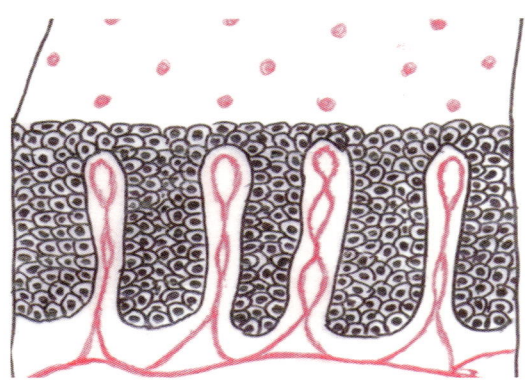

Fig. 5.29: Atypical metaplasia—punctation formation

lateral compression of stromal papillae. The papillae do not fuse with each other as in normal metaplastic process. The vascular network within each villus persists and undergoes marked proliferation.

Depending upon the stage of the metaplastic process, at which neoplastic transformation takes place, the pre-existing vascular capillary network may become tortuous and compressed vertically to varying degrees, or form basket-like network by the neoplastic epithelium, giving rise to different colposcopic findings such as punctations, mosaic and acetowhite epithelium.

Punctations

Neoplastic transformation early in metaplasia will have vessels extending close to the surface (Fig. 5.29). This end-on visualization of intraepithelial capillaries is seen in a stippled pattern as red dots producing the colposcopic pattern of punctations.

Punctations may be fine or coarse. Fine punctations are seen in minor lesions (Fig. 5.30) and widespread fine punctations are generally seen in inflammatory conditions. In major histopathological abnormalities, punctations are usually localized, coarse and irregularly spaced because of the capillary dilatation and increased intercapillary distance (Figs 5.31, 5.32A and B). Punctations are significant when they are found in an area of acetowhite epithelium inside the transformation zone.

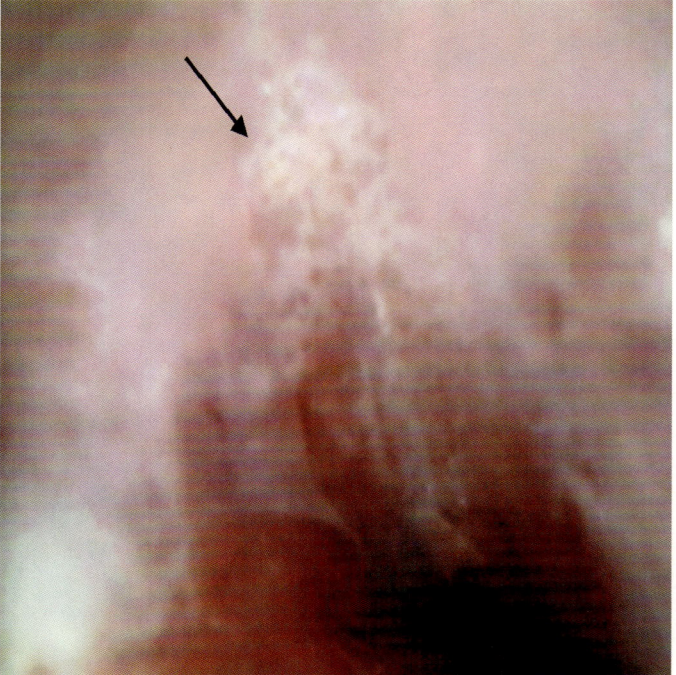

Fig. 5.30: After acetic acid application: Flat AW epithelium with fine, regular punctations over anterior lip

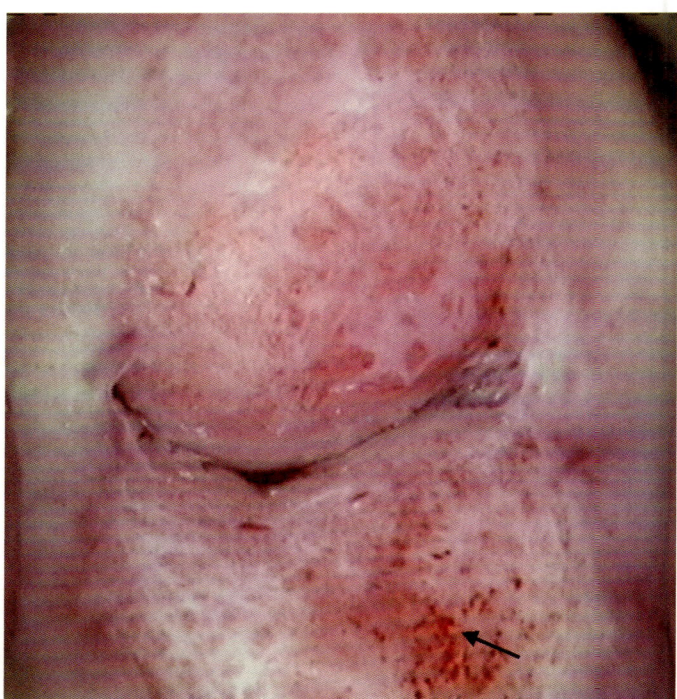

Fig. 5.31: Coarse, irregularly placed punctations on anterior and posterior lips

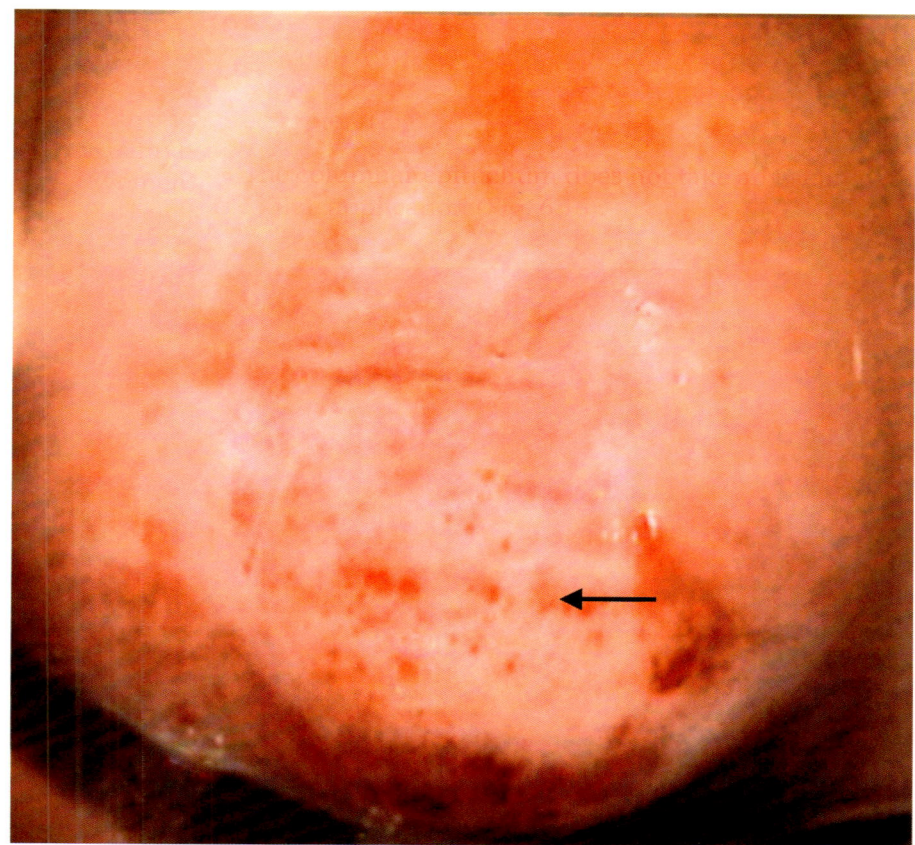

Fig. 5.32A: After application of acetic acid: Dense AW lesion with coarse, irregularly placed punctations over posterior lip

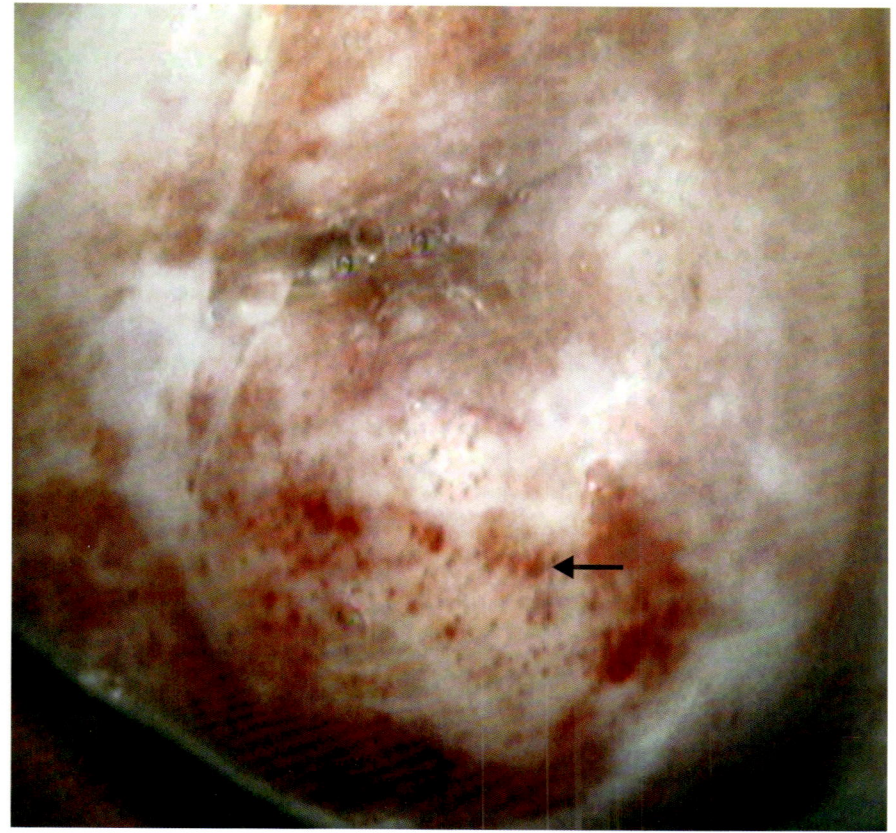

Fig. 5.32B: Same cervix (Fig. 5.32A) under green filter

Mosaic

Atypical transformation at a later stage of metaplasia, when vessels had been pushed to half way down the epithelium, would result in blocks or buds of atypical epithelium surrounded by ramifications of blood vessels which gets compressed by the proliferating atypical epithelium, producing a basket weave structure around the blocks of abnormal epithelium (Fig. 5.33).

These tiles of white epithelium separated by red partitions, give a honeycomb appearance, resulting in the abnormal colposcopic finding of mosaic appearance. Because of severe compression, some of the capillaries eventually disappear resulting in increased inter-capillary distance which may be colposcopically seen as irregular punctations or mosaic.

Mosaic may appear fine (Figs 5.34A and B) or coarse (Figs 5.35A and B) according to the size and shape of the tiles that may be regular or irregular depending upon the degree of underlying abnormality.

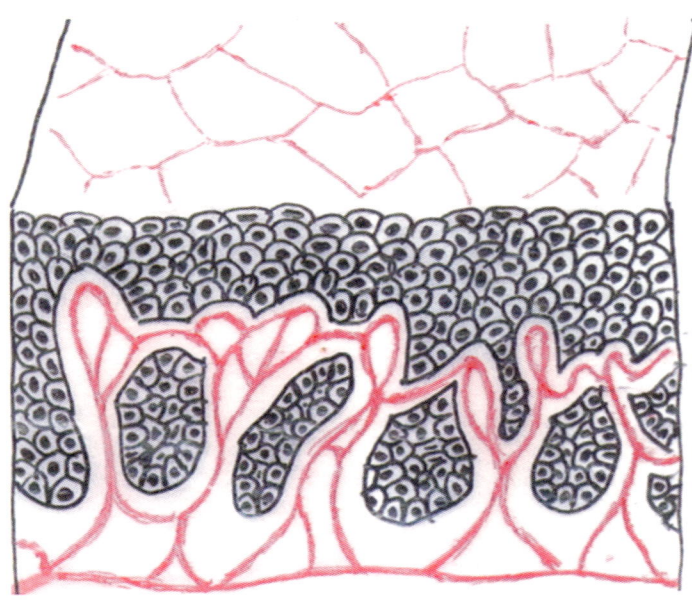

Fig. 5.33: Atypical metaplasia—mosaic formation

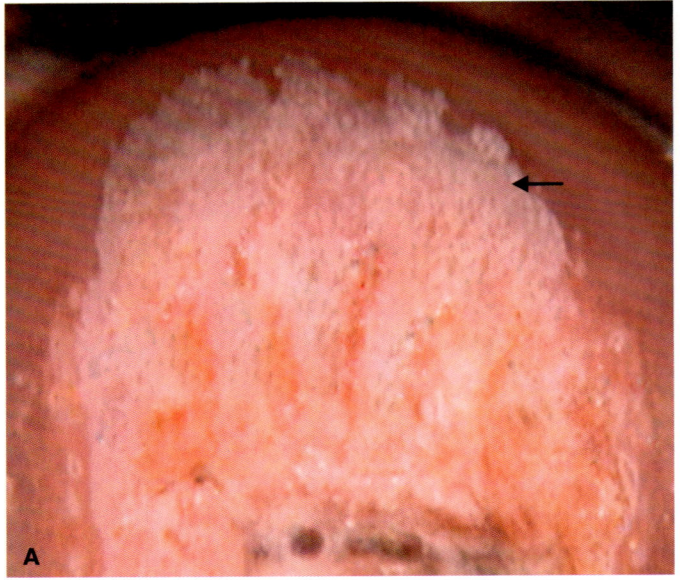
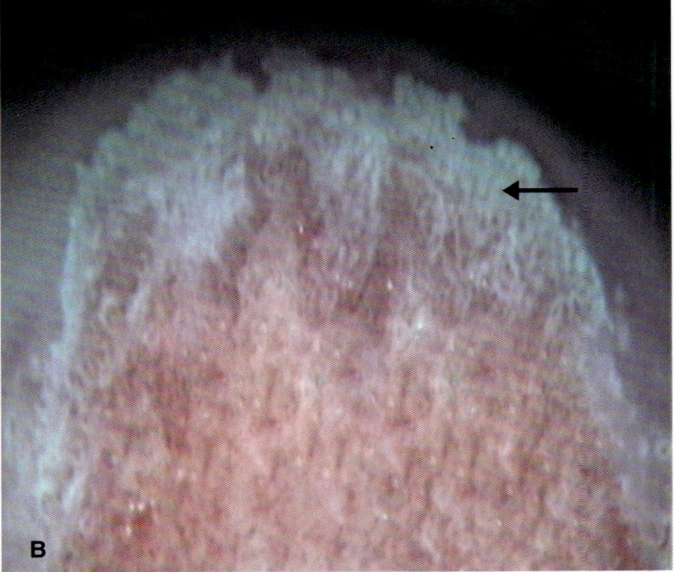

Fig. 5.34: Gr 1 AW epithelium with fine regular mosaic over outer part of anterior lip: (A) After application of acetic acid and (B) under green filter

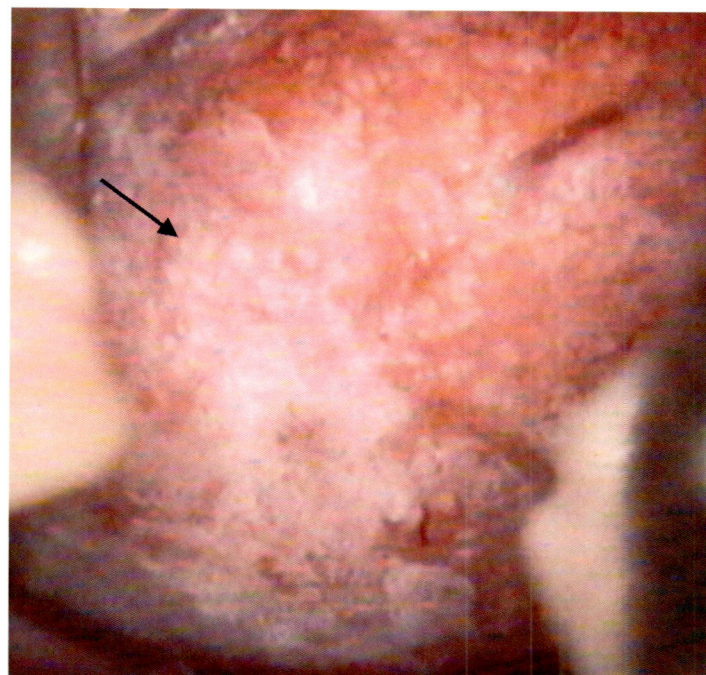

Fig. 5.35A: AW epithelium with coarse mosaic

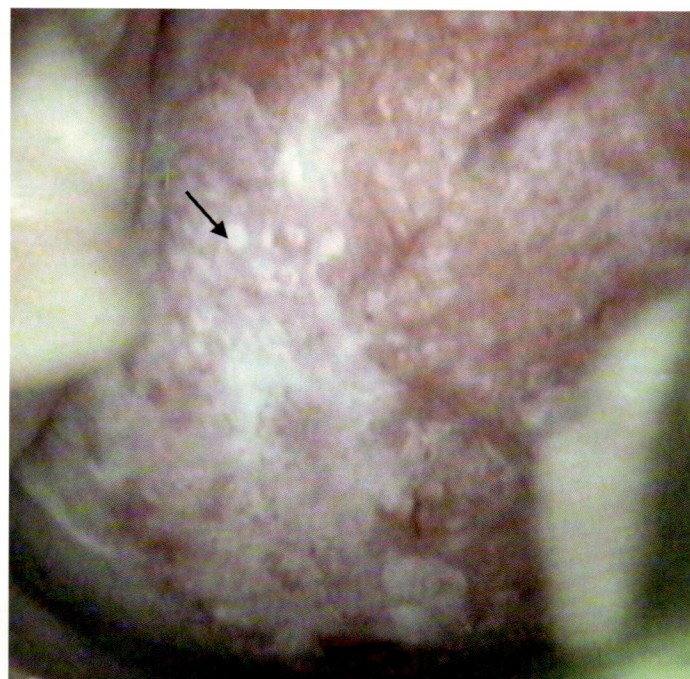

Fig. 5.35B: Same cervix
(Fig. 5.35A) under green filter

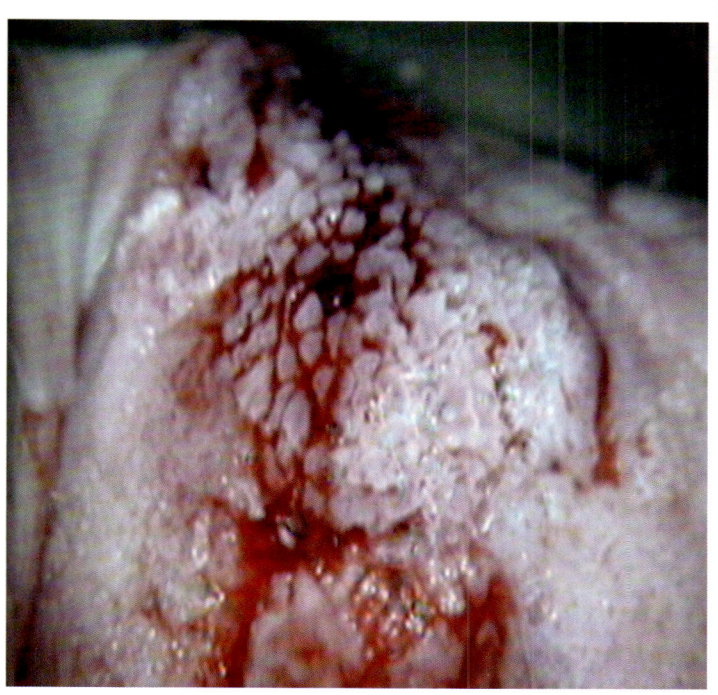

Fig. 5.35C: Dense AW epithelium and coarse
irregular mosaic seen under green filter

Acetowhite Epithelium

When neoplastic alteration occurs late in metaplasia after all the capillaries have been pushed down from the papillae, only AW epithelium is produced (Fig. 5.36).

It is a focal colpscopic lesion visible after application of acetic acid as a transient change.

Acetic acid causes tissue edema and superficial coagulation of intracellular proteins, thereby reducing the transparency of the epithelium. When this happens the subepithelial capillaries are less easily visible and the epithelium itself appears white. This occurs because of one or more factors such as increase in number of cell layers, increased cellularity, increased N:C ratio, and increased nuclear density.

Acetowhite change can be seen in immature metaplastic epithelium, regenerating epithelium, subclinical papilloma viral infection, pre-neoplastic and neoplastic lesions.

Degree of acetowhiteness is directly proportional to the severity of underlying histological abnormality.

Surface contour of AW epithelium may be flat (Figs 5.37 to 5.39) or may have micropapillary projections or brain like microconvolutions (Fig. 5.40).

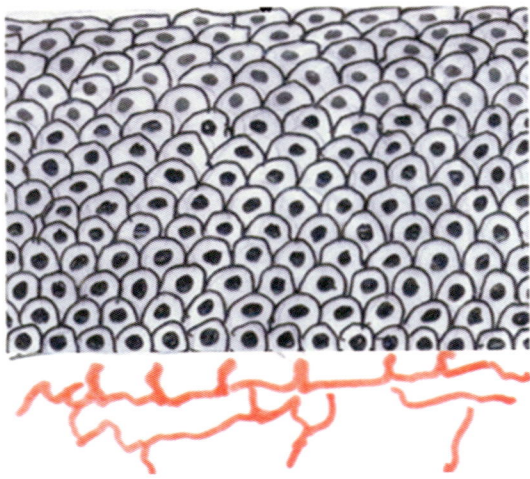

Fig. 5.36: Atypical metaplasia—abnormal epithelium giving rise to only acetowhite epithelium

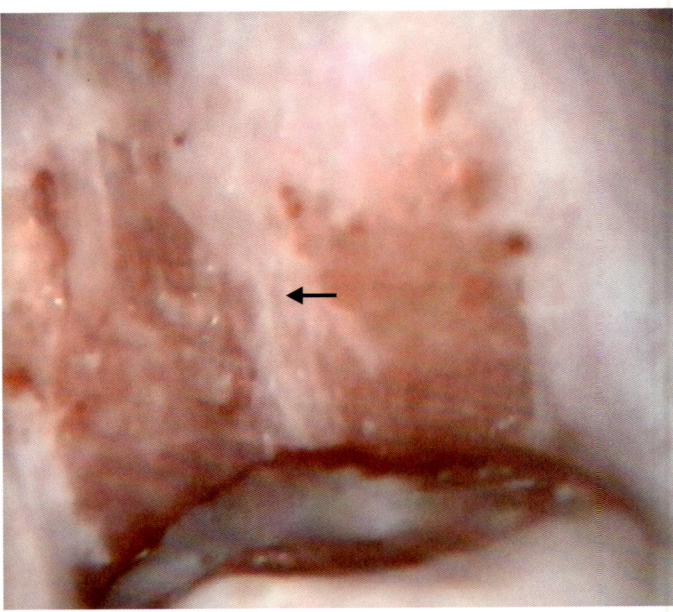

Fig. 5.37: After application of acetic acid: Flat AW lesion on anterior lip near external os with feathery margins

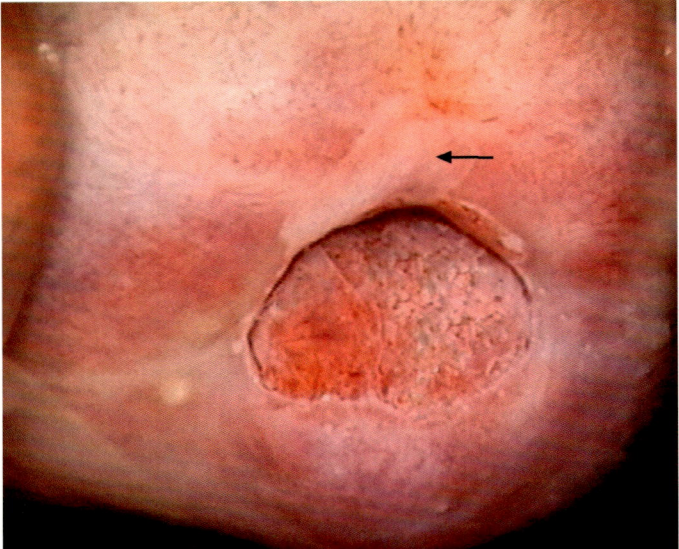

Fig. 5.38A: After the application of acetic acid: Flat AW lesion on anterior lip

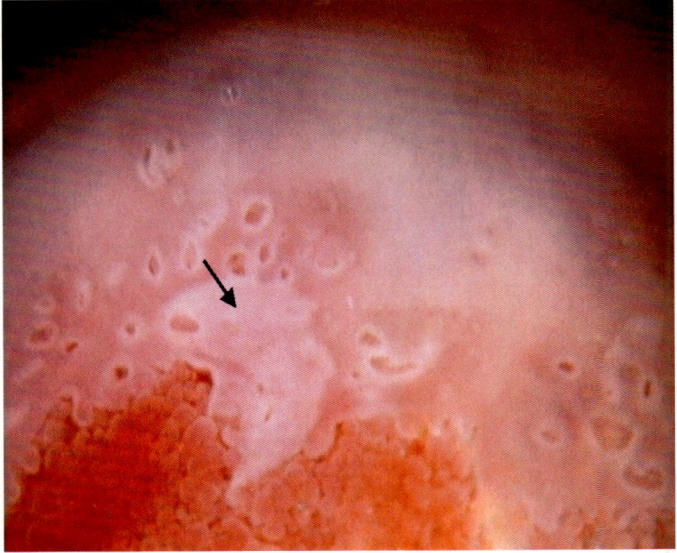

Fig. 5.38B: After application of acetic acid: Flat AW lesion with sharp borders on anterior lip along with many gland openings

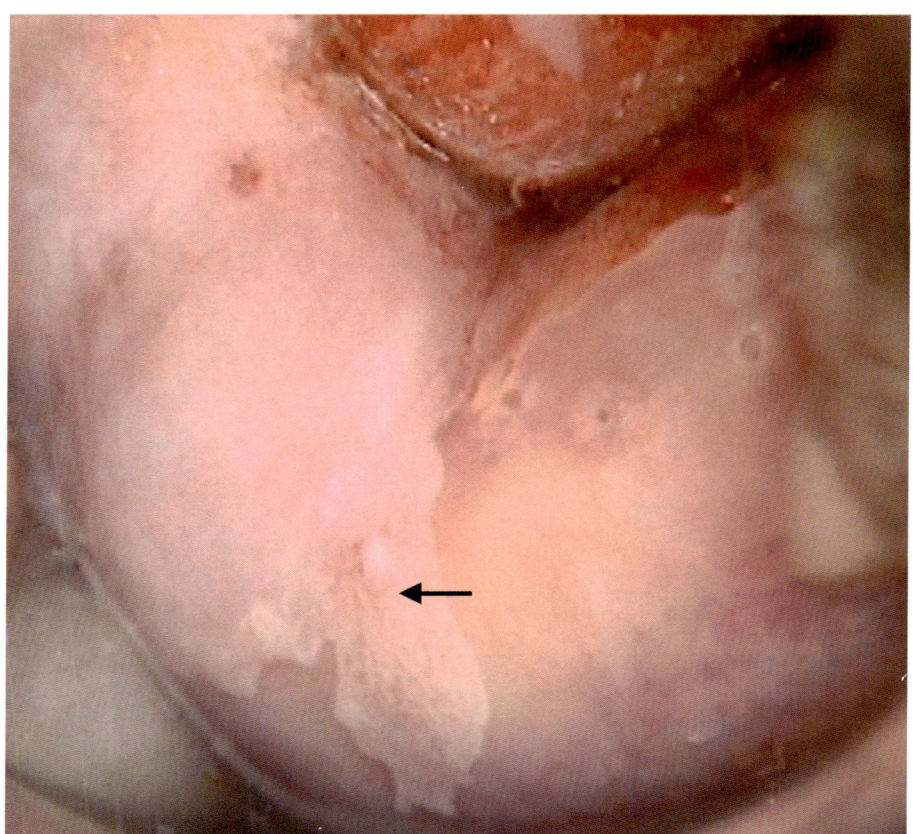

Fig. 5.39: AW lesion with distinct raised sharp margin on posterior lip at 6 O' clock. Lesion on right lateral side is of lesser grade

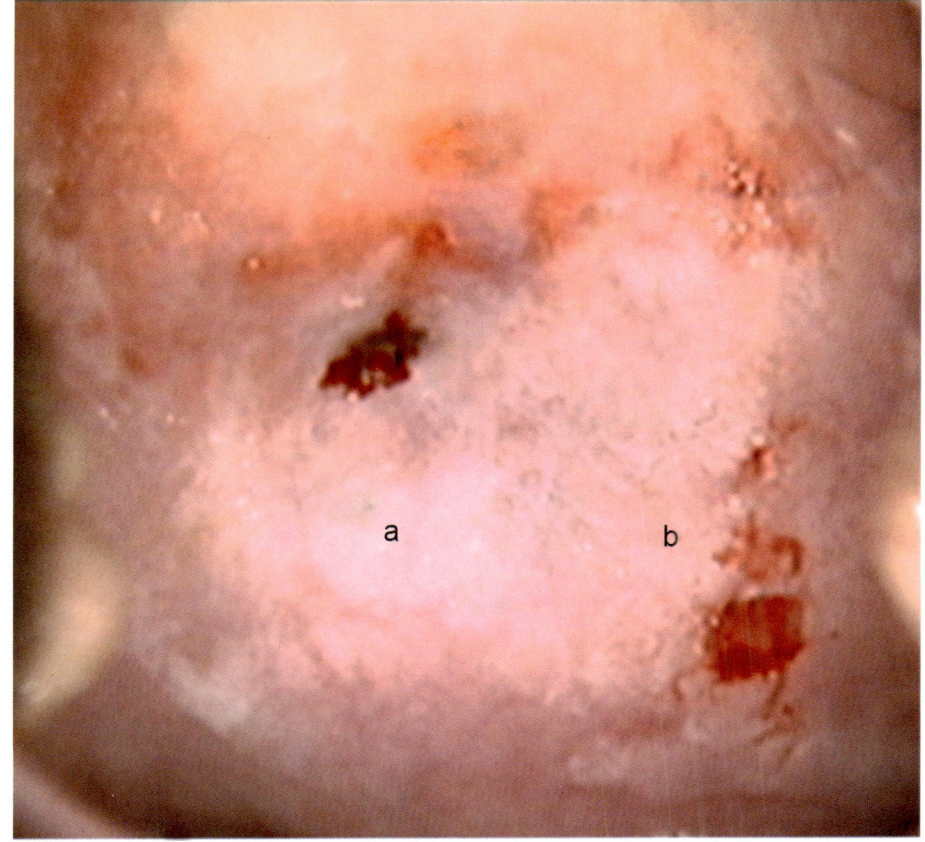

Fig. 5.40: Dense AW epithelium in the centre (a) along with micropapillary surface on left side (b)

Leukoplakia (Keratosis)

It is the white epithelium which can be seen with naked eye before the application of acetic acid. This is due to hyperkeratosis and parakeratosis resulting in keratin on the surface and may overlie normal as well as abnormal epithelium (Fig. 5.41). It may be thin which is usually not significant (Fig. 5.42) or thick with irregular surface usually seen in pronounced atypical lesions (Figs 5.43 and 5.44). These lesions are significant when they are located inside transformation zone. All these lesions must be biopsied as they may overlie and hide malignant lesions.

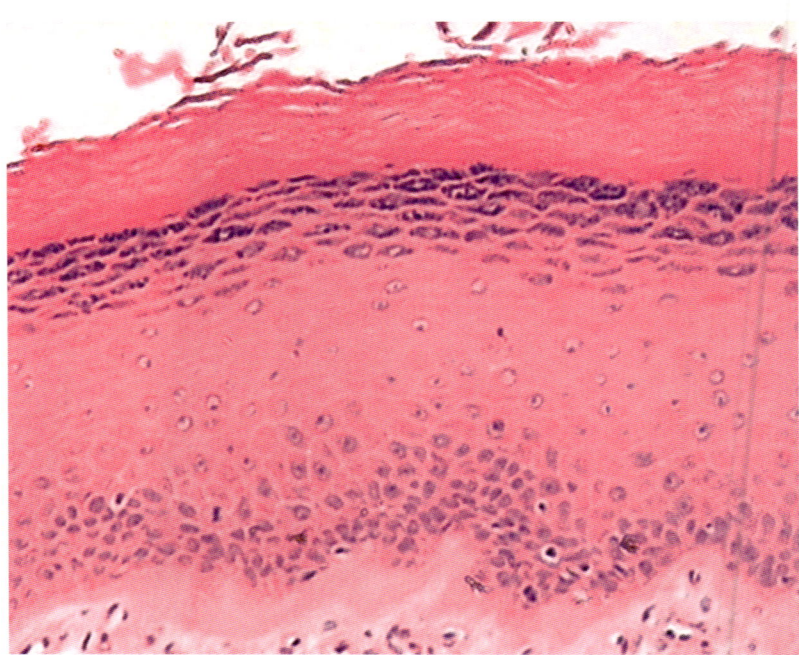

Fig. 5.41: Microphotograph of keratosis— epithelium covered with thick keratin layer

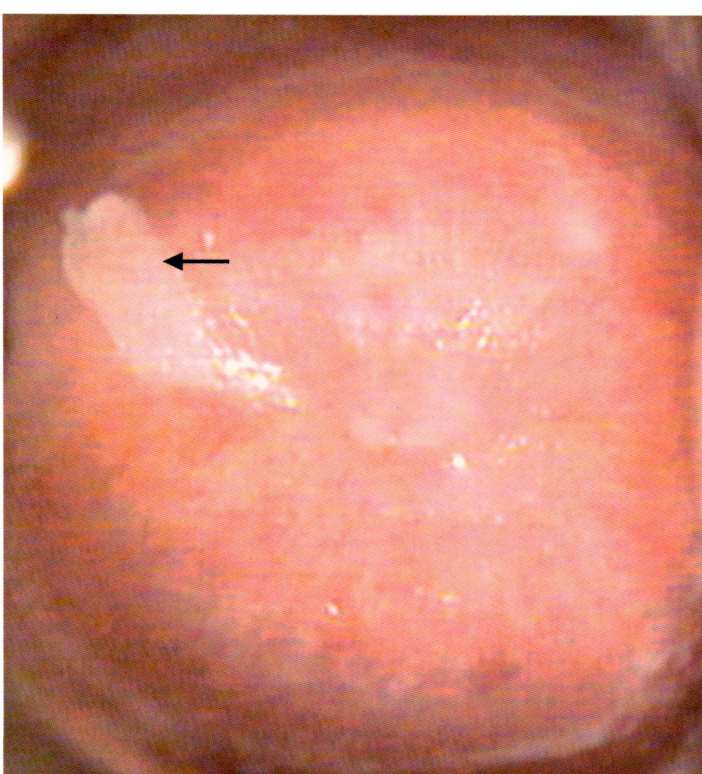

Fig. 5.42: Thin white epithelium seen before application of acetic acid— keratosis

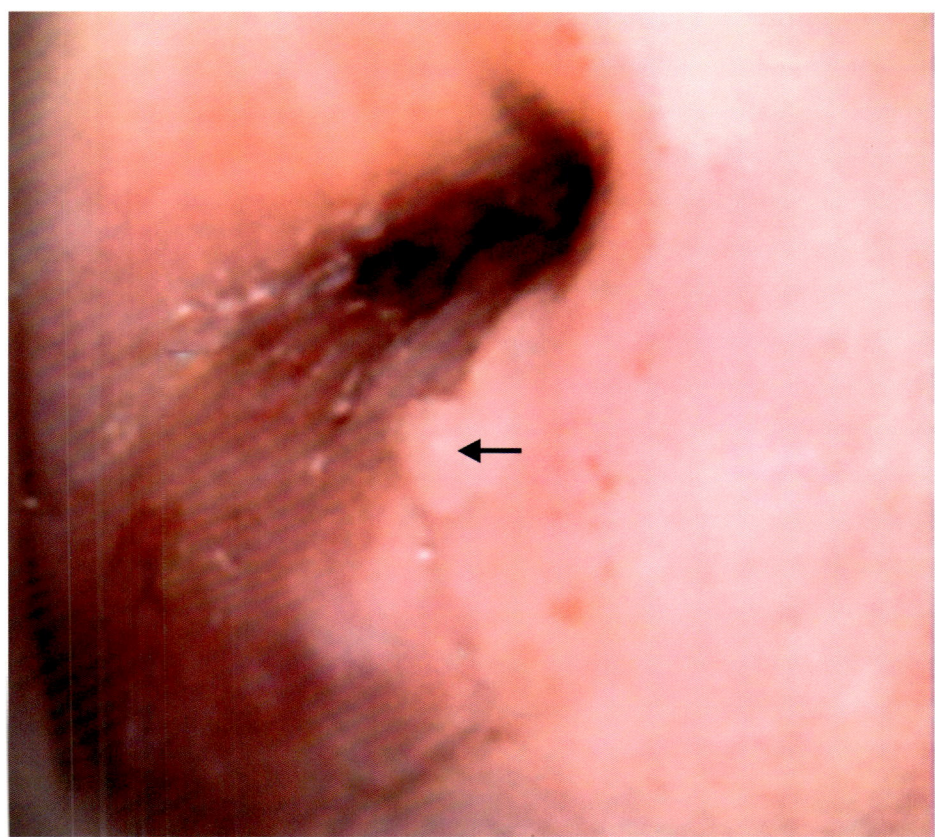

Fig. 5.43: Thick, raised white epithelium with irregular surface seen before application of acetic acid—keratosis

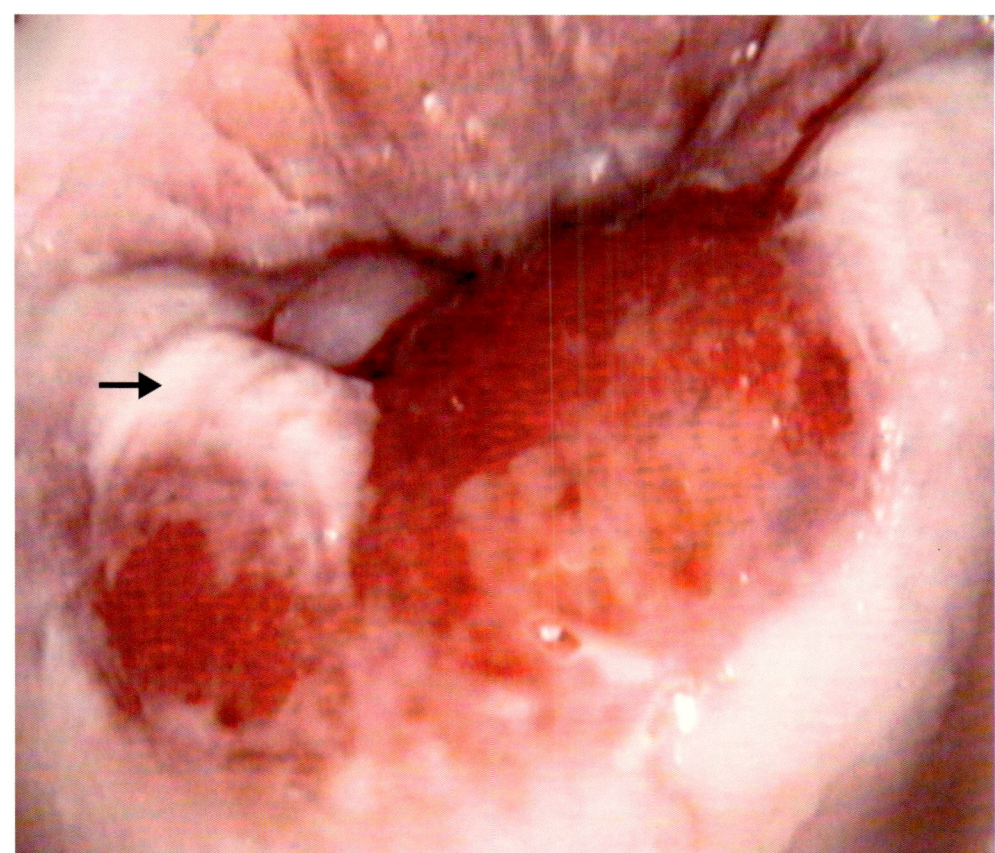

Fig. 5.44: Thick, raised white epithelium with irregular surface seen before application of acetic acid along with decubitus ulcer in a case of prolapse uterus

Reverse Mosaic

Reverse mosaic is another abnormality that may be seen colposcopically on rare occasions. It indicates the beginning of atypical metaplasia. Little red islands representing the tips of former grape-like papillae are seen surrounded by white metaplastic squamous epithelium (Figs 5.45 and 5.46) which has filled the clefts and folds between villi of columnar epithelium. This appearance is short lived and soon changes to either punctation or mosaic when atypical epithelium proliferates further.

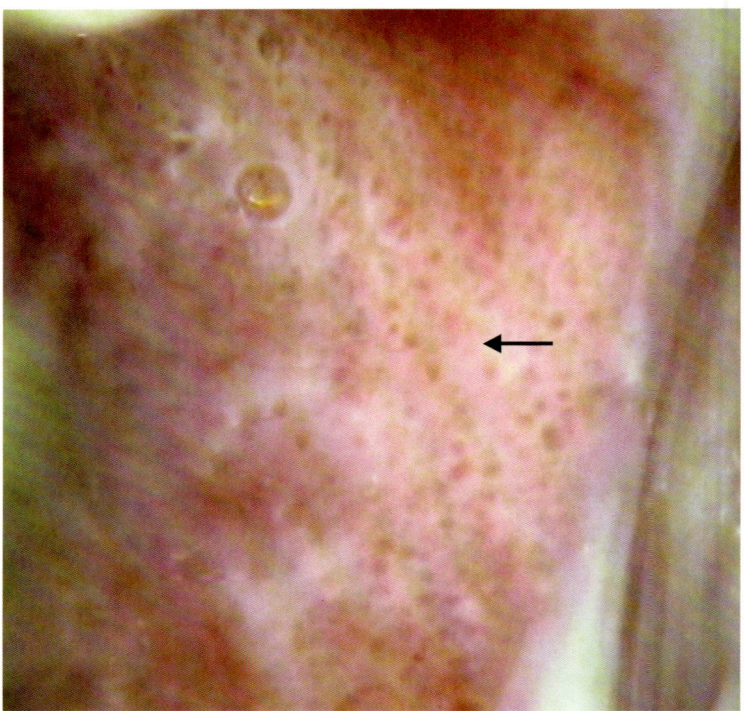

Fig. 5.45: After application of acetic acid: Reverse mosaic seen as red islands surrounded by white partitions

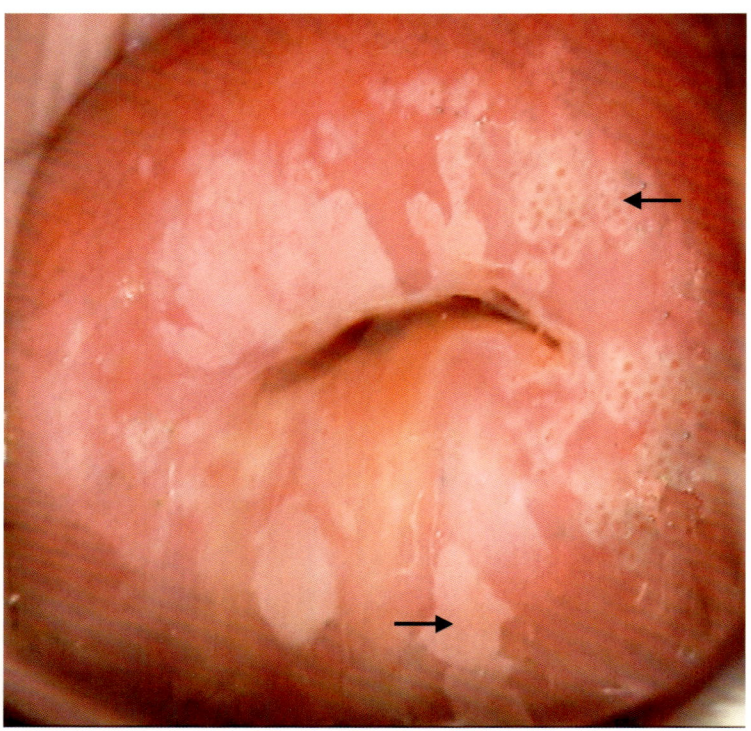

Fig. 5.46: Reverse mosaic seen over anterior lip along with many tongues of grade 1–2 acetowhite epithelium

Atypical Vessels

These are abnormal vessels which appear as a result of neovascularization following the release of tumor angiogenetic factor and abnormal rapid proliferation of cells forcing vessels to acquire different bends and shapes indicating invasion.

They appear colposcopically as irregular vessels with marked variation in caliber, course, and branching pattern such as cork-screw, or spaghetti formation (Figs 5.47A and B).

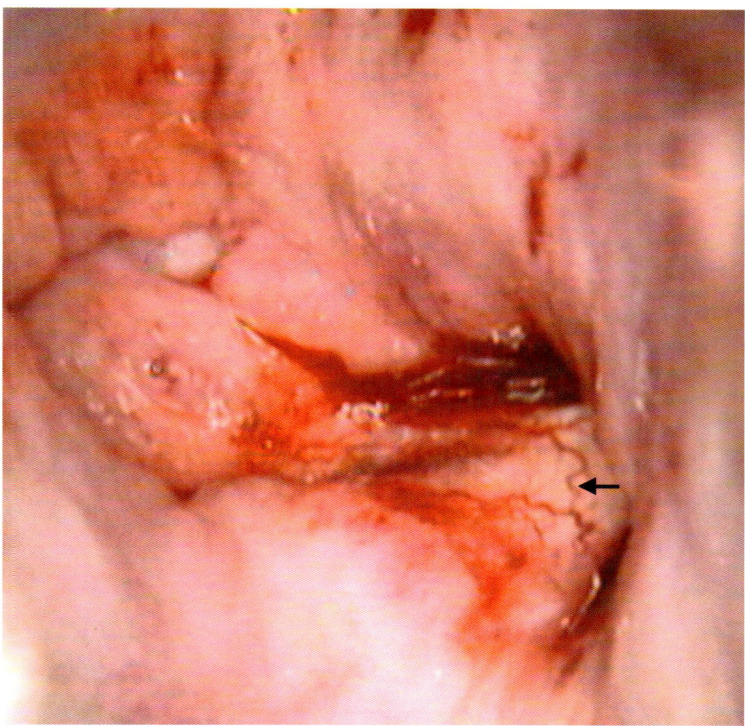

Fig. 5.47A: Atypical vessels seen along with irregular surface contour

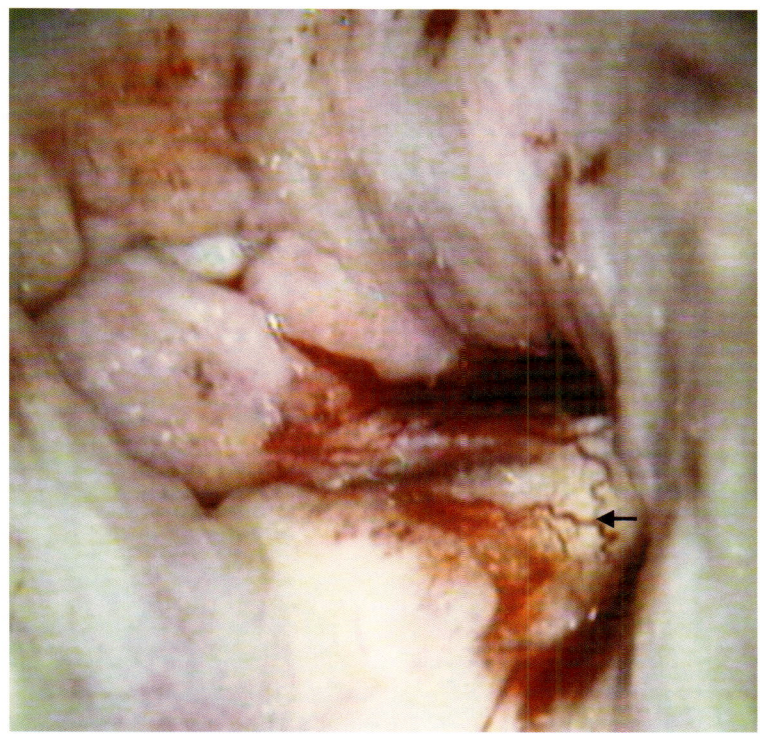

Fig. 5.47B: Same cervix under green filter

Iodine-Negative Epithelium

Normal squamous epithelium which contains glycogen becomes mahogany brown in color after application of Lugol's iodine.

Epithelium which lacks glycogen such as columnar epithelium, immature metaplastic epithelium, and dysplastic epithelium do not take up iodine stain. Patchy iodine uptake (Fig. 5.48) is usually seen in lesser grade lesions in comparison to distinct yellow color lesions (Fig. 5.49). Atrophic epithelium and inflamed epithelium are lightly stained.

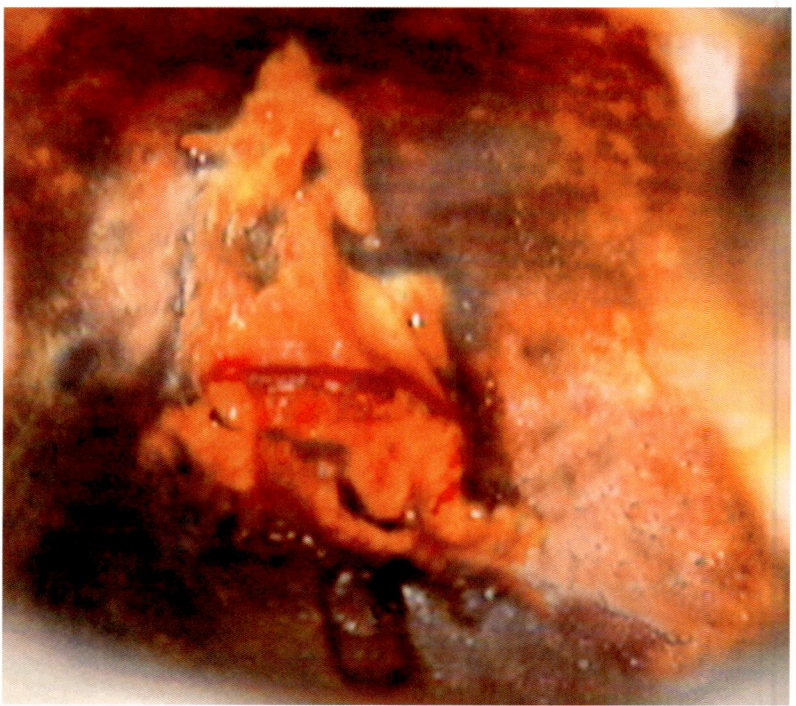

Fig. 5.48: Patchy iodine uptake

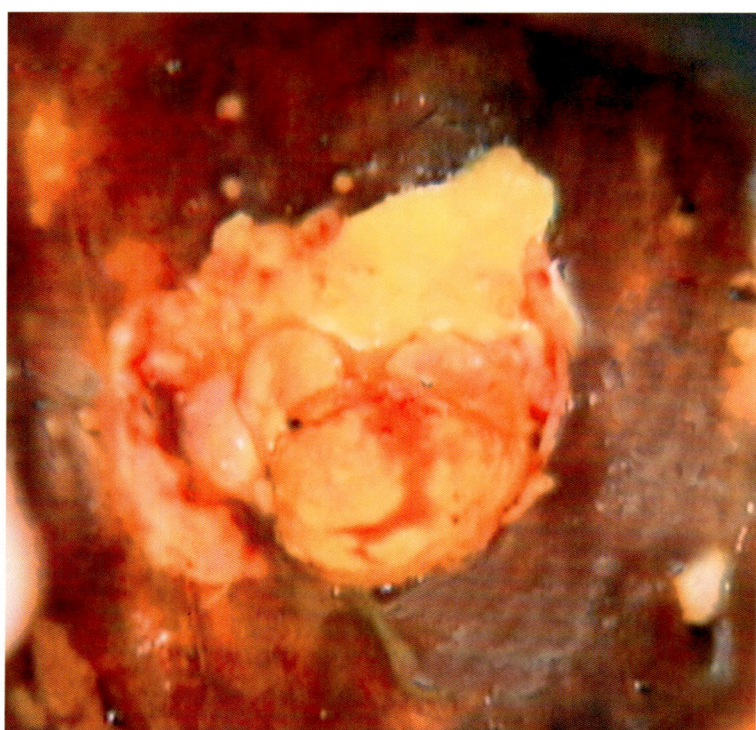

Fig. 5.49: After application of Lugol's iodine: Abnormal epithelium seen as distinct yellow color area

Normal Cervix and the Variants

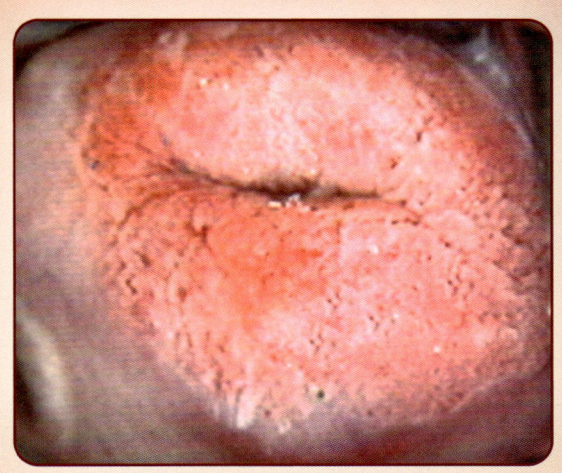

Chapter Outline

During organogenesis of lower female genital tract, cervix and upper part of the vagina are derived from mullerian ducts (columnar component), while the lower part of the vagina is derived from the genital sinus ridge (squamous component).

During intrauterine life, gradually the initial mullerian columnar epithelial lining of the vagina and most of the ectocervix get converted by metaplasia into squamous epithelium and is known as original squamous epithelium. Columnar epithelium lining the endocervical canal persists. Junction of both the epithelia is called original squamocolumnar junction (OSCJ).

The SC junction usually coincides with the external os of the cervix at the time of birth (Fig. 6.1A), but its location is not static and changes in different phases of life. During menarche and 1st pregnancy, it comes on to the cervical portio (Figs 6.1B and C), where it stays throughout a woman's menstruating life. This deceptive movement is caused by the high estrogen levels, which increase the mass of mesenchymal elements in the stroma, resulting in eversion of cervix. With the withdrawal of estrogens in the postmenopausal state, the SCJ recedes into the endocervical canal (Fig. 6.1D) and may not be visible on the ectocervix.

Structure of cervical epithelium and underlying stroma is dependent on the hormonal status, which is reflected in the colposcopic appearance as well as the cytological picture during different phases of life.

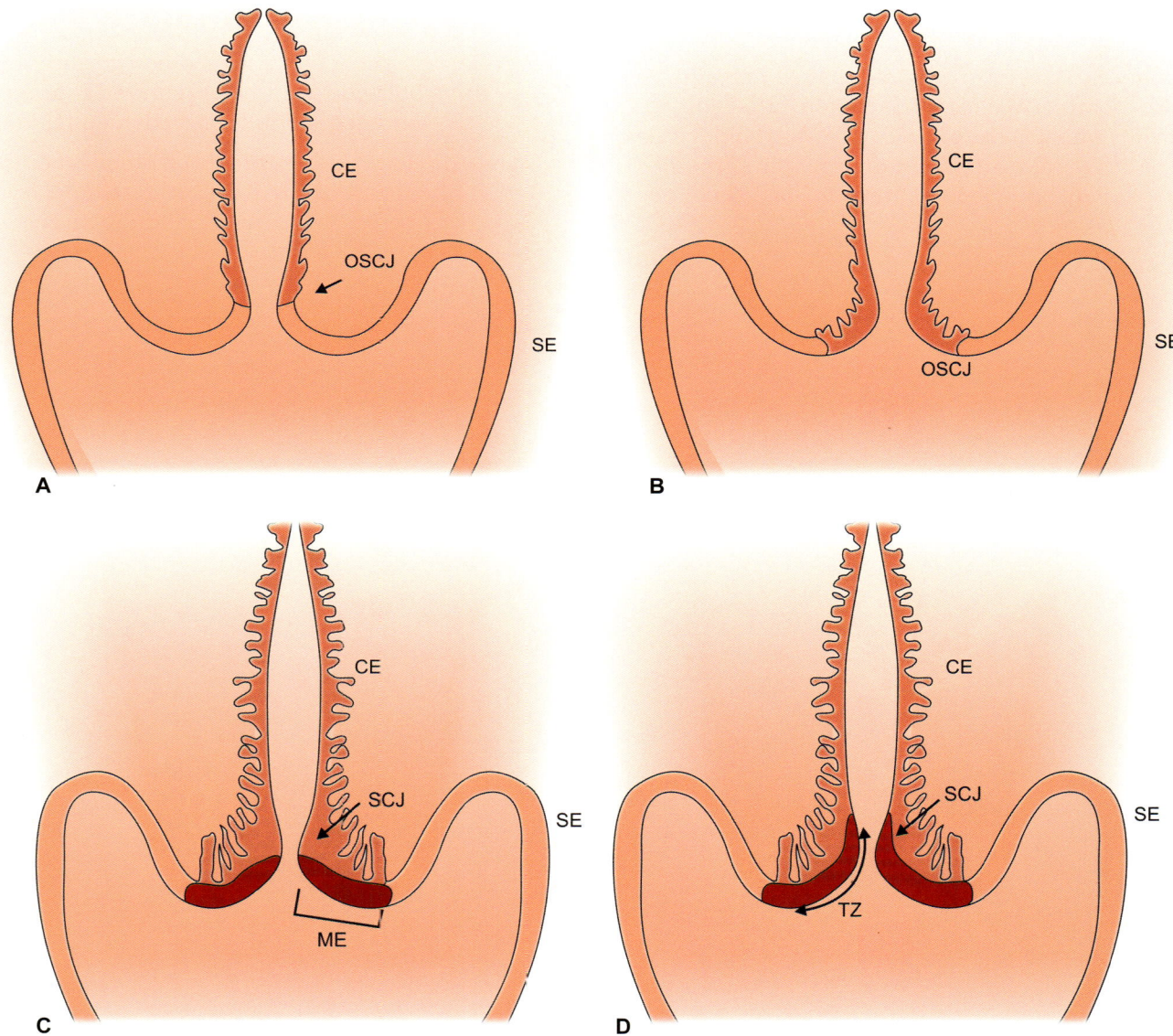

Fig. 6.1: Location of SCJ (A) at birth, (B and C) Reproductive age, (D) Postmenopausal age

NORMAL CERVIX IN REPRODUCTIVE PHASE

Ectocervical Epithelium

Normal cervix in reproductive phase is lined by non-keratinized squamous epithelium. Generally, it is 16–20 layers thick and consists of basal, parabasal, intermediate and superficial layers (Figs 6.2 and 6.3).

Basal layer attached to the basal lamina consists of single layer of small cells disposed perpendicularly. Parabasal layer is two to three cells thick and consists of round cells larger than basal cells. As the cell layers move up, cellular differentiation and maturation takes place which is indicated by increase in cell size, increase in cytoplasmic mass and reduction in nuclear size. Character of the cytoplasm also changes. Accumulation of glycogen takes place in the middle and upper layers of epithelium and keratin is acquired in superficial layers. Cellular character is better defined in cytological smears.

Vasculature: Terminal vessels of the cervix have four zones (Fig. 6.4); the deepest comprising of a plexus of freely anastomosing vessels in the stroma. Arising from this zone are the palisade-like vessels running perpendicular or obliquely and terminating under the epithelium in a basal network parallel to the surface. From this basal plexus, terminal capillaries of the subepithelial tissue arise to form capillary loops just below and indenting the epithelium. It is the capillaries of the fourth zone which can be seen through the colposcope during reproductive life. Normally terminal vessels do not go beyond the lower one-third of the squamous epithelium.

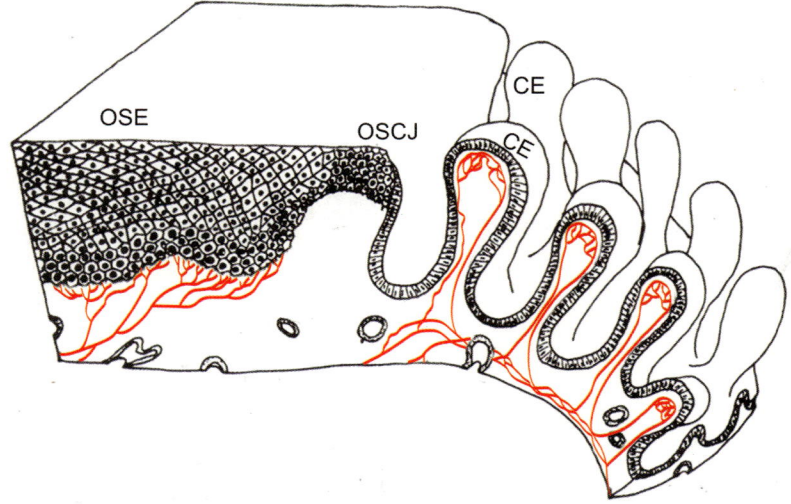

Fig. 6.2: Schematic diagram of squamous epithelium and columnar epithelium
OSE Original squamous epithelium, CE Columnar epithelium, OSCJ Original Squamocolumnar junction

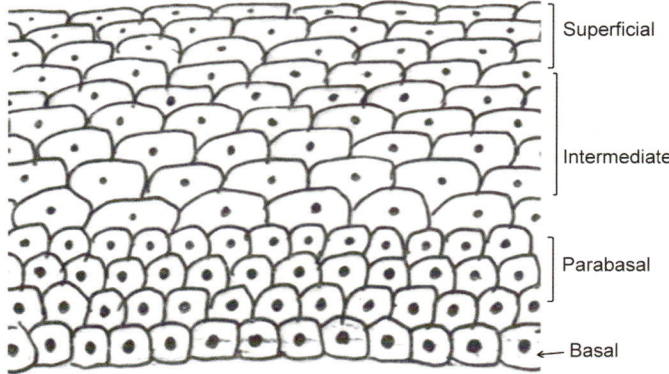

Fig. 6.3: Normal squamous epithelium showing basal, parabasal, intermediate and superficial cell layers

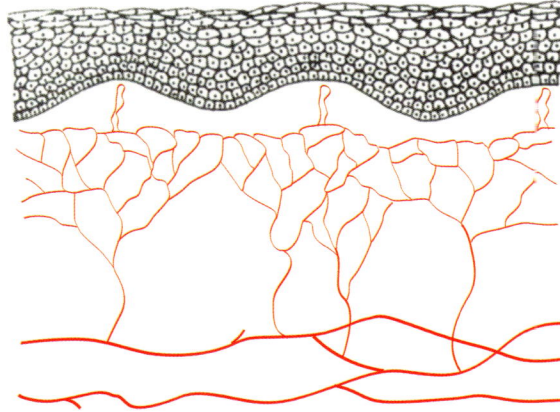

Fig. 6.4: Schematic diagram: Vasculature of squamous epithelium

Colposcopy: Original squamous epithelium on the ectocervix looks translucent, flat, homogeneous, and uniformly pink in color (Fig. 6.5). Vasculature of normal squamous epithelium is seen in the form of network or hair pin capillaries (Figs 6.6 to 6.8).

Acetic acid has no effect on original squamous epithelium. After iodine application, it becomes mahogany brown in color.

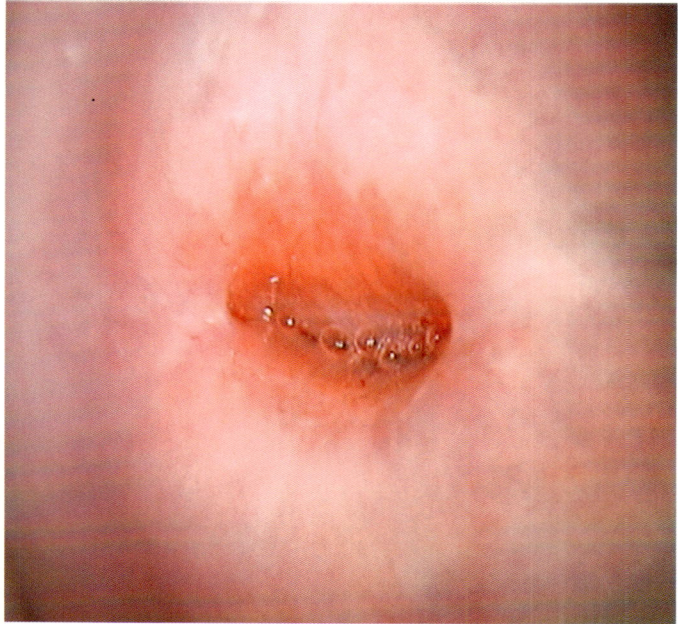

Fig. 6.5: Normal cervix with translucent, flat, homogeneous, and uniformly pink original squamous epithelium. Part of red, velvety columnar epithelium seen near external os

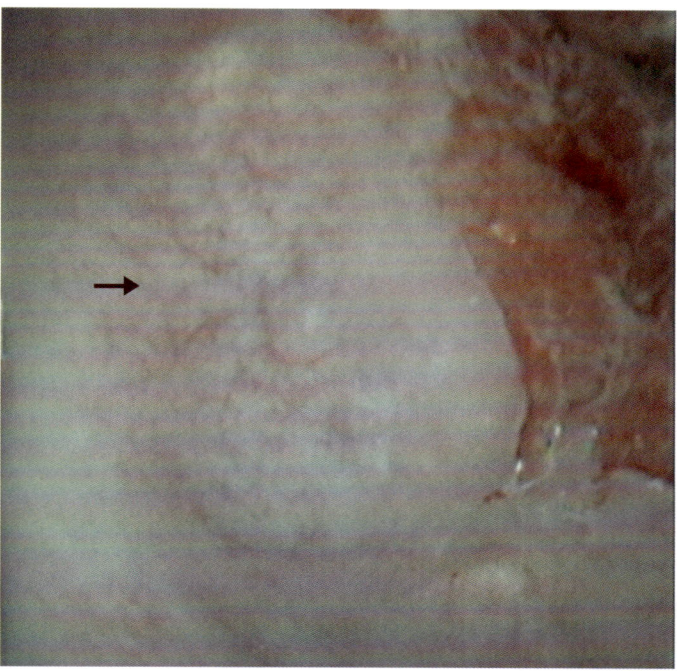

Fig. 6.6: Under green filter: Normal network and hair pin capillaries of OSE

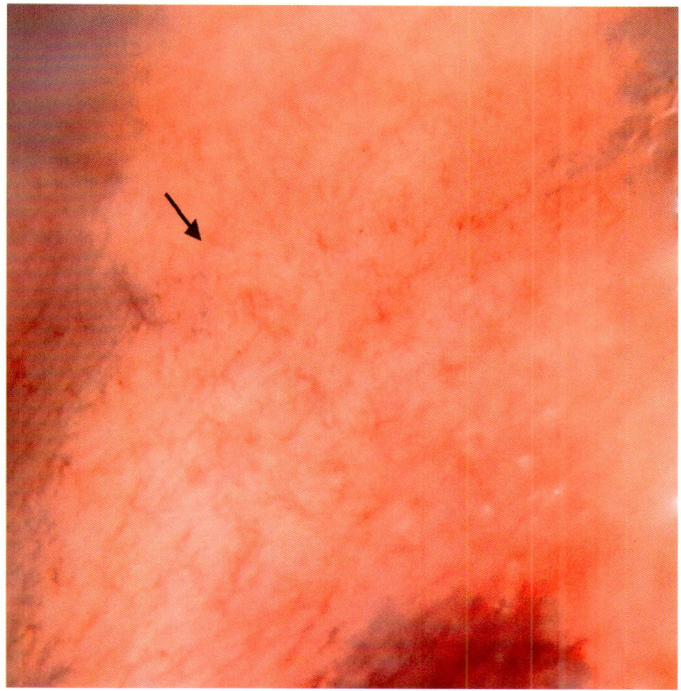

Fig. 6.7: OSE with normal network and hair pin capillaries under high magnification

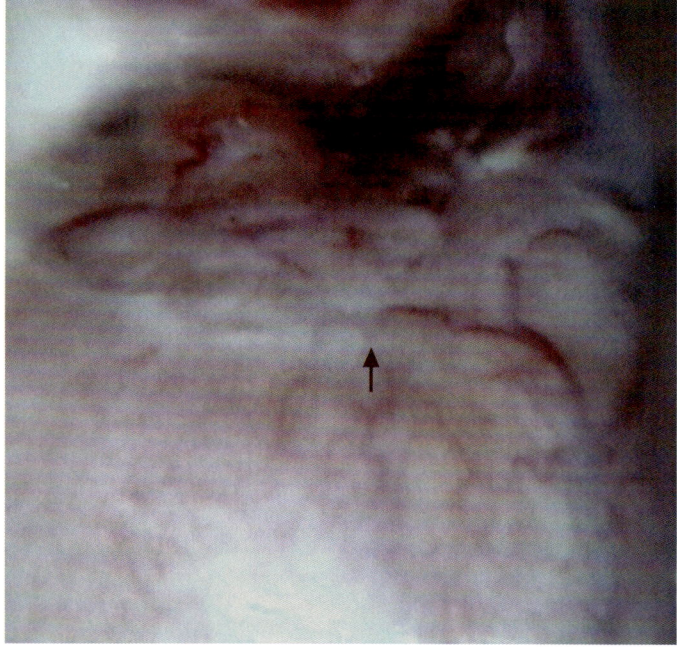

Fig. 6.8: Under green filter: Normal network and hair pin capillaries of OSE along with dichotomously dividing uniform caliber vessels of normal TZ

Endocervical Epithelium

Normal endocervical mucosa is lined by single layer of mucin secreting, ciliated columnar epithelium lining the villi. The core of villi contains loose connective tissue and fine capillaries.

The epithelium dips into the underlying connective tissue as crypts which on cross-section appear like glands.

Vasculature: Terminal vessels of columnar epithelium consist of inter-twining capillaries forming a multi-channel network at the top which has an ascending and descending capillary (Fig. 6.9).

Colposcopy: After saline application, columnar epithelium lining the endocervix gives a red velvety appearance (Fig. 6.10). Adjacent to SC junction, it has a papillary configuration. Each papilla shows a terminal capillary loop.

After acetic acid application, it assumes grape-like appearance near SC junction (Fig. 6.11) while shows ridges or folds inside endocervical canal (Fig. 6.12).

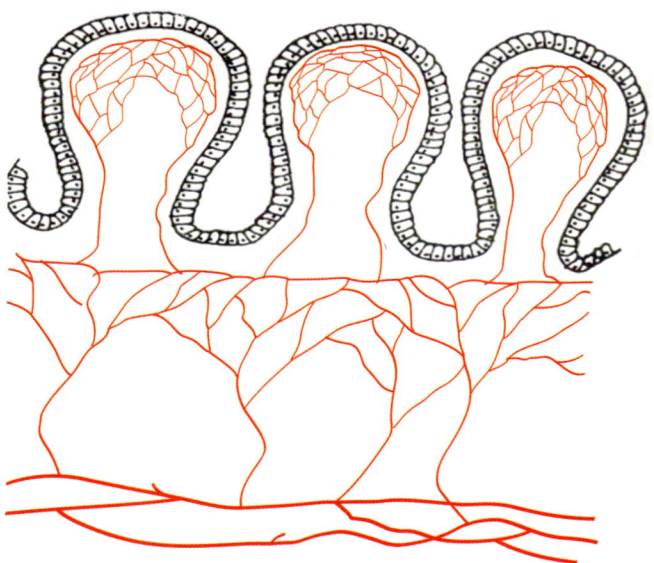

Fig. 6.9: Schematic vasculature of columnar epithelium

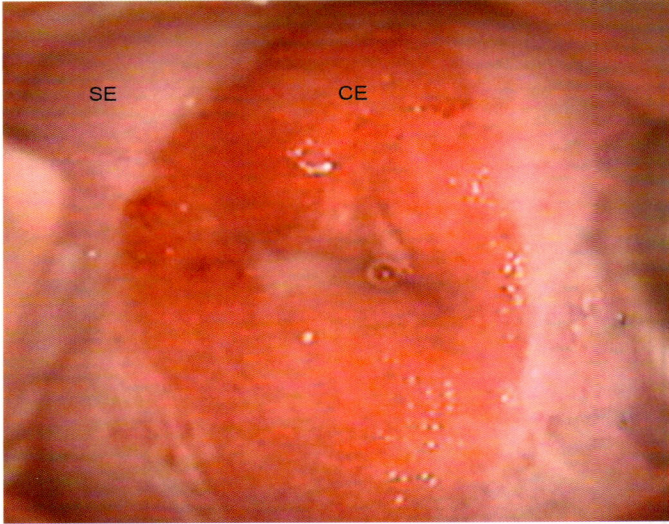

Fig. 6.10: Red, velvety columnar epithelium (CE) around external os along with part of squamous epithelium (SE) at periphery

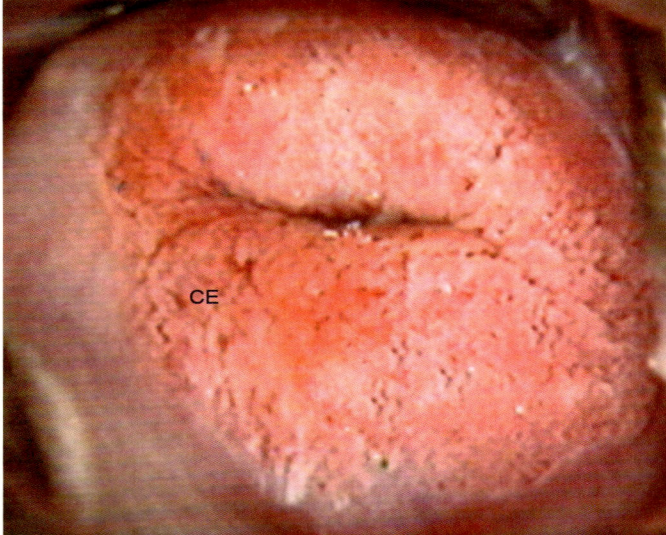

Fig. 6.11: After acetic acid application: Grape-like columnar epithelium

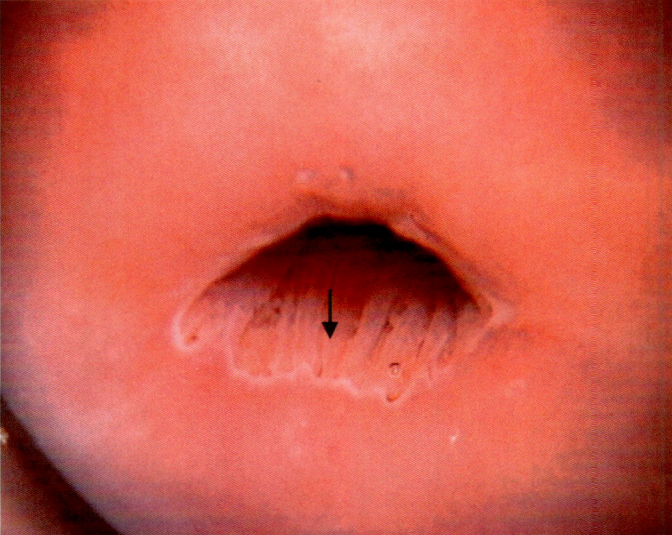

Fig. 6.12: Ectropion showing lower end of endocervix with columnar epithelium as ridges or folds

When the columnar epithelium comes onto the ectocervix it is called ectopy, also called erythroplakia or congenital erosion (Figs 6.11, 6.13 and 6.14). This is seen commonly in reproductive phase of life, during pregnancy, oral contraceptive use and also in diethylstilbestrol exposed females. In multiparous women, columnar epithelium of lower end of endocervical canal may be visible with the widely opened bivalve speculum, while withdrawing the speculum. It is due to old bilateral tears of external os and is known as the ectropion (Fig. 6.15).

The columnar epithelium does not take any stain with iodine application (Fig. 6.16).

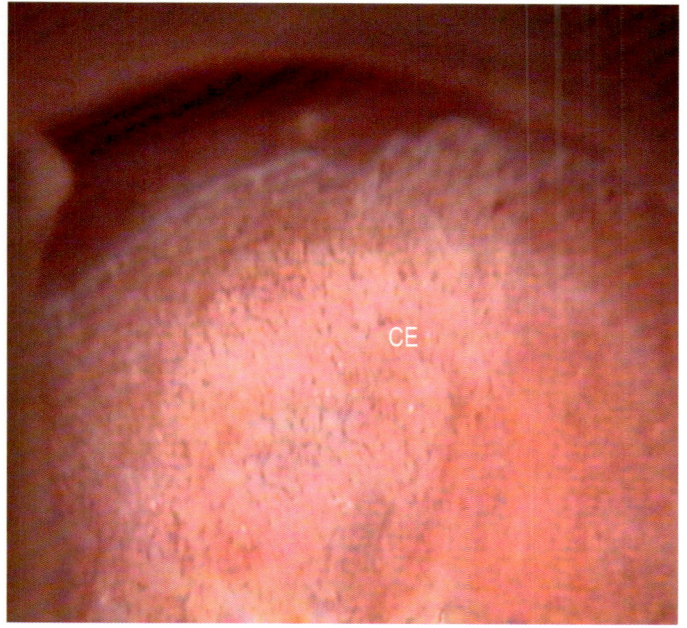

Fig. 6.13: After acetic acid application: Grape-like columnar epithelium over ectocervix— ectopy

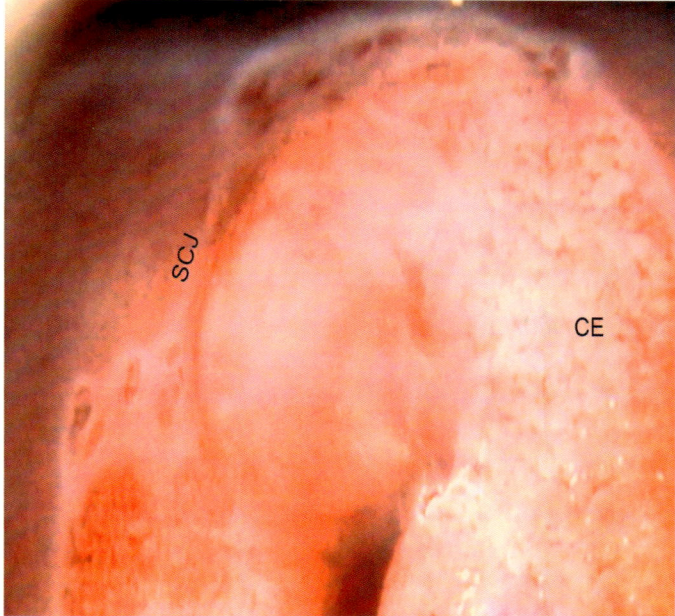

Fig. 6.14: Ectopy with sharp squamocolumnar junction and grape-like columnar epithelium

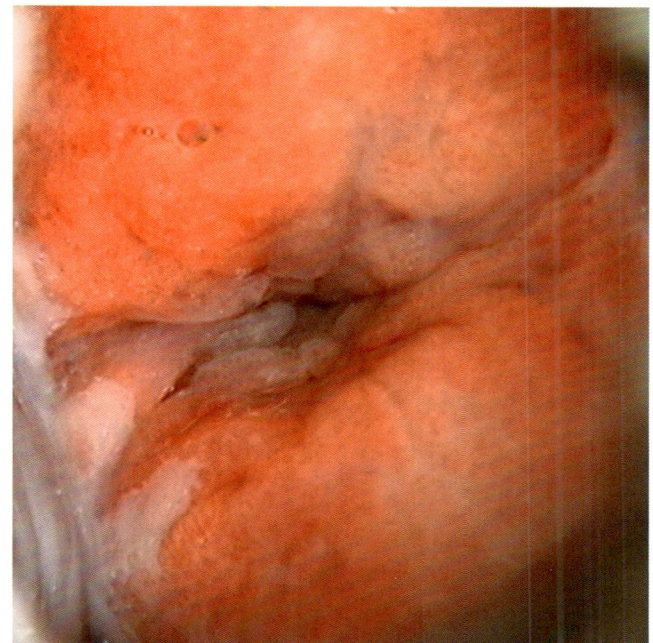

Fig. 6.15: Ectropion: Lower end of endocervical canal visible due to old bilateral tears of external os

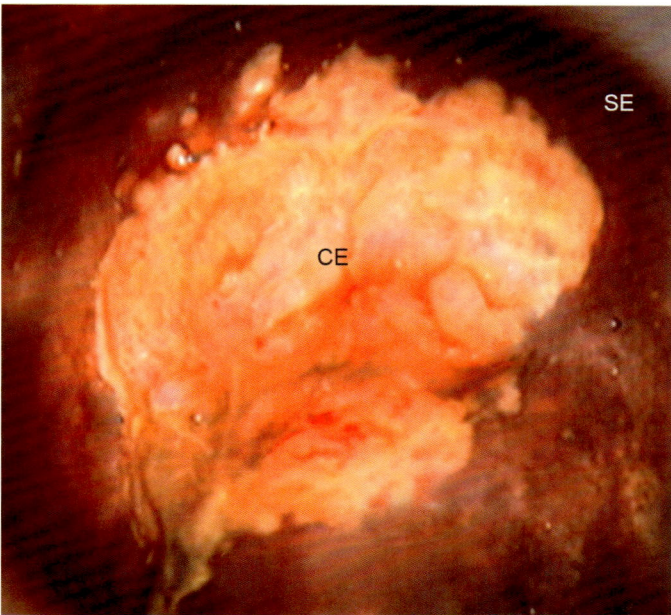

Fig. 6.16: After application of Lugol's iodine: Columnar epithelium is iodine negative while glycogenated squamous epithelium is stained mahogany brown

Squamocolumnar Junction and Transformation Zone (TZ)

Interface of original squamous epithelium and endo-cervical epithelium, called squamocolumnar junction normally coincides with external os at birth. At the time of attaining menarche, with the estrogen mediated proliferation of cervical stroma and eversion of external os, squamocolumnar junction may come on to the ectocervix. This junction is of paramount importance as the metaplastic process starts here leading to the formation of transformation zone. Metaplasia is an ongoing process. It is most active during intrauterine life, menarche and first pregnancy when high levels of estrogen are present. Thus squamocolumnar junction is not static. It keeps moving in a cephalic direction.

Colposcopy: The transformation zone in a normal cervix may depict variable findings depending on the extent and stage of metaplastic process that it has undergone. Area of early metaplastic change is seen as loss of translucency of the tips of villi of columnar epithelium seen as white dots in between (Fig. 6.17) whereas immature metaplasia is seen as tongues of mild acetowhite areas within the columnar epithelium, as isolated islands progressing from distal to more proximal zones or may be completely covering the original columnar epithelium (Figs 6.18 and 6.19A). Immature metaplasia is characteristically iodine negative (Fig. 6.19B).

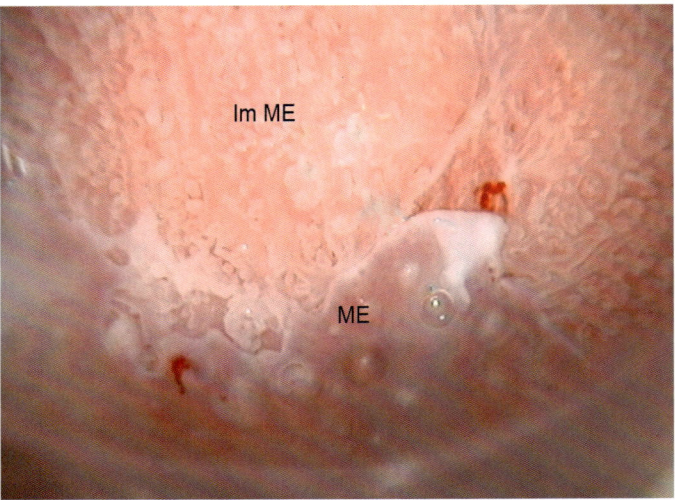

Fig. 6.17: Various stages of metaplasia seen as white dots as well as smooth tongues and more advanced over outer part of TZ

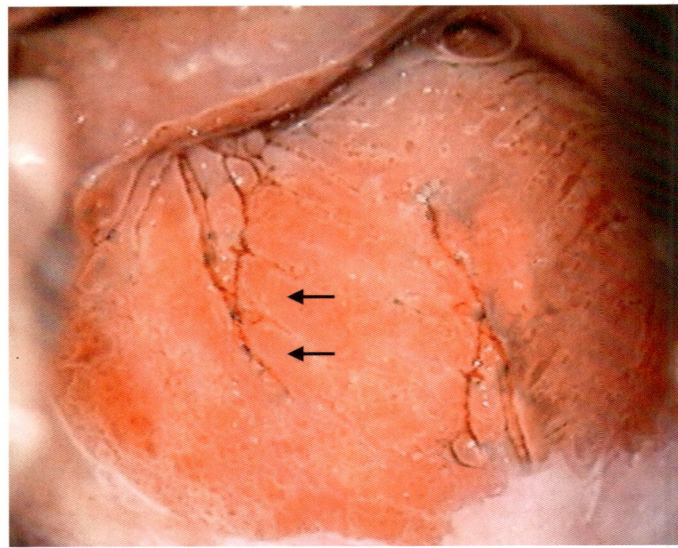

Fig. 6.18: Various stages of metaplasia seen as smooth tongues of immature metaplastic epithelium over posterior lip of cervix. Outer part shows more advanced metaplastic epithelium

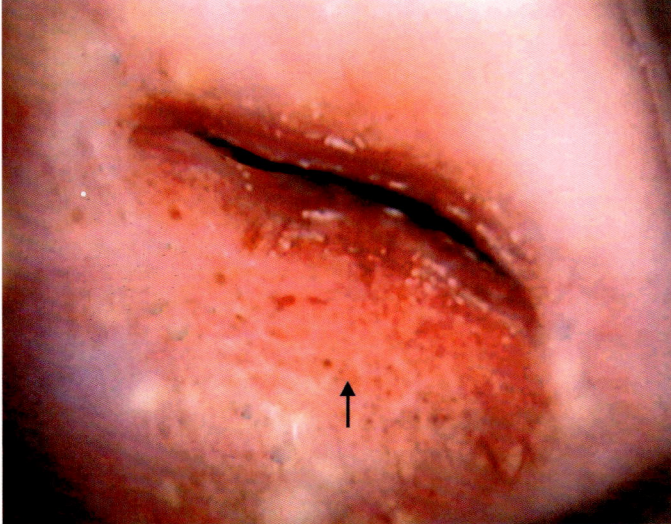

Fig. 6.19A: Various stages of metaplasia seen over posterior lip of cervix, anterior lip shows mature metaplastic epithelium

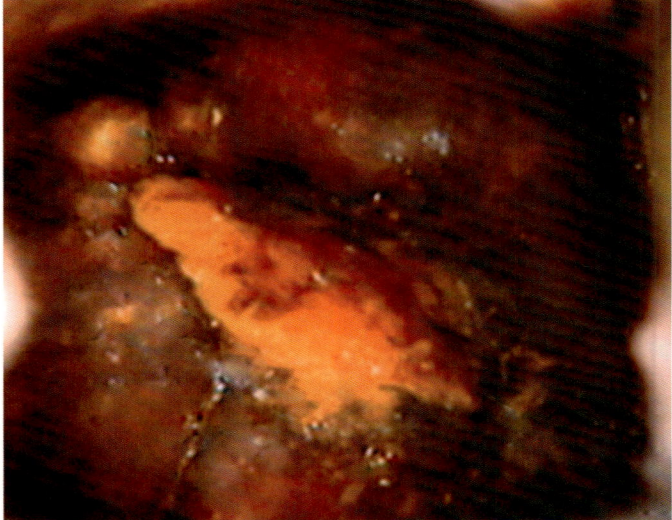

Fig. 6.19B: Same cervix showing iodine negative immature metaplastic epithelium while mature is iodine positive

The fully mature metaplasia appears smooth like original squamous epithelium, except for the presence of gland openings and nabothian cysts (Figs 6.20 and 6.21).

Nabothian follicles are translucent cysts elevated above the adjacent epithelium. When new they are bluish in color and turn yellowish on becoming old (Figs 6.22 and 6.23).

Gland opening is seen as red crater surrounded by a white ring. Five grades of gland openings can be recognised, which reflect the degree of atypical epithelium. Various grades of gland openings can be appreciated in Figs 6.20 and 6.21.

Gr. I: Gland opening without a surrounding ring, seen as a red crater.

Gr. II: A narrow indistinct white ring surrounds the G.O.

Gr. III: White ring surrounding the G.O. is distinct but unelevated.

Gr. IV: White ring surrounding the G.O. is distinct and elevated.

Gr. V: Solid gland opening.

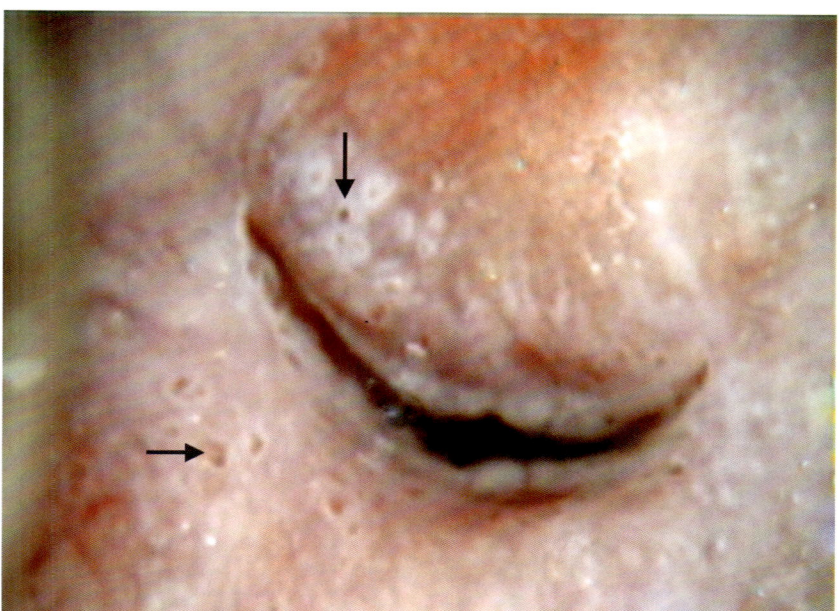

Fig. 6.20: Transformation zone showing various grades of gland openings (grades II–IV)

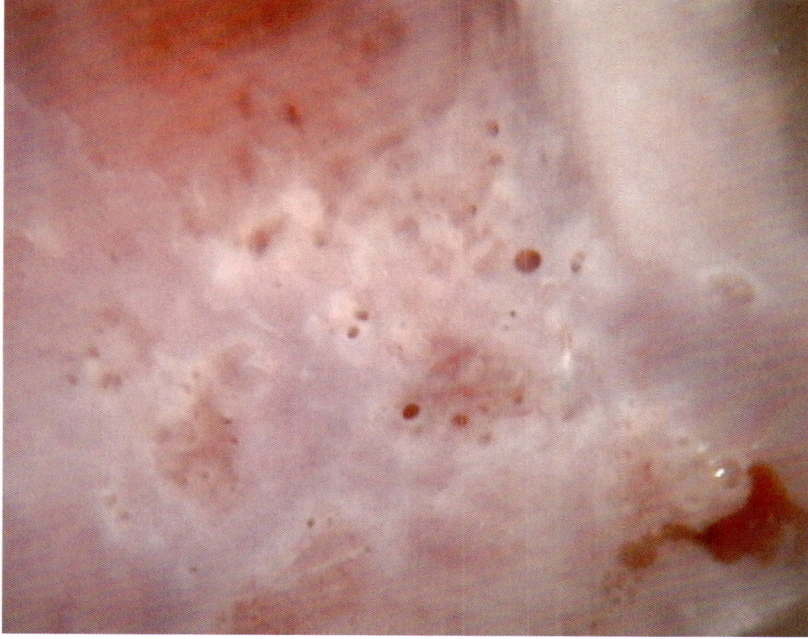

Fig. 6.21: Transformation zone showing gland openings, mostly grades 1–2

Inner or cephalic limit of TZ, i.e. the new squamo-columnar junction (between metaplastic squamous and columnar epithelia) is defined by the presence of normal columnar epithelium (Fig. 6.22). Outer limit of TZ is defined by the presence of gland openings and/or nabothian cysts (Figs 6.22 and 6.23).

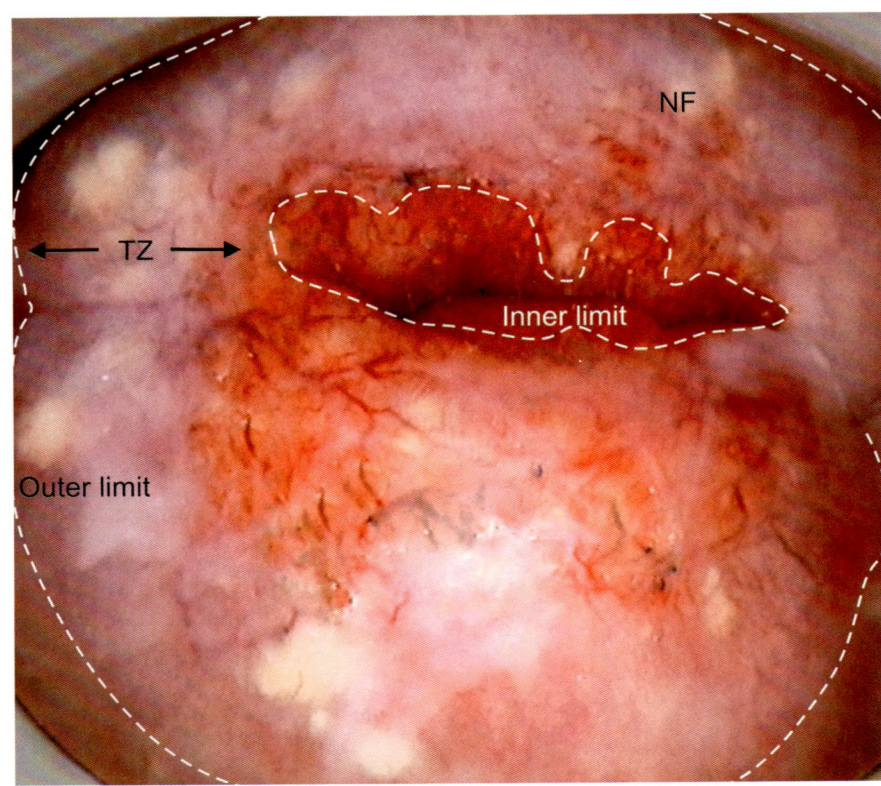

Fig. 6.22: After acetic acid application—various stages of metaplasia along with old yellowish nabothian follicles

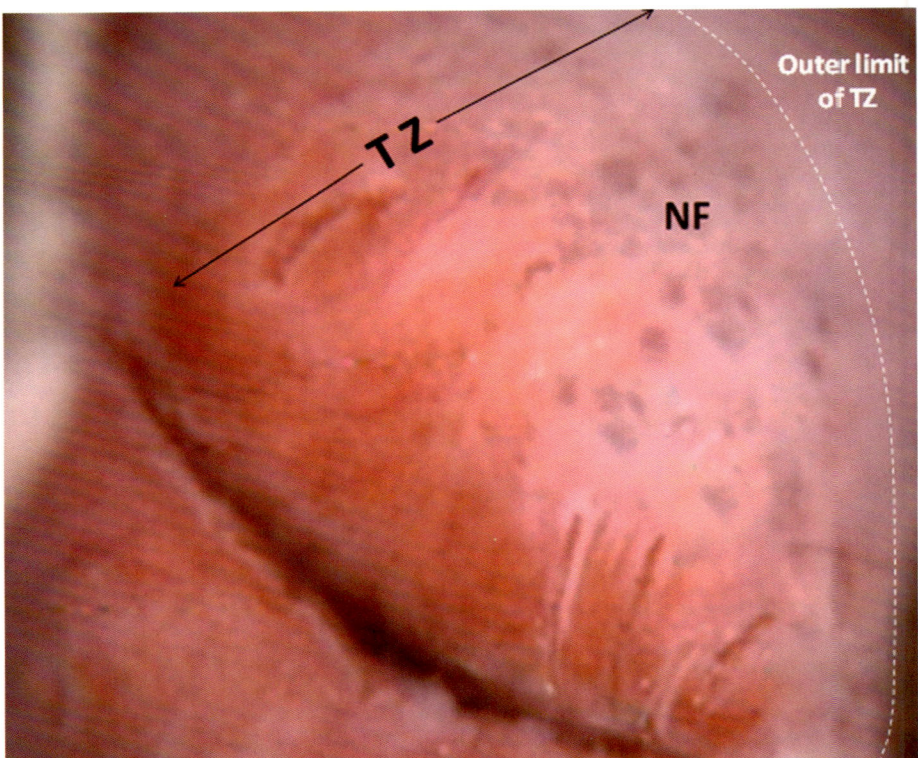

Fig. 6.23: Transformation zone—mature metaplastic epithelium with multiple bluish nabothian follicles at outer end and immature epithelium at inner end

At times, SC junction may be seen forming an aceto-white concentric ring around the os (Fig. 6.24) because of the presence of immature cells. SC junction is not static. During reproductive life, it keeps moving up in a cephalic direction as a result of metaplasia.

Vascular pattern of transformation zone is like that of original squamous epithelium, i.e. network and hair-pin capillaries. One more type of blood vessel may be seen in association with nabothian follicles. These are dilated vessels but of uniform calibre and divide dichotomously into a network of delicate capillaries (Figs 6.25 and 6.26).

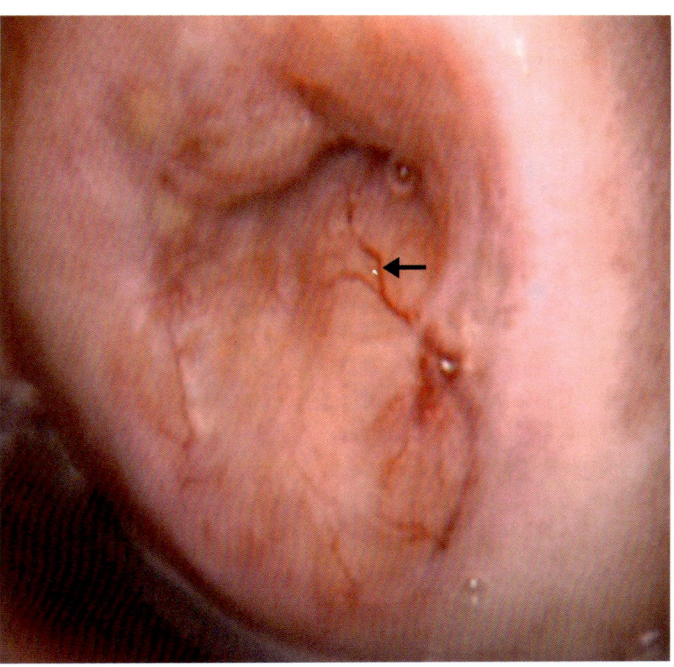

Fig. 6.24: Immature metaplastic epithelium forming concentric ring around columnar epithelium

Fig. 6.25: Transformation zone with normal, dilated, uniform caliber and dichotomously dividing vessels

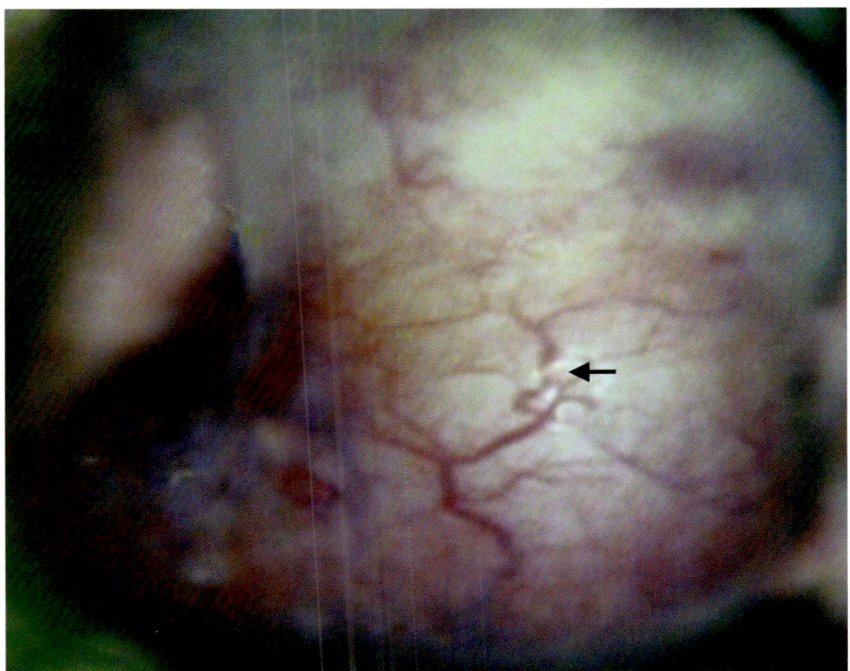

Fig. 6.26: Under green filter: Nabothian cyst with overlying normal, dilated, dichotomously dividing vessels

CERVIX IN PREGNANCY

Cervical epithelium is highly sensitive to alterations in hormonal levels. Increased estrogen levels in pregnancy give rise to increased vascularity and hypertrophy of the fibromuscular stroma of cervix, increasing the cervical volume, which in turn causes eversion of endocervical canal and the squamocolumnar junction comes to lie on to the ectocervix.

This change starts from early pregnancy and continues till about 36th week. Everted endocervical epithelium exposed to acidity of vagina undergoes dynamic phase of squamous metaplasia especially during first pregnancy. Endocervical columnar epithelium also responds by proliferating and folding into polypoid projections.

Colposcopy: Colposcopic examination in pregnancy is difficult. Because of vaginal laxity, vaginal walls prolapse through the speculum interfering with the view. To remove this difficulty, large-sized speculum should be used and their blades can be covered by condom cut at the tip. Endocervical mucus is tenacious and proper visualization of endocervix is difficult.

5% acetic acid can be used to overcome the problem of excessive mucus. However, colposcopic examination is mostly satisfactory, because of everted endocervical canal. Highly vascular cervical epithelium gets easily traumatized further compromising the view.

In pregnancy, colposcopic findings are one grade higher than the non-pregnant cervix for a given pathology; therefore, experience is needed to interpret the colposcopic findings during pregnancy.

Cervix is bluish in color. Ectopy is a very common finding in pregnancy. Increased vascularity accentuates the effect of acetic acid reaction. Extensive immature metaplasia may show acetowhitening (Fig. 6.27). Fine mosaic or punctation may also be seen within the acetowhite areas of physiologic metaplasia (Fig. 6.28). Microglandular hyperplasia of the columnar epithelium may be seen. After acetic acid application, very large papillae can be seen two to three times larger than in non-pregnant state. After Lugol's iodine, squamous epithelium becomes dark brown, almost black in color.

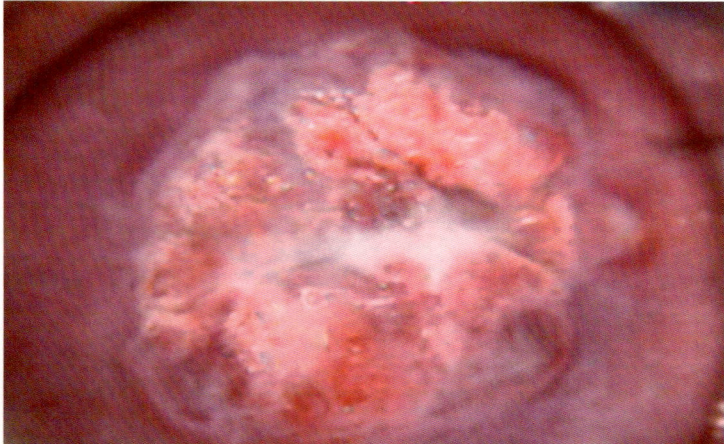

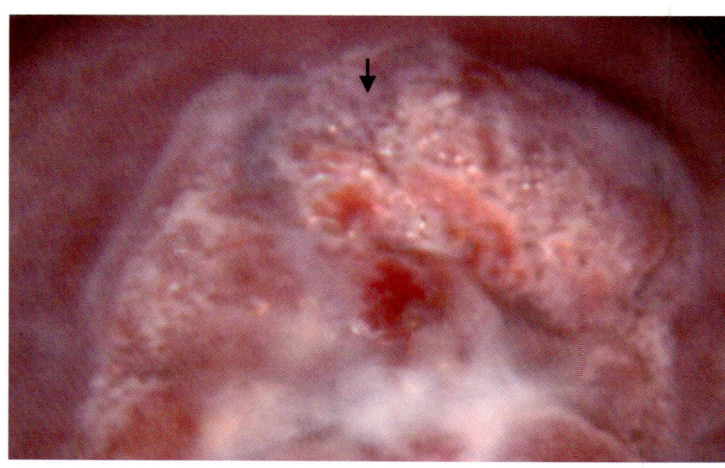

Fig. 6.27: Cervix in pregnancy with ectopy and acetowhite epithelium all around

Fig. 6.28: Cervix in pregnancy—acetowhite epithelium and mosaic at 12 O' clock

During pregnancy, the stroma of the cervix may undergo focal decidual change which appears as a raised plaque or a pseudopolyp (Fig. 6.29A). This polypoid surface irregularity with prominent vascularity (Fig. 6.29B) may mimic a high grade lesion or cancer. These reactions or changes in the cervix are present in about 20% of normal pregnant women. They are benign lesions. Bleeding is a common symptom and may occur at any stage of pregnancy. Any suspicious lesion should be biopsied.

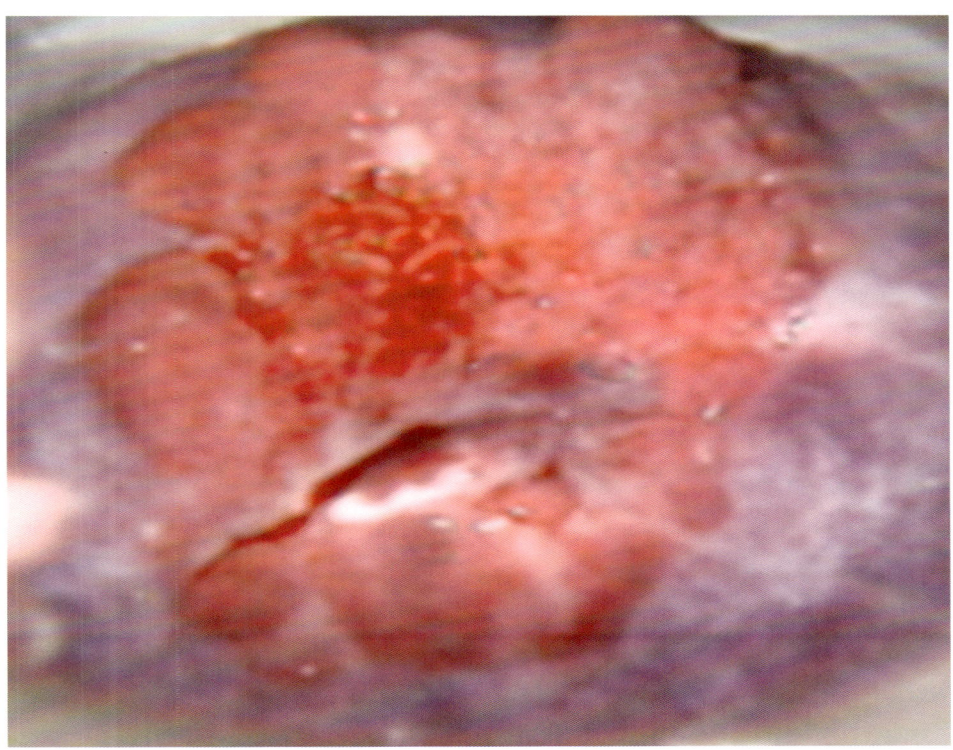

Fig. 6.29A: Cervix in pregnancy bluish in color showing ectopy with pseudopolyps

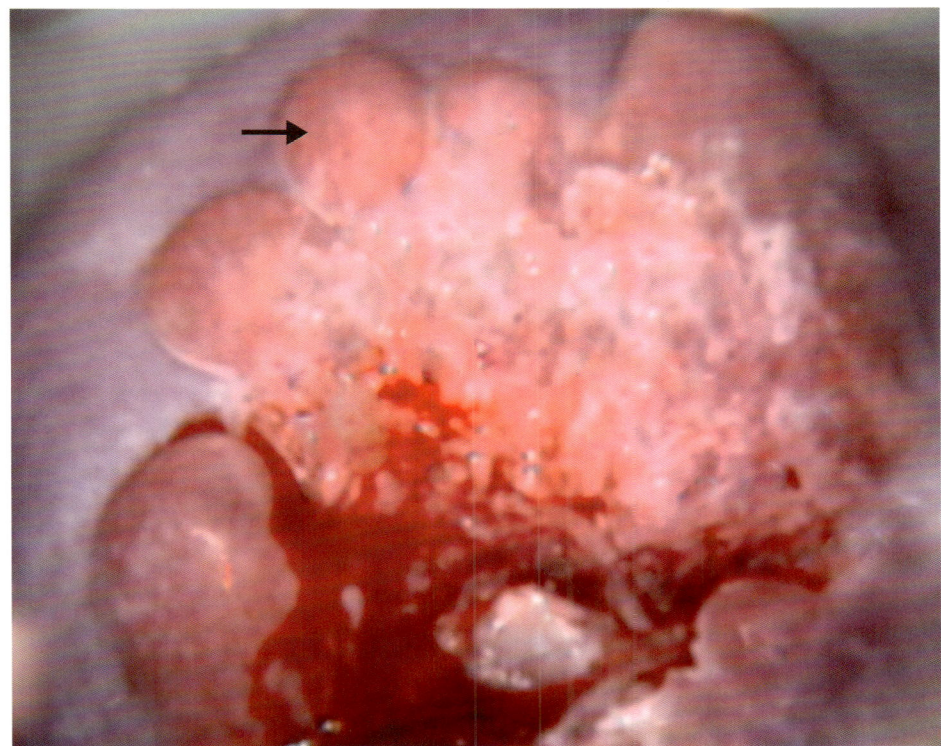

Fig. 6.29B: Same cervix after application of acetic acid showing friability and pseudopolyps

POSTMENOPAUSAL CERVIX

With advancing age, decreased hormonal levels affect cervical stroma which diminishes in amount along with decrease in vascularity. Vessels become narrow and fragile. Squamous epithelium reduces in thickness and is mainly composed of basal and parabasal layer. Glycogen content is also diminished drastically, altering the normal bacterial flora and making the epithelium more prone to infection.

Colposcopy: Cervix appears pale in color because of diminished vascularity (Fig. 6.30). Squamocolumnar junction recedes higher inside the endocervical canal and is mostly not visible. Columnar epithelium becomes flat, smooth and only rarely shows papillae, gets easily traumatized during endocervical evaluation (Fig. 6.31).

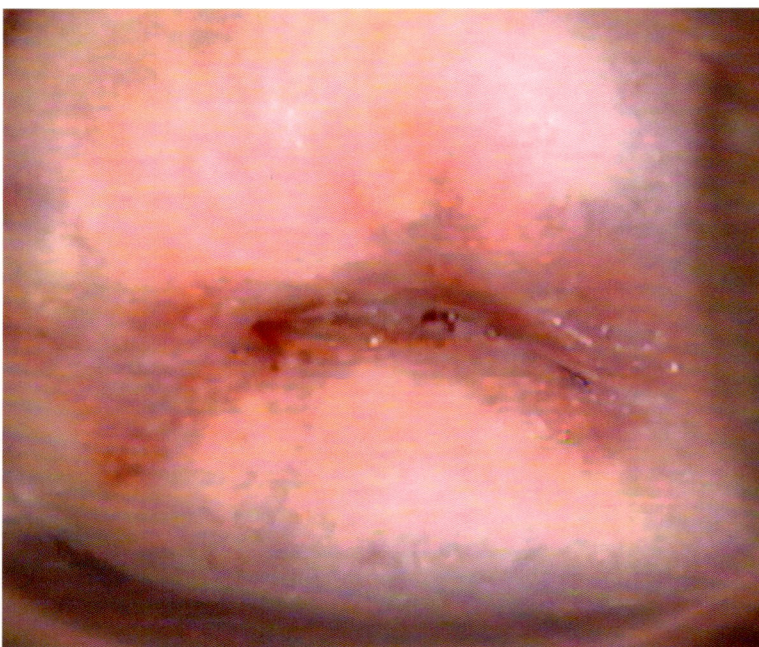

Fig. 6.30: Postmenopausal cervix—pale in color with SCJ receded in endocervix

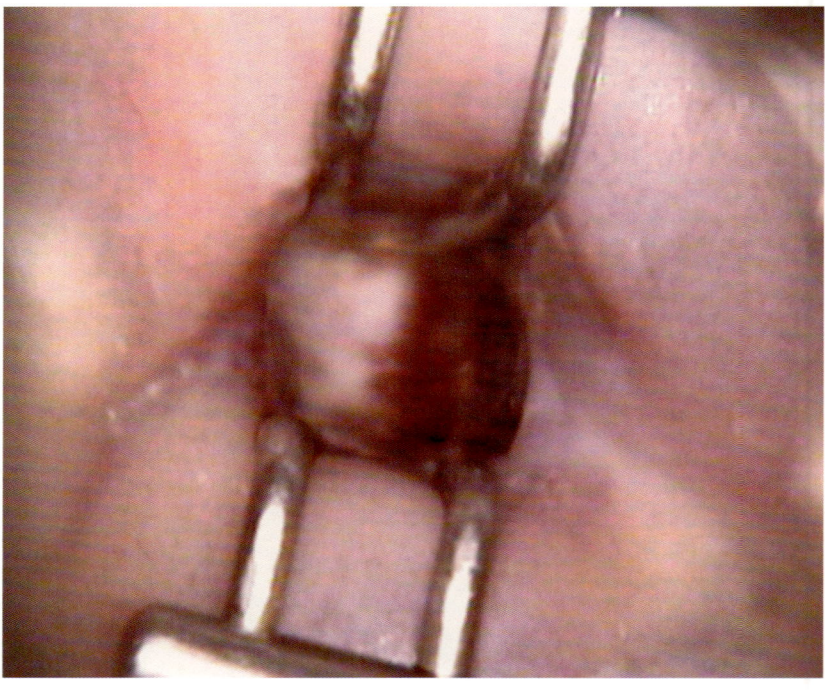

Fig. 6.31: Postmenopausal cervix—columnar epithelium in endocervix gets traumatized easily

Thin epithelium can be very easily traumatized. Subepithelial hemorrhages may be seen (Fig. 6.32). Sometimes spider-like vessels of the deeper zone may be visualized because of reduced thickness of the epithelium.

After iodine application, squamous epithelium which is deficient in glycogen becomes pale brown in color (Fig. 6.33).

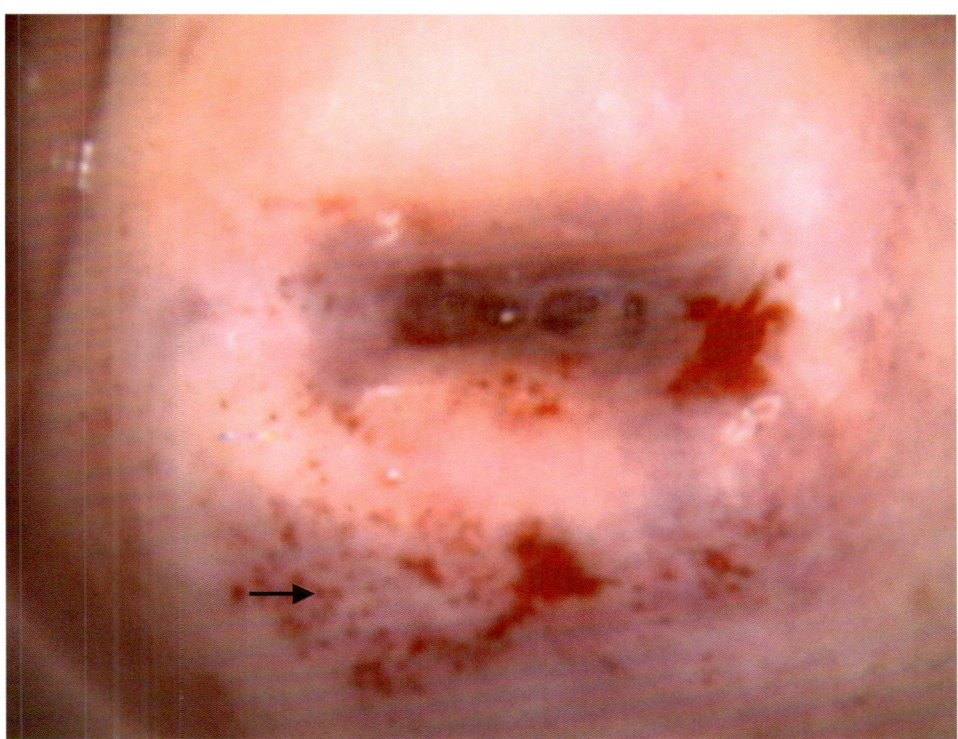

Fig. 6.32: Postmenopausal cervix with traumatic subepithelial hemorrhage

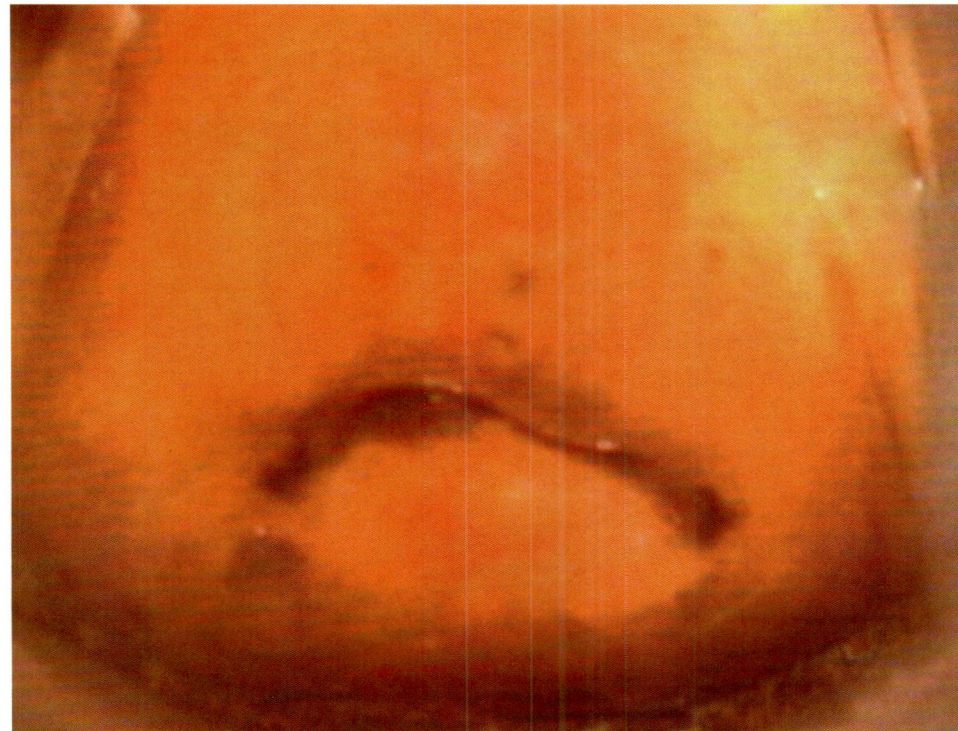

Fig. 6.33: Postmenopausal cervix after Lugol's iodine—pale in color due to reduced glycogen content

REGENERATIVE EPITHELIUM

After the conservative treatment for cervical in-trae-pithelial neoplasia such as ablative procedures, loop electrosurgical excision or conization, proper follow-up by cytology and colposcopy is mandatory.

During this healing period, many confusing appearances are encountered. Hence colposcopic examination should be avoided after such procedures till healing is complete which takes approximately 4–6 months.

Colposcopy: During healing process, neovascularization occurs which may be seen as fine punctations that may be arranged in radiating lines from the external os. After sometime, these punctate lines disappear and are eventually replaced by subepithelial fibrosis (Fig. 6.34), seen as white areas before application of acetic acid. Usually there is no change on acetic acid application.

At times mild acetowhiteness can be present which has to be differentiated from the residual CIN (Fig. 6.35). Such an area does not take iodine stain as well. In such a situation, colposcopist may also take a biopsy which easily differentiates the two conditions.

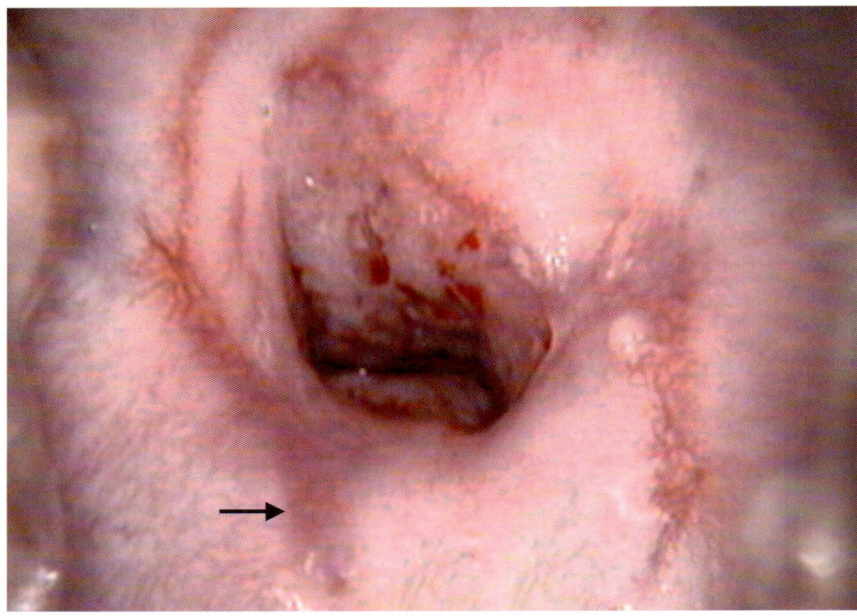

Fig. 6.34: Regenerative epithelium showing neovascularization and subepithelial fibrosis

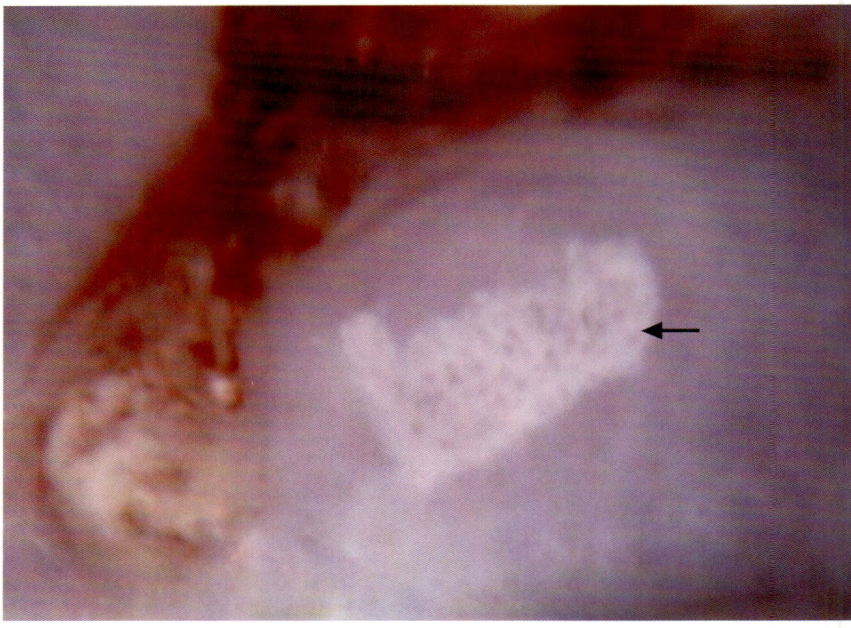

Fig. 6.35: Cervix showing regenerated epithelium as localized acetowhite epithelium and punctations

Inflammatory Lesions

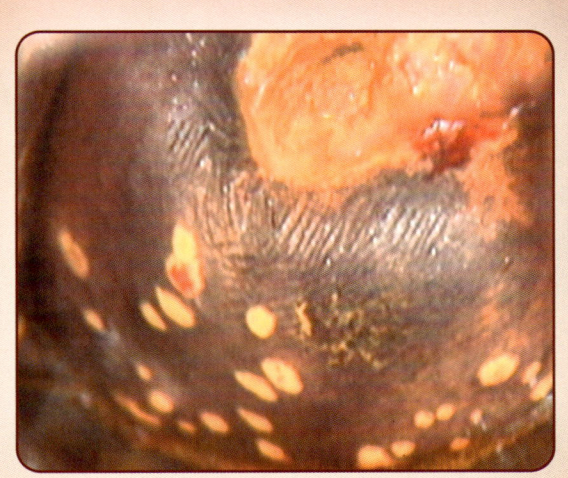

Chapter Outline

INTRODUCTION

Inflammation plays an important part in causing various lesions in the cervix and vagina. Though squamous epithelium lining the cervix is quite resistant, its peculiar anatomical predisposition to repeated trauma and exposure to various inflammatory agents makes it vulnerable.

Response to different inflammatory agents is generally non-specific and at times it may be difficult to pin-point the etiology.

Inflammation can be caused by bacteria (mixed or polymicrobial), protozoa, fungus, viruses, trauma, radiation, chemical agents (gel or creams) or foreign bodies (IUCD or retained tampons).

Inflammatory lesions are mostly symptomatic with pruritic or non-pruritic, purulent or non-purulent, malodorous or non-odorous and frothy or non-frothy discharge. They may also be associated with lower abdominal pain, backache or dyspareunia.

Conditions should be identified and differentiated from cervical neoplasia and treated. Biopsy should be taken whenever in doubt.

Examination of external genitalia, vagina and cervix for vesicles, shallow ulcers and bimanual palpation for tenderness or masses should be done in detail to diagnose these conditions.

Non-specific Acute Inflammation

Earliest changes take place in the connective tissue which shows edema and congestion with dilatation of superficial vessels.

Later, polymorphonuclear cells infiltrate the connective tissue and then the overlying epithelium and endocervical crypts. At this stage, there is desquamation of epithelium with degeneration of epithelial cells resulting in vessels coming close to the surface. Desquamation of deeper layers may lead to ulcer formation in severe infection.

Colposcopy: In acute inflammation, abnormal cervical discharge may be seen exuding from external os. It may be copious and non-specific (Fig. 7.1) or pus-like in bacterial infection (Fig. 7.2). However, some infections like monilia and trichomonas present with characteristic cervical discharge (described in respective sections).

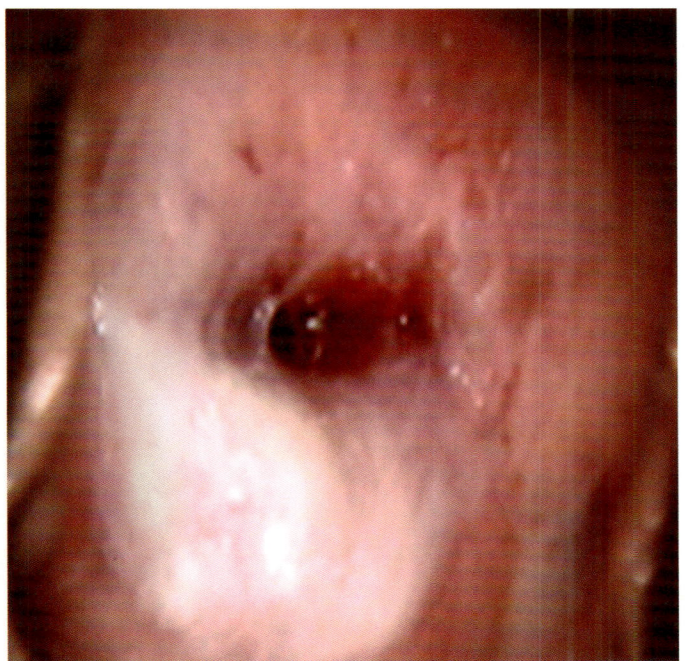

Fig. 7.1: Acute cervicitis with non-specific cervical discharge

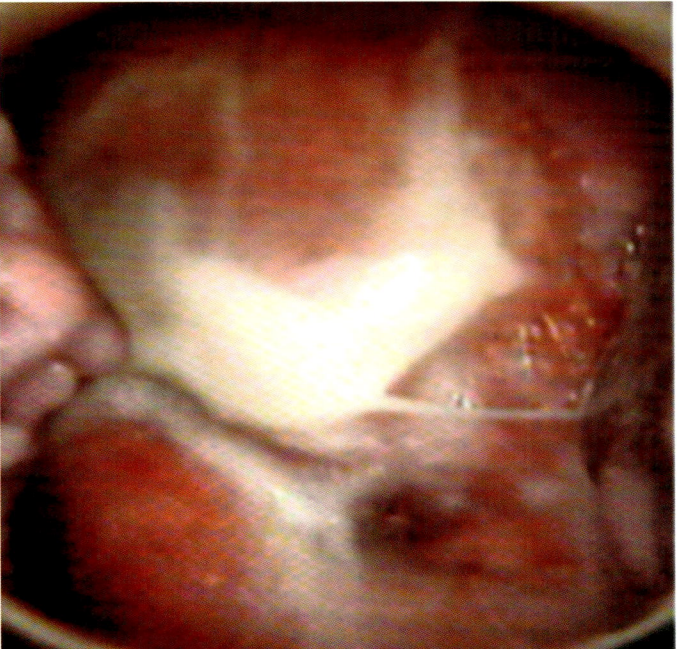

Fig. 7.2: Copious purulent discharge in bacterial infection

Cervicitis is generally associated with vaginitis also. In acute cervicovaginitis, cervix and vagina show congestion in the form of intense red color which can even be appreciated on naked eye examination. Study of vasculature shows increase in vascularity seen as increase in number as well as calibre of terminal vessels (Fig. 7.3). Intercapillary distance may appear decreased partly because of increase in number of terminal vessels and partly because of dilatation of pre-existing vessels.

Cervix may show fine, regular, diffuse punctations. Punctations have a tendency to coalesce and form larger deep red areas (Fig. 7.4). Changes in acute inflammation of cervix are diffuse in nature and often involve ectocervix even beyond transformation zone.

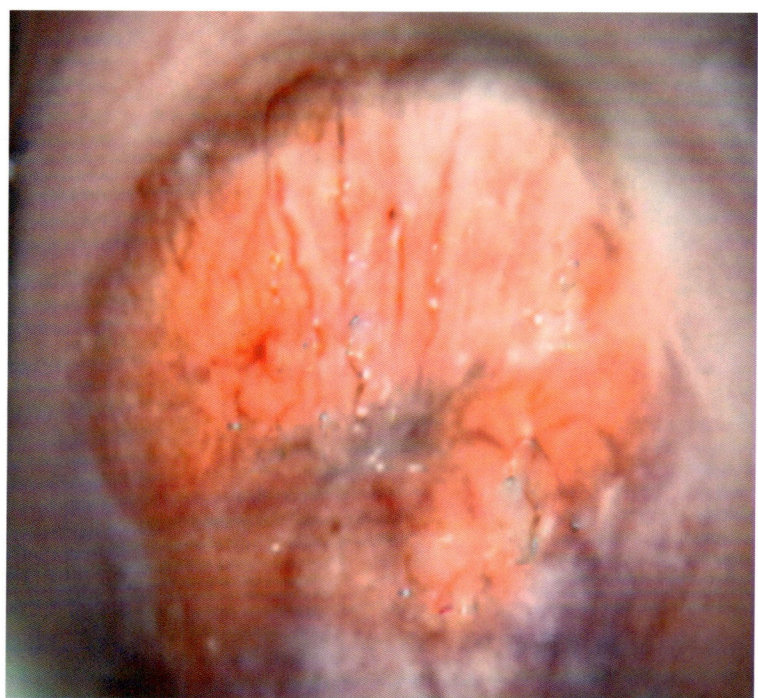

Fig. 7.3: Acute cervicitis with increased vascularity

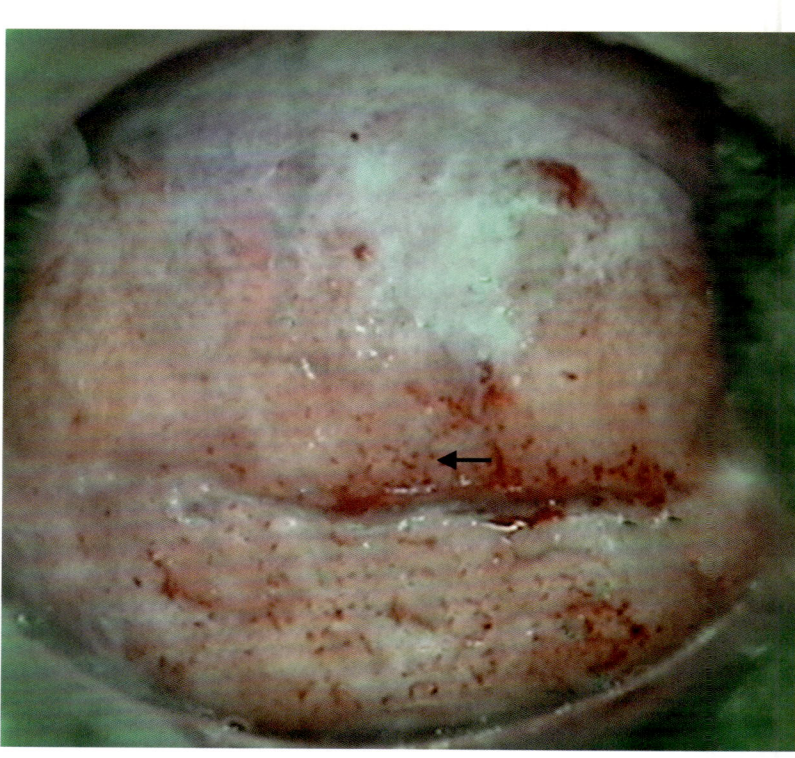

Fig. 7.4: Fine regular diffuse punctation seen in acute cervicitis

In severe infection, there may be small yellow necrotic areas of microabscess formation (Figs 7.5 and 7.6), that may be surrounded by red halo hyperemic stroma. Acetic acid application does not produce any change in acute cervicovaginitis.

Lugol's iodine application imparts granular appearance or patchy uptake due to the presence of small glycogen free areas which are iodine negative (Figs 7.7 and 7.8). In severe inflammation, iodine application gives diffuse orange red color due to the absence of glycogen and increased underlying vascularity.

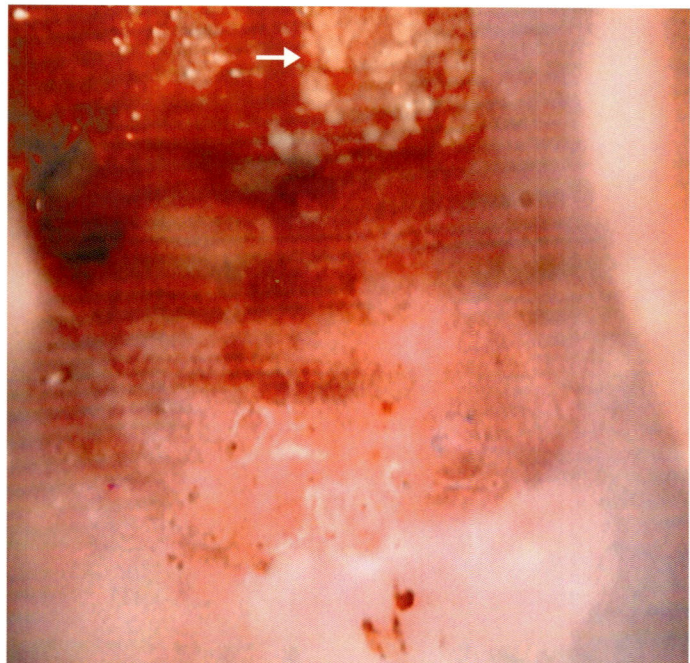

Fig. 7.5: Yellow necrotic areas seen near os over anterior lip with increased vascularity

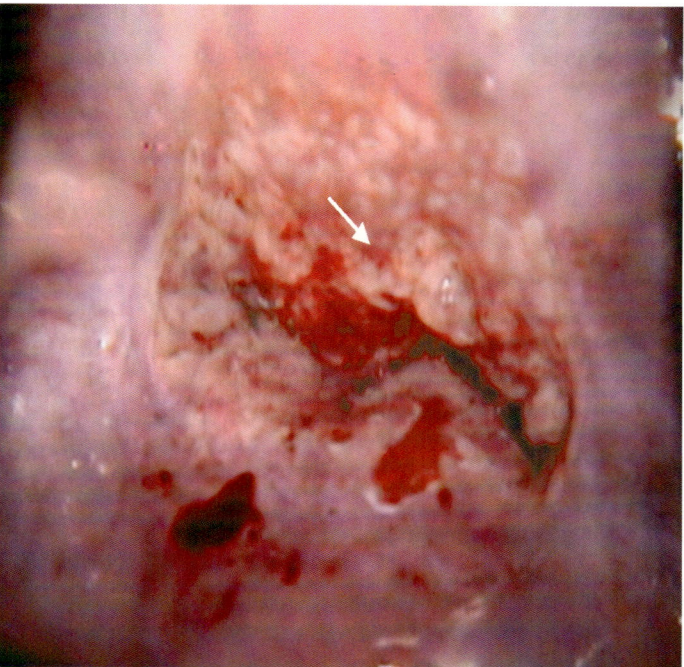

Fig.7.6: Yellow necrotic areas seen over anterior lip with increased vascularity, punctations and ulceration over posterior lip

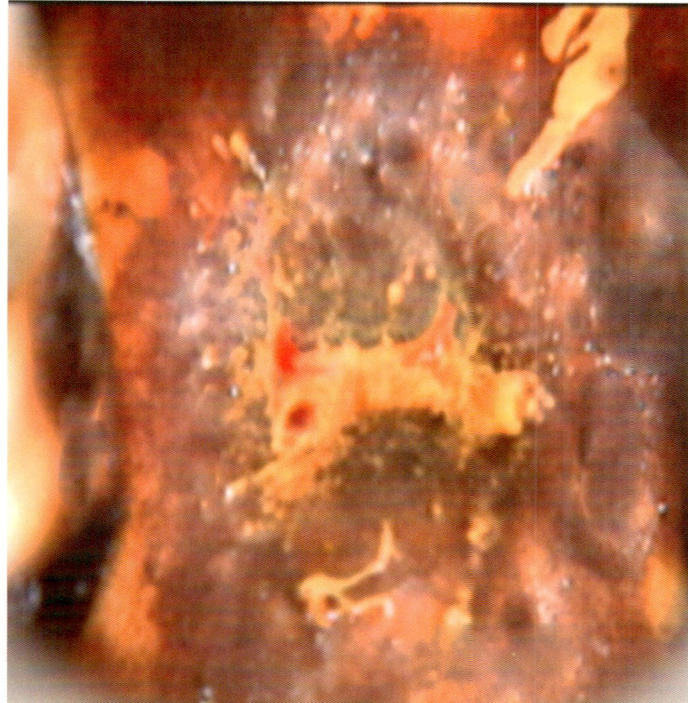

Fig. 7.7: Diffuse iodine negative areas in acute cervicitis

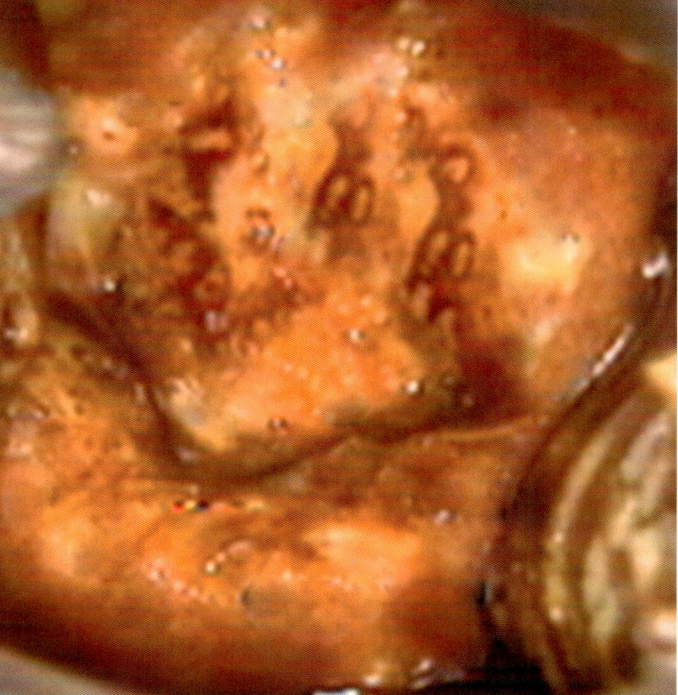

Fig. 7.8: Patchy iodine uptake in cervicitis

Chronic Inflammation

Chronic inflammation is characterized by presence of lymphocytes and histiocytes. Infiltration is diffuse at first and later forms foci around dilated capillary vessels just under the epithelium.

Colposcopy: In chronic inflammation, white punctations are seen against a pink background (Figs 7.9 and 7.10). This is called follicular cervicitis occurring as a result of formation of lymphoid follicles in the stroma.

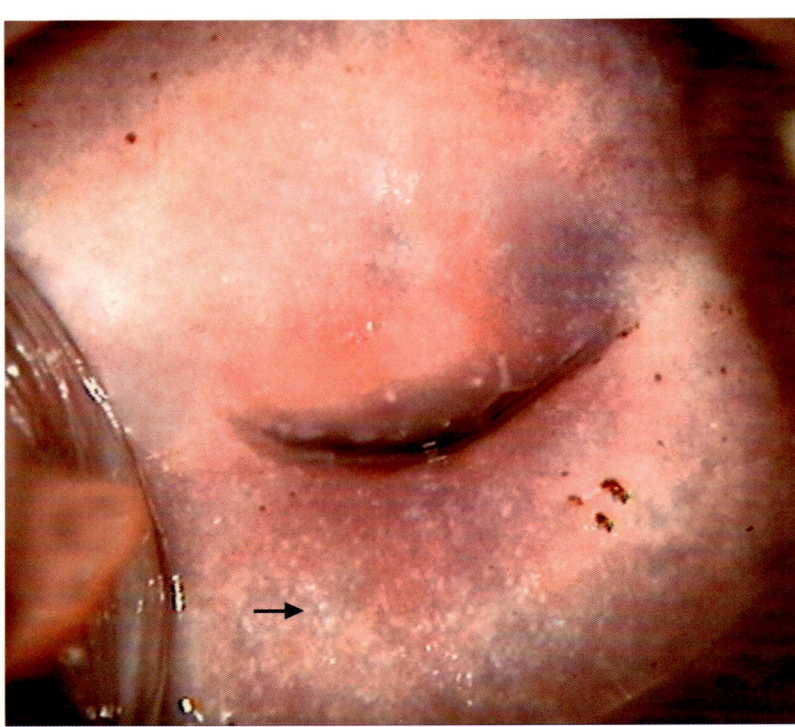

Fig. 7.9: Diffuse granular white punctations in chronic cervicitis

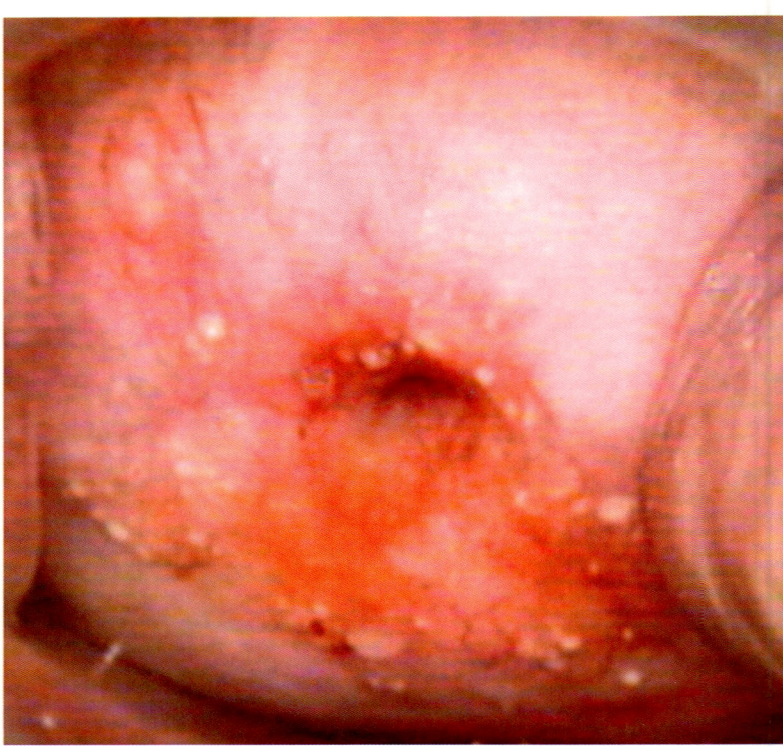

Fig. 7.10: Follicular cervicitis with diffuse white punctations and increased vascularity

Inflammatory findings may at times be confused with cervical intraepithelial neoplasia, however, one can differentiate by the facts that punctations are fine and regular in inflammation. Findings are not restricted to transformation zone only (Fig. 7.11). If still in doubt, biopsy should be taken.

Chronic inflammation may cause recurrent ulceration and healing of cervix, resulting in distortion of the cervix due to healing by fibrosis (Fig. 7.12).

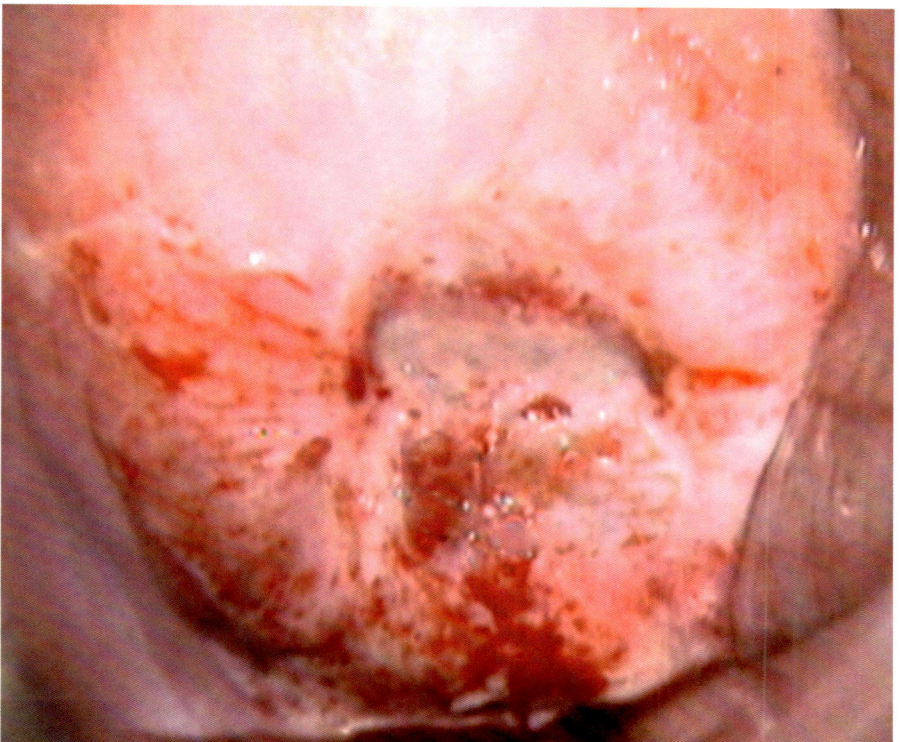

Fig. 7.11: Cervix shows increased vascularity, widespread punctations and ulceration beyond transformation zone mainly over posterior lip. Discharge can be seen exuding from endocervix

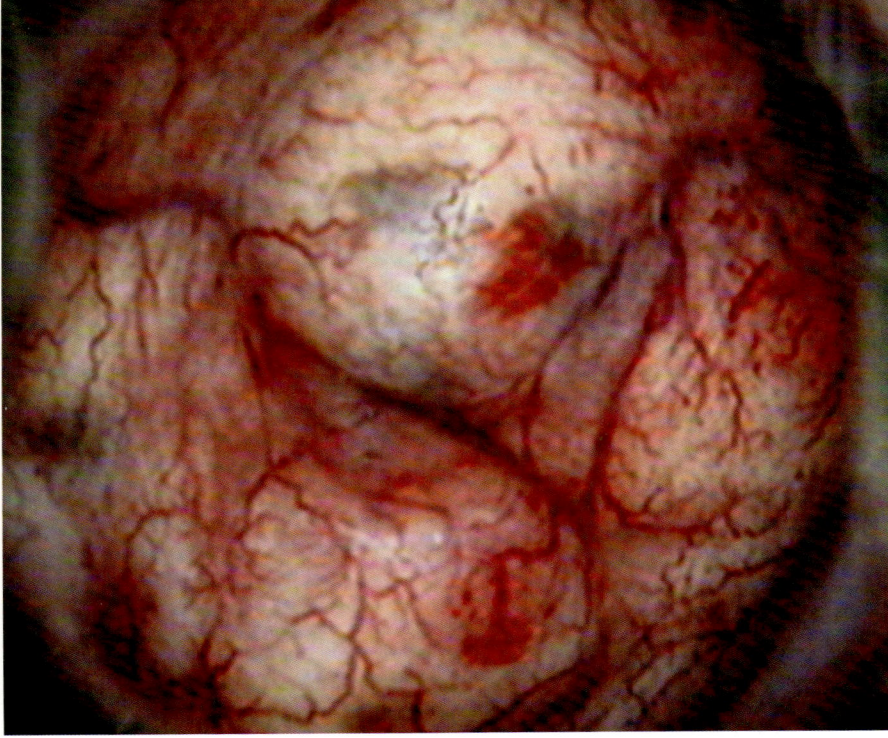

Fig. 7.12: Healed cervix after chronic cervicitis causing distortion of cervix, increased vascularity but no abnormal vessels

BACTERIAL INFECTIONS

Bacterial infections most commonly associated with cervicitis are *Chlamydia trachomatis, Gardnerella vaginalis* and *Neisseria gonorrhoeae*.

Chlamydia trachomatis (CT)

It is an obligate intracellular bacterial microorganism and has a predilection to attach and invade columnar epithelium. It can cause cervicitis along with salpingitis, urethral syndrome and Bartholin's abscess. Oral contraceptive use giving rise to ectopy and thus more exposed endocervical epithelium is more commonly associated with the *Chlamydia* infection.

Colposcopy: Shows no specific pattern but exophytic follicular cervicitis has been found very commonly associated with *CT* infection (Fig. 7.13). In a study conducted at Safdarjung hospital, follicular cervicitis was found to be associated with *CT* infection in 31% cases. Other features which have also been found to be associated with this infection are fragile epithelium and congested cervix, hypertrophic and congested ectopic columnar epithelium and mucopurulent discharge at the os (72%).

Several researchers have reported an increased incidence of *CT* colonization/seropositivity in cases of CIN and even invasive cervical cancer. It needs further evaluation as *Chlamydia* infection is amenable to antibiotic therapy and associated abnormal cytology has been reported to be reversible after appropriate therapy.

Gardnerella vaginalis

It is the most important cause of bacterial cervico-vaginitis.

Smear is characterized by the presence of epithelial cells showing degeneration with heavy background of bacilli. Such a condition is called *Bacterial vaginosis*. Epithelial cells with numerous bacilli clinging to its surface are called "clue cells" which are pathognomonic of *Gardnerella* infection.

Colposcopic appearance is that of a non-specific inflammation.

Neisseria gonorrhoeae

These are small gram-negative diplococci, sometimes seen in the cytoplasm of epithelial cells but cannot be diagnosed cytologically as other organisms may appear similar. Diagnosis is confirmed by culture.

Cervix may show profuse creamy yellow pus-like discharge (Fig. 7.14). No specific pattern is seen on colposcopy.

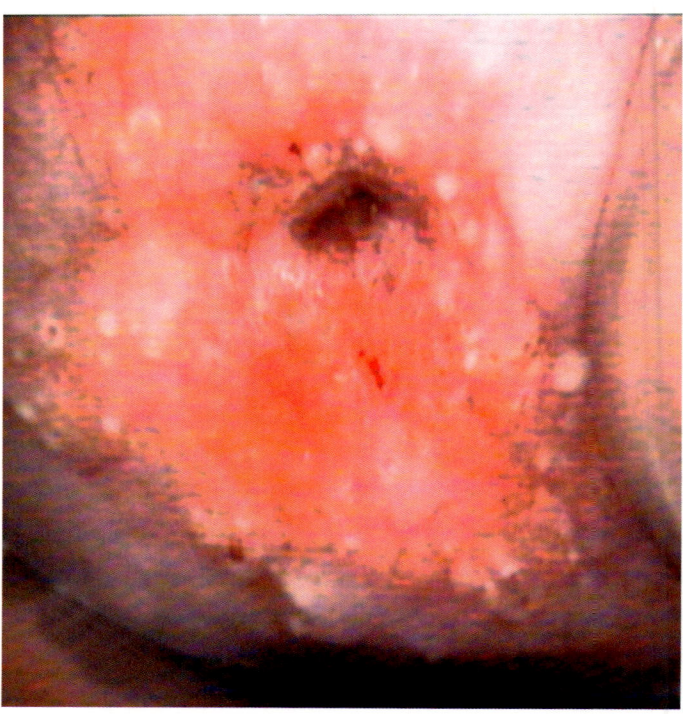

Fig. 7.13: Follicular cervicitis along with increased vascularity

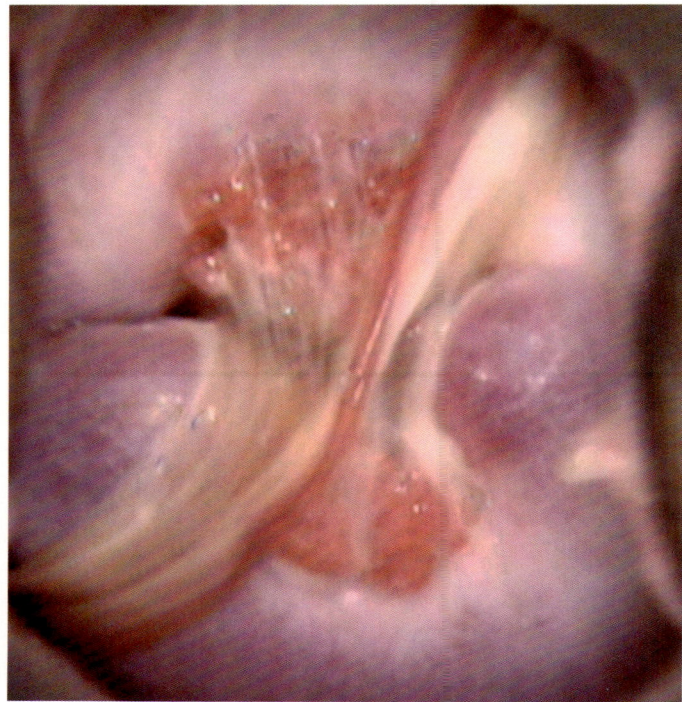

Fig. 7.14: Profuse creamy yellow pus-like discharge

Tuberculosis

Cervical lesion is rare. It can present as cervicitis or ulcerative lesion (Figs 7.15 to 7.17) which may have to be differentiated from invasive carcinoma.

Actinomyces

Lower genital tract may sometimes show presence of actinomyces. Generally, these colonies do not evoke inflammatory reaction but pose potential danger of causing pelvic inflammatory disease. In a study conducted at Safdarjung hospital, *Actinomyces* was found in the cervical smears of 28% of women using intrauterine device over a long period.

Colposcopically, no specific pattern is identified.

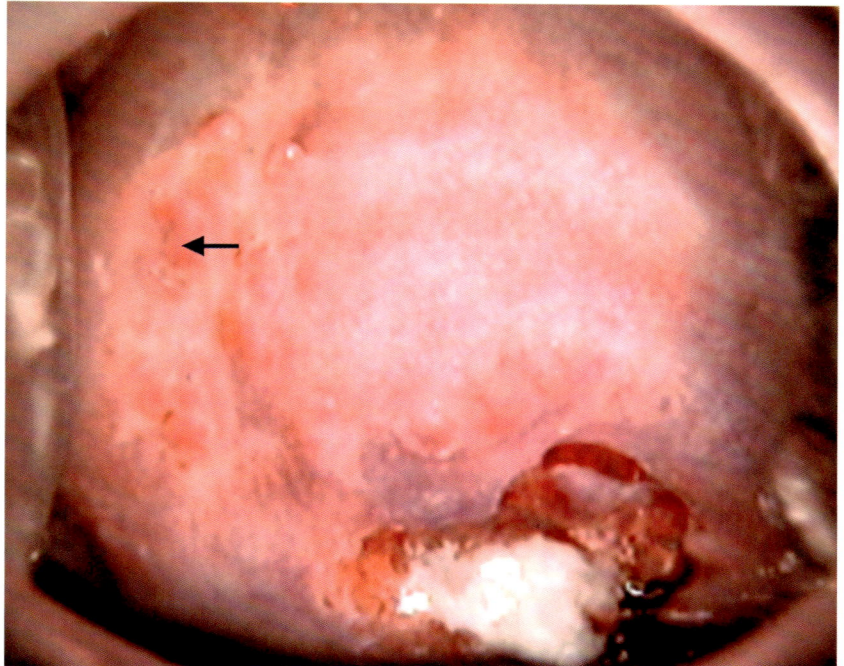

Fig. 7.15: Confirmed case of tubercular endometritis and cervicitis showing acute cervicitis with ulcers in anterolateral fornix

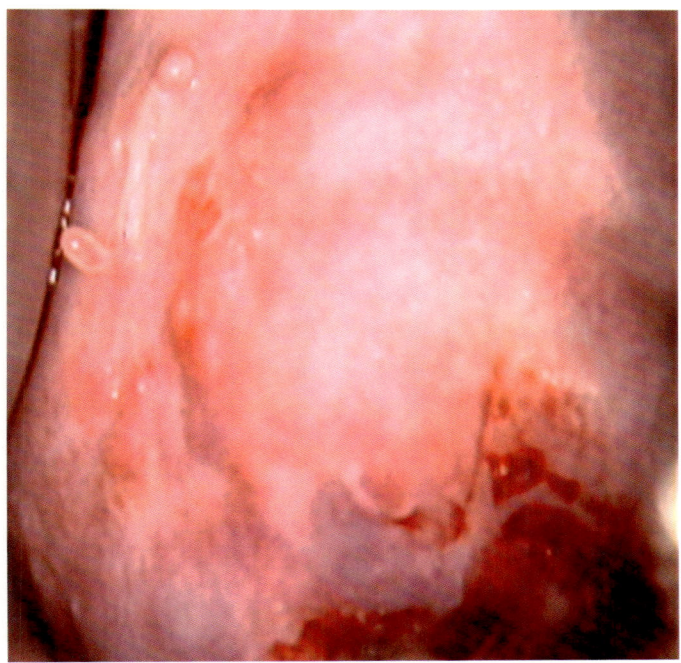

Fig. 7.16: Same cervix under higher magnification

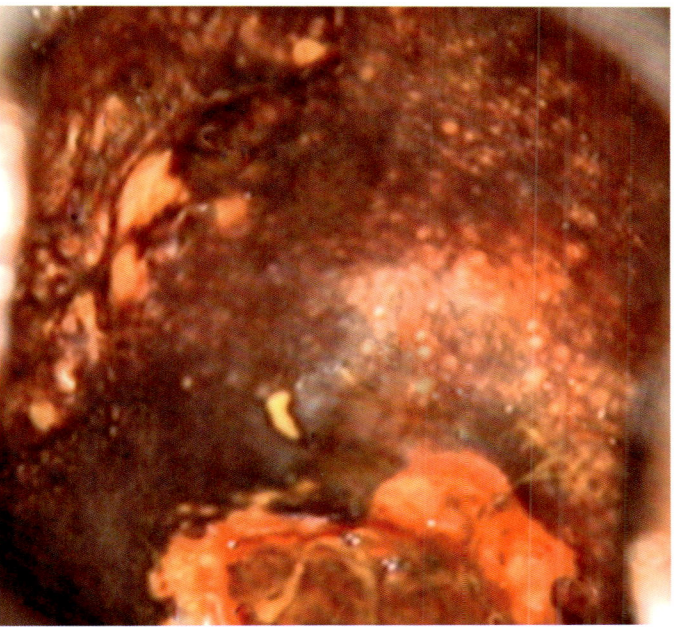

Fig. 7.17: Same cervix showing patchy iodine uptake and granular appearance of cervix

PROTOZOAL INFECTIONS

Trichomonas vaginalis

It is a flagellated protozoan and is the most common cause of sexually transmitted cervicovaginal infection.

Colposcopy: Discharge in acute trichomonal infection is thin, yellowish-green, frothy in appearance and foul smelling (Fig. 7.18). However, in chronic infection, discharge may be absent.

After saline application, cervix may show diffuse fine punctations seen as red stippling against a pink background (Fig. 7.18).

At higher magnification, characteristic vascular pattern of *Trichomonas* infection can be better appreciated which is produced by hairpin capillaries that extend high up into the stromal papillary processes and show two or more crests at the top of the loop. These double crested vessels give fork-like appearance (Fig. 7.19) or are seen as diplococci with end on view.

In severe infection, cervix may show strawberry appearance due to the presence of widespread large red patches. This is because of concentrated areas of

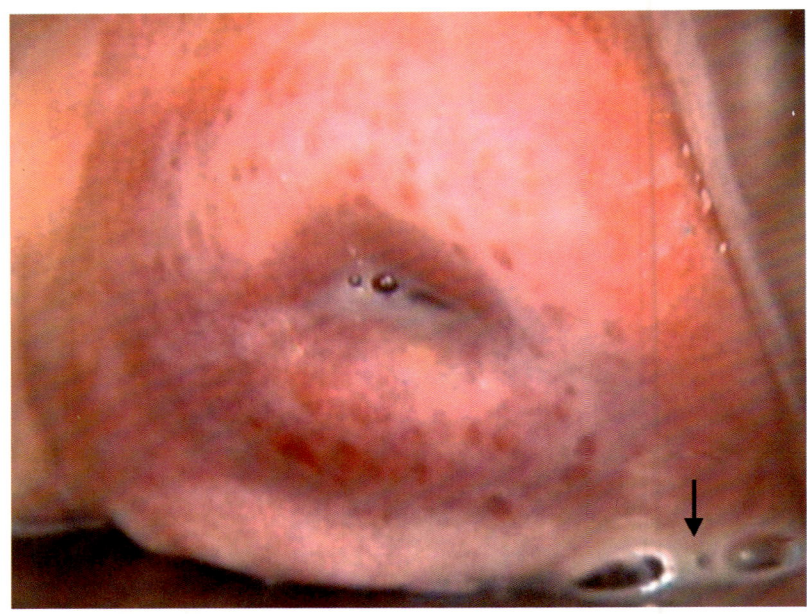

Fig. 7.18: Strawberry appearance of cervix due to diffuse punctations along with typical greenish frothy discharge

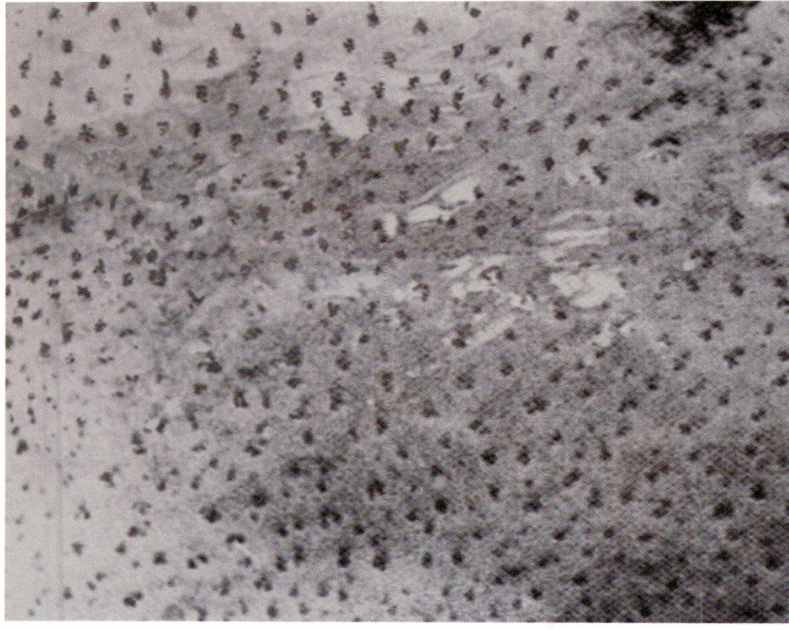

Fig. 7.19: Double crested vessels with forked appearance in *Trichomonas* infection

large dilated vessels in underlying stroma (Fig. 7.20). These patches are poor in glycogen content and do not take up iodine stain, producing a typical leopard appearance (Fig. 7.21).

Kolstad has described the angioarchitecture of *Trichomonas vaginalis* according to the severity of infection in three grades:

I. Scattered double-crested capillaries (DCC)

II. Massive occurrence of DCC either in circumscribed or diffuse pattern

III. Massive occurrence of DCC both in circumscribed and diffuse pattern.

Double crested vessels disappear after specific treatment of the infection. Trichomonal infection is characterizd by marked degenerative cellular changes, dirty background and presence of parasites in the smear.

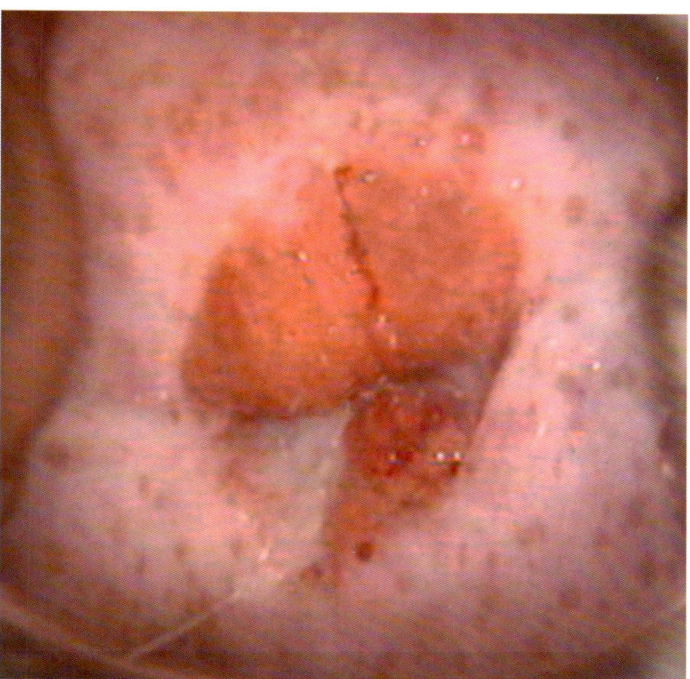 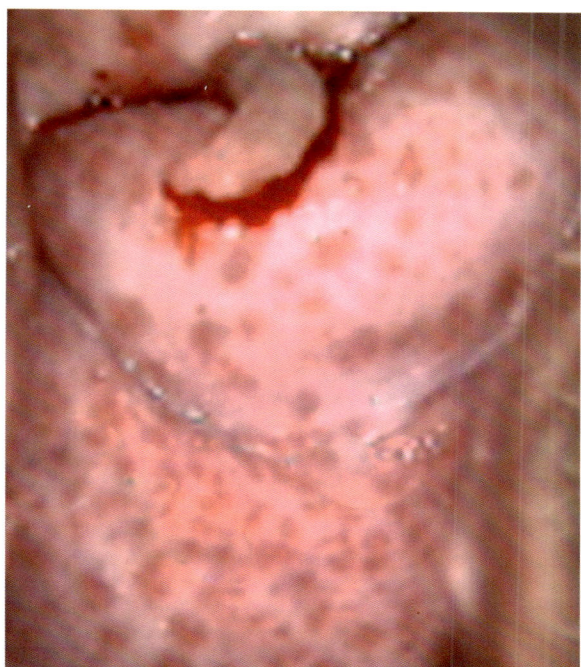

Fig. 7.20: Strawberry appearance due to diffuse punctations

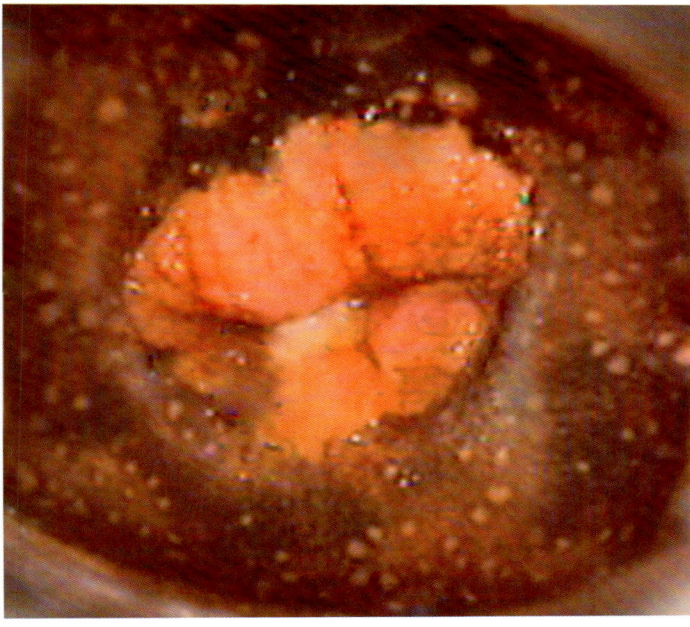 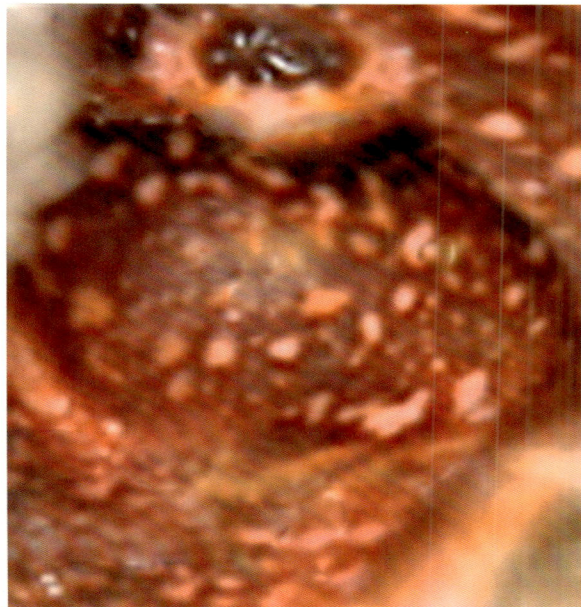

Fig. 7.21: Leopard appearance due to diffuse iodine negative patches

FUNGAL INFECTIONS

Candida Albicans

It is yeast-like fungus, a commensal of lower genital tract in up to 50% of women without any symptomatic evidence of the disease. Infection is commonly seen in diabetes, pregnancy, patients using corticosteroids, chemotherapy, oral contraceptive users and in immunosuppressed patients.

Discharge is typically thick, cheesy, curd-like but may be thin and watery also.

Colposcopy: It is non-specific. Mucosa is diffusely hyperemic and bleeds readily. Sometimes white punctations are seen against red field (Fig. 7.22).

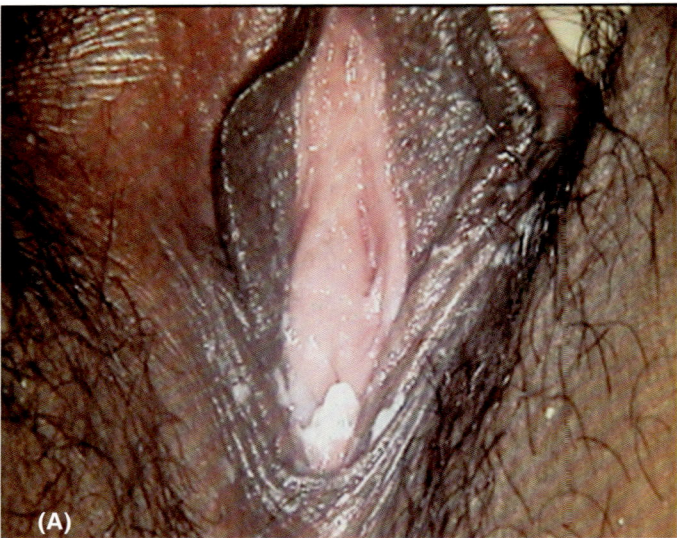

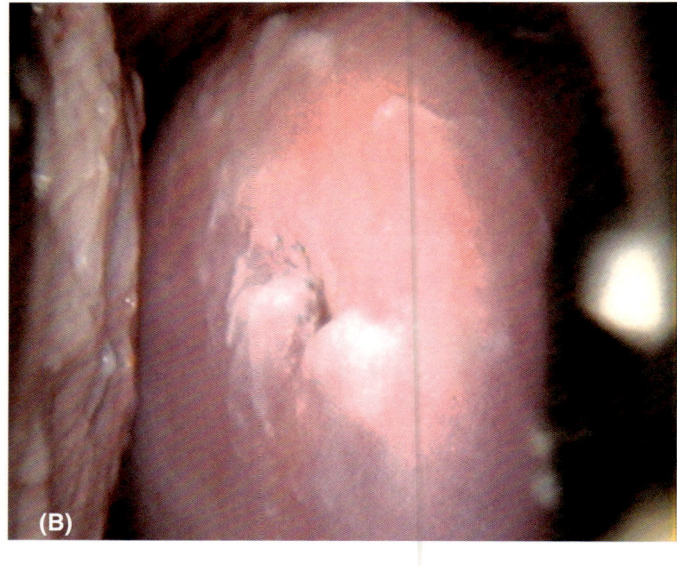

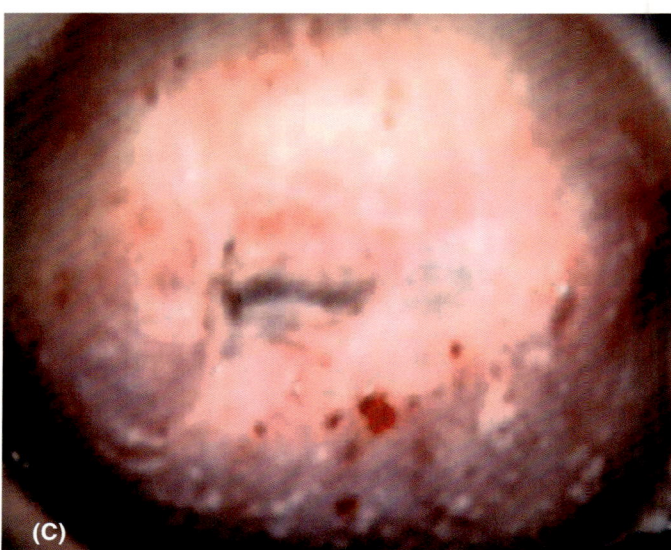

Fig. 7.22: Candidal infection: (A) Discharge at vulva; (B) Discharge at cervix; (C) White punctations with increased vascularity

VIRAL INFECTIONS

Herpes Simplex Virus

Herpetic lesions are seen mostly on vulva, vagina and only at times over the cervix. The lesion starts as an intraepithelial vesicle filled with fluid. Later numerous neutrophils infiltrate and get enmeshed in fibrinous exudate, vesicle enlarges and top layers of epithelium covering it disintegrate leading to ulcer formation.

Base of ulcer is covered with fibrinous exudate and polymorphs. Cellular changes of herpes infection like multinucleation and nuclear molding can be seen in epithelial cells and even stromal cells.

Colposcopy: In acute stage, cervix shows generalised hyperemia. There may be vesicles filled with clear fluid which usually persist for few days only and then break open leaving very painful shallow ulcers which heal later (Figs 7.23 to 7.25).

Cytology is confirmatory showing large, multinucleated infected cells containing dense cytoplasm. Later viral particles may be seen condensed in the center of nucleus as intracellular inclusion which is surrounded by a clear halo.

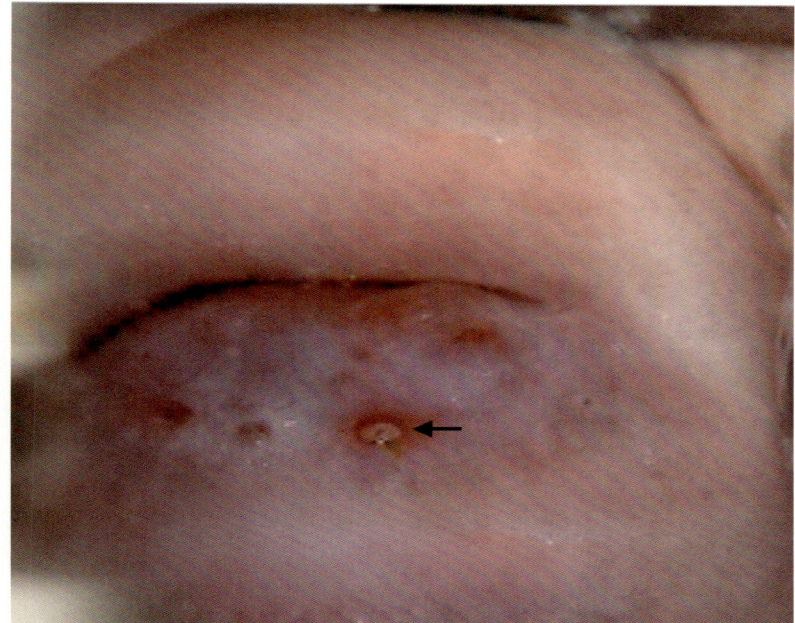

Fig. 7.23: Shallow herpetic ulcer along with increased vascularity

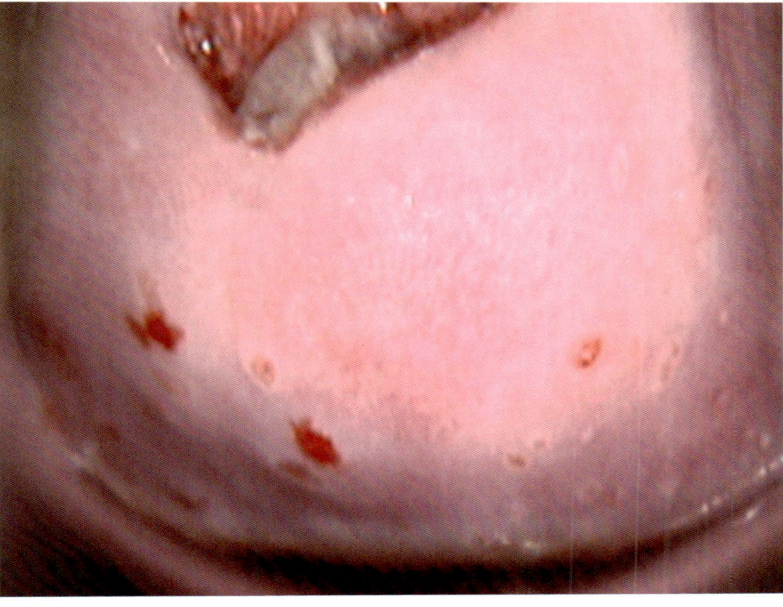

Fig. 7.24: Multiple ulcers over posterior lip of cervix away from TZ

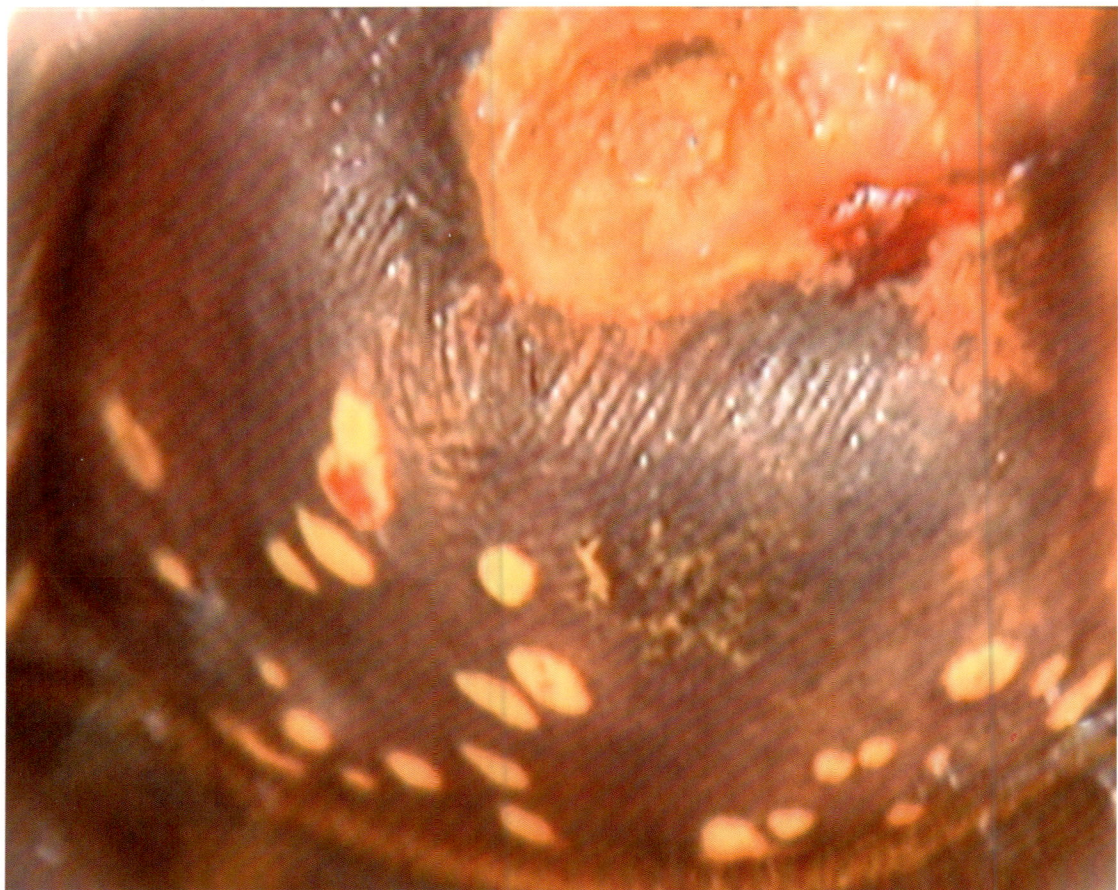

Fig. 7.25: Same cervix (Fig. 7.24) after Lugol's iodine application

Human Papillomavirus Infection

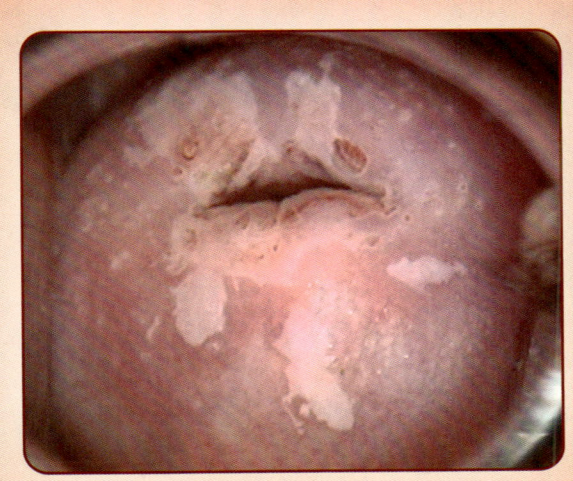

Chapter Outline

INTRODUCTION

Over the last three decades, various epidemiological and clinical studies have established the role of human papillomavirus (HPV) infection as the prime etiologic agent in the causation of cervical cancer.

More than 120 different types of HPVs have been characterized based on the genetic sequence of the outer capsid protein L1. These viruses (virions) are quite similar structurally, but demonstrate significant specificity with regard to the anatomic location of the epithelium they infect and the type of lesion that they produce. The majority are epitheliotropic and produce focal epithelial proliferations at the site of infection. Approximately 30 different types of HPV have been characterized in the infectivity of anogenital tract. These have been associated with a spectrum of anogenital disease ranging from codylomata acuminata to invasive cervical carcinoma.

Two oncogenic risk groups have been classified depending upon the lesions they produce (Table 8.1).

VIRAL GENOME

HPV virus is a double-stranded circular DNA virus of diverse phylogeny. The papillomavirus genome is a DNA molecule of 8000 base pairs contained in spherical protein coat or capsid (Fig. 8.1). It is organized into 3 major functional regions (Fig. 8.2):

- 'Early' region with genes encoding for proteins involved in viral replication, transcription control, and cellular transformation (E1–E8).
- 'Late' region with genes encoding for structural capsid proteins involved in viral assembly (L1, L2).
- 'Upstream' regulatory region (URR) that regulates transcription from early and late regions, and also controls production of viral proteins and infection particles.

Table 8.1: HPV types and oncogenic risk

Risk group	HPV types	Associated lesions
Low	6, 11, 42, 44, 53, 54, 61, 82, 83, 81	Commonly benign lesions, condylomata accuminata Occasionally low grade lesions
High	16, 18, 31, 33, 35, 39, 45, 51, 52, 56, 58, 59, 66, 68	High grade lesions (CIN 2,3) Invasive cancer of cervix, vulva, penis or anus

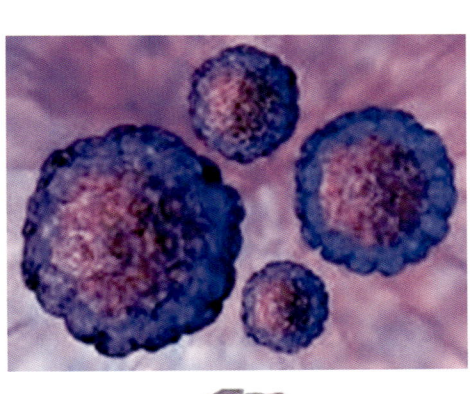

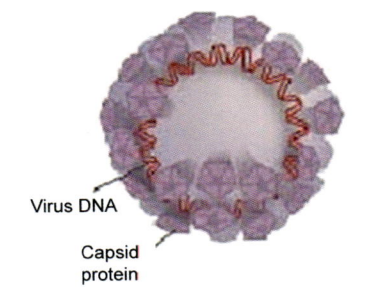

Fig. 8.1: HPV

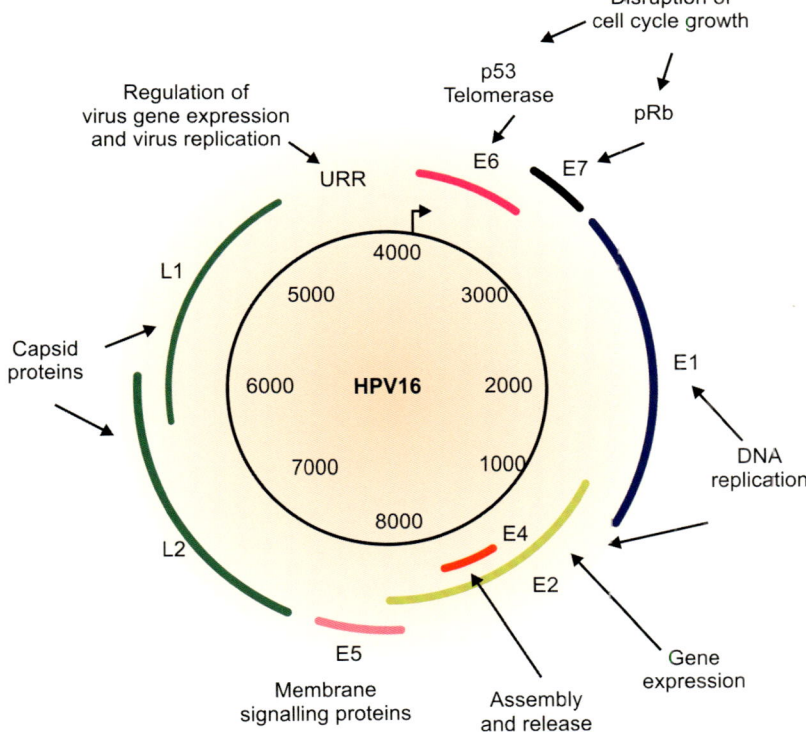

Fig. 8.2: Papillomavirus genome

VIRAL EFFECT & HPV-INDUCED CARCINOGENESIS

The two primary oncogenes of high-risk HPV types are E6 and E7. These two genes are expressed early in the HPV life cycle, and their products alter the host-cell metabolism to favor neoplastic development, by forming complexes with and degrading the host proteins involved in cell cycle regulation, viz. p53 and pRb respectively.

In healthy cells p53 and pRb act as negative regulators or check points to prevent abnormal cell division. In infected cells, however, these control pathways are absent due to the formation of inactive p53-E6 and pRb-E7 complexes. This regulatory loss prevents apoptosis

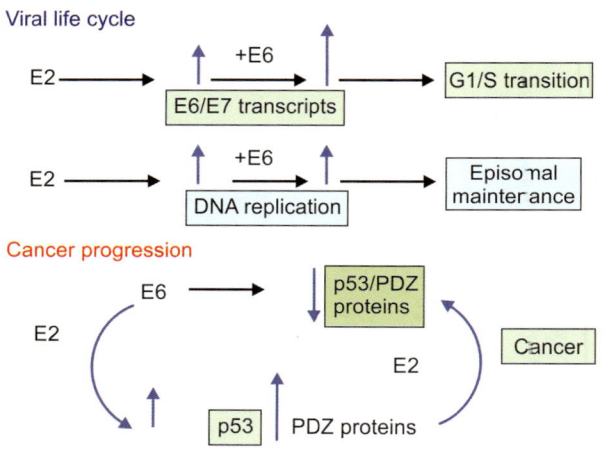

Fig. 8.3: Viral effect

of the infected host epithelial cells. In addition, E6 and E7 proteins may cause chromosomal destabilization, and inhibit cyclin dependent kinase inhibitors and host interferons, probably contributing to the development of cancer (Fig. 8.3).

The HPV lesions infection is frequently observed in young women, especially in their 20s and 30s, because of active metaplastic process occurring in transformation zone. The virus can replicate in the nucleus of immature cells with major mitotic activity.

HPV infections are initiated when the virus gains access to cervical epithelial surface through micro-abrasions during sexual intercourse (Fig. 8.4). HPV targets the basal cells in the stratified squamous epithelium and the metaplastic cells at the squamocolumnar junction of the cervix. HPV may also infect the glandular epithelium of the endocervix, resulting in glandular neoplasia.

After entering the cell, virus gets integrated in the nucleus and sheds its protein coat. The circular DNA remains episomal in location in latent infection. It persists through cell division by low level DNA replication without significant transcriptional activity. It can persist there in this state for varying periods of time remaining latent which can be diagnosed by molecular methods only.

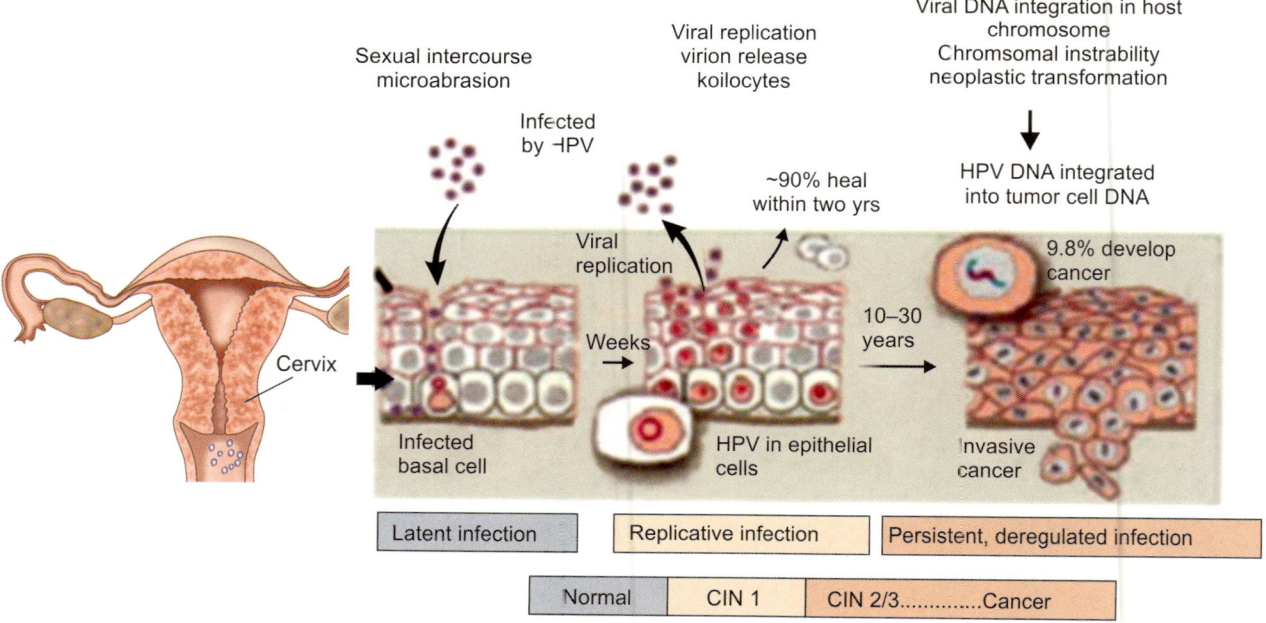

Fig. 8.4: HPV-induced carcinogenesis

After episomal infection is established, low grade or high grade lesion may be produced depending upon the HPV subtype (Low/High risk). Viral gene expression does not occur in basal and parabasal cells. They are expressed only when viral integrated host cells start to differentiate and mature as the cells move upwards. The degree of expression of HPV E6 and E7 is highly correlated with the type of cervical lesion: in low-grade lesions, E6 and E7 are expressed at low levels in the basal cells and higher levels in the upper layers of the epithelium; whereas in high-grade lesions E6 and E7 are expressed at high levels throughout the epithelium, and the HPV DNA is more likely to integrate into the host-cell chromosome, increasing cellular proliferation and the risk of malignancy. Viral replication results in the formation of novel viral particles that are released at the surface of the epithelium (Fig. 8.4).

Cervix reacts to HPV infection by proliferation and hyperplasia rather than degeneration and inflammation seen in response to other infective agents. First sign of active expression occurs within the parabasal layer causing increased cell division (acanthosis) and capillary overgrowth (papillomatosis).

If transcriptional control of viral genome in the basal and parabasal cells fails, expression of viral oncogenes in these replicating cells may induce chromosomal instability and thus initiate transformation. When the HPV is high risk, it interferes with DNA replication of cells, the viral genome gets integrated into the host cells chromosome and expression of viral oncogenes occur, producing high grade lesions and even invasive cancer.

Many important cofactors such as immune status of the host and personal factors like multiple sexual partners, contraceptive methods, smoking, alcohol, drugs, nutritional status and other sexually transmitted infections regulate the interaction between the cell and the virus and thus the resultant disease expression and eventual outcome.

NATURAL HISTORY OF HPV INFECTION

Course of genital HPV infection is extremely variable. The infection may remain latent which is the commonest consequence. Latent infection is widely distributed in the genital squamous epithelium. This infection is either cleared quickly through either the innate immune system or other mechanisms. 80% of new HPV infections clear within 1 year, and approximately 90% clear within 2 years. Clearance of infection is more rapid in younger women in comparison to those over 30 years of age.

Among persistent infections, 25-30% may develop areas of morphological changes, and progress, giving rise to subclinical or clinical lesions. Neoplastic transformation, premalignant or malignant may occur anywhere in the genital tract but is more common in cervix. Infections persisting for longer than 2 years become chronic, leading to low-grade cellular abnormalities called LSIL/CIN 1, majority of which may resolve spontaneously. Some Persistent HPV infection may progress to High grade cellular abnormalities (HSIL/CIN2, 3), a small proportion of which may spontaneously regress. If left undetected and untreated, years or decades later CIN2 or 3 can progress to cervical cancer (Fig 8.5).

Factors such as smoking, infection with C. *trachomatis*, herpes simplex virus, HIV and immune-suppressed individuals, are associated with an increased risk of persistent infection and clinical manifestations such as genital warts, CIN or invasive cancer.

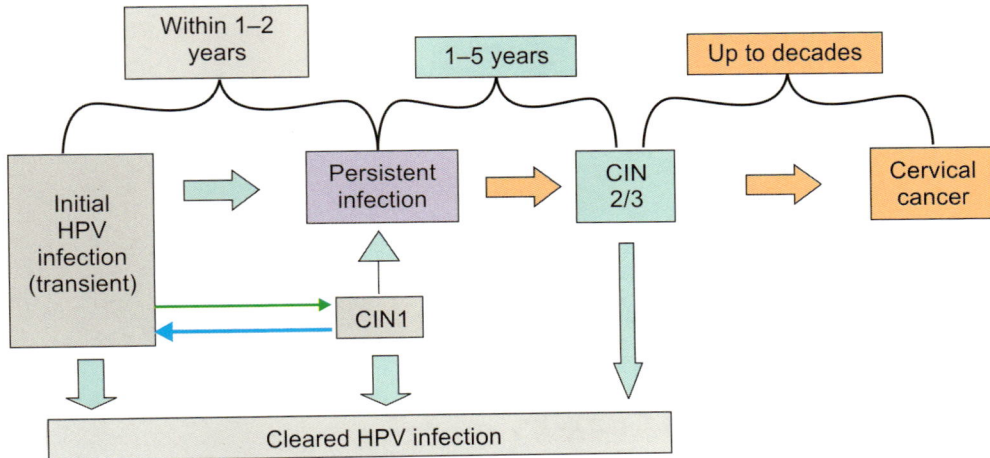

Fig. 8.5: Natural history of HPV infection

COLPOSCOPY

HPV produces extremely variable patterns, ranging from macroscopic florid lesions to clinically inapparent minimal lesions. These lesions may not remain confined to transformation zone. However, lesions inside the transformation zone are more significant because of their oncogenic potential.

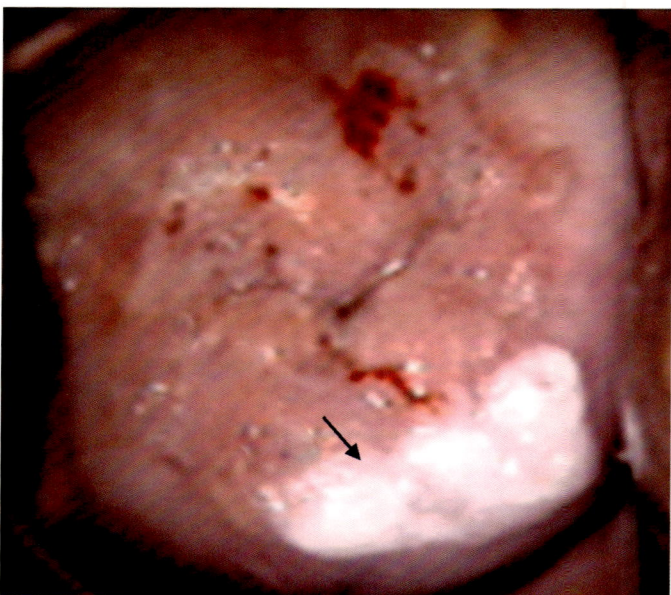

Fig. 8.6A: Thick keratotic lesion with lobulated surface surrounded by AW epithelium

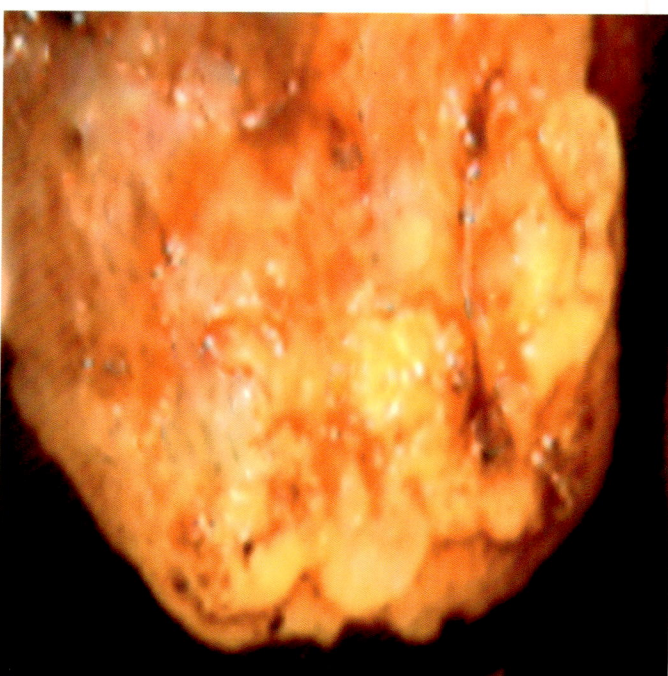

Fig. 8.6B: Same lesion after Lugol's iodine application—no iodine uptake

I. Exophytic/Productive Lesions

Florid, Macroscopic Variety

These can be seen with naked eye also. In such lesions, there is acanthosis, parakeratosis and pronounced papillomatosis. Sometimes there may be nuclear enlargement also. Connective tissue along with blood vessels invaginates into the overlying epithelium giving rise to formation of papillary processes.

Colposcopy: Papillae may appear raised, verrucous with bulbous or rounded projections with keratosis (Figs 8.6A, B and 8.7). It may also show step ladder pattern (Fig. 8.8).

After acetic acid application, epithelium shows a thick white surface with papillary projections, each of which may show a capillary loop. Presence of capillary loop in each papilla is the most reliable diagnostic feature (Figs 8.9A, B and 8.10) and is best seen after acetic acid effect is wearing off.

At times, vascular pattern is bizarre in shape and caliber. This has to be differentiated from invasive carcinoma which may also produce finger-like projections. But in carcinoma, the vascular pattern will be highly atypical. Projections will vary in size and may coalesce with one another.

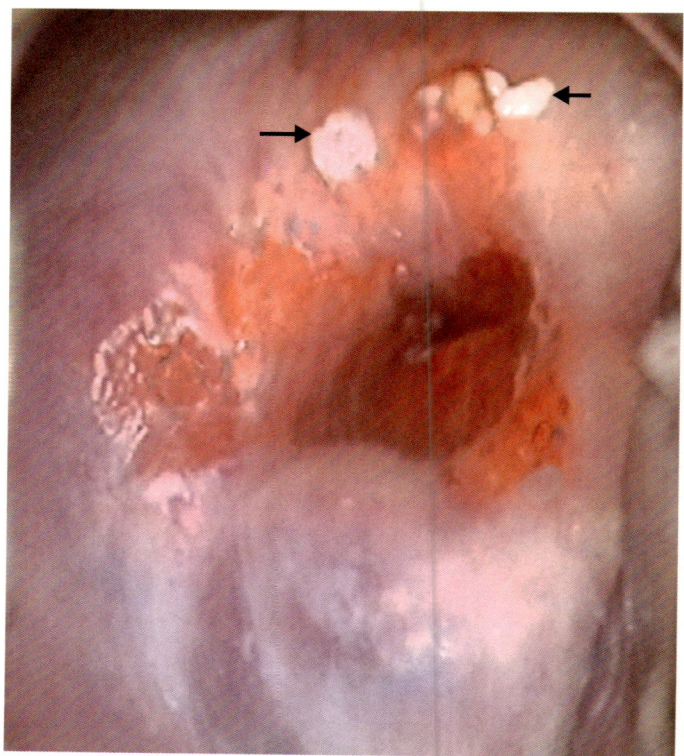

Fig. 8.7: Raised keratotic spiky lesion over anterior lip

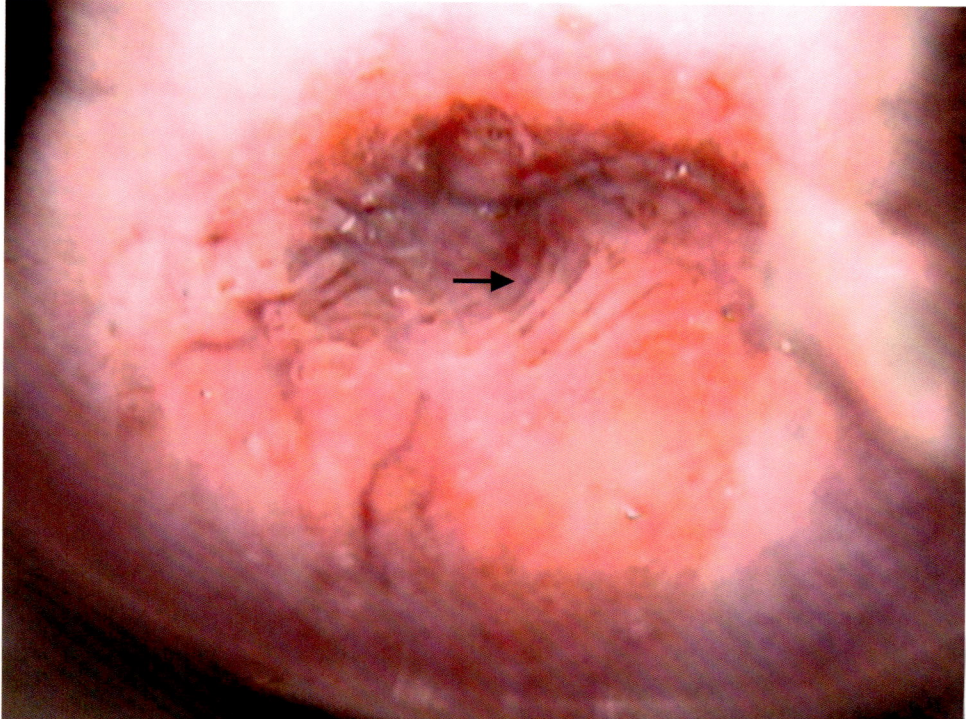

Fig. 8.8: HPV infection: Stepladder pattern on posterior lip after acetic acid application

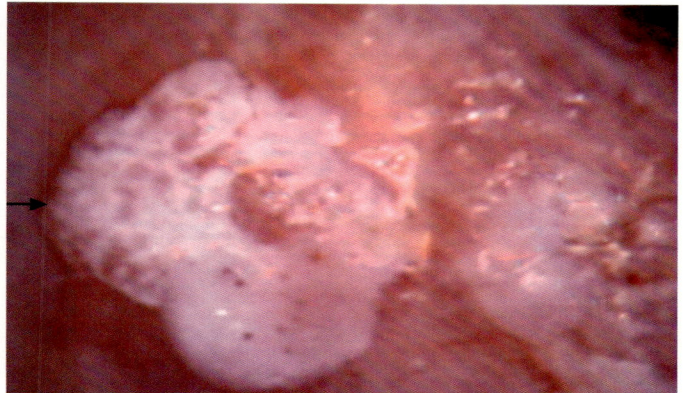

Fig. 8.9A: Raised thick white lesion. Each papilla showing a capillary loop

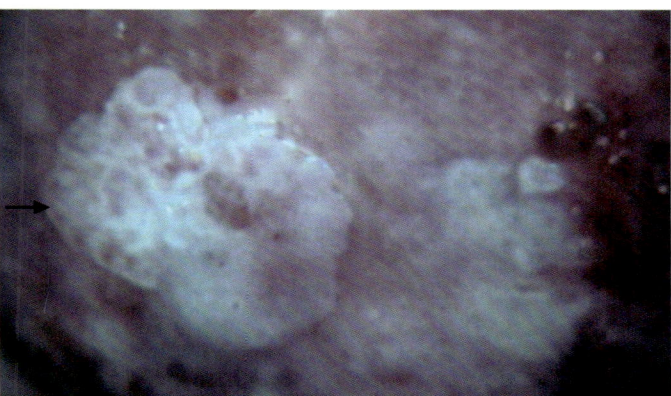

Fig. 8.9 B: The same lesion under green filter

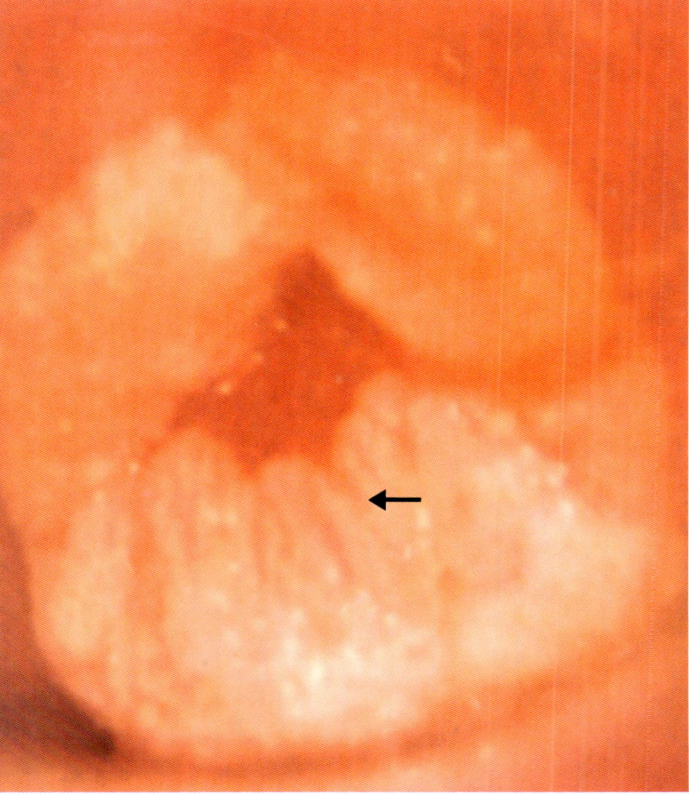

Fig. 8.10: HPV infection (florid/macroscopic) papilliferous circumoral white lesion with rounded projections and central capillary loop visible in papillae

Early/Micropapillary Lesions

Such lesions cannot be easily seen on naked eye examination. Papillomatosis is not pronounced and histology is dominated by marked acanthosis. Epithelium proliferates forming projections termed as Asperities.

Colposcopy (Figs 8.11. to 8.17)**:** Well demarcated white keratotic lesion with irregular and spiky surface is seen. These finger-like projections called asperities usually do not show capillary loops.

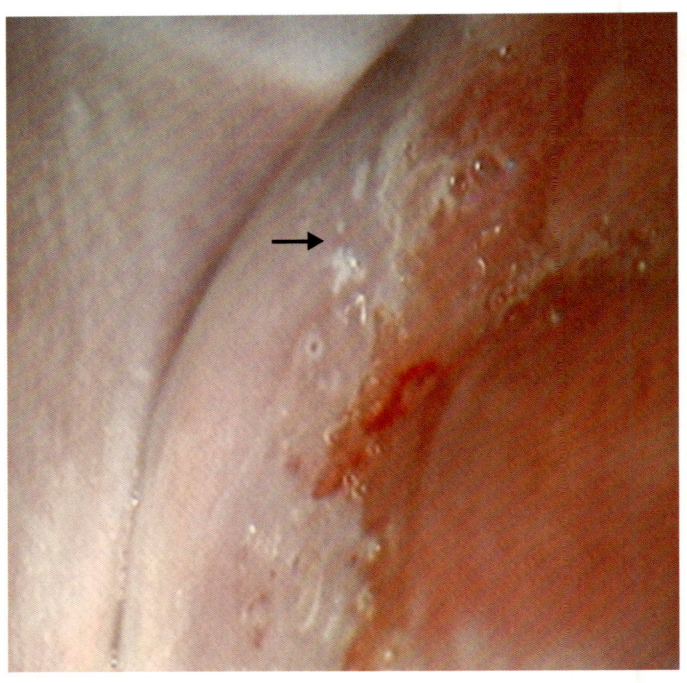

Fig. 8.11: Cervix showing asperities at outer margin of ectopy

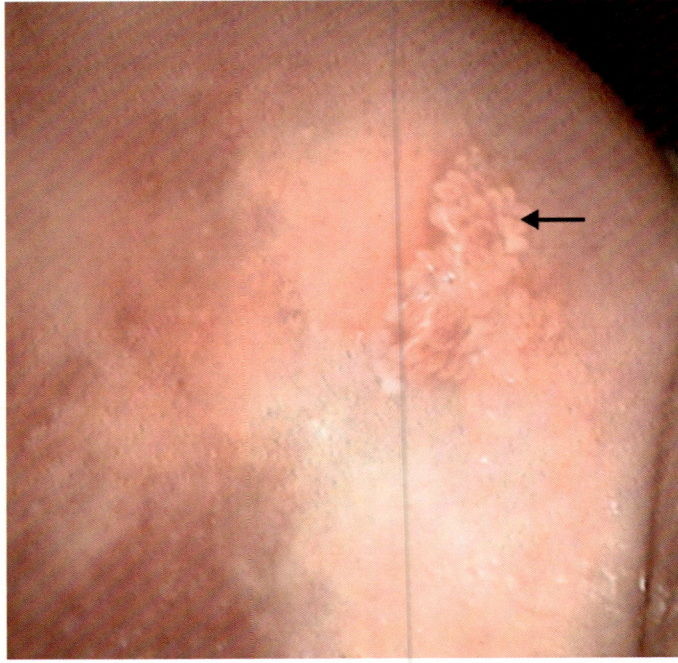

Fig. 8.12: Cervix after application of acetic acid, showing asperities with central vessel

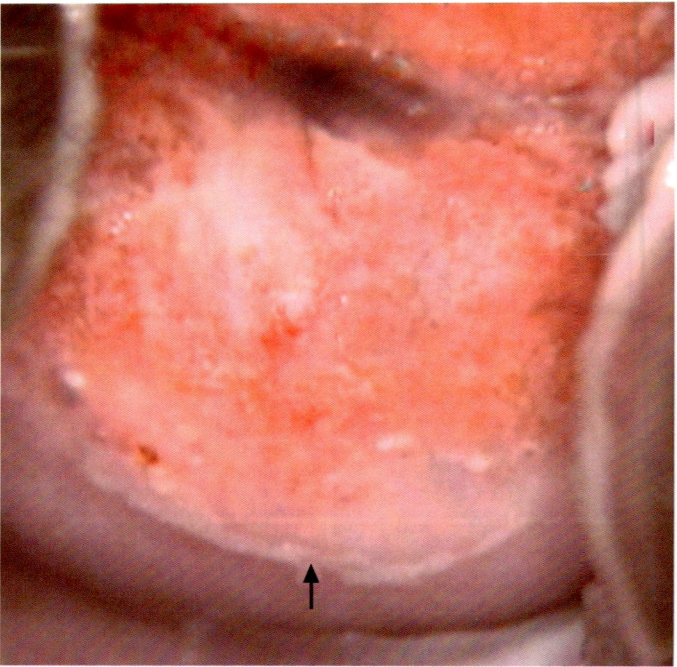

Fig. 8.13A: Cervix after application of acetic acid, showing keratotic grade 1 AW lesion over posterior lip

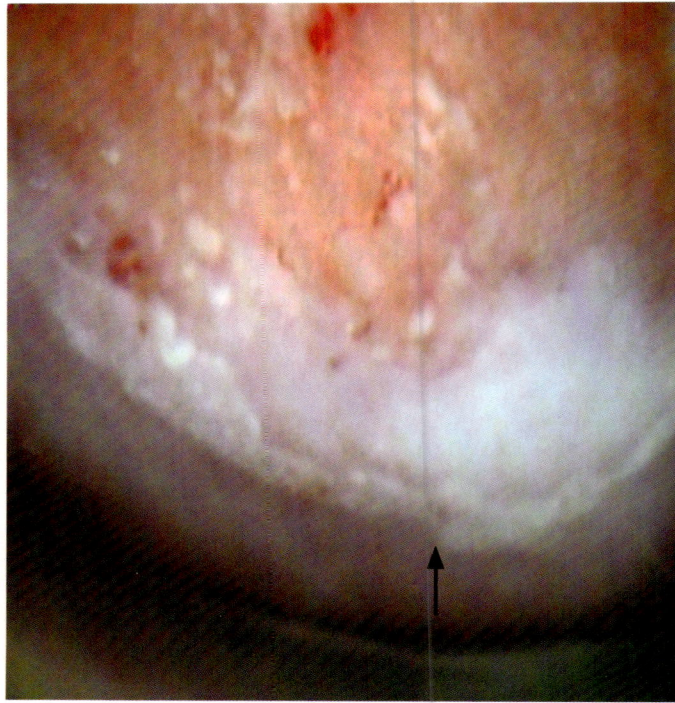

Fig. 8.13B: Same cervix under green filter

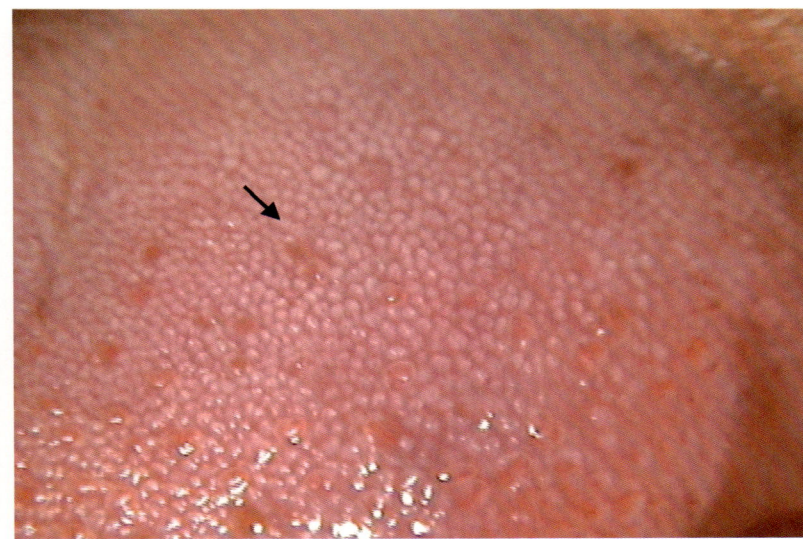

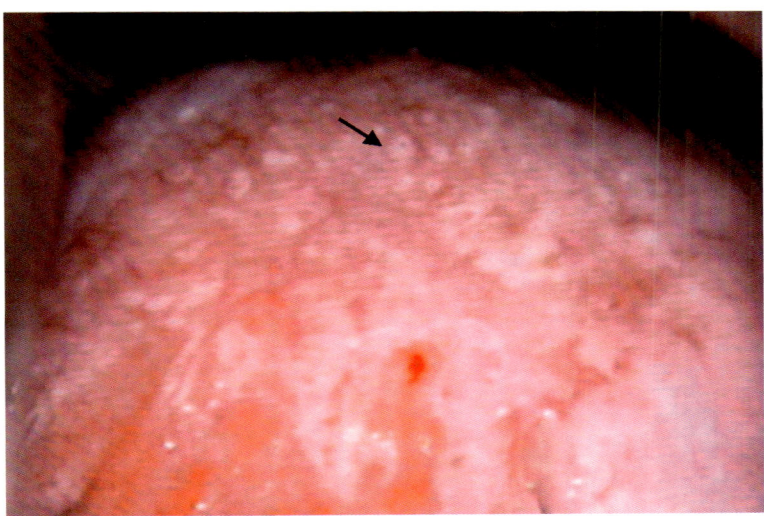

Fig. 8.14: A part of cervix under high magnification showing asperities beyond TZ

Fig. 8.15: Anterior lip of cervix after application of acetic acid showing asperities

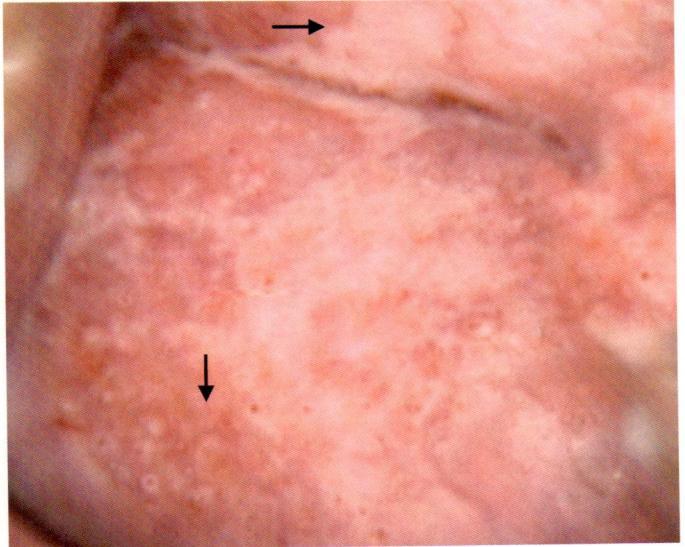

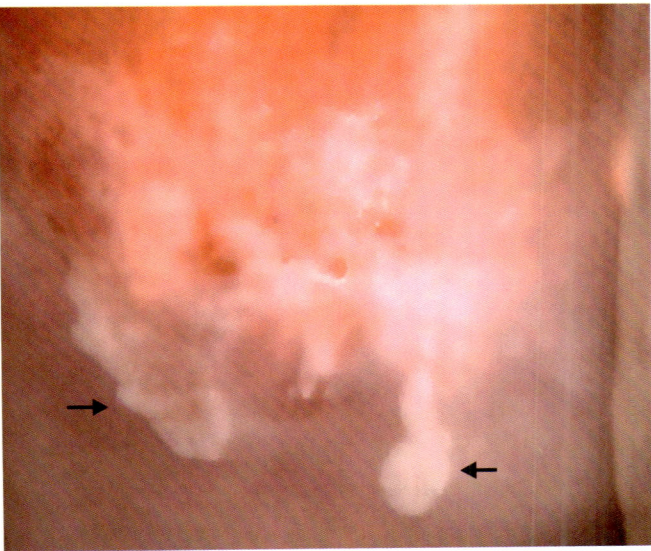

Fig. 8.16: After application of acetic acid: Asperities scattered all over, AW lesion seen near os reaching in endocervix

Fig. 8.17: After application of acetic acid: White keratotic lesion with irregular spiky surface, extending up to fornix

At times angiogenesis within multiple papillae can be seen as capillary loops of regular caliber with punctate-like appearance (Fig. 8.18) or ill-defined mosaic-like pattern containing large central vessel. Such a picture may be because of associated CIN (Figs 8.19A and B). The differentiation has to be made by histopathology.

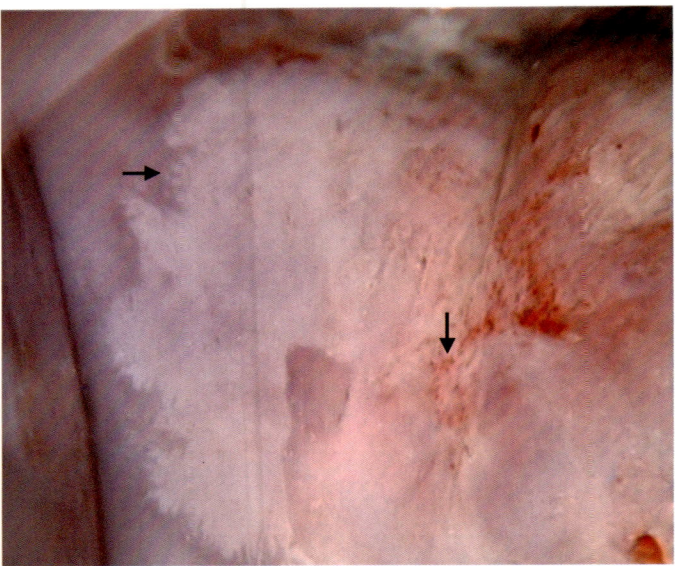

Fig. 8.18: Cervix after application of acetic acid showing mosaic and punctate-like appearance at places

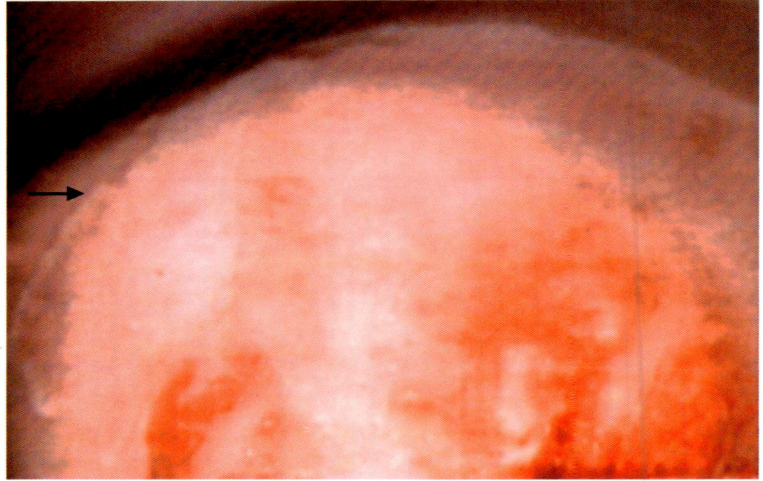

Fig. 8.19A: After application of acetic acid: Grade 1 AW epithelium and mosaic with spiky margins

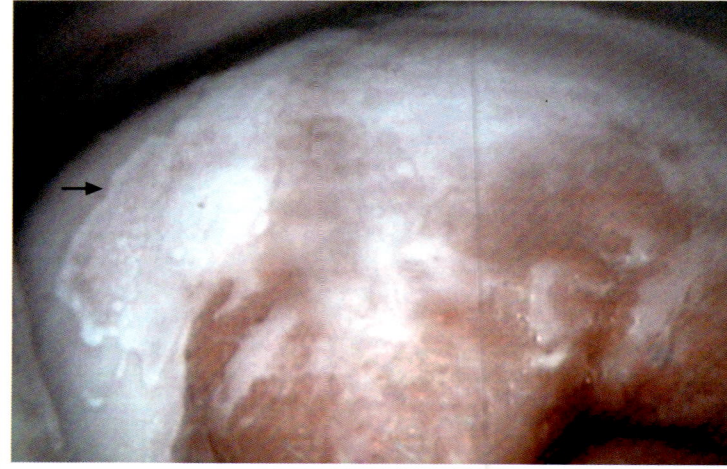

Fig. 8.19B: Same cervix under green filter

II. Flat or Inverted lesions

These lesions cannot be seen by naked eye and are diagnosed colposcopically, hence, termed as *subclinical papilloma viral infection* **(SPI).**

This type of condyloma shares many morphological features of an intraepithelial neoplasia with which it is frequently associated.

Colposcopy: SPI may be seen as flat, acetowhite lesion (Figs 8.20 to 8.23) or white punctations (Fig. 8.24).

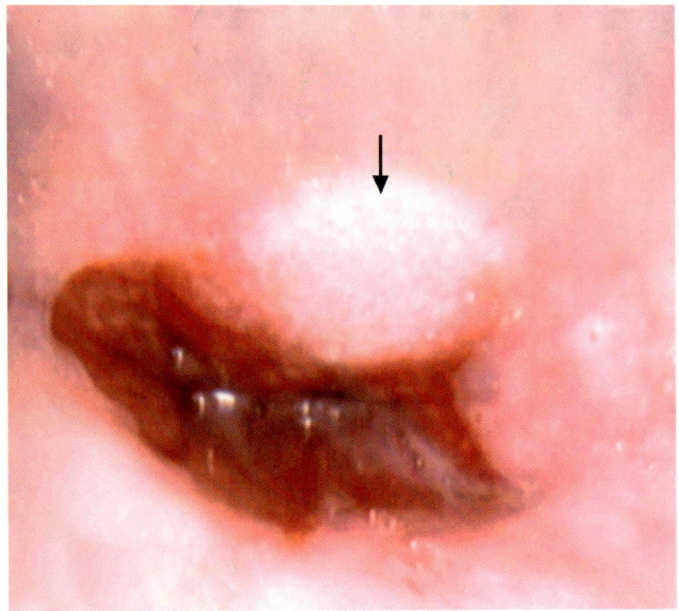

Fig. 8.20A: After acetic acid application: Flat, AW lesion over anterior lip

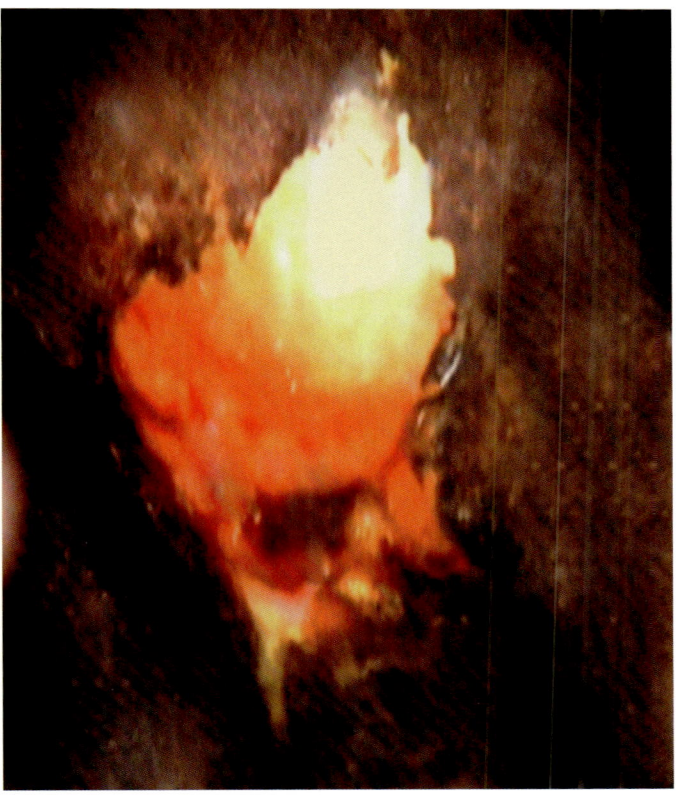

Fig. 8.20B: Same cervix after Lugol's iodine

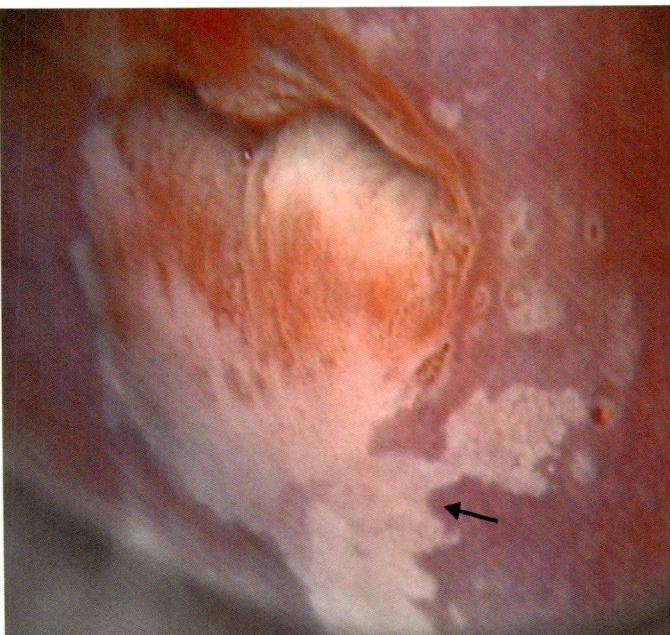

Fig. 8.21: After application of acetic acid: Flat AW epithelium reaching beyond TZ

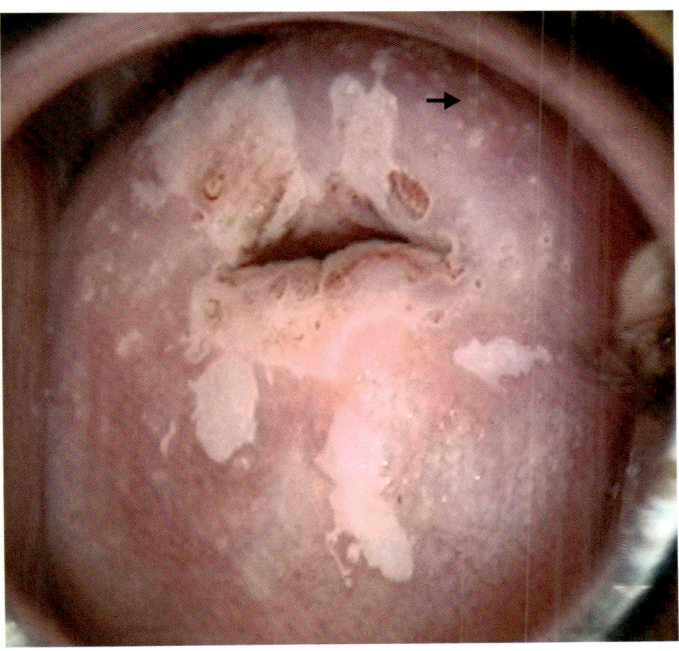

Fig. 8.22: After application of acetic acid: Asperities over anterior lip and tongues of flat AW epithelium all over

Regular fine mosaic or punctation may be seen (Figs 8.25 and 8.26). This is the most common of HPV lesions and is very difficult to differentiate from CIN 1.

Coarse and irregular mosaic or punctations indicate the presence of CIN.

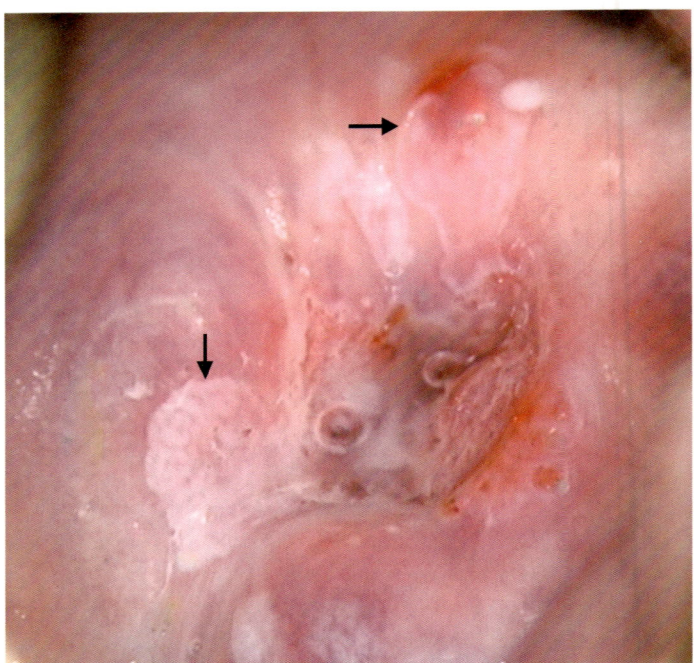

Fig. 8.23: After application of acetic acid: Tongues of flat AW epithelium over anterior and posterior lips

Fig. 8.24: After application of acetic acid: White punctations (arrow) seen along with gland openings

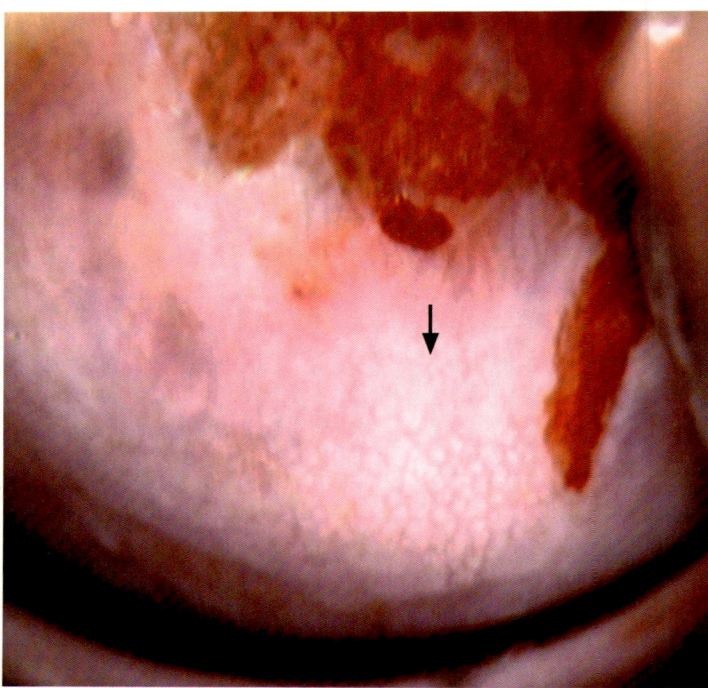

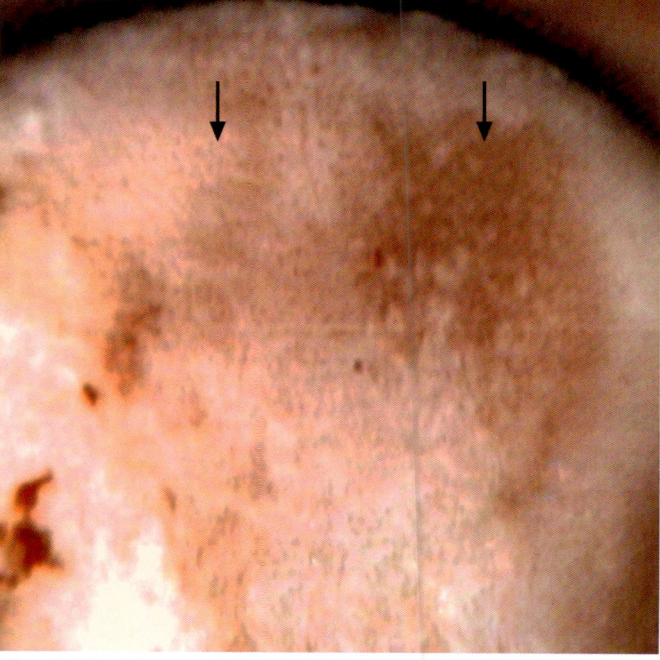

Fig. 8.25: AW epithelium with mosaic over posterior lip beyond TZ

Fig. 8.26: After application of acetic acid: Widely scattered punctations and mosaic

DETECTION OF HPV INFECTION

HPV infection may be detected as under:
- **Latent infection:** By molecular hybridization techniques
- **Subclinical lesions:** By colposcopy, cytology, and histopathology
- **Clinical lesions:** Condylomata observed by naked eye.

Unlike other DNA viruses, conventional cell cultures cannot detect HPV.

Molecular Hybridization Techniques

Techniques that do not use amplification:
- Dot blot, Southern blot
- In situ hybridization

Techniques that use amplification:
- Signal amplification (HPV DNA detection by type II hybrid capture)
- Target amplification (PCR for genotyping)
- Transcription mediated amplification of E6/E7 mRNA

Dot blot and Southern blot techniques use radioactive system and take too long to get the results. They detect the presence of HPV DNA in exfoliated broken cells. Both are highly sensitive and specific methods. However, when used in tissues they are costly and difficult. Therefore, they are used only for research and have been replaced by polymerase chain reaction (PCR) and the hybrid capture system (HCS), the newer in vitro probe tests that have proven to be accurate for epidemiologic and clinical use.

In situ hybridization uses biopsy material fixed in paraffin that makes denaturalization difficult. It detects HPV DNA held in the nucleus of infected cells or in the episomal status. It is a highly specific technique but sensitivity is low.

Hybrid capture 2 HPV DNA test (HC2) is an in vitro nucleic acid hybridization assay that uses complex/branched probe technology to amplify the signal generated by the probe. This is the method used currently for detection of HPV DNA in cervical mucosa. It can screen 14 high-risk types of HPV DNA frequently found in genital tract (16, 18, 31, 33, 35, 39, 45, 51, 52, 56, 58, 59, 66, 68). However, it cannot determine the specific HPV genotype present.

PCR assay amplifies the target nucleic acid. It identifies the HPV subtypes and is highly sensitive because of its inherent capacity to detect very small amount of DNA. It can identify the specific viral type present as well as quantify the viral load, although viral load has not been shown to be clinically useful. However, strict laboratory procedures and control are critical in decreasing contamination related false positivity and involve high cost.

The molecular tests that detect non-integrated viral DNA in the cells give good sensitivity but have poor specificity. In addition, some of them cross-react with low risk types as well as non-oncogenic HPV types giving false positive results

E6E7 mRNA HPV assay: More advance molecular methodology has now been introduced to identify genetic level over-expression that indicates viral gene integration into a host cell genome representing viral persistence. E7 is a major transforming oncogene during early stage and E6 at a later stage of carcinogenesis. Inhibition of these genes affects apoptosis and decreased cell viability. Detection of HPV E6 and E7 expression can be done by a transcription-mediated amplification-based assay, which allows the detection of E6/E7 mRNA transcripts of 14 high-risk HPV types (16, 18, 31, 33, 35, 39, 45, 51, 52, 56, 58, 59, 66, 68). However, the test does not discriminate between the 14 high-risk HPV types.

This assay does not show cross-reactivity with any tested high-risk HPV types or with normal flora and opportunistic organisms that may be found in cervical samples. Thus E6E7 mRNA HPV assay has been found to have equal sensitivity (95%) as HC2 but is much more specific, the positive predictive value being > 90% compared to 15–25% with HC2.

Specimen Collection and Storage

Material is obtained using a conical brush (Fig. 8.27) to remove the endo- and exo-cervical cells. It can also be obtained by the woman herself. The material is transferred into a special tube which can be kept up to

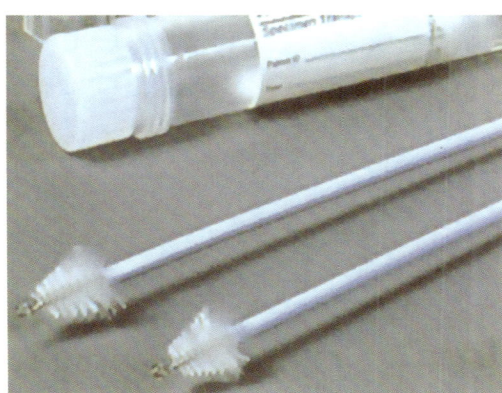

Fig. 8.27: Conical brush used for HPV testing

15 days at room temperature. The test can also be performed on residual cells from a liquid based cytology specimen (Reflex DNA testing).

ROLE OF HPV DNA TESTING

HPV DNA testing has been incorporated into screening, management and follow-up programs. Its use is recommended for the following indications:

1. As an adjunct to Pap smear for cervical cancer screening in women over 30 years of age to screen for the presence or absence of high-risk HPV types. Dual screening program combining cytology and HPV testing minimizes the anticipated lower specificity of HPV testing, at the same time its increased sensitivity allows the extended screening intervals. It is not recommended in women below 30 years of age due to high prevalence of transient HPV infection in younger woman.
2. To screen patients with ASC-US cervical cytology results to determine the need for referral for colposcopy.
3. As a follow-up of the conservative treatment for preinvasive disease.

The flowchart (Fig. 8.28) outlines the management of women with combined cytology and hrHPV DNA screening results. Those who test positive for HPV DNA with cytology of ASC-US or more should be immediately referred for colposcopy. If both are negative, she can have regular screening at intervals of **3/5** years. However, HPV positive and cytology negative women need further follow-up as high levels of anxiety in such women can lead to unnecessary over-treatment, if not counseled properly. Depending upon the facilities available, triaging can be done with HPV 16/18 genotyping, E6/E7 mRNA testing for further colposcopy referral.

HPV VACCINATION

HPV vaccination is a major breakthrough in prevention of cervical cancer with the potential to eradicate more than 70% of Ca Cx worldwide. Two types of vaccines have been prepared, prophylactic and therapeutic.

Therapeutic vaccine (immunotherapy) is based on expression of E6 and E7 HPV oncogenes. It eliminates existing HPV infection but is still under trial.

Prophylactic vaccine (immunization) is based on expression of L1 capsid protein of the virus assembled into virus like particles (VLPs) which are used as

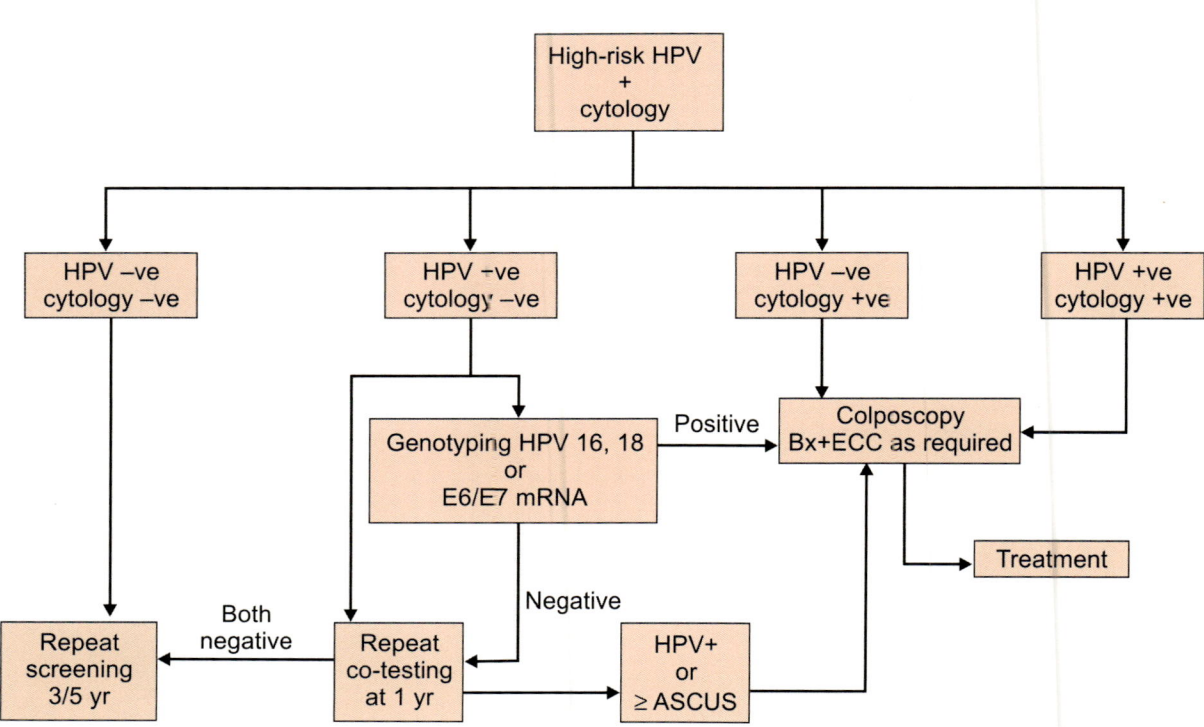

Fig. 8.28: Management of HPV DNA test results

antigen for immunization. It prevents HPV infection to occur, through generation of high levels of 'neutralizing' antibodies. VLPs of L1 capsid proteins are DNA-free but similar in both structure and immunogenicity to authentic papilloma virions. These are highly immunogenic, non-infectious and non-oncogenic.

Two HPV vaccines are currently available in India; a HPV- 6/11/16/18 vaccine Gardasil®, and a HPV- 6/18 AS04-adjuvanted vaccine Cervarix®. 2010. Both vaccines provide excellent protection against HPV-16 and -18 and their related cervical outcomes.

The HPV- 6/11/16/18 vaccine is a quadrivalent vaccine (referred to as HPV4) that also provides protection against non-oncogenic HPV types -6 and -11 which can cause genital warts and CIN 1 (Fig. 8.29).

The HPV-16/18 AS04-adjuvanted vaccine (referred to as HPV2) has a proprietary AS04 adjuvant system which has been shown to enhance humoral and B cell responses compared to the same antigens adjuvanted with aluminium, and provide greater cross-protection efficacy against 10 non-vaccine oncogenic HPV types (–31, –33, –35, –39, –45, –51, –52, –56, –58, –59) and thus reduce morbidity and mortality related to non-16/18 related cervical cancer disease.

Recommendations for Use

Vaccination with HPV2 or HPV4 is recommended by various international and national obstetrics and gynecological societies for prevention of cervical cancers and precancers. Both vaccines might provide protection against some other HPV-related cancers in addition to cervical cancer, although there are currently only data sufficient to recommend HPV4 for protection against vulvar and vaginal cancers and precancers. HPV4 is recommended also for prevention of genital warts.

ACIP recommends routine vaccination of females aged 11 or 12 years with 3 doses of either HPV2 or HPV4. The vaccination series can be started beginning at age 9 years.

Vaccination is recommended for females aged 13 through 26 years who have not been vaccinated previously or who have not completed the 3-dose series. If a female reaches age 26 years before the vaccination series is complete, remaining doses can be administered after age 26 years. Ideally, vaccine should be administered before potential exposure to HPV through sexual contact.

Dosage, Administration and Schedules

The dosing and administration schedules are the same for HPV4 and HPV2. Each dose is 0.5 mL, administered intramuscularly, preferably in a deltoid muscle. The vaccines are administered in a 3-dose schedule. The second dose is administered 1 to 2 months after the first dose, and the third dose is administered 6 months after the first dose.

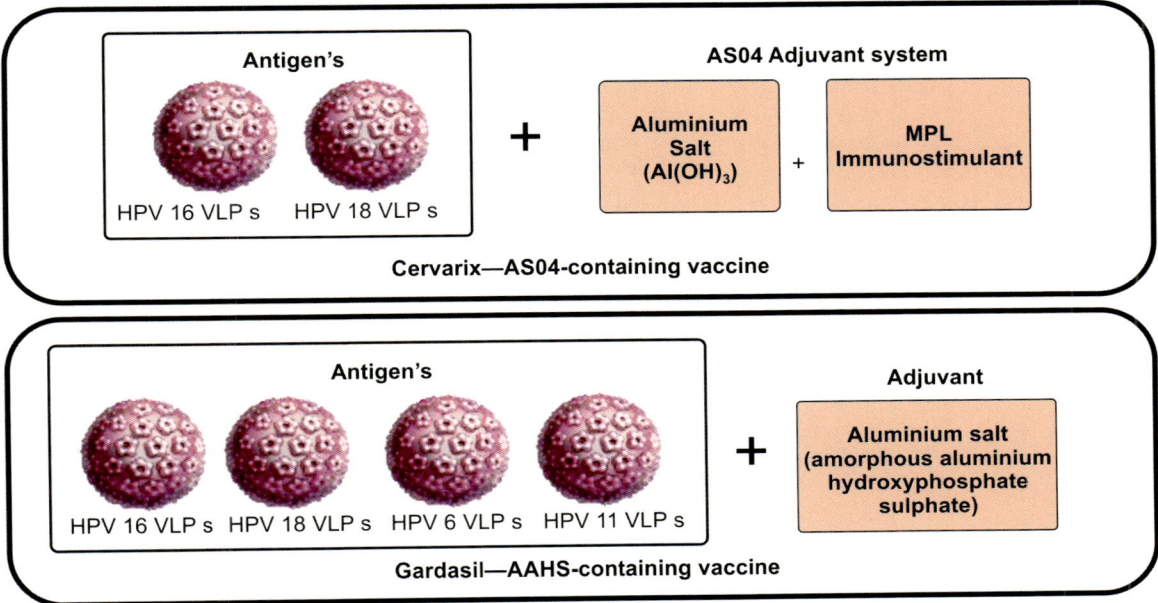

Fig. 8.29: Composition of two HPV vaccines. MPL (monophosphoryl lipid A) is a purified lipopolysaccharide from a bacterial wall and is a powerful stimulant of the immune system

The minimum interval between the first and second dose of vaccine is 4 weeks and between the second and third dose is 12 weeks. The minimum interval between the first and third dose is 24 weeks. Doses received after a shorter-than-recommended dosing interval should be readministered. If the HPV vaccine schedule is interrupted, the vaccine series does not need to be restarted. Coadministration of a different inactivated or live vaccine, either simultaneously or at any time before or after HPV vaccine, is permitted because neither HPV vaccine is a live vaccine.

Whenever feasible, the same HPV vaccine should be used for the entire vaccination series. No studies address interchangeability of HPV vaccines. However, if the vaccine provider does not know or have available the HPV vaccine product previously administered, either HPV vaccine can be used to complete the series to provide protection against HPV 16 and 18. For protection against HPV 6 or 11-related genital warts, a vaccination series with less than 3 doses of HPV4 might provide less protection against genital warts than a complete 3-dose HPV4 series.

Special Situations

Females who have abnormalities on their cervical cancer screening results are likely to be infected with one or more genital HPV types. With increasing severity of Papanicolaou (Pap) findings, the likelihood of infection with HPV 16 or 18 increases, and benefits of vaccination decrease. Vaccination is still recommended for such females, because vaccination can provide protection against infection with HPV vaccine types not already acquired. Females should be advised that vaccination will have no therapeutic effect on an existing HPV infection or abnormal Pap test.

Prevaccination assessments (e.g. Pap testing or screening for high-risk HPV DNA, type-specific HPV tests, or HPV antibody) to establish the appropriateness of HPV vaccination are not recommended at any age.

A history of genital warts or clinically evident genital warts indicates infection with HPV, most often HPV 6 or 11. Vaccination is still recommended for such females because vaccination can provide protection against infection with HPV vaccine types not already acquired. Females should be advised that vaccination will have no therapeutic effect on an existing HPV infection or genital warts.

Lactating women can receive HPV vaccine.

HPV2 and HPV4 are not live vaccines, and can be administered to females who are immunosuppressed (from disease or medications). However, the immune response and vaccine efficacy might be less than that in immunocompetent persons.

Precautions and Contraindications

HPV vaccines are not recommended for use in pregnant women. If a woman is found to be pregnant after initiating the vaccination series, the remainder of the 3-dose series should be delayed until completion of pregnancy. Pregnancy testing is not needed before vaccination. If a vaccine dose has been administered during pregnancy, no intervention is needed.

HPV vaccines can be administered to persons with minor acute illnesses. Vaccination of persons with moderate or severe acute illnesses should be deferred until after the patient improves.

Syncope can occur after vaccination and has been observed among adolescents and young adults. To avoid serious injury related to a syncopal episode, vaccine providers should consider observing patients for 15 minutes after they are vaccinated.

HPV vaccines are contraindicated for persons with a history of immediate hypersensitivity to any vaccine component. HPV4 is produced in *Saccharomyces cerevisiae* (Baker's yeast) and is contraindicated for persons with a history of immediate hypersensitivity to yeast. Prefilled syringes of HPV2 have latex in the rubber stopper and should not be used in persons with anaphylactic latex allergy. HPV2 single dose vials contain no latex.

Cervical Intraepithelial Lesions

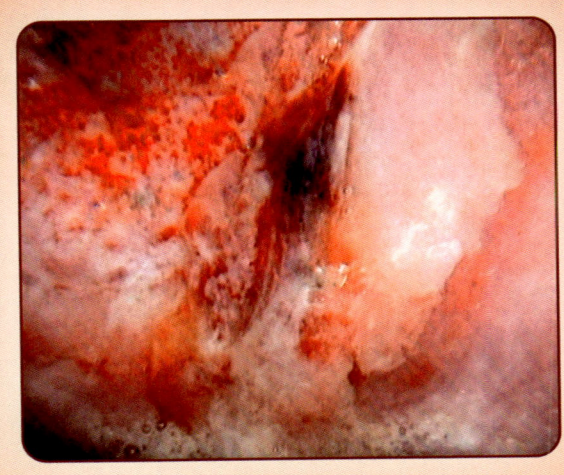

Chapter Outline

Invasive carcinoma of cervix is preceded by a series of random cellular changes that remain confined within the epithelium and are termed as intraepithelial lesions which may involve the squamous or glandular epithelium.

SQUAMOUS INTRAEPITHELIAL LESIONS (SILs)

It is believed that metaplastic cells during immature metaplastic stage may acquire neoplastic potential and give rise to abnormal growth of epithelium near squamo-columnar junction. Thereafter it may spread to involve larger areas of transformation zone. Intraepithelial changes generally stop short at the squamo-squamous junction of the transformation zone and do not involve original squamous epithelium unless invasion takes place.

Cervical intraepithelial neoplasia (CIN) is a histologic term that was coined by Richart in 1975 and replaced the older term dysplasia. He clubbed severe dysplasia and carcinoma in situ into CIN 3 because cytologically, histologically and biologically it is difficult to differentiate severe dysplasia from carcinoma in situ.

Depending upon the severity of the abnormal changes and degree of loss of maturation and differentiation, CIN has been categorized into three grades. In CIN 1, cellular changes are limited to lower third, in CIN 2 up to middle third and in CIN 3 whole thickness of the epithelium is involved. In the recent past, HPV and CIN 1 have been clubbed together as low grade lesions and a two tier classification has been introduced for cytologic as well as histologic nomenclature of squamous intraepithelial lesions (Table 9.1). However, it is important to understand that cytologic LSIL is not equivalent to histologic CIN 1 and cytologic HSIL is not equivalent to histologic CIN 2, 3.

Abnormal growth of the epithelium in SIL is characterized by increased number of cell layers, loss of maturation and polarity. Cells acquire neoplastic characteristics in nuclei and cytoplasm.

DNA content of the cell increases, nuclei show enlargement leading to increased nuclear: cytoplasmic ratio, hyperchromatism, increased mitotic activity and abnormal mitotic figures. Cytoplasmic differentiation suffers resulting in decreased glycogen content.

Epithelium shows cellular density leading to increased number of nuclei per unit area, which together with increased DNA content is seen colposcopically as various grades of acetowhite epithelium according to degree of abnormality.

Cohesiveness between the cells is also decreased making the epithelium prone to minor trauma (Fig. 9.1). Sometimes surface keratinization may also be seen.

Table 9.1: Different terminologies of squamous intraepithelial lesions

Histologic terminologies			Cytologic terminology
Dysplasia terminology	*CIN terminology*	*New histologic terminology*	*Bethesda system cytologic terminology*
Atypia	HPV related changes	Low grade CIN	LSIL
Mild dysplasia	CIN 1		
Moderate dysplasia	CIN 2	High grade CIN	HSIL
Severe dysplasia	CIN 3		
Carcinoma in situ			

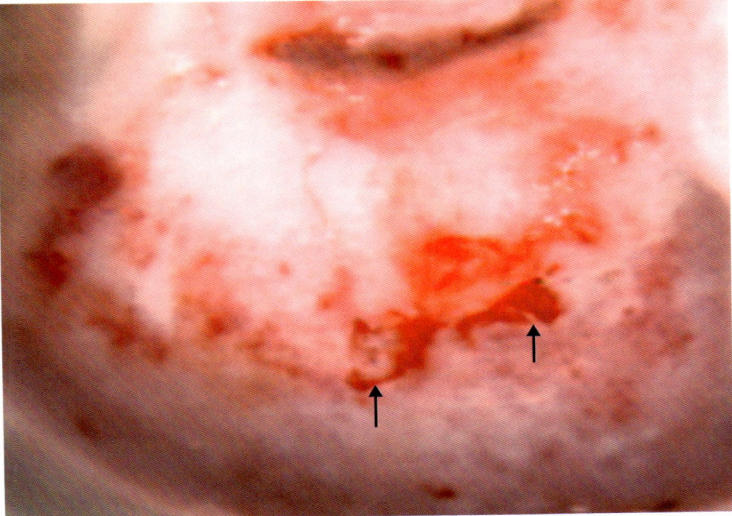

Fig. 9.1: After application of acetic acid: AW epithelium along with abrasion due to decreased cohesiveness (Rag sign)

Underlying connective tissue stroma is edematous. There is localized proliferation of vessels leading to increase in the number as well as the caliber, resulting in congestion and formation of tortuous loops of varying size. These vessels may push through the covering epithelium reaching just beneath the surface and dilate at the top due to lateral compression by abnormally proliferating cells (Fig. 9.2), seen colposcopically as punctations. At times the vessels form a network like basket weave around the blocks of abnormal cells (Fig. 9.3) and give rise to mosaic appearance on colposcopy. Disorderly proliferation of the cells later may distort the adjacent stroma. Consequently, stromal papillae along with the capillary loop may get compressed and disappear giving rise to increased intercapillary distance.

All these changes in the vascular network along with the epithelial changes can be seen colposcopically as hyperemia, various grades of punctations, mosaic and acetowhite epithelium in combination or isolation.

Squamous intraepithelial abnormalities have been categorised into different grades depending upon the severity of the abnormal changes and degree of loss of maturation and differentiation.

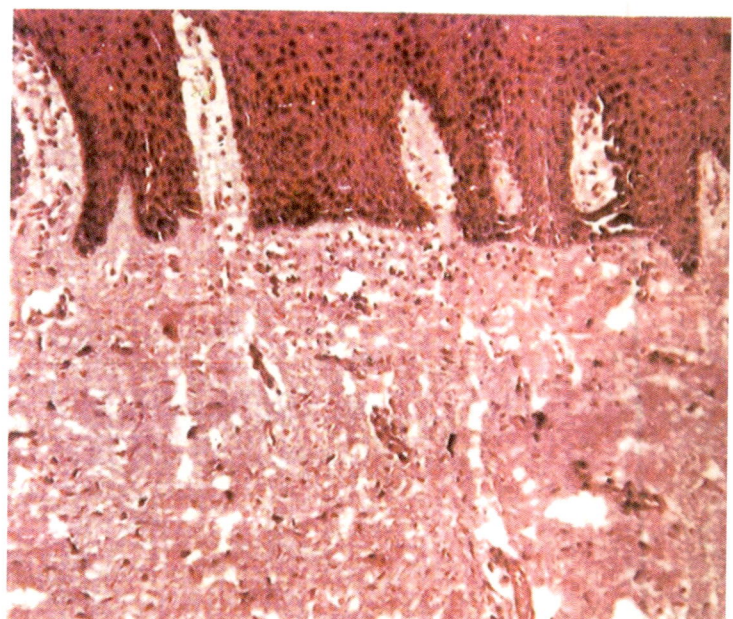

Fig. 9.2: Microphotograph: Connective tissue stromal papillae along with capillaries are seen pushing into covering squamous epithelium reaching almost to the surface. Increased intercapillary distance is seen. Entire thickness of epithelium is undifferentiated. Basal lamina is intact

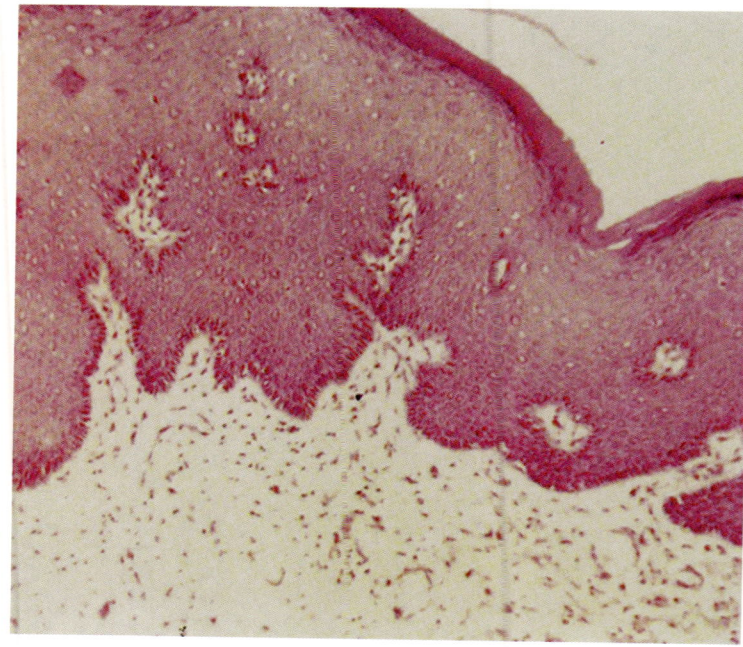

Fig. 9.3: Microphotograph: Connective tissue stromal papillae in the epithelium are forming a network around the blocks of abnormal epithelium. Entire thickness of epithelium is undifferentiated. Basal lamina is intact

Colposcopy: For colposcopic diagnosis of CIN, the area of interest is transformation zone as this is the zone of cellular unrest. Atypical transformation zone is recognized by presence of abnormal vasculature, acetowhitening, surface contour, margins and the iodine negativity and a score is given according to modified Reid's colposcopic index.

Colposcopy defines the type of the lesion whether low or high grade, maps the extent of the lesion and localises the site of biopsy.

Low Grade Lesions (Reid's Score 0–2)

In the early stages, the undifferentiated cells are limited to the lower one-third of the epithelium (Fig. 9.4). Many times low grade changes may be associated with inflammation also. Such epithelial changes regress after appropriate treatment of infection.

After saline application, cervix usually does not show any abnormality but sometimes foci of fine and regularly placed punctations, hyperemic area (Fig. 9.5A) may be seen.

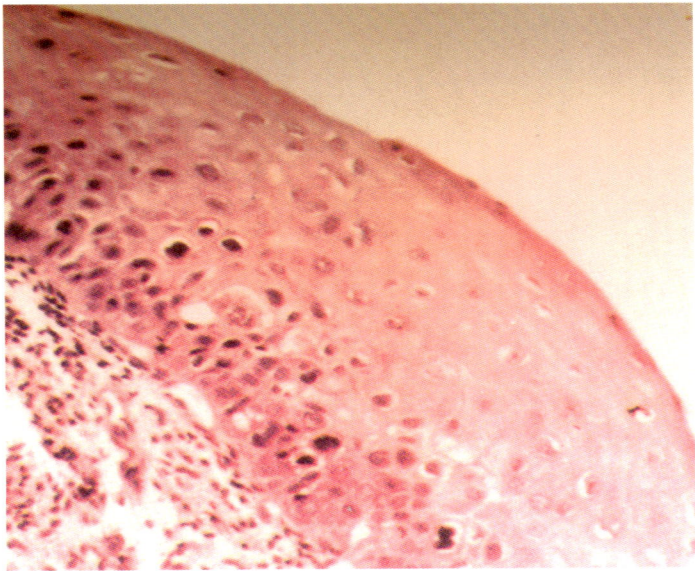

Fig. 9.4: Microphotograph: Lower one-third of epithelium shows loss of polarity, hyperchromatic, large irregular nuclei and prominent mitotic figures. The middle and upper layers mostly show normal maturation and orderly arrangement of cells

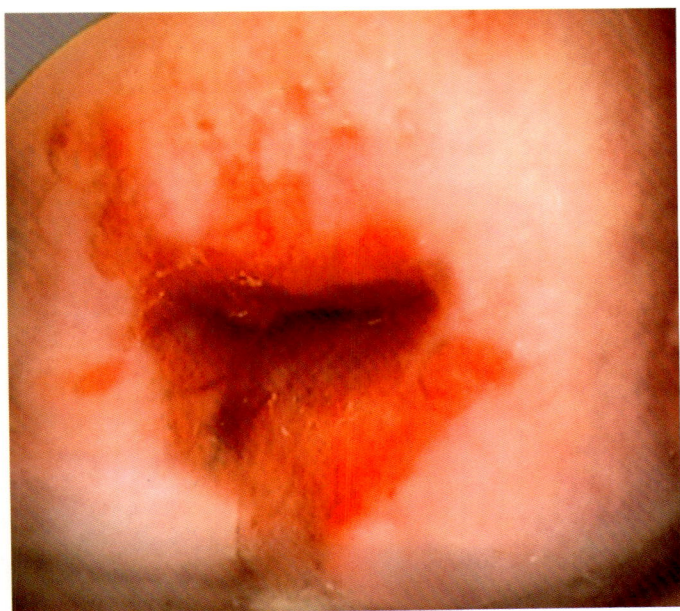

Fig. 9.5A: After saline application. Hyperemia over anterior lip

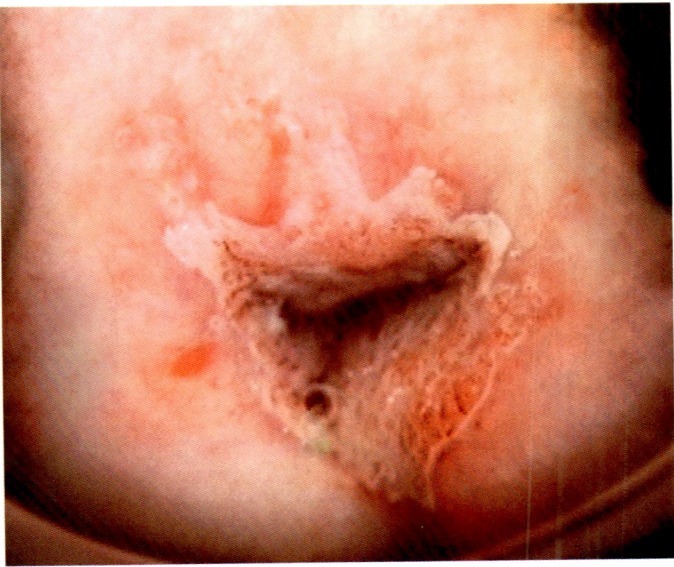

Fig. 9.5B: Same cervix after acetic acid: Grade 1 AW epithelium and fine punctations over anterior lip

After application of acetic acid, white lesions appear with flat surface, indistinct or hazy borders (Fig. 9.5B, 9.6A to C and 9.7A and B). Acetowhite change occurs slowly, lasts for a short time and fades quickly. Such pattern may also be seen with metaplastic epithelium, and regenerative epithelium.

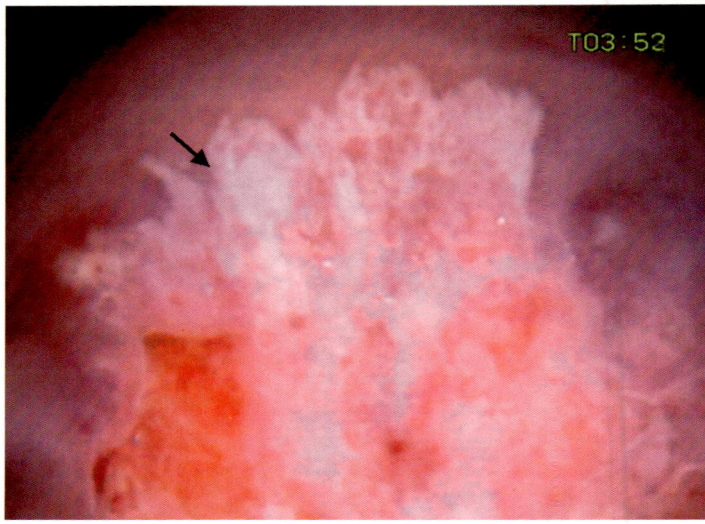

Fig. 9.6A: AW epithelium with flat surface and indistinct borders over anterior lip

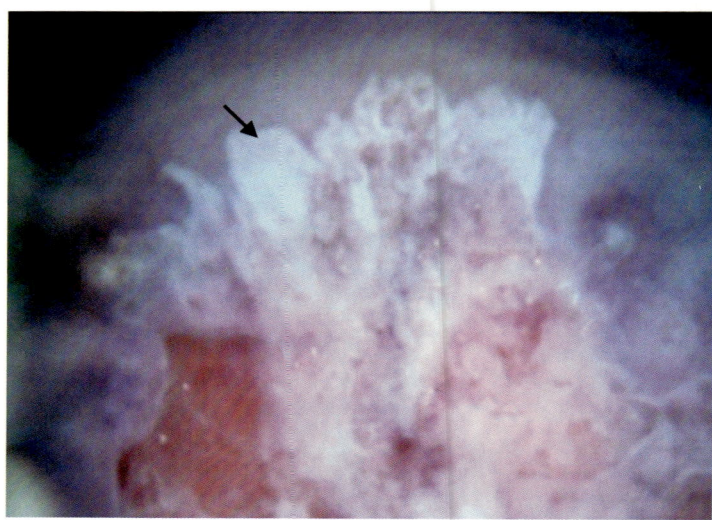

Fig. 9.6B: Same cervix under green filter

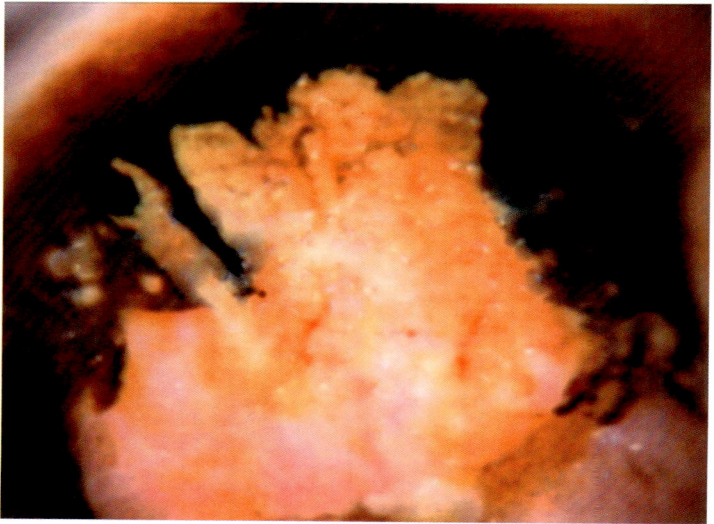

Fig. 9.6C: Same cervix—no iodine uptake by abnormal area

Acetowhitening associated with metaplasia is translucent and less dense with indistinct margins. The acetowhite area of metaplasia blends with the normal epithelium. The tongues of metaplasia point towards the extenal os centripetally. The acetowhite lesions associated with CIN are invariably located closer to or abutting the squamocolumnar junction. These spread centrifugally pointing away from the external os. Biopsy should be taken for confirmation of the final diagnosis.

Vascular pattern is either inconspicuous or may show fine and regular mosaic or punctation (Figs 9.8A, B and 9.9A, B and 9.10).

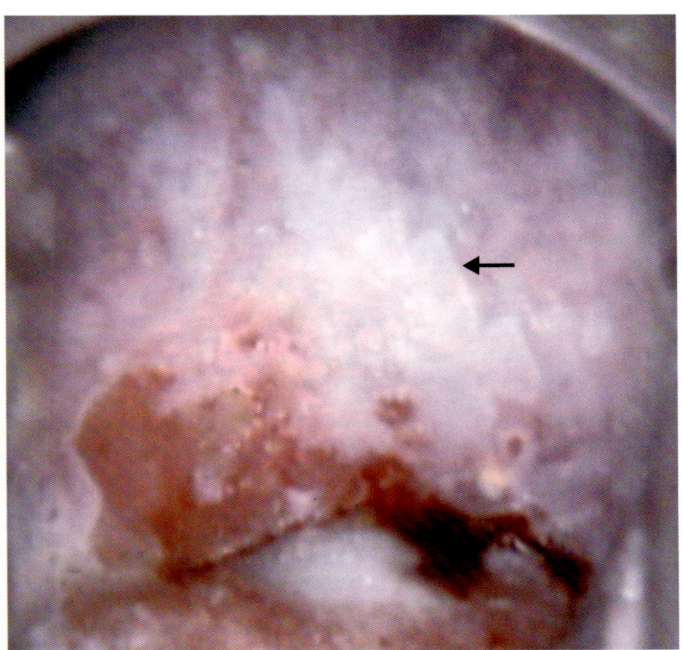

Fig. 9.7A: After acetic acid application: Shiny white lesion with flat surface and indistinct borders over anterior lip

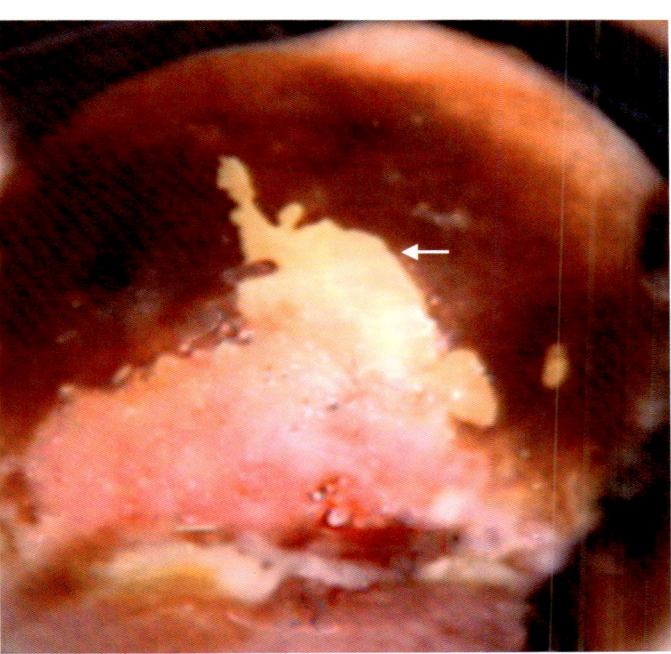

Fig. 9.7B: Same cervix after Lugol's iodine application—iodine negative lesion

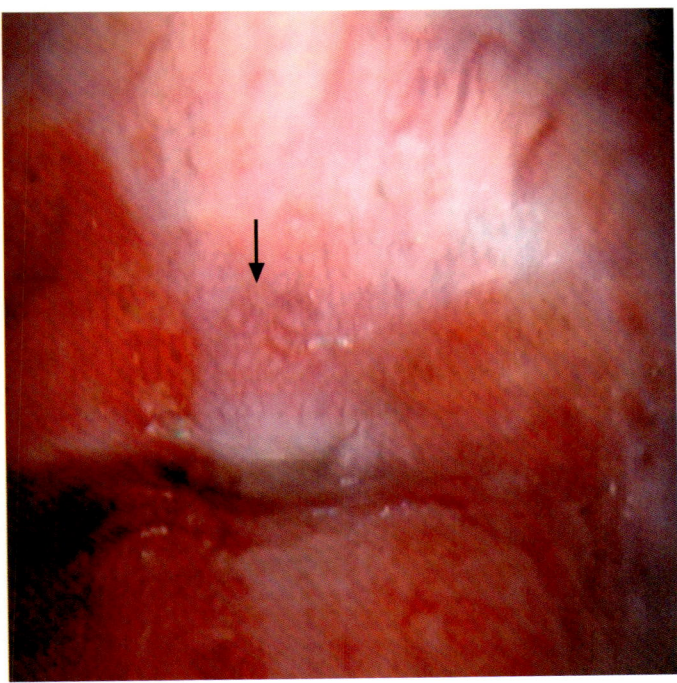

Fig. 9.8A: Grade 1 AW epithelium with regular mosaic

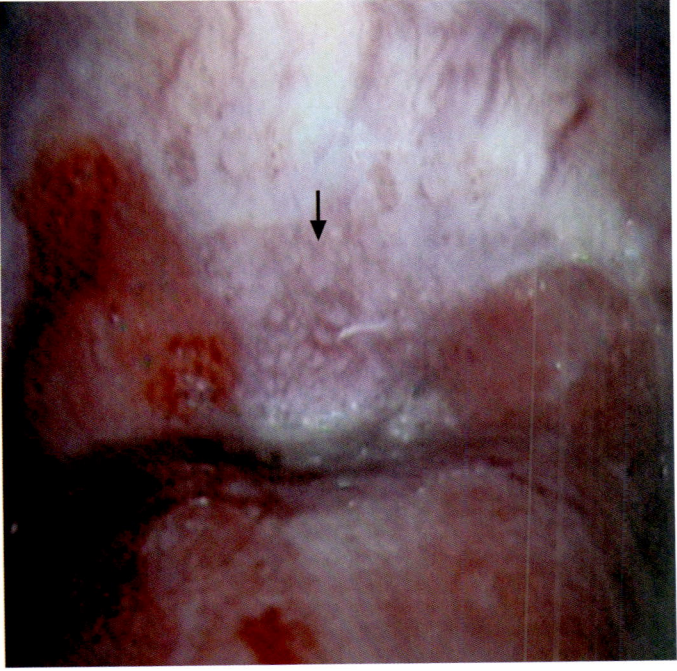

Fig. 9.8B: Same cervix under green filter

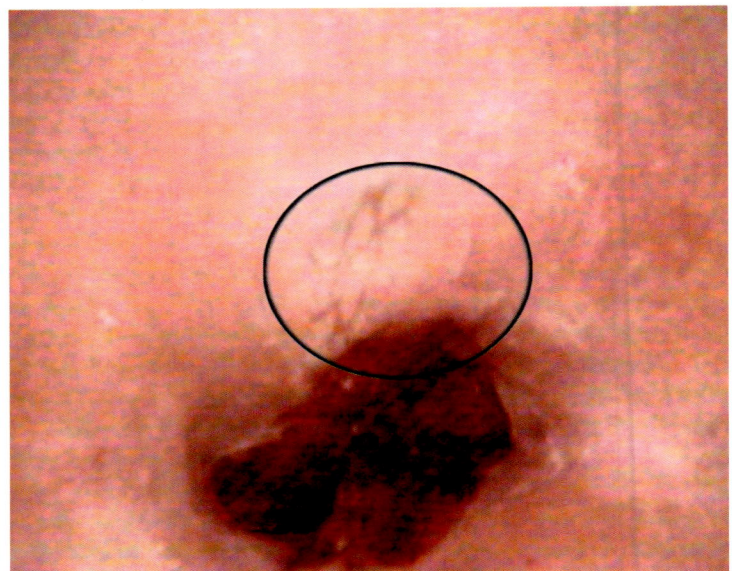

Fig. 9.9A: Grade 1 AW epithelium with fine mosaic

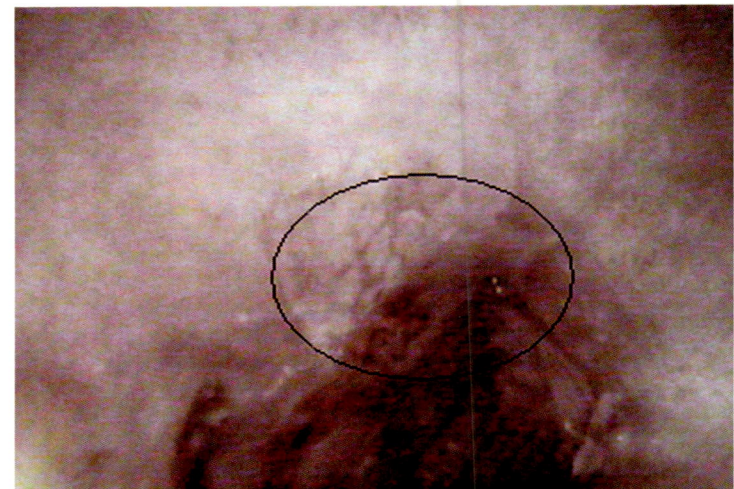

Fig. 9.9B: Same cervix (Fig. 9.9A) under green filter

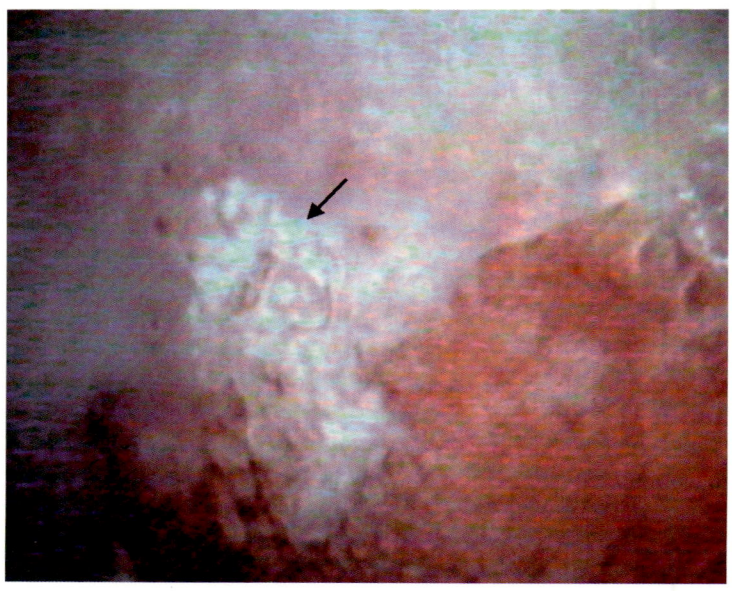

Fig. 9.10: AW epithelium with irregular mosaic inside TZ

Colposcopic Lesions with Reid's Score 3–5

Numbers of undifferentiated cell layers are more than that of CIN 1, occupying up to two-third of the epithelial thickness. Cell maturation suffers comparatively more and proceeds only up to the level of parabasal cells (Fig. 9.11).

Colposcopy: After saline application, localized hyperemia (Fig. 9.12A) or coarse punctations may be seen. After acetic acid application, white lesion which appears has flat surface but sharp and distinct margins.

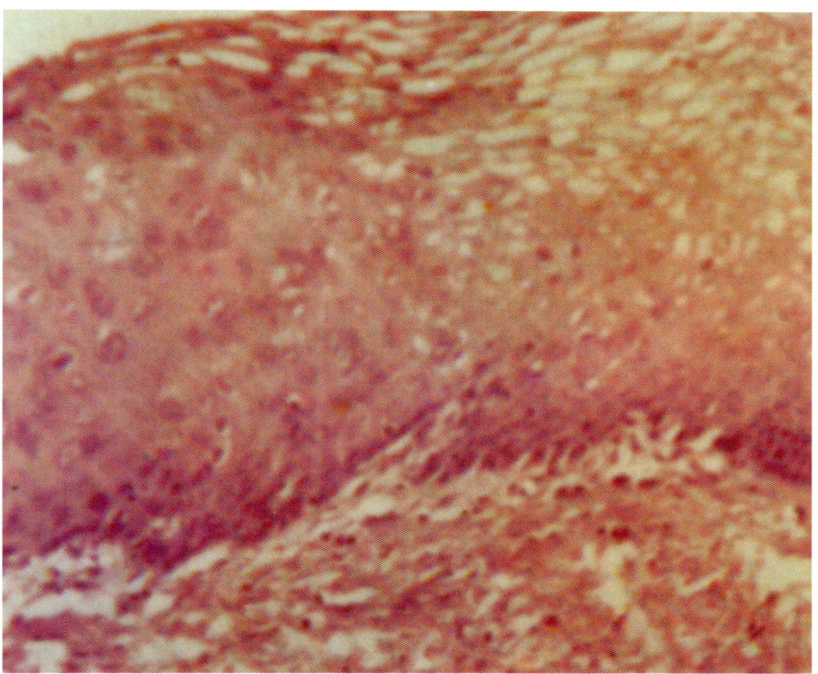

Fig. 9.11: Microphotograph: Co-existing CIN 1 and 2 — on extreme left, basal two-thirds of the epithelium is undifferentiated. The abnormality is decreasing and occupying only one-third as it is joining the normal squamous epithelium. Nuclear enlargement, loss of stratification and maturation can be very well appreciated

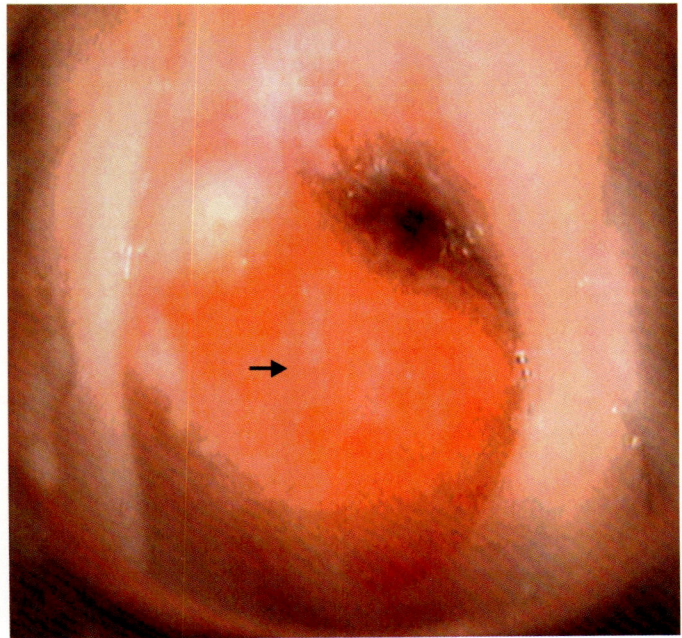

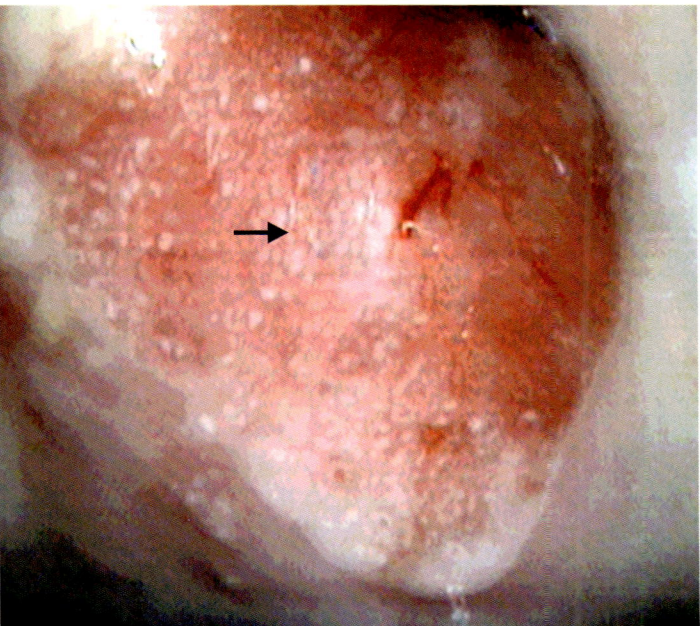

Fig. 9.12A: After saline application showing hyperemia over posterior lip

Fig. 9.12B: Same cervix following acetic acid: Grade 2 AW epithelium with coarse mosaic

Lesions appear quickly, last for several minutes and fade slowly (Figs 9.13 to 9.17A) and are iodine negative (Fig. 9.17B). Coarse punctations and mosaic may be seen (Figs 9.12B and 9.16). Intercapillary distance usually remains normal. These lesions mostly correspond to CIN 1–CIN 2 pathology. Sometimes different grades of acetowhite epithelium can be found in the same lesion.

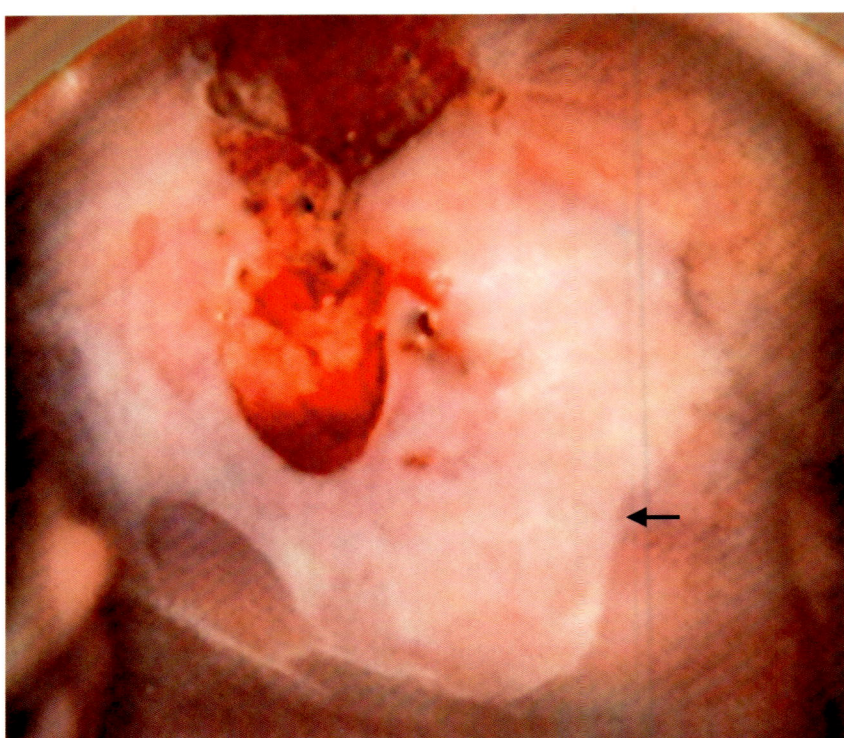

Fig. 9.13: AW epithelium with flat surface and sharp margins

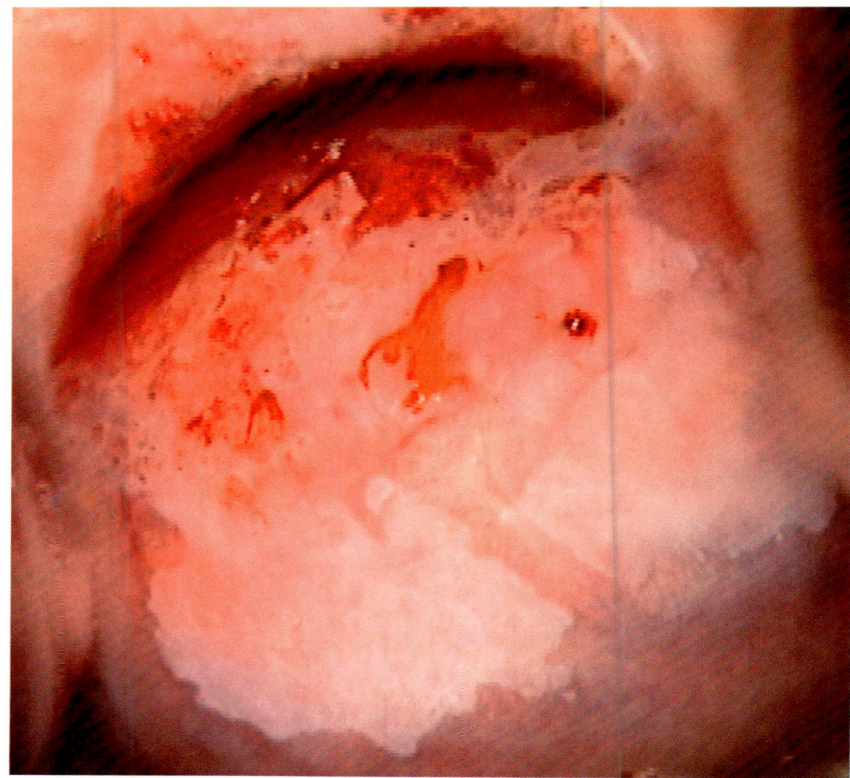

Fig. 9.14: AW epithelium with flat surface and sharp borders

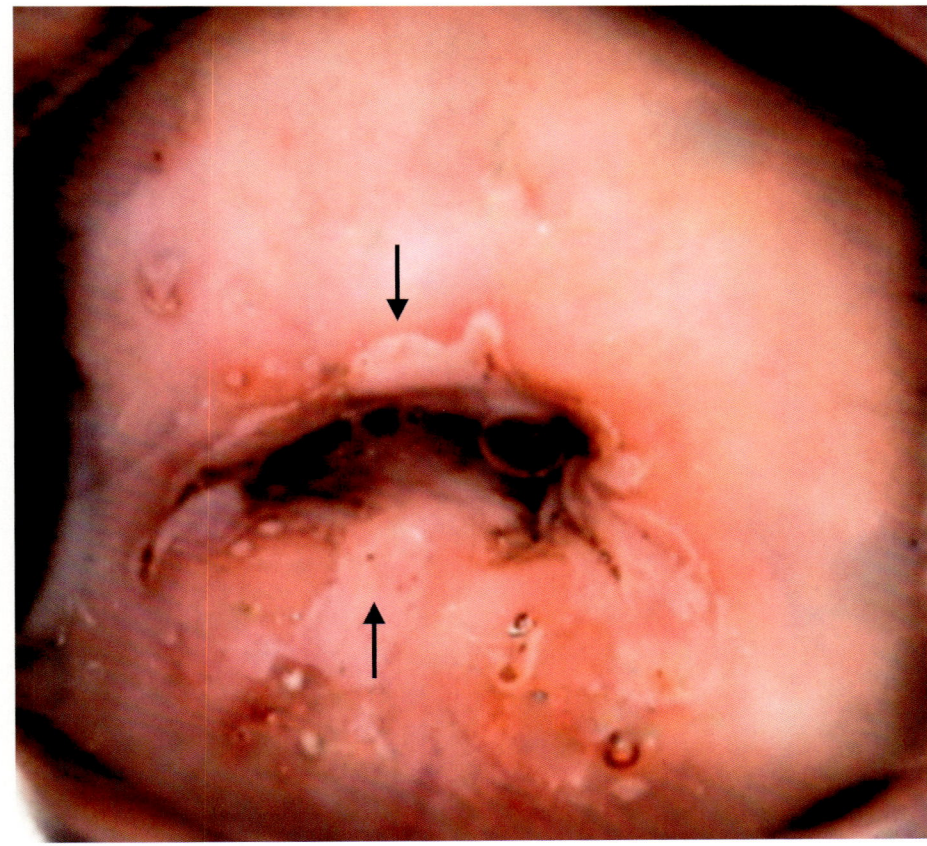

Fig. 9.15: AW epithelium with sharp border reaching inside endocervix over anterior lip; grade 1 epithelium seen over posterior lip

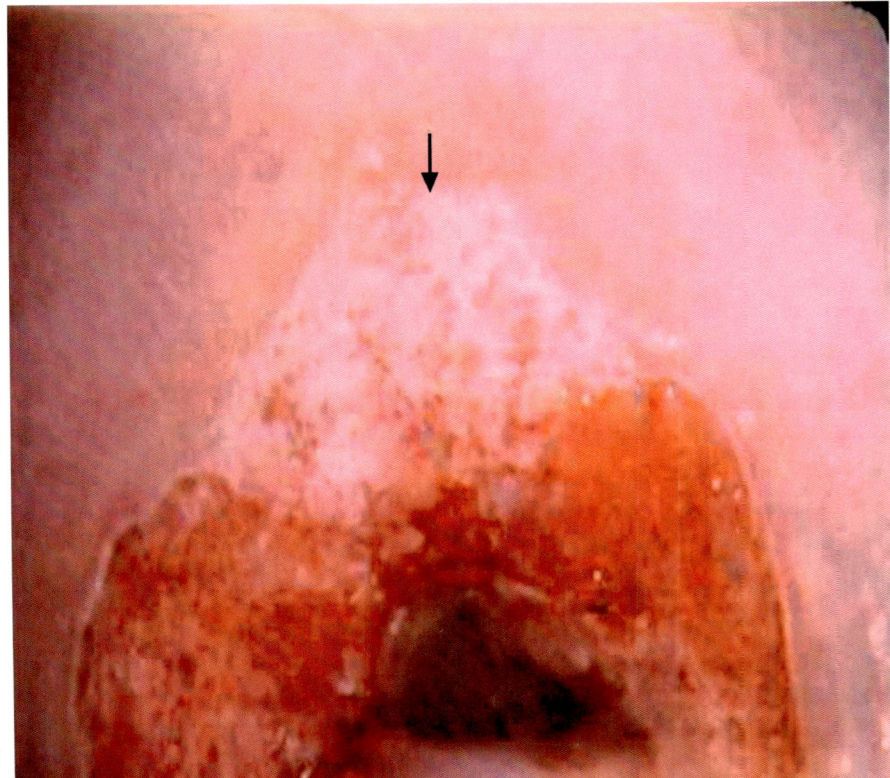

Fig. 9.16: Dense acetowhite ephithelium at 11–1 O'clock with coarse punctations

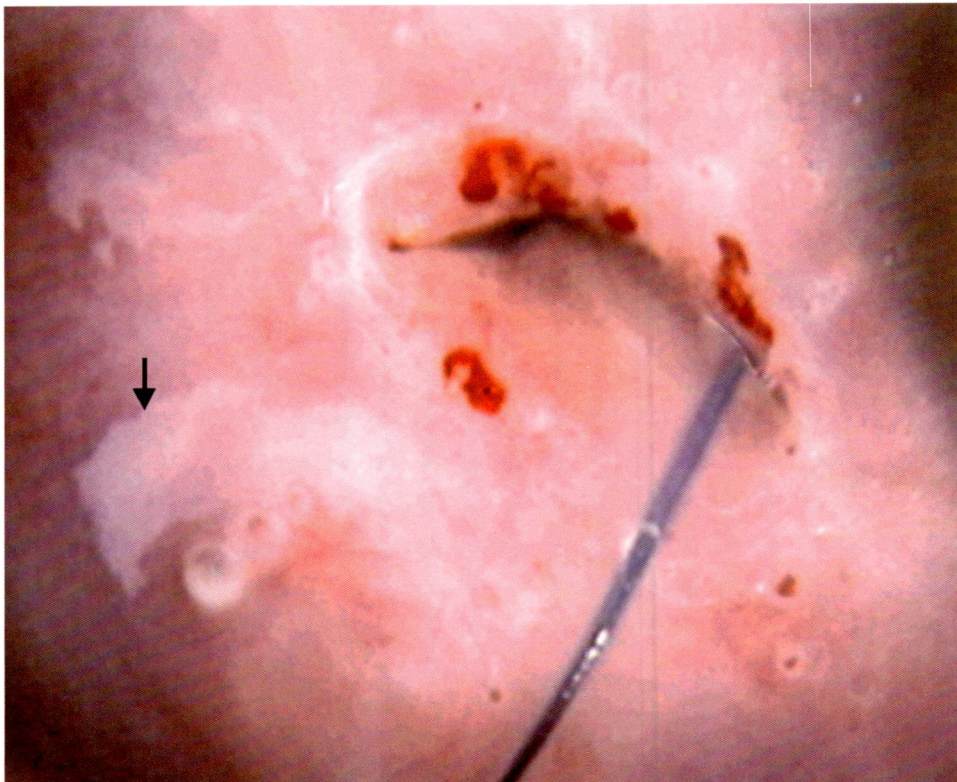

Fig. 9.17A: AW epithelium with flat surface and sharp borders over posterior lip but with indistinct border over anterior lip

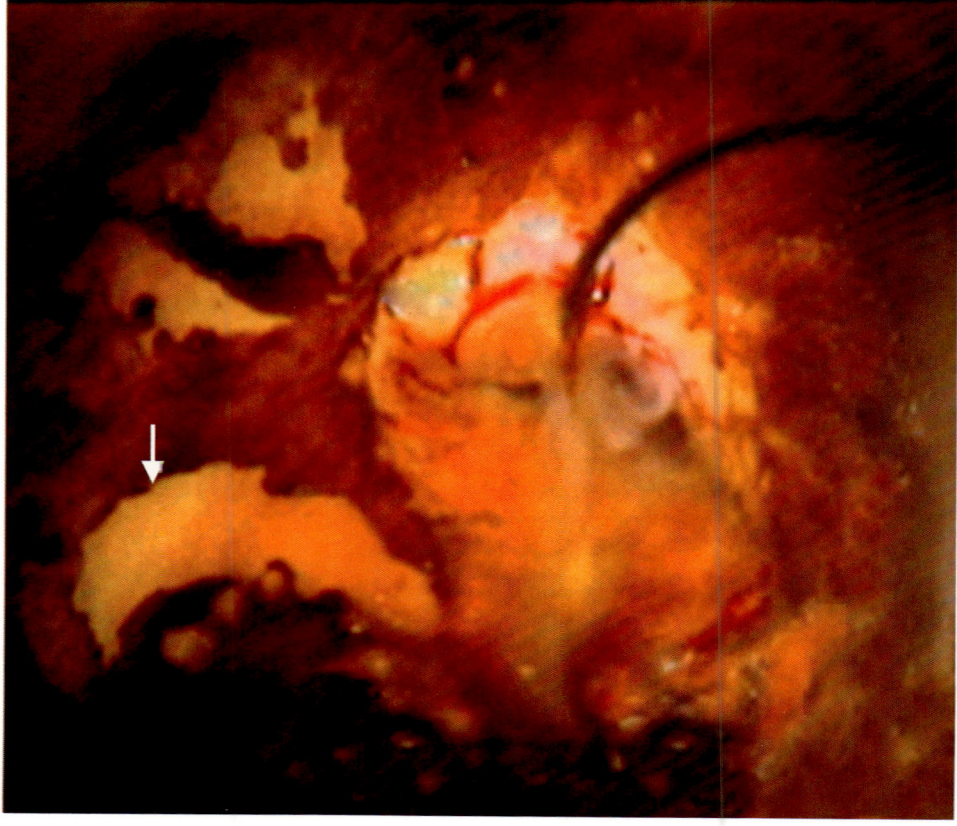

Fig. 9.17B: Same cervix— iodine negative

High Grade Lesions (Reid's Score 6–9)

It includes severe dysplasia as well as carcinoma in situ of the older terminology. Cellular abnormality is much more advanced and involves the full thickness of the epithelium.

CIN may involve the underlying crypts as well. Undifferentiated cells reach the topmost layer of the epithelium. Normal horizontal stratification of this surface layer is lost. No cell maturation takes place.

Colposcopy: Following saline application local hyperermia (Fig. 9.18A). After application of acetic acid, lesions appear very quickly, stay for a longer time and fade slowly.

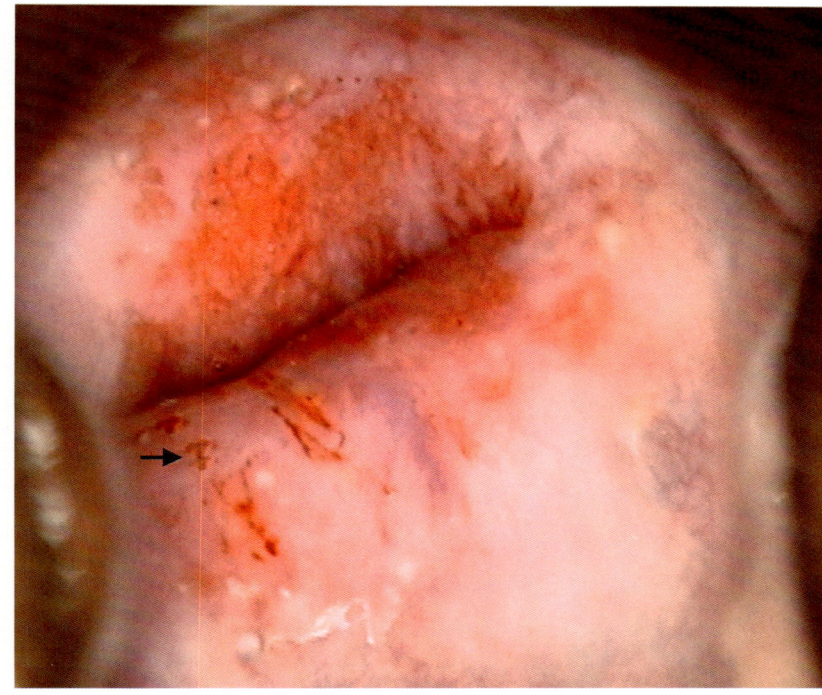

Fig. 9.18A: Hyperemia surrounding external os with coarse irregular punctations over anterior as well as posterior lip

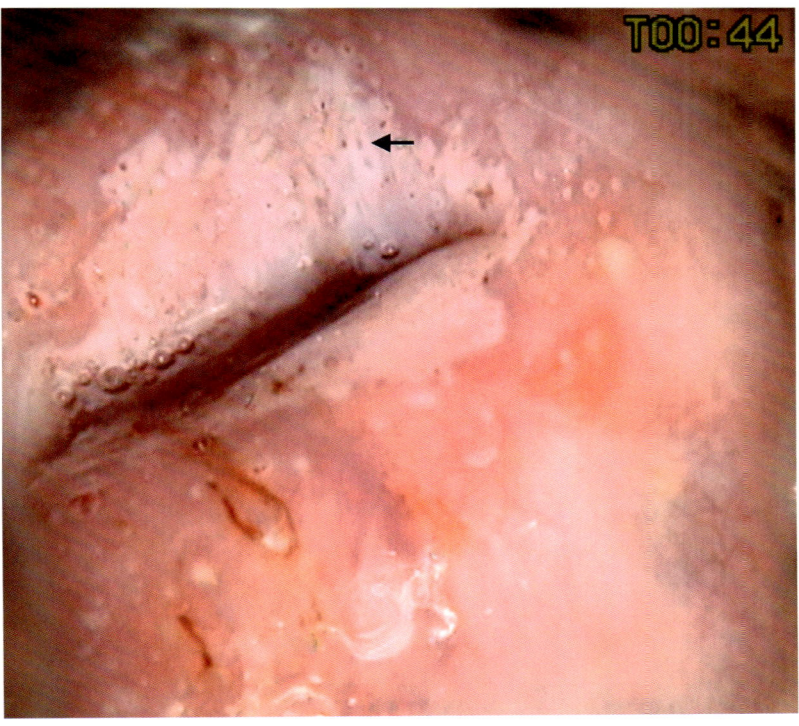

Fig. 9.18B: Same cervix after acetic acid application: Dense AW epithelium with raised surface over anterior lip reaching inside endocervix along with many cuffed gland openings

Lesions are ivory or oyster white in color with raised or may be uneven surface and have very sharp raised or rolled up margins (Figs 9.18B, 9.19 and 9.20). Cuffed gland opening may also be present. Vascular pattern is abnormal in the form of coarse and irregular mosaic or punctation (Fig. 9.24). Intercapillary distance is markedly increased.

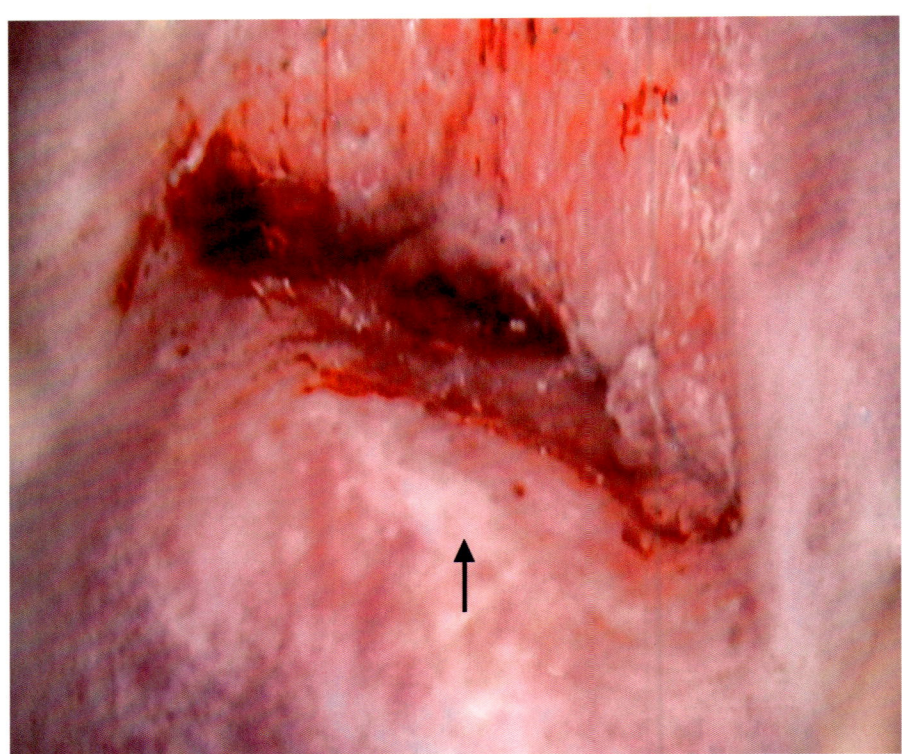

Fig. 9.19: AW epithelium with raised surface and cuffed gland opening inside TZ

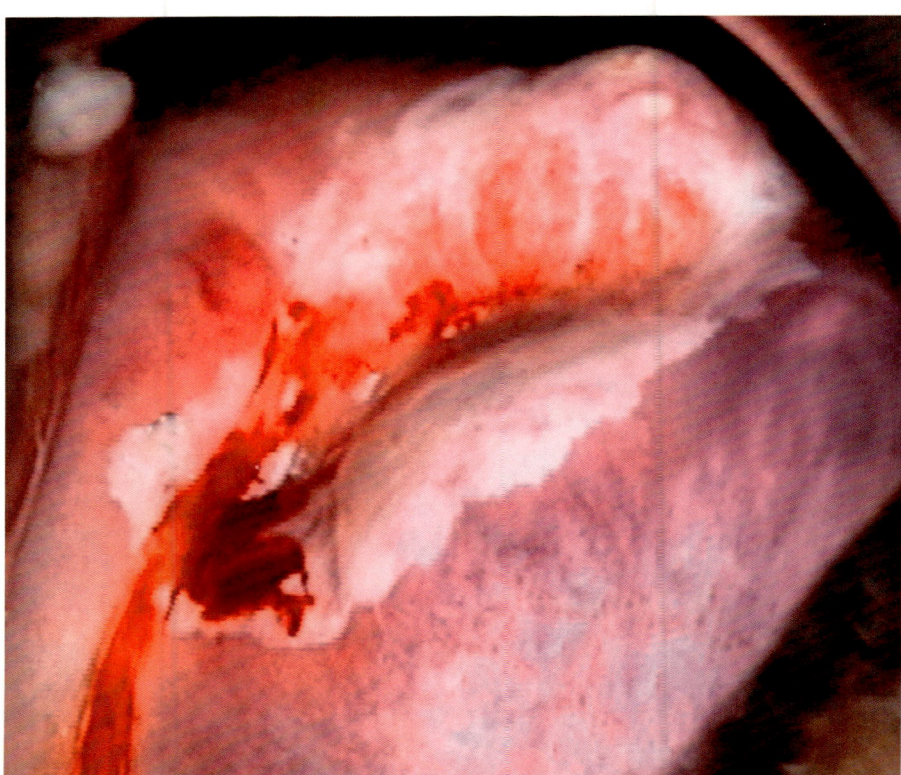

Fig. 9.20: Dense AW epthelium with raised surface and sharp margins

Higher grade central lesion may show internal borders when surrounded by peripheral low grade lesion. Such finding is known as **inner border sign** which is a sharp AW demarcation within a less opaque AW area (Figs 9.21 to 9.23) which is mostly associated with significant high grade lesions.

One grade of CIN does not occupy the transformation zone uniformly. Usually the caudal portion of the lesion is of a lower grade, while portion near squamo-columnar junction is of a higher grade (Fig. 9.21C). This is why it is extremely important to visualize and sample the upper limit of the lesion.

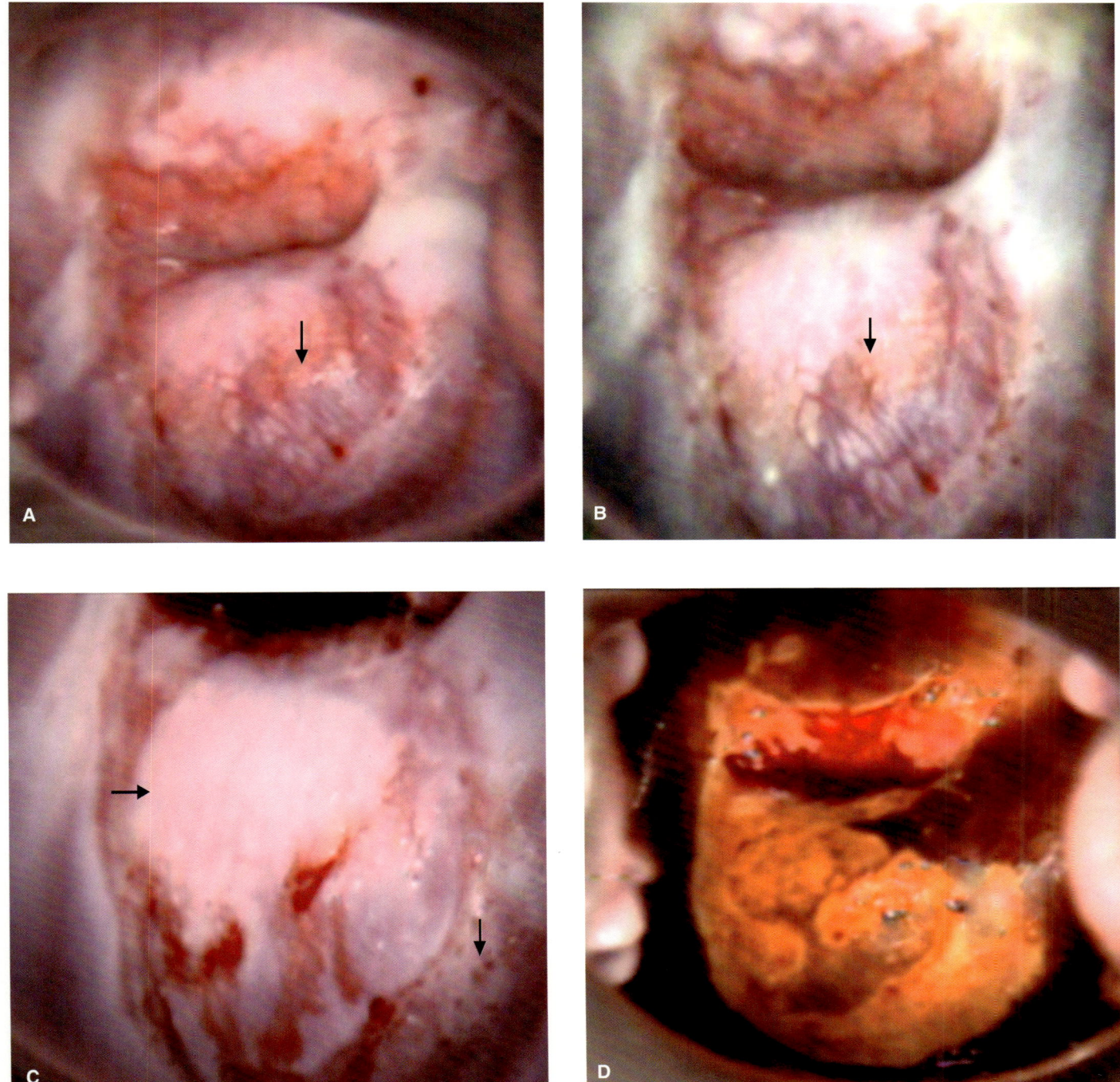

Fig. 9.21: (A) After saline: Local hyperemia and mosaic-like vasculature, (B) under green filter with mosaic-like vasculature, (C)after acetic acid: thick raised AW epithelium with sharp internal border and coarse punctations, (D) after iodine application: no iodine uptake

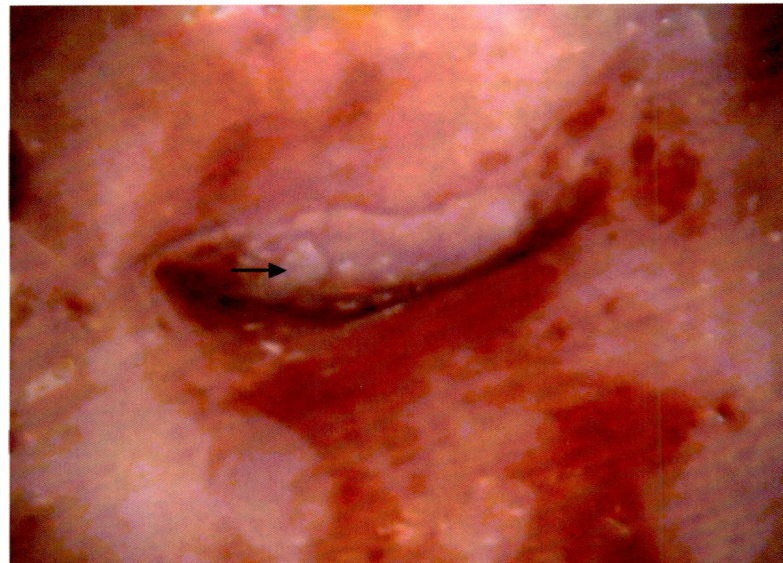

Fig. 9.22: Dense high grade AW lesion with inner border surrounded by peripheral low grade lesion reaching inside endocervix

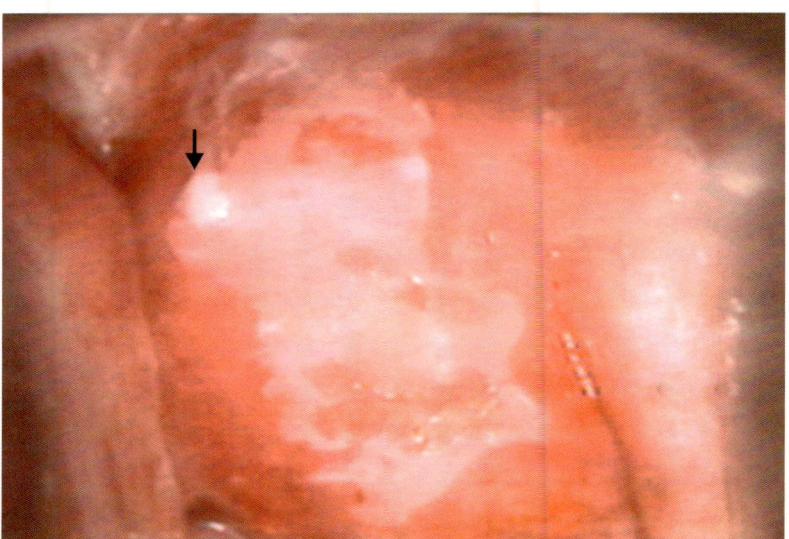

Fig. 9.23: Dense AW epithelium with raised surface and inner border surrounded by thinner epithelium

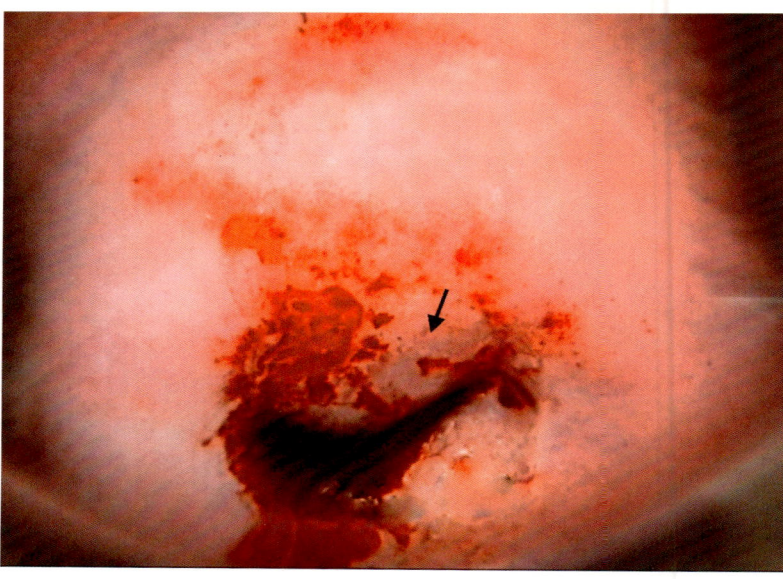

Fig. 9.24: AW epithelium with coarse punctations reaching inside endocervix

Major lesions may show **ridge sign** also (Fig. 9.25). At times in CIN, only keratosis can be found on the cervix overlying the abnormal epithelium and that is why all keratotic lesions must be biopsied especially when they are surrounded by AW epithelium (Fig. 9.26).

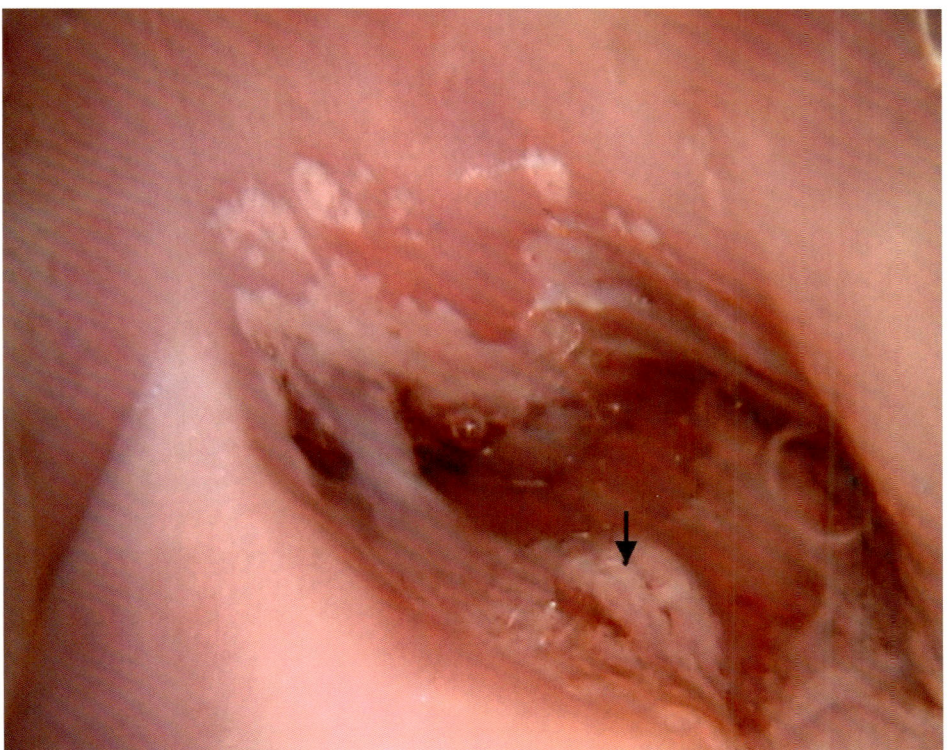

Fig. 9.25: Thick opaque epithelium on the anterior lip near SCJ between 9 to 11 O' clock. Posterior lip shows thick opaque AW epithelium growing as ledge near SCJ (ridge sign) at 6 O' clock

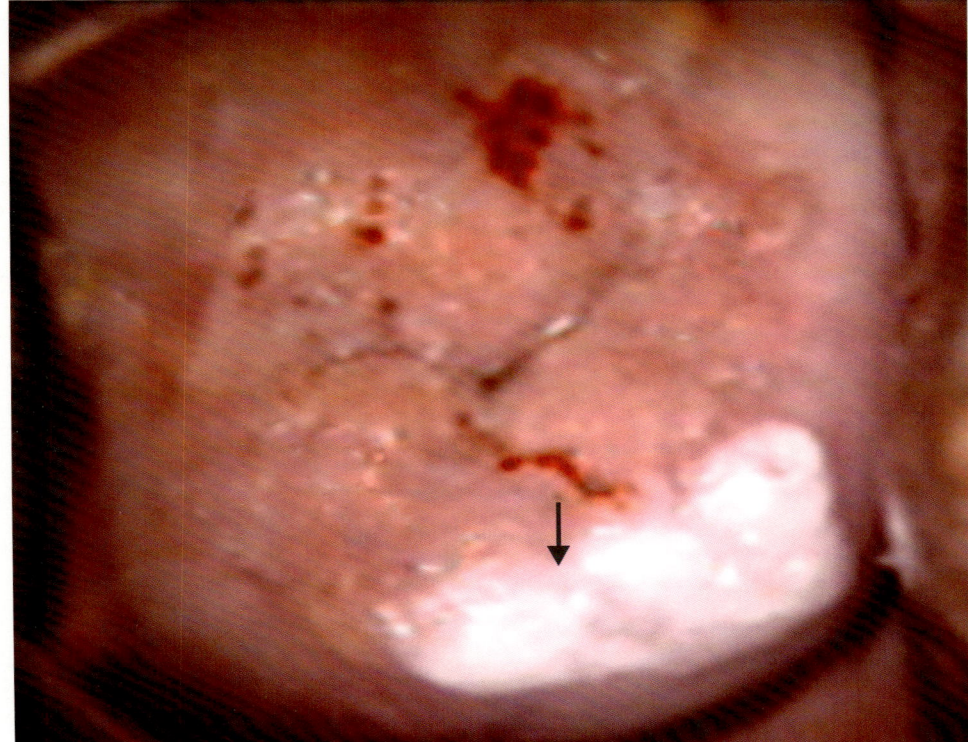

Fig. 9.26: Thick keratotic lesion with lobulated surface surrounded by AW epithelium

GLANDULAR INTRAEPITHELIAL LESIONS

Similar to squamous epithelium, cervical glandular epithelium may show a spectrum of intraepithelial changes ranging from mild to severe abnormalities known as glandular intraepithelial neoplasia (GIN), which is divided into low grade and high grade GIN. Low grade lesions include atypical glandular changes associated with inflammation, post-radiotherapy, and mild atypical hyperplastic changes less severe than adenocarcinoma in situ (AIS). High grade CIGN includes AIS only.

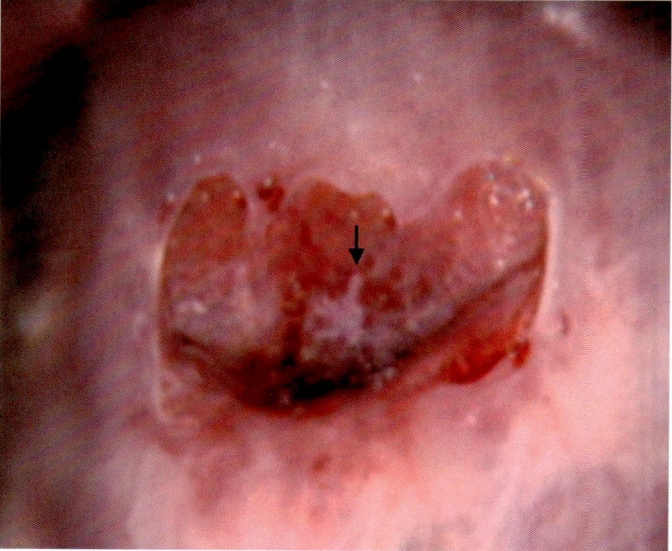

Fig. 9.27: Isolated elevated AW lesion over columnar epithelium not contiguous with SCJ

Adenocarcinoma in situ of cervix is much less common in comparison to its squmous counterpart and is found mainly in younger women. The use of endocervical brush has increased its detection.

These lesions may be multifocal in origin and a significant number of cases are associated with concurrent high grade squamous lesions. The abnormality mostly involves surface epithelium alone and may sometimes have associated involvement of crypt epithelium. It is rare to find crypt abnormality alone.

Adenocarcinoma in situ is detected easily when associated with squamous lesion or occasionally when present on the ectocervix. But detection is difficult when the lesion occurs alone as the lesions can be found beneath normal metaplastic or dysplastic epithelium. They can lie lateral to a squamous lesion, between two squamous lesions or above the squamous in mixed lesions and lie higher within the endocervix in pure glandular variety.

Colposcopic Appearances

In comparison to squamous lesions, the glandular lesions are difficult to recognize colposcopically as there is no characteristic colposcopic appearance for glandular abnormalities. The lesion may be recognized by the presence of wide gland openings or discrete patches of large fused papillae of varying size somewhat acetowhite that may be confused with immature metaplasia, condylomata or microglandular hyperplasia.

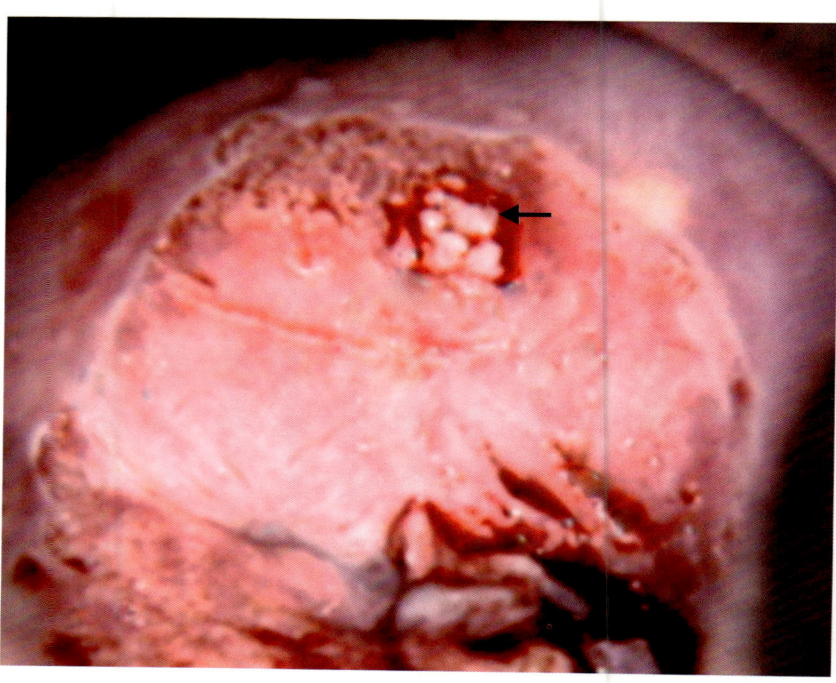

Fig. 9.28: Isolated block of papillary like fusion surrounded by metaplastic epithelium

For differentiating such lesions, Cecil Wright has described the following colposcopic criteria:

1. Lesion location over columnar epithelium not contiguous with SCJ (Fig. 9.27)
2. Large fused papillary excrescences (Fig. 9.28)
3. Single or multiple dots at the tips of papillary projections produced by looped vessels (Fig. 9.29)
4. Papillary processes with scalloped edges and budding
5. Flat patchy red and white areas (Fig. 9.30)
6. Atypical vessels resembling waste-thread, tendril, root, and character writing (Fig. 9.31)
7. Large gland or crypt openings (Fig. 9.32)

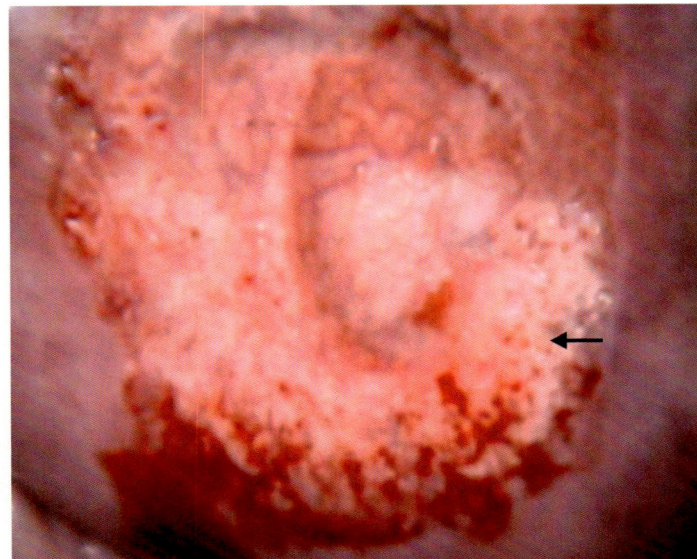

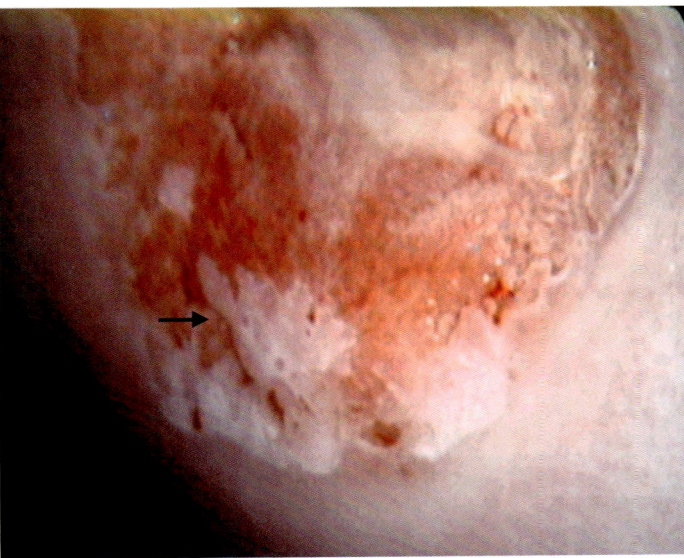

Fig. 9.29: Papillary like fusions with multiple dots at the tips of papillary projections suggestive of GIN

Fig. 9.30: Flat variegated red and white area between 5 and 7 O' clock (ACIS on biopsy)

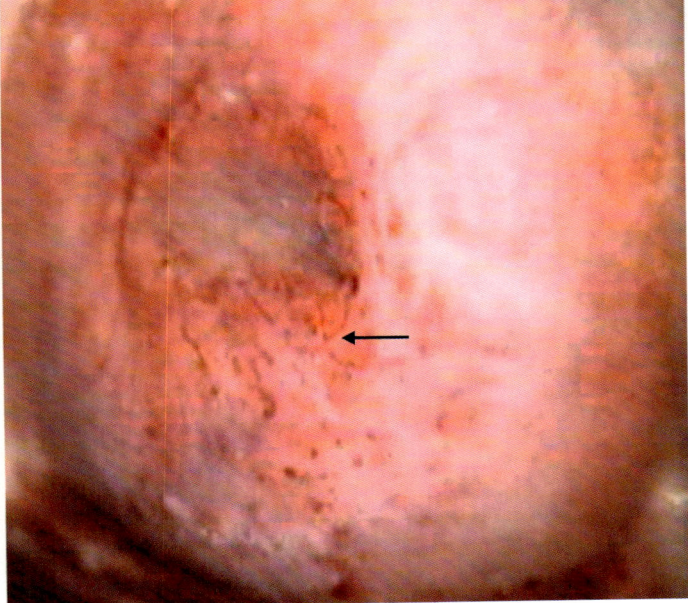

Fig. 9.31: Waste-thread like vessels seen over the posterior lip near SC junction

Thus one should have a high index of suspicion for glandular lesions, if the abovementioned findings are seen in the presence of cytological picture of atypical glandular cells/AGC favoring neoplasia/AIS (Figs 9.27 to 9.33).

Mostly diagnosis of adenocarcinoma in situ is made by histopathology of directed biopsy or in cone biopsy specimens. The grading of lesion is determined by the degree of cellular abnormality. Early invasion is more difficult to diagnose because newly formed malignant glands do not easily give the impression of infiltration, unlike changes in the early stromal invasion in squamous cell carcinoma.

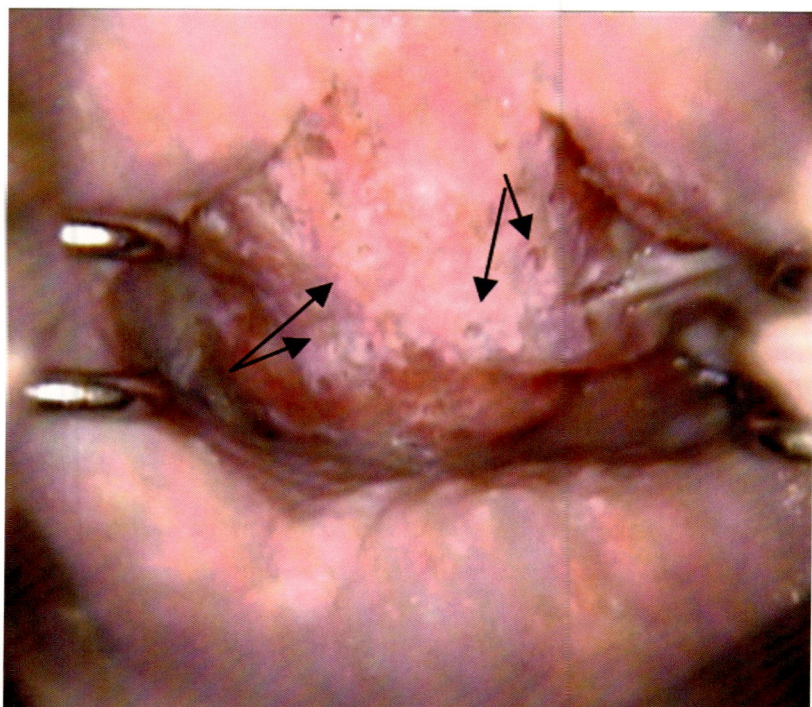

Fig. 9.32: Large gland openings in acetowhite area inside endocervical canal suggestive of GIN

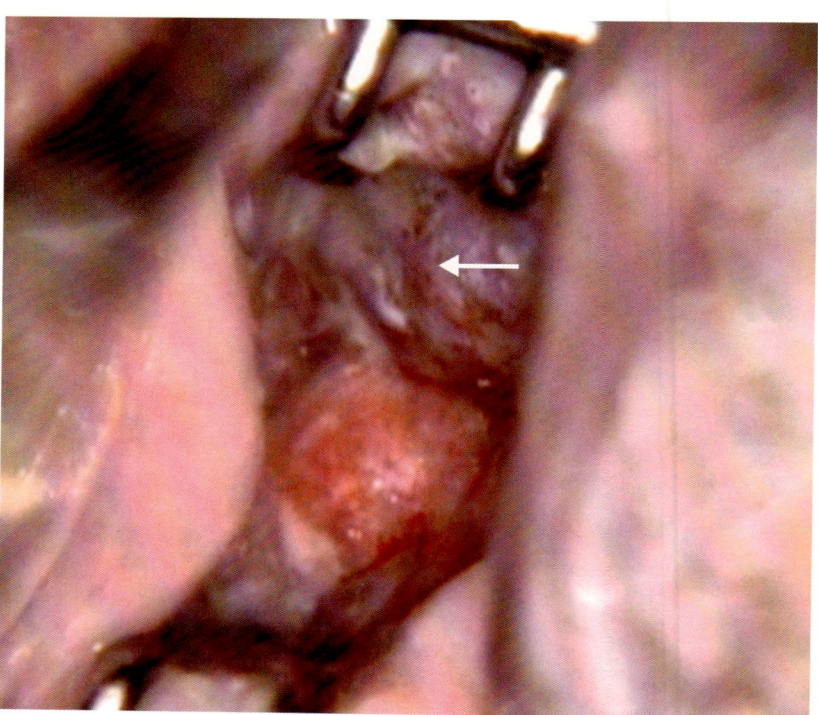

Fig. 9.33: Endocervix showing coarse punctations and AW epithelium scattered all over suggestive of adenocarcinoma, proven on endocervical curettage biopsy

Invasive Lesions

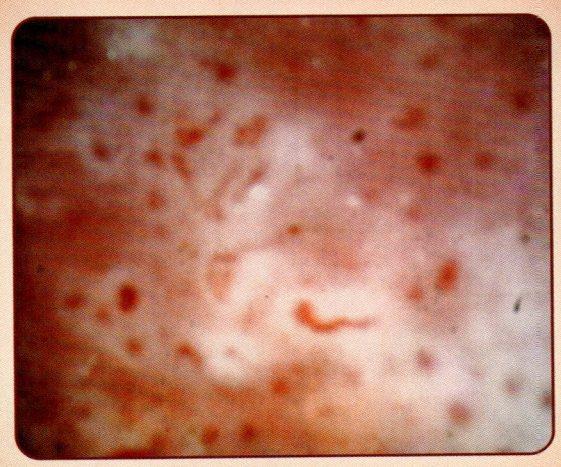

Chapter Outline

Macroscopically, clear cut invasive lesion can be easily identified by naked eye on per speculum examination and does not require colposcopy for its diagnosis (Fig. 10.1). But for the diagnosis of early stromal invasive and microinvasive lesions, use of colposcopy is of great value.

As already described earlier, invasion is mostly preceded by cervical intraepithelial neoplasia, which lies dormant for some length of period that may vary from one year to as long as 20 years and then progresses to invasive carcinoma. In intraepithelial stage, basement membrane of the epithelium remains intact. As invasion occurs, the basement membrane is breeched by neoplastic cells which divide and invade the underlying connective tissue stroma.

After invasion occurs, neoplastic cells proliferate rapidly in a disorderly manner. To meet the increased nutritional requirement of the rapidly proliferating epithelium, tumor angiogenetic factor (TAF) is released which gives rise to neovascularization. These newly formed vessels give rise to localized hyperemia and decrease in intercapillary distance initially. As the disorderly proliferation of cancer cells continue, some of the vessels disappear resulting in increased intercapillary distance and even large avascular area. Disappearance of large number of capillaries at times may cause ischemic necrosis of tissue leading to ulceration. Irregular blocks of neoplasic cells cause abnormal proliferation and distortion of vascular pattern resulting in formation of atypical blood vessels.

In invasive carcinoma, there is abnormal proliferation of epithelium as well as the connective tissue stroma. Colposcopic pattern depends upon the predominance of the proliferating component in an area. Edema or fibrosis of connective tissue may predominate in exophytic or endophytic lesions respectively altering the colposcopic appearance. Neoplastic cells have abundance of proteins in nuclei as well as cytoplasm and become oyster white after application of acetic acid. They lack in glycogen and are iodine negative. Keratinizing squamous cell carcinoma also give rise to keratin formation.

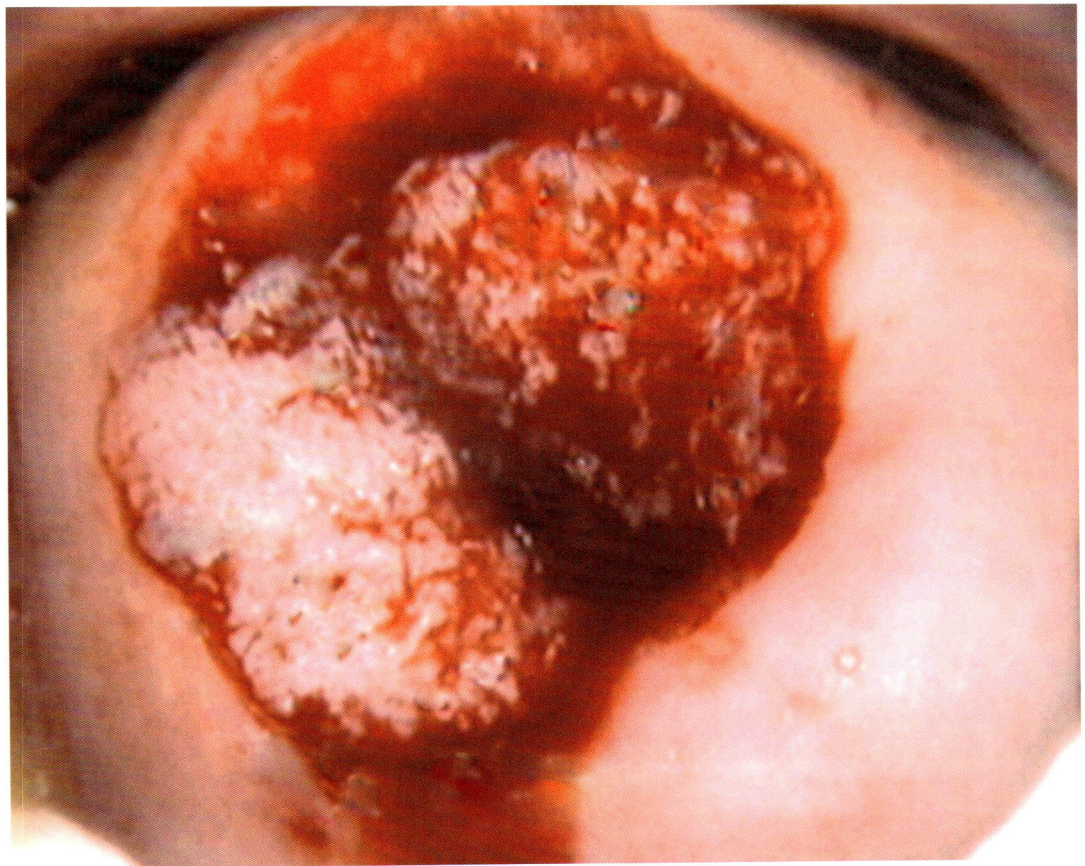

Fig. 10.1: Proliferative growth of cervix on naked eye examination

Colposcopy

Main aim of colposcopy is to take biopsy from the most abnormal area to rule out invasion. Several studies show that most severe lesions may not always demonstrate the most abnormal findings, and approximately 50% cases of microinvasive cancers may be missed on colposcopy. At times even focal invasive cancer may be difficult to distinguish (Figs 10.2A and B).

To differentiate between preinvasive and invasive lesions, one must take into account surface contour, color tone, clarity of demarcation, intercapillary distance and the vascular pattern altogether (Figs 10.3A to C).

IFCPC 2011 terminology criteria for possible invasion include atypical vessels and additional findings: fragile vessels, irregular surface, exophytic lesion, necrosis, ulceration, and tumor/gross neoplasm.

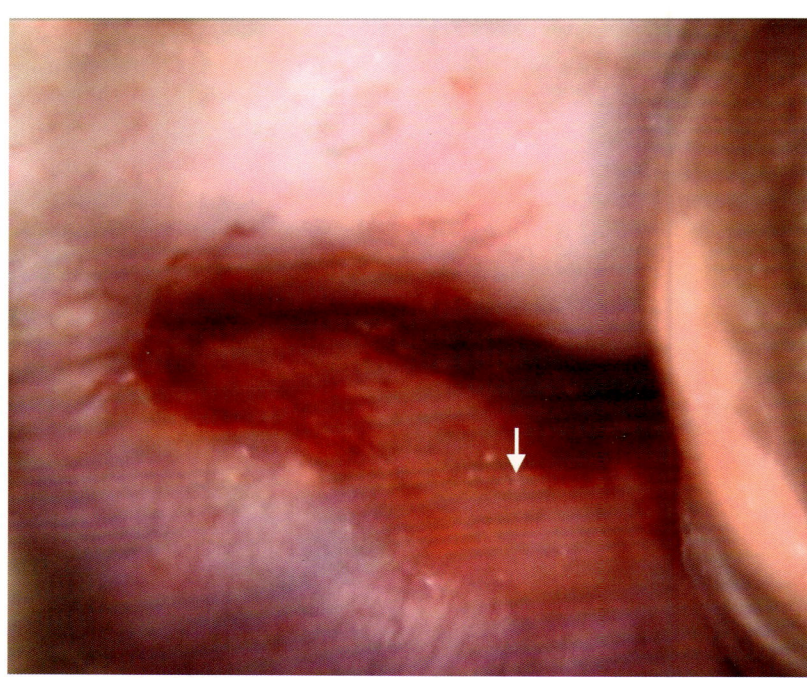

Fig. 10.2A: After normal saline: Focal raised area and hyperemia over posterior lip

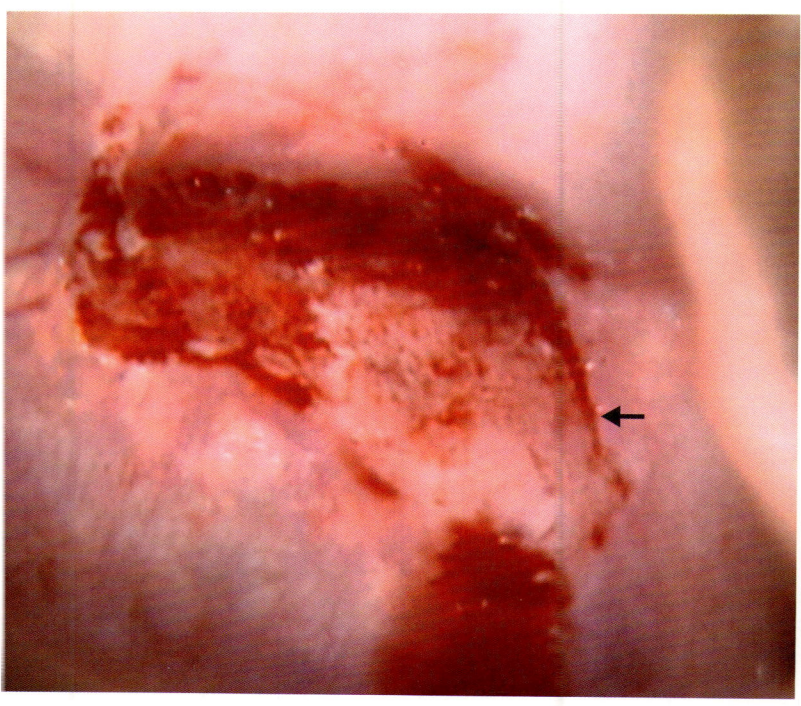

Fig. 10.2B: Same cervix after acetic acid: Thick AW epithelium, coarse punctations and fragile vessels

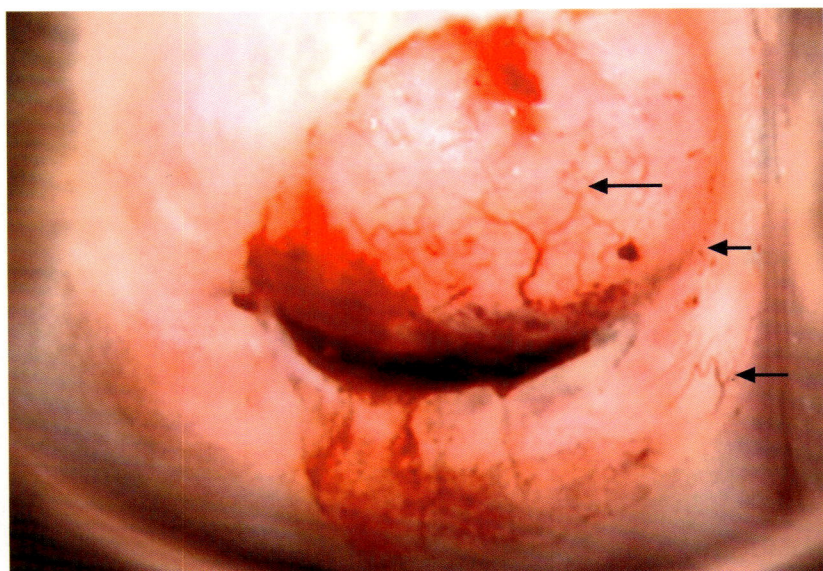

Fig. 10.3A: After saline application: Atypical vessels and coarse punctations

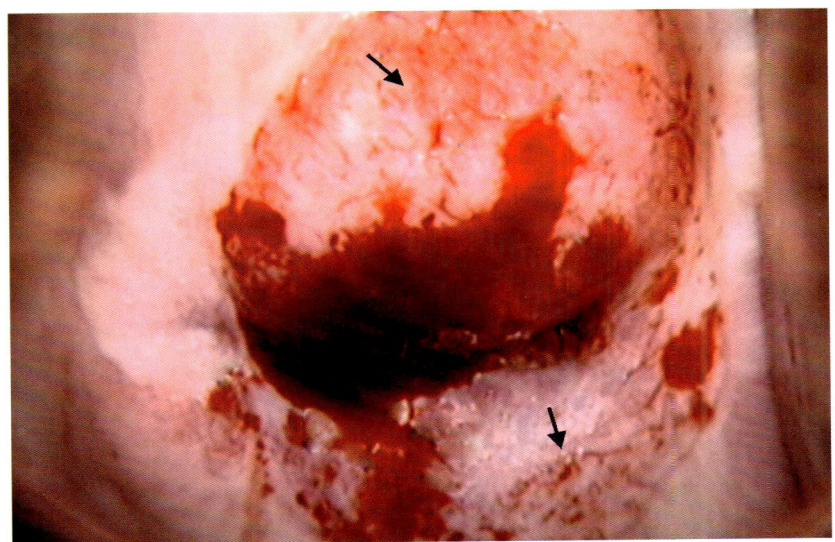

Fig. 10.3B: Same cervix after acetic acid application: Dense AW epithelium, atypical vessels and coarse punctations

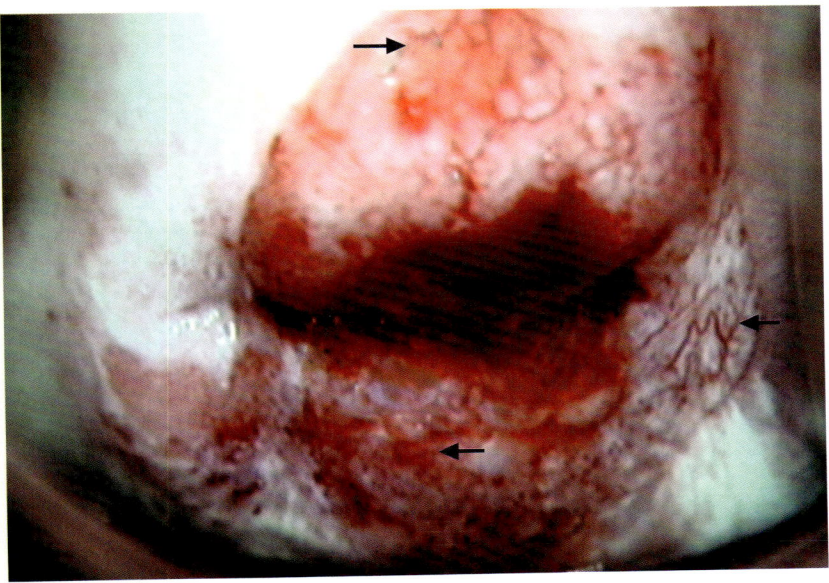

Fig. 10.3C: Under green filter: Coarse mosaic on anterior lip, coarse punctations on posterior lip. Many atypical vessels are also seen

SQUAMOUS CELL CARCINOMA

Colposcopic appearance differs in exophytic and endophytic lesions.

Exophytic Form

In exophytic form, the lesion is soft, surface contour is irregular, breech of mucosal integrity may be there, Intense acetowhite epithelium along with vascular abnormalities may also be seen (Figs 10.4A to C). Later, surface may show ulceration and necrosis (Figs 10.5 and 10.6). Lesions bleed very easily on minor touch because of friability of the vessels (Fig. 10.7).

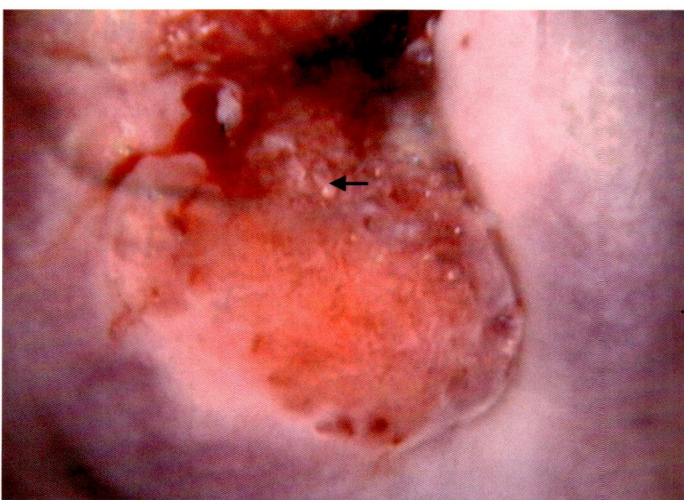

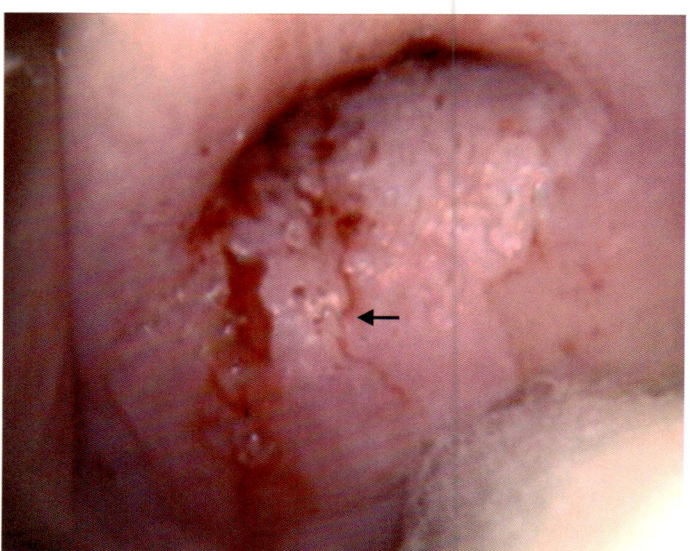

Fig. 10.4A: After saline application: Slightly irregular surface near os, hyperemia over posterior lip

Fig. 10.4B: Same cervix after acetic acid: Thick acetowhite lesion with grade 3–4 gland openings and atypical vessels

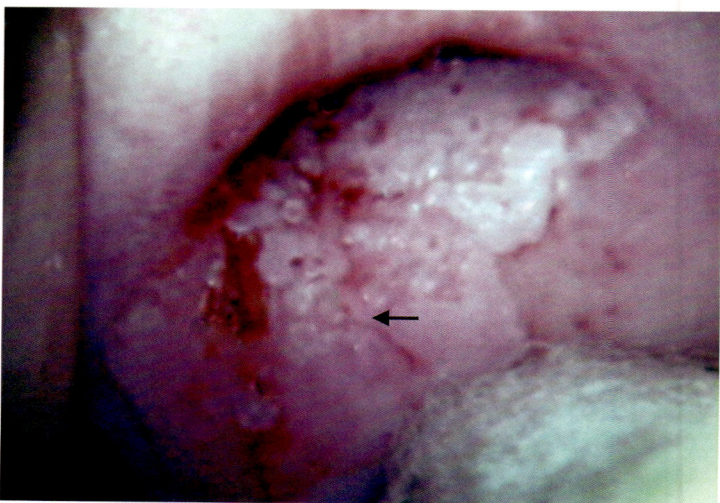

Fig. 10.4C: Same cervix under green filter

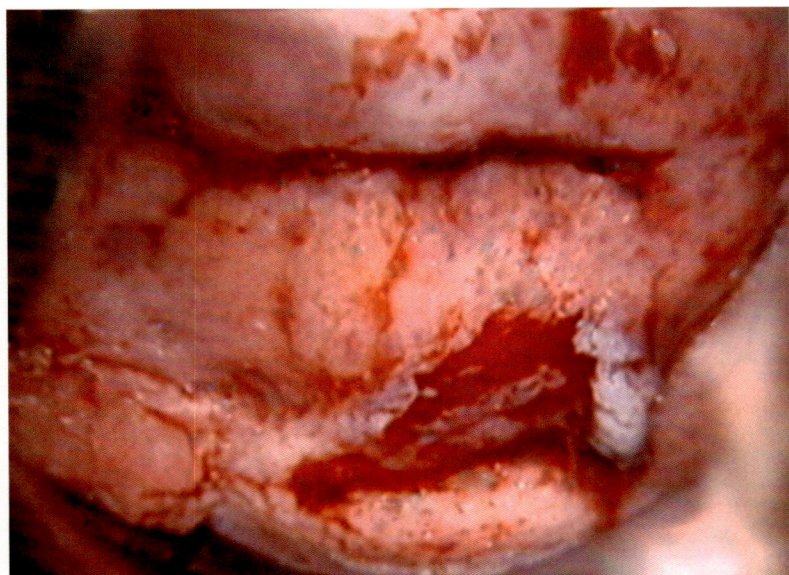

Fig. 10.5: Ulcerative lesion with acetowhite epithelium and atypical vessels

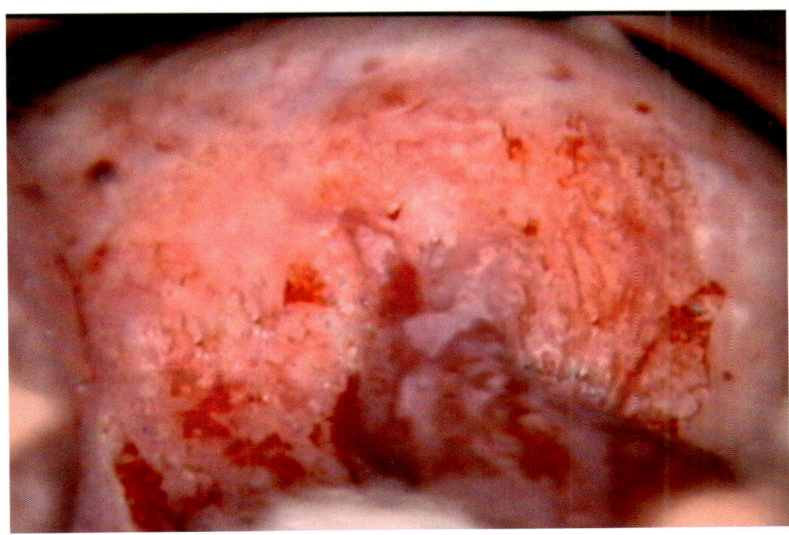

Fig.10.6: Ulcerative lesion, AW epithelium and atypical vessels, bleeding on touch

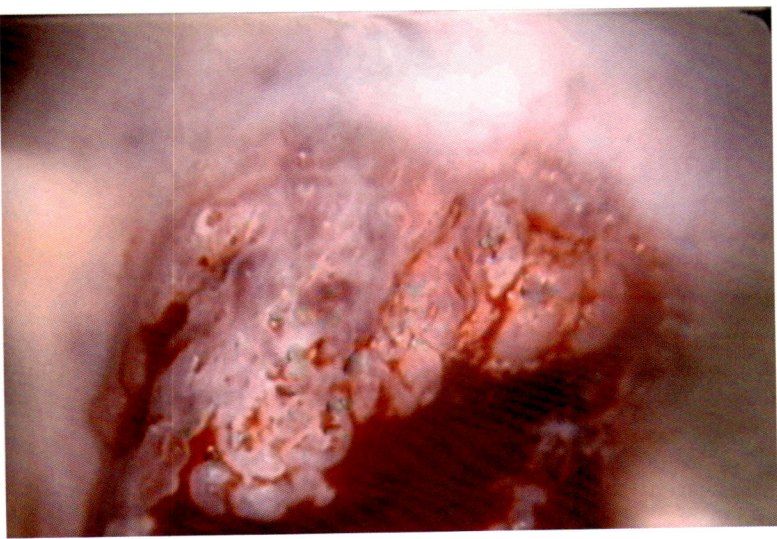

Fig. 10.7: Soft, exophytic growth with irregular surface contour, AW epithelium and atypical, friable vessels

Endophytic Form

In **endophytic form**, lesion is hard and cervix is retracted. Very thick acetowhite area may be seen (Figs 10.8A and B). Vascular abnormalities may or may not be seen in endophytic lesions. Sometimes thick, irregular keratosis can be seen overlying the neoplastic lesions (Figs 10.9A and B).

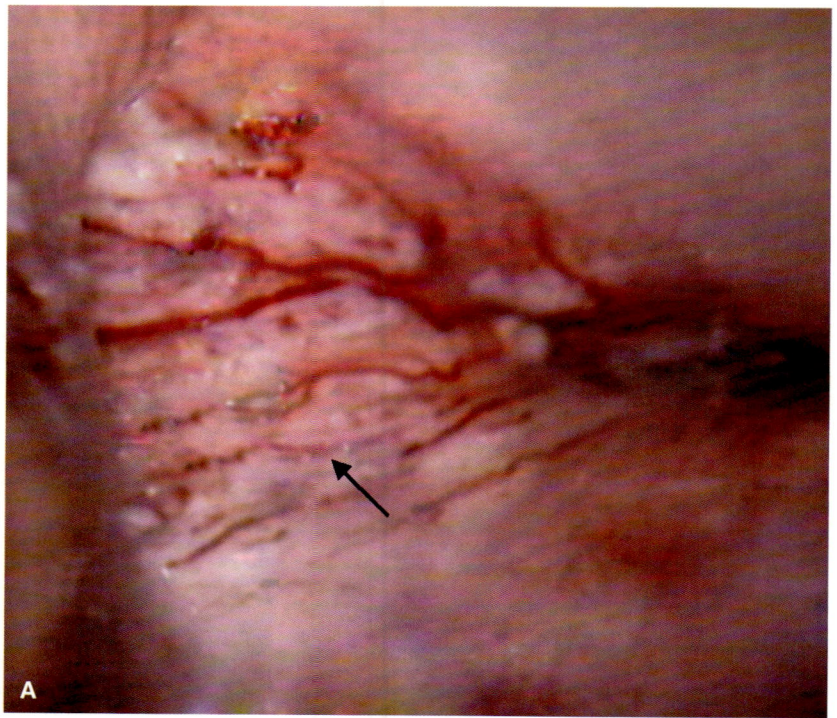

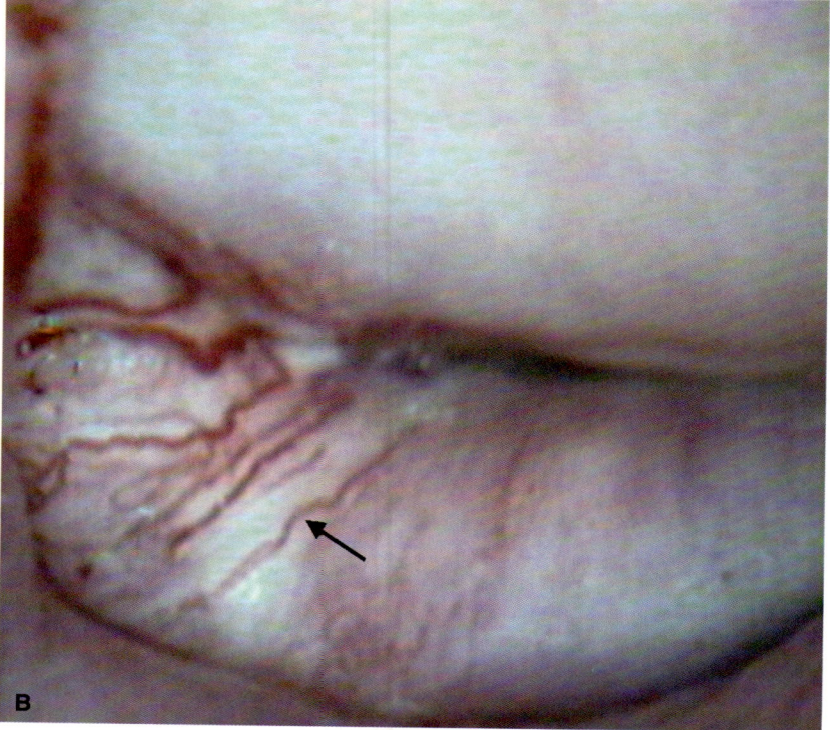

Figs 10.8A and B: After acetic acid application: Endophytic lesion with thick irregular acetowhite lesion, atypical vessels in localized area on right lateral part of the cervix

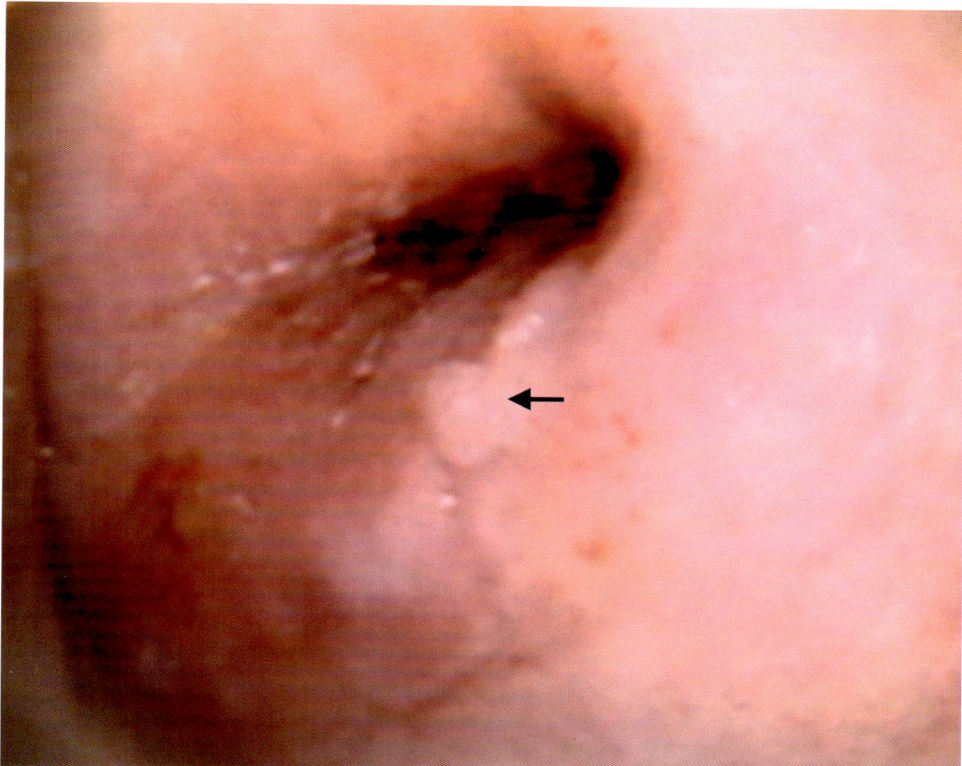

Fig. 10.9A: After saline application: Thick keratosis over posterior lip

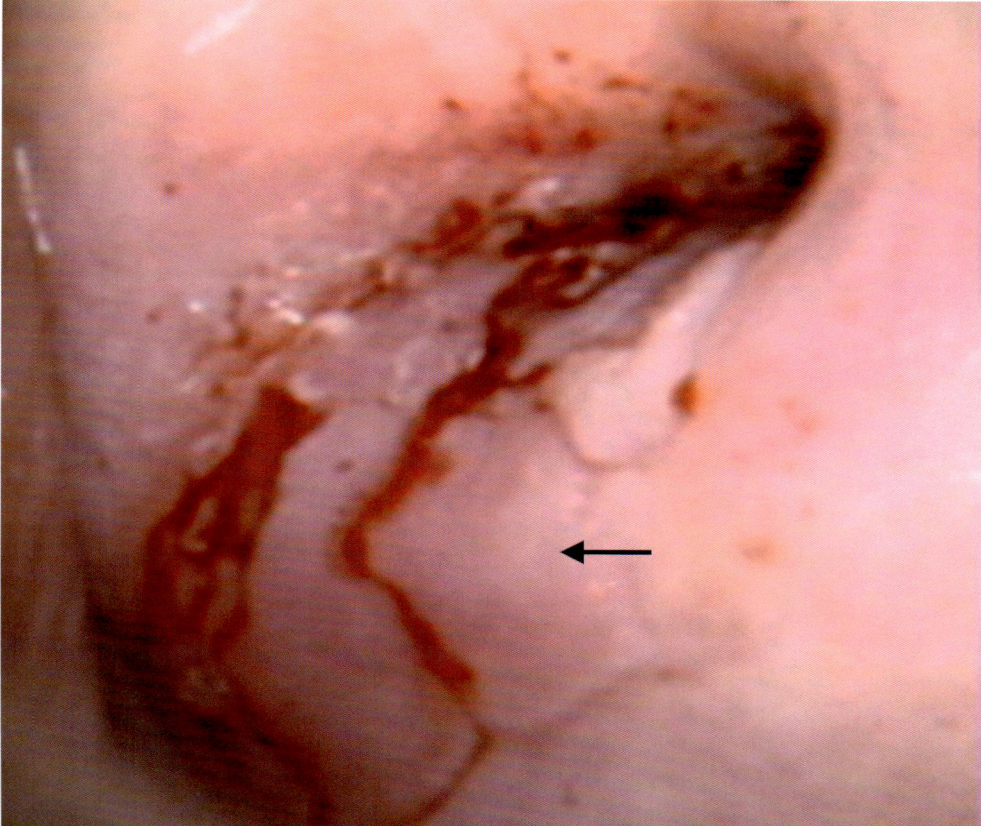

Fig. 10.9B: Same cervix after acetic acid: Thick AW epithelium, coarse punctations and fragile atypical vessels

Atypical Vessels

Atypical vessels are the hallmark of invasion and are almost always found only in invasive cancer. Atypical blood vessels are strikingly irregular in size, calibre, shape, course and mutual arrangement. These may be horizontal superficial vessels running parallel to the surface having irregular course with sharp, irregular bends, may show constrictions and dilatation and may appear or disappear abruptly.

Vessels are usually placed at a greater distance than normal, at times having irregular and large avascular fields. They do not have dichotomus tree-like branching. There is no steady decrease in diameter of the dividing branches which may also have sharp and irregular bends (Fig. 10.8). Bizarre vessels in the form of spaghetti, corkscrew or comma shapes may be seen (Figs 10.10 to 10.13).

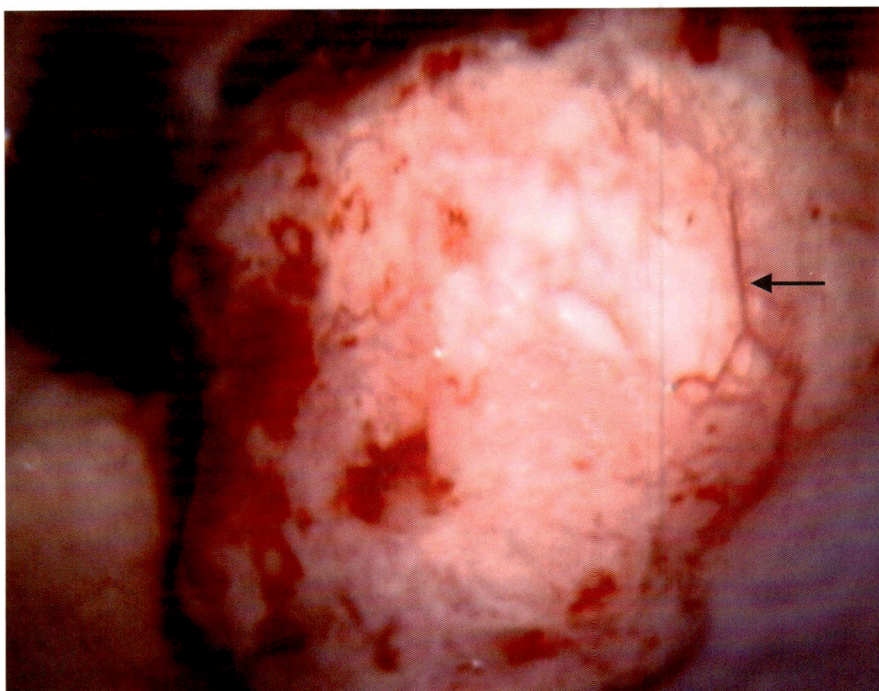

Fig. 10.10A: After saline application: Part of the cervix showing hard growth with AW epithelium and atypical vessels

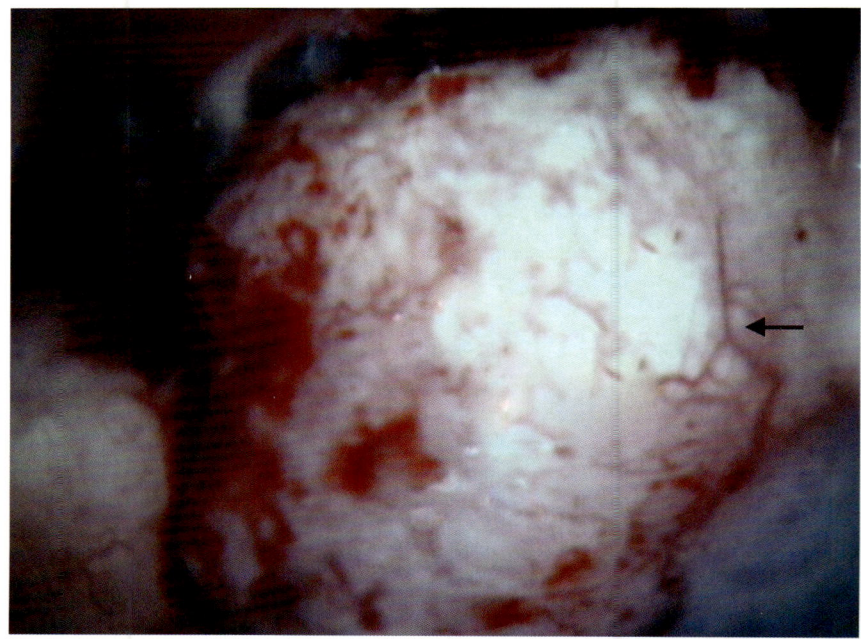

Fig. 10.10B: Same cervix under green filter

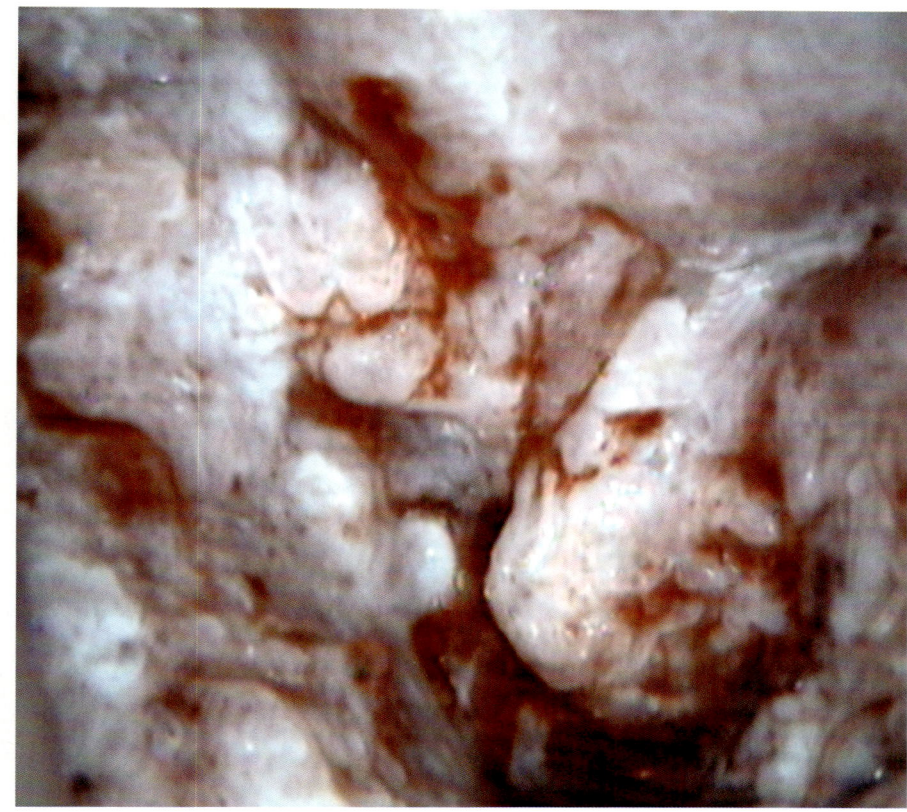

Fig. 10.11: Exophytic growth under green filter showing irregular surface contour, dense AW epithelium, coarse punctations and atypical vessels

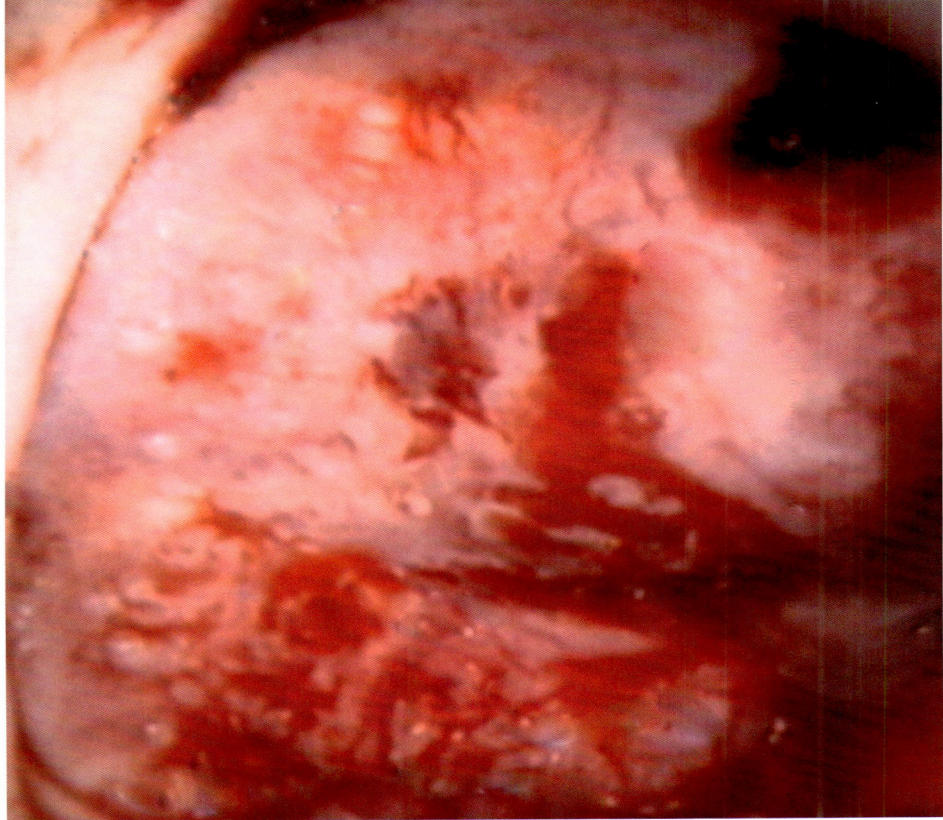

Fig. 10.12: Atypical vessels seen in various shapes

When atypical vessels make their appearance in an extensive area of mosaic or punctation in a CIN lesion, it indicates early invasion (Fig. 10.14).

Vascular atypia is more common in well-differentiated squamous cell carcinoma than poorly differentiated lesions and adenocarcinoma, wherein early stages intercapillary distance usually remains normal and vessels may not show any atypical pattern. Sometimes vascular changes of early invasive cancer may be very difficult to recognize. There may not be any discernible pattern of vessel arrangement.

Microinvasion is a histological diagnosis depending upon the depth of invasion. It cannot be diagnosed on colposcopy only.

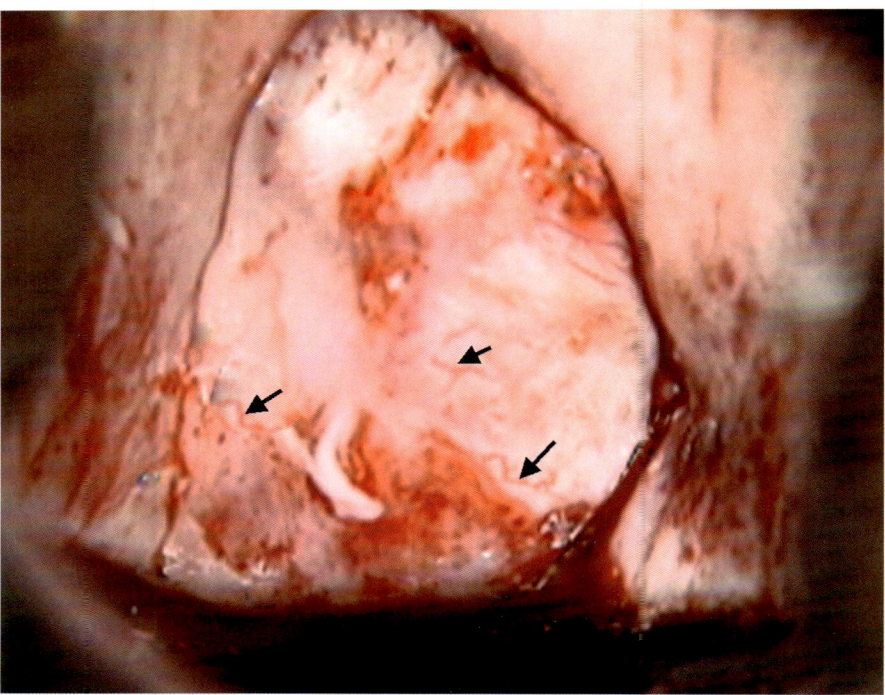

Fig. 10.13: Cervix with irregular surface contour, dense AW epithelium atypical vessels and rag sign

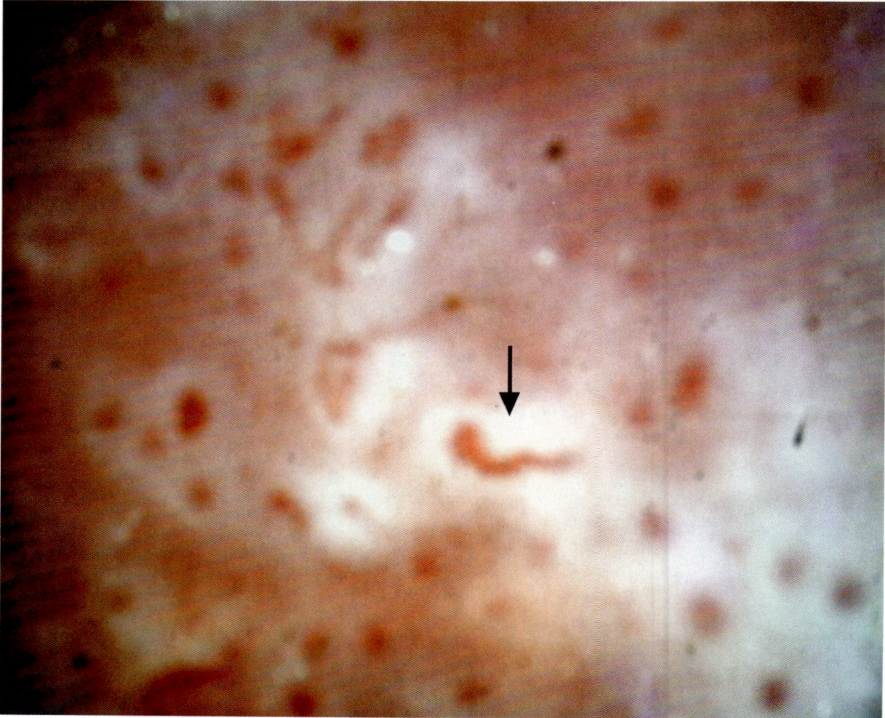

Fig. 10.14: Coarse punctations with atypical comma-shaped vessel

ADENOCARCINOMA

Adenocarcinoma does not show any characteristic colposcopic appearance. Like invasive squamous carcinoma atypical vessels, irregular surface contour may be seen. Sometimes enlarged papillae of columnar epithelium which are adherent to each other may be seen (Fig. 10.15). Appearance may resemble exophytic condyloma but the vascular pattern is abnormal (Figs 10.16 and 10.17). In such cases, biopsy is confirmatory.

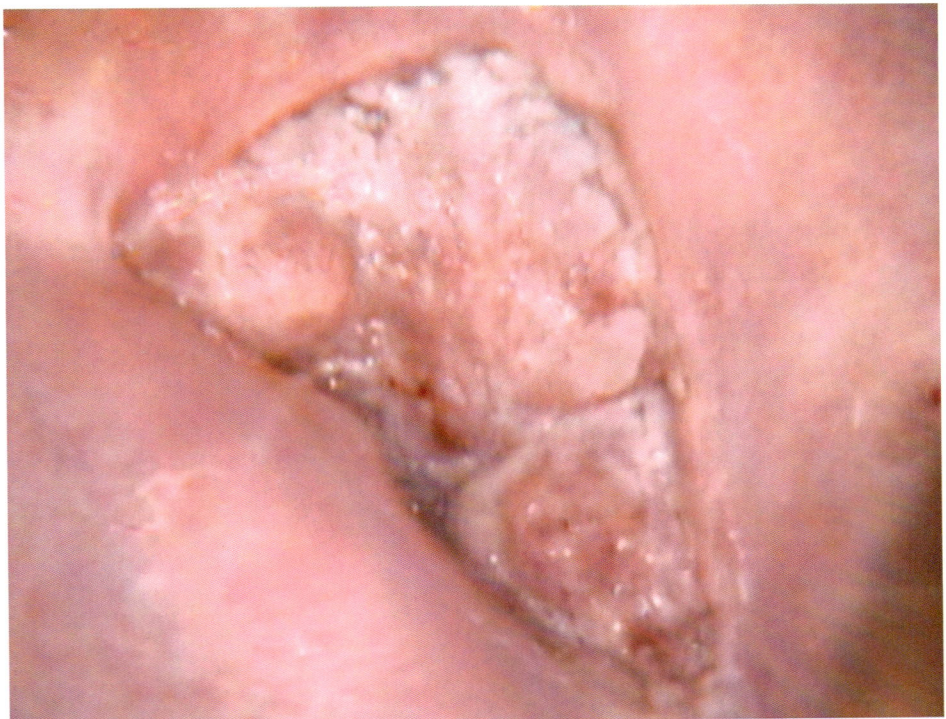

Fig. 10.15: Large dense AW, fused papillary excrescences of a cervical adenocarcinoma

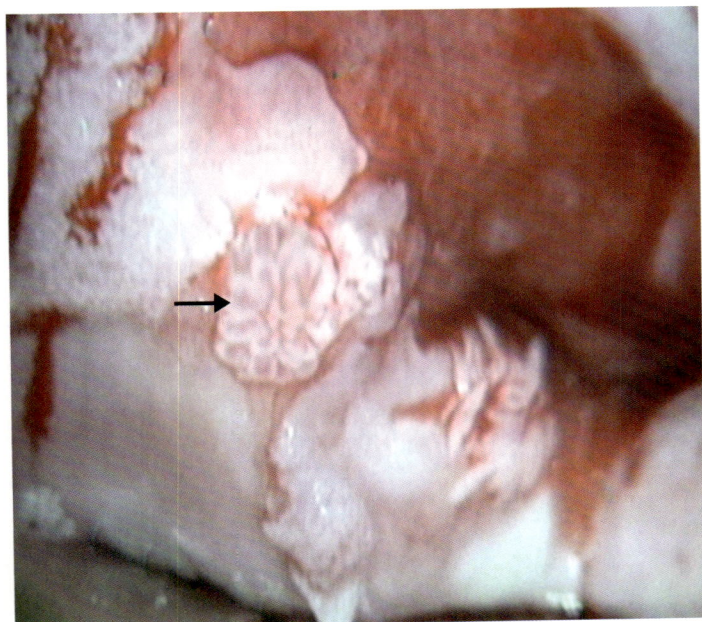

Fig. 10.16: Wart-like lesion showing finger-like projections with central vessel and acetowhite epithelium with friable vessels

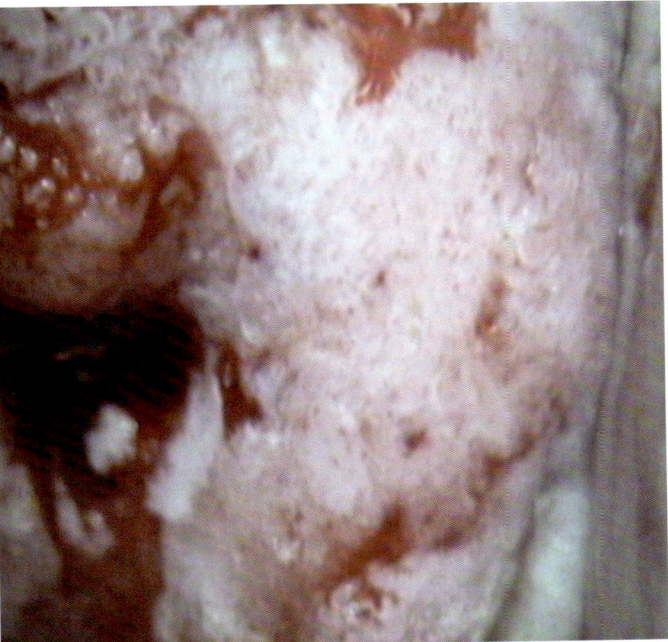

Fig. 10.17: Warty growth with AW epithelium and atypical vessels

In adenocarcinoma, false negative cytology rate is high as abnormal cells when present only in the crypts deep to the surface may not be seen in the smear. The cells are also difficult to be recognized.

POST-IRRADIATION CHANGES

After radiotherapy for cervical cancer, a close follow-up has to be done by cytology and colposcopy to diagnose residual disease or recurrence. Radiotherapy affects the mucosa of whole of vagina and cervix. After healing, there is epithelial atrophy with appearance of abundant tiny capillaries underneath the atrophic epithelium, which are dilated vessels.

Colposcopy: Although colposcopy is infrequently used after irradiation of cervix, it serves as an effective means for detecting and localizing local recurrence. Following irradiation, initially the tumor shrinks in size and there is decrease in intercapillary distance. Sometimes fibrous scar tissue appears which stands out as white area with smooth surface and usually does not show any blood vessel.

After complete healing, vagina and cervix may show hyperemia. Petechial hemorrhage may also be seen. Later large irregular and dilated vessels may be seen which may at times be bizarre also, but are usually widely scattered. Acetic acid application does not produce any change in this atrophic epithelium. Many a times cervix may not be visible because of frequent conglutination of vagina.

Recurrence of cancer cervix may occur after many years (Figs 10.18A and B). Therefore these patients require prolong follow-up.

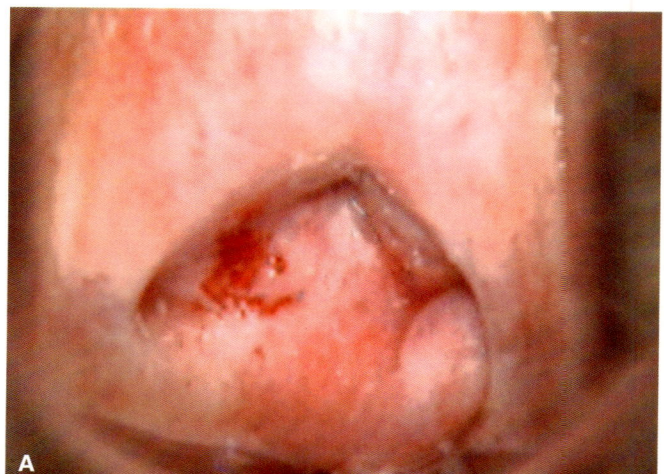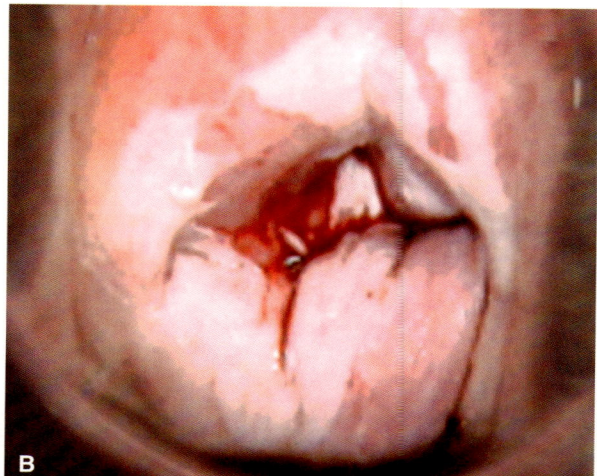

Fig. 10.18: Cervix showing post-radiotherapy recurrence after 4 yrs— (A) showing eroded epithelium at one place, (B) dense, thick, raised AW epithelium with sharp margins surrounding the os and inside endocervix also

Minimizing
Colposcopy Errors

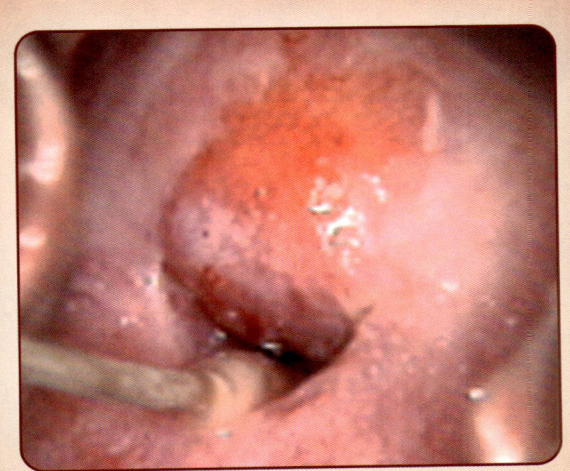

Chapter Outline

Colposcopy has provided tremendous benefit in early detection of lesions of lower genital tract and their management. Aim of colposcopy is to detect high grade lesions of the cervix, know the extent of the lesion and rule out invasive cancer before conservative management. But like any other diagnostic procedure, this is also not fool-proof and has limitations and many problems, confronted even by the most skilled observer. These limitations cannot be over-looked and may pose a dilemma to the observer as well as lead to errors in the diagnosis.

The diagnostic accuracy of colposcopy depends upon the ability of the examiner to recognize different lesions and grade them according to known scoring systems, which depends upon appropriate training and experience. Thus, the colposcopic assessment and histological diagnosis do not always correlate.

In our experience, positive predictive value of a colposcopic impression of CIN 3 is over 75%. However, the positive predictive value declines with lower grades of CIN.

To achieve best results, one should have thorough knowledge of pathogenesis and natural history of disease. For high degree of accuracy and minimizing errors, one must acquire good training, experience and follow established colposcopic protocols and practice. Besides this one should use good clinical judgment also.

SOURCES OF ERRORS

One should be aware of various sources of errors and know methods to minimize them. Errors can result from:

1. Misinterpretation of colposcopic lesions:
   - Over-diagnosis
   - Under-diagnosis
   - Colposcopy performed during regenerative phase
2. Incomplete colposcopic examination:
   - Inadequate colposcopy
   - Incomplete visualization of SCJ
   - Failure to detect vaginal lesions
   - False SCJ
3. Physiological conditions affecting colposcopic pattern:
   - Menopause
   - Pregnancy
4. Errors associated with biopsy technique:
   - Inappropriate biopsy site
   - Inadequate biopsies
   - Undirected biopsy
5. Other sources

Among the potential errors of colposcopy, misinterpretation of lesion and incomplete visualization are the most important, poor biopsy technique and inadequate biopsy follow close behind. Most importantly, one should maintain the standard of care by updated knowledge and following guidelines.

Misinterpretation of Colposcopic Lesion

Expertise in colposcopy can be measured by the accuracy with which one can predict the histology of a colposcopically defined lesion. Though final diagnosis must always be established by histopathological examination especially before considering any ablative procedure, one should not always accept the histological diagnosis uncritically.

Misinterpretation of patterns is the most common error in colposcopy. Prerequisite for interpretation of colposcopic image requires a thorough knowledge of pathophysiology of disease because every colposcopic image is a reflection of specific tissue pattern resulting from interaction of surface epithelium and stroma.

Over-Diagnosis

It would be easy, if all acetowhite and all non-glycogenated epithelia were abnormal. But, unfortunately it is not so. As a general rule, the colposcopist is more likely to over-diagnose than to under-diagnose a particular lesion. It is generally thought that an atypical transformation zone (ATZ) may harbor a neoplastic lesion and should be biopsied.

Grade 1 lesions: It has been seen that grade 1 lesions seen as flat, mild acetowhite lesions with feathery margins, with or without fine, regular punctations or mosaic, are more likely to be over diagnosed (Figs 11.1 and 11.2).

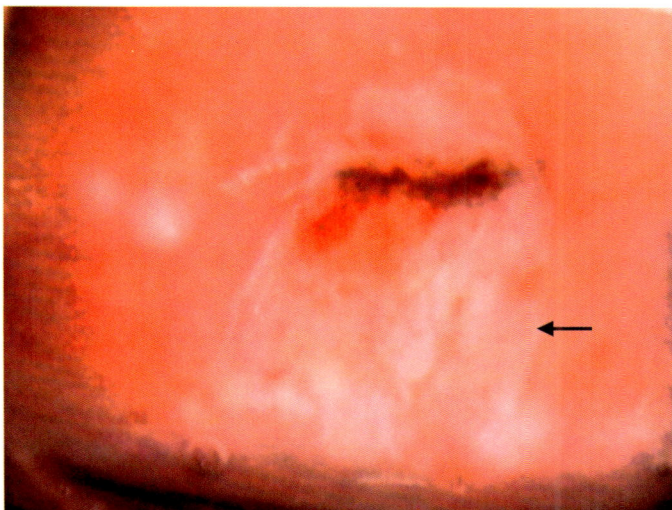

Fig. 11.1: Grade 1 AW epithelium with feathery margins

Such a picture may also be seen in immature or active metaplastic epithelium, a common finding specially in young women (Fig. 11.3); regenerative epithelium following surgical procedures as CO_2 laser, cryosurgery, electro-coagulation diathermy or trauma which may persist for many months or even years; subclinical papilloma virus infection; and congenital transformation zone; all being benign or physiological conditions which may present as atypical transformation zone with mild acetowhiteness. These all may be difficult to distinguish from early grades of CIN without biopsy. Such lesions must be biopsied, if in doubt especially by the beginner.

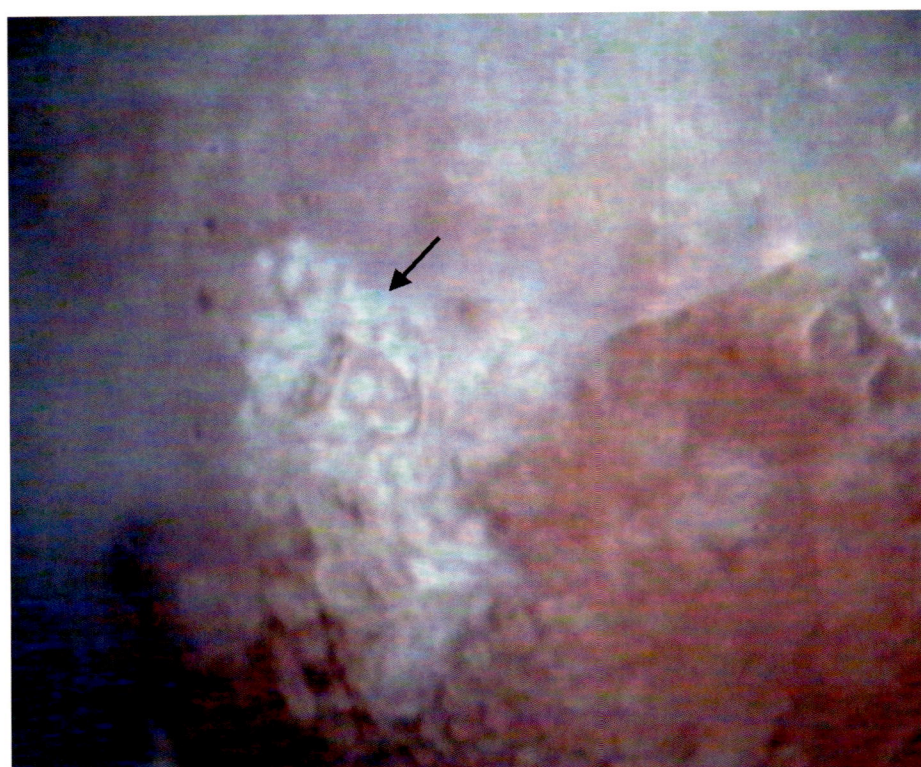

Fig. 11.2: Grade 1 AW epithelium with fine mosaic

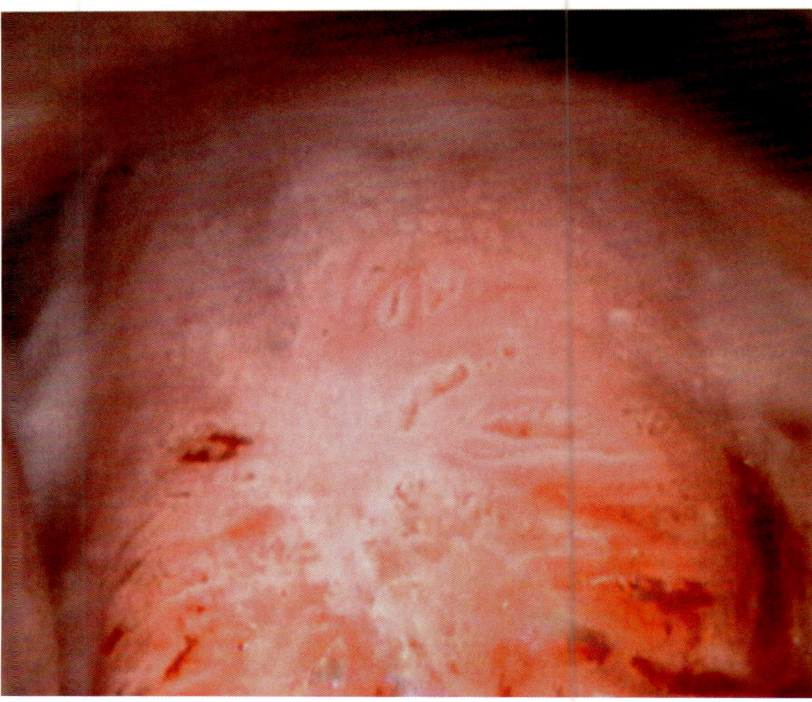

Fig. 11.3: Immature metaplastic epithelium with whitish hue

Majority of grade 1 lesions on colposcopy are found to be benign lesions. However, rarely these may turn out to be high grade CIN on biopsy, but such lesions generally have associated abnormal cytology result also. Thus grade 1 lesions on colposcopy in presence of inflammatory Pap smear may be just observed and biopsied only if the lesion persists. Low grade colposcopic lesions should not be treated by "see and treat" approach without prior biopsy. Radical treatment should always be avoided, if in doubt about the diagnosis. One must also do self-auditing of clinical as well as colposcopic findings.

Vascular pattern may also lead to a confusing picture at times. Multiple papillae of exophytic condyloma may have angiogenesis in the form of multiple coiled loops or more obliquely or horizontally directed vessels which can mimic papillary adenocarcinoma or squamous cell carcinoma (Fig. 11.4). Regularity of vessel spacing and uniformity of calibre is absent in malignancy. In such a situation, only histopathology can differentiate.

At times irregular contour of damaged cervix and large number of irregularly running vessels of chronic cervicitis may be confusing. In such a case, one should take all the findings together, not in isolation and score the findings before coming to final conclusion (Fig. 11.5).

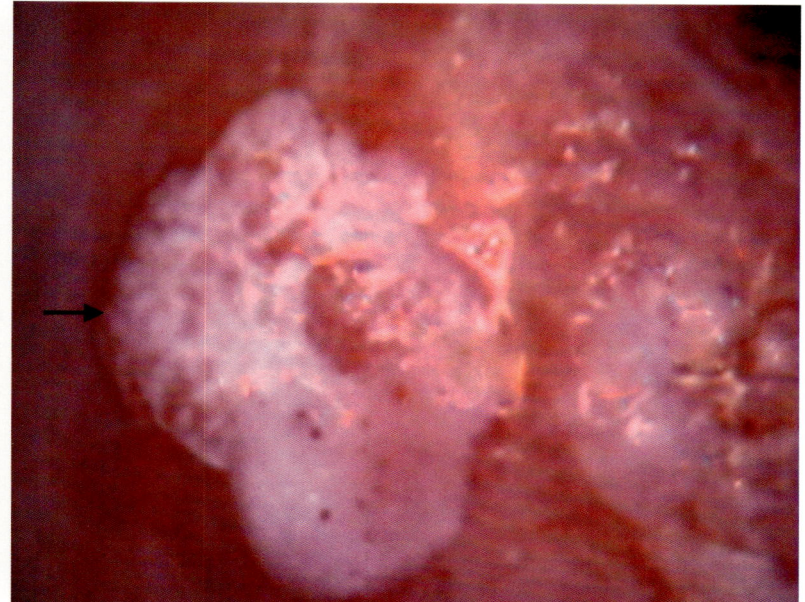

Fig. 11.4: Raised thick AW lesion with vessels in papillae and grade 2 gland openings

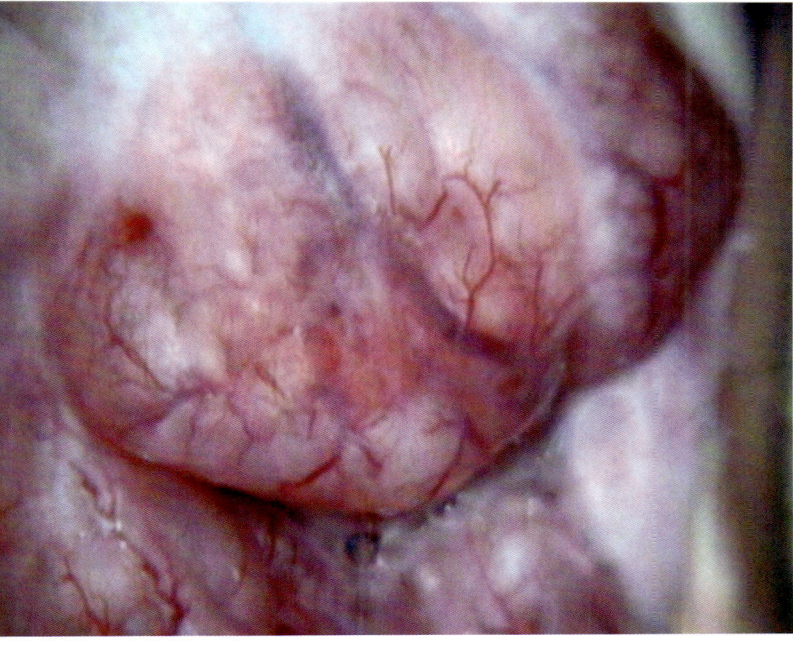

Fig. 11.5: Irregular contour of cervix with prominent vessels

Under-Diagnosis

Under-diagnosis of a lesion is a grave error especially when one misses invasive cancer. This happens when one does not adhere to standard protocol, fails to visualize endocervical canal or vaginal extent, or fails to take biopsy from the most abnormal area. The importance of various colposcopic images, grade for grade, in terms of signifying neoplasia is listed in the following order:

1. **Atypical blood vessels:** Appearance of atypical vessels in transformation zone is the hallmark feature of invasion.
2. **Acetowhite epithelium:** This is second important colposcopic image because it carries not only an intrinsic association with CIN but also provides the background in which vascular changes must be evaluated.

Higher grade of acetowhite epithelium should be given more importance in comparison to lower grade of vascular abnormalities (Fig. 11.6). Multiple grades of AW epithelium in a single patient require multiple biopsies (Fig. 11.7).

3. **Mosaic and punctations:** These are significant only when present in the background of acetowhite epithelium.
4. **Leukoplakia:** It is less important as it usually reflects HPV but it may be covering an underlying high grade lesion.

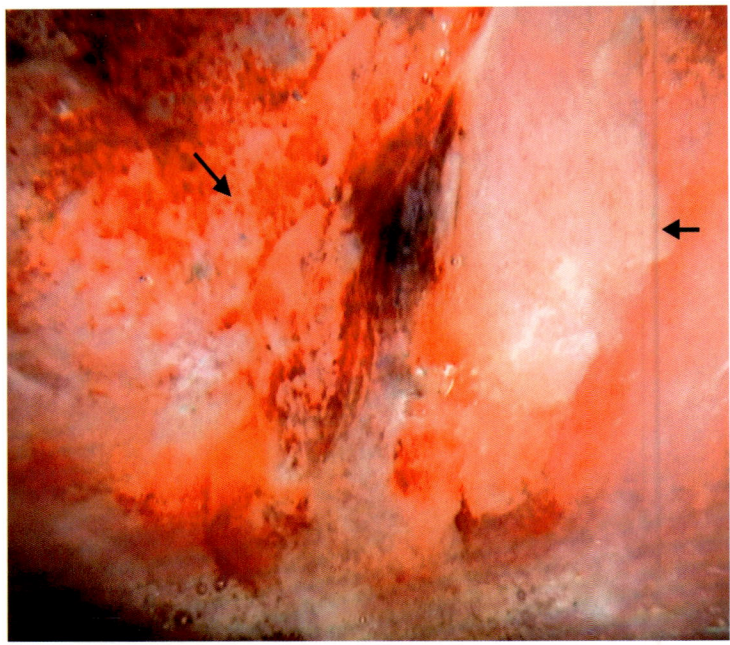

Fig. 11.6: Punctations at 8–10 O' clock and dense acetowhite lesion of higher grade at 3–5 O' clock

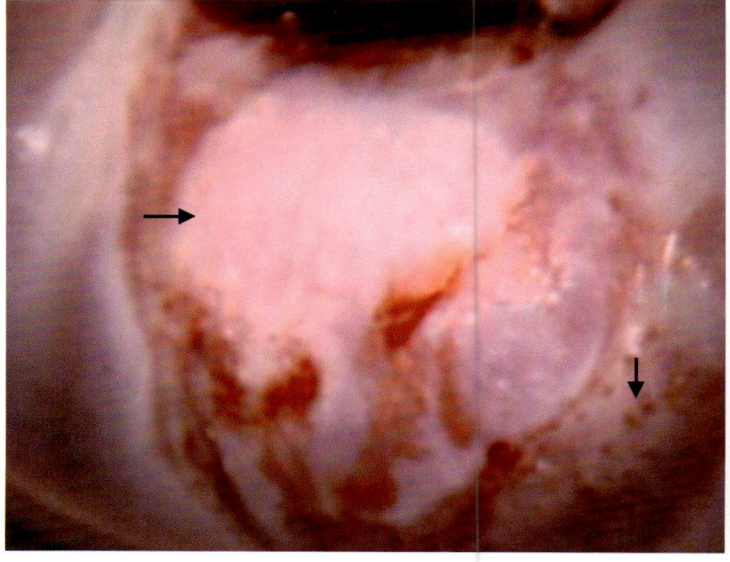

Fig. 11.7: Grade 3 AW epithelium with internal margin, surrounded by grade 2 epithelium on left side, irregular punctations at 4–5 O' clock. Multiple biopsies are required as central lesion with internal border is of higher grade

Colposcopy Performed during Regenerative Period of Epithelium

Colposcopy should be avoided during regenerative period of epithelium because one may find confusing findings during this period (Fig. 11.8).

Incomplete Colposcopic Examination

Another common error in colposcopy is making the diagnosis without completely visualizing the cervix. 10–15% of colposcopies done for abnormal smears are incomplete due to inadequate colposcopy or non-visibility/incomplete visibility of SCJ.

Inadequate Colposcopy

Colposcopic examination is inadequate, if visualization of cervix is obscured for any reason. Some examples are illustrated: Presence of endocervical polyp (Fig. 11.9), big retention cyst blocking the external os (Fig. 11.10), stenosed external os (Fig. 11.11) or post-irradiation/post-surgical conglutination of vagina/cervix.

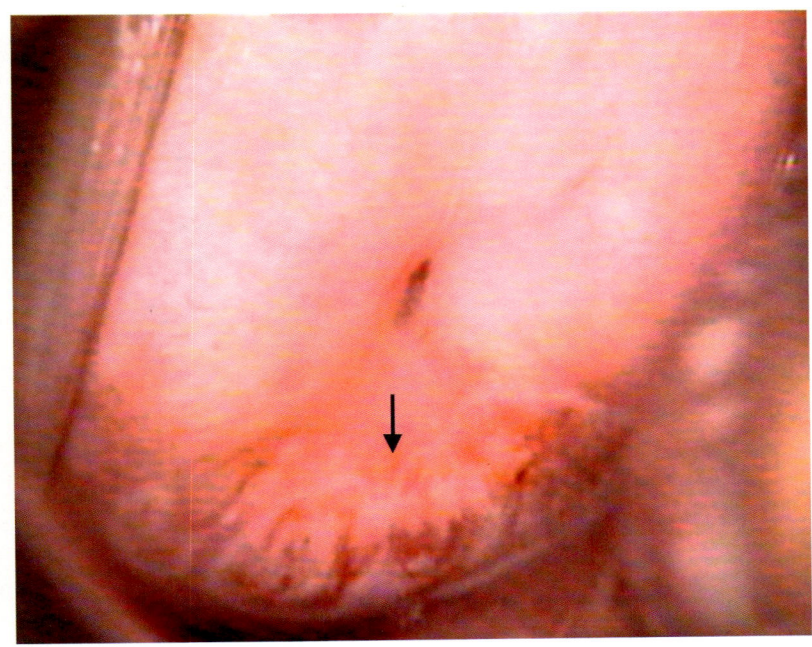

Fig. 11.8: Post-traumatic regenerative epithelium seen as grade 1 acetowhite epithelium and punctations, away from transformation zone

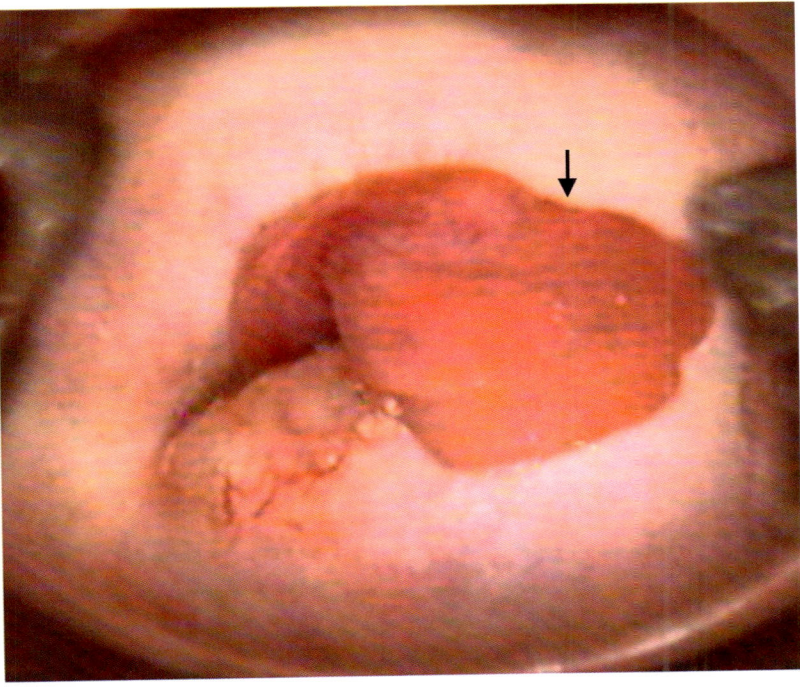

Fig. 11.9: Inadequate colposcopy—endocervical polyp at external os

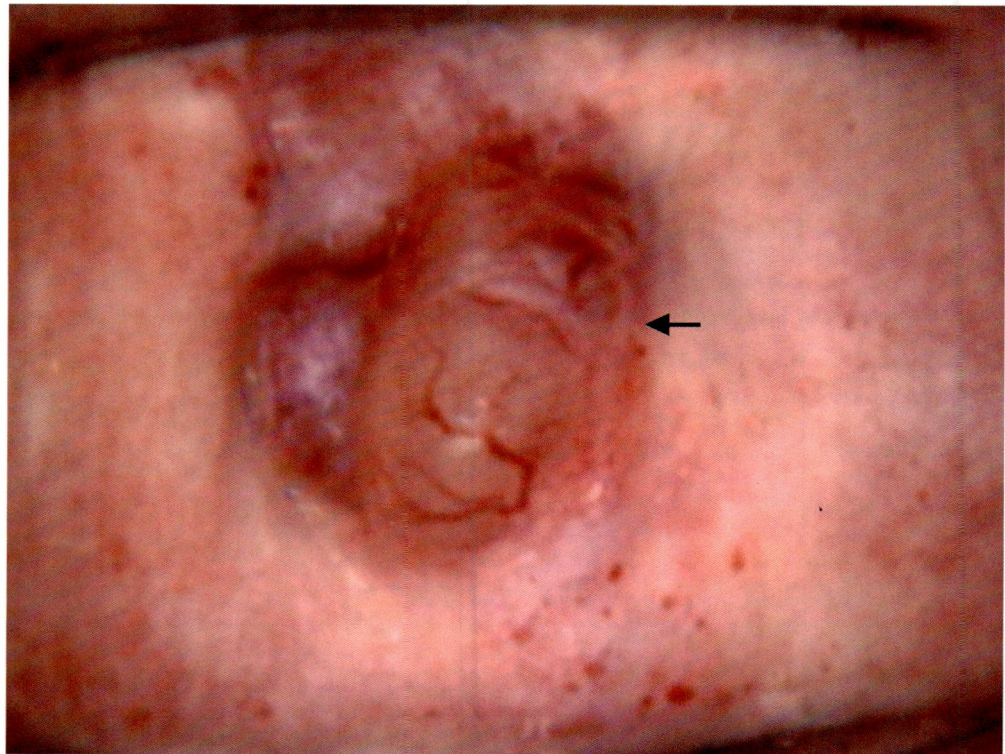

Fig. 11.10: Inadequate colposcopy—big nabothian cysts blocking external os

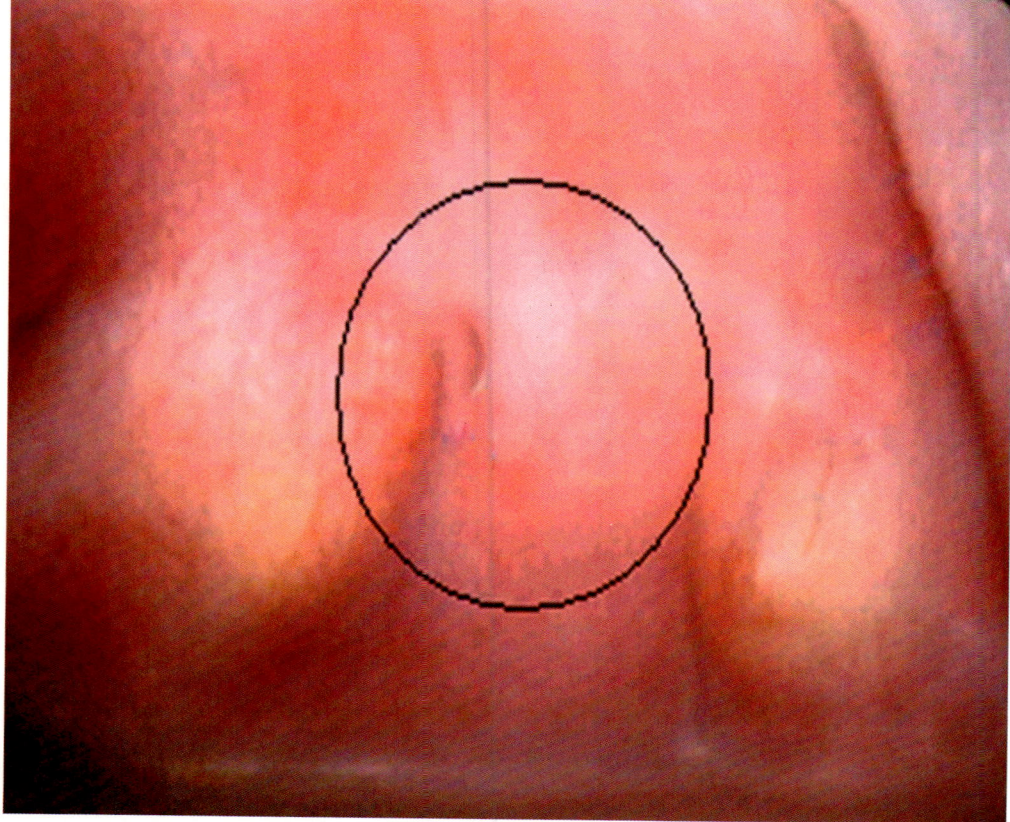

Fig. 11.11: Inadequate colposcopy—pinhole external os along with big nabothian cyst

Incomplete Visibility of SCJ

The incomplete visibility of SCJ can also lead to errors in colposcopic interpretation, if attention is not paid to it. The abnormal lesion is seen extending high in the canal and SCJ is not visible in cases illustrated in Figs 11.12 and 11.13. SCJ may also not be visible following irradiation or postsurgical procedure of cervix (Fig. 11.14).

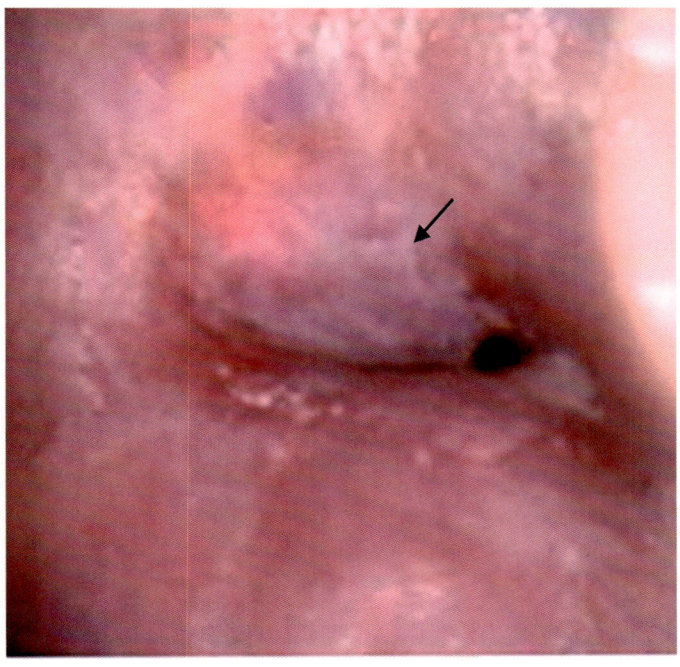

Fig. 11.12: Upper margin of lesion is inside the endocervical canal and not seen

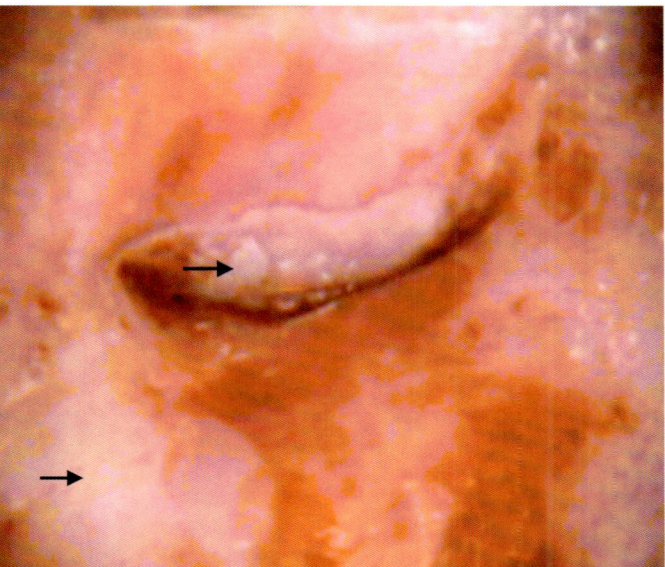

Fig. 11.13: Cervix shows grade 1 AW epithelium over posterior lip and grade 2 epithelium with a denser lesion inside with internal margins on the anterior lip which is reaching inside endocervix. Biopsy showed high grade lesion. Later LEEP diagnosed microinvasive carcinoma

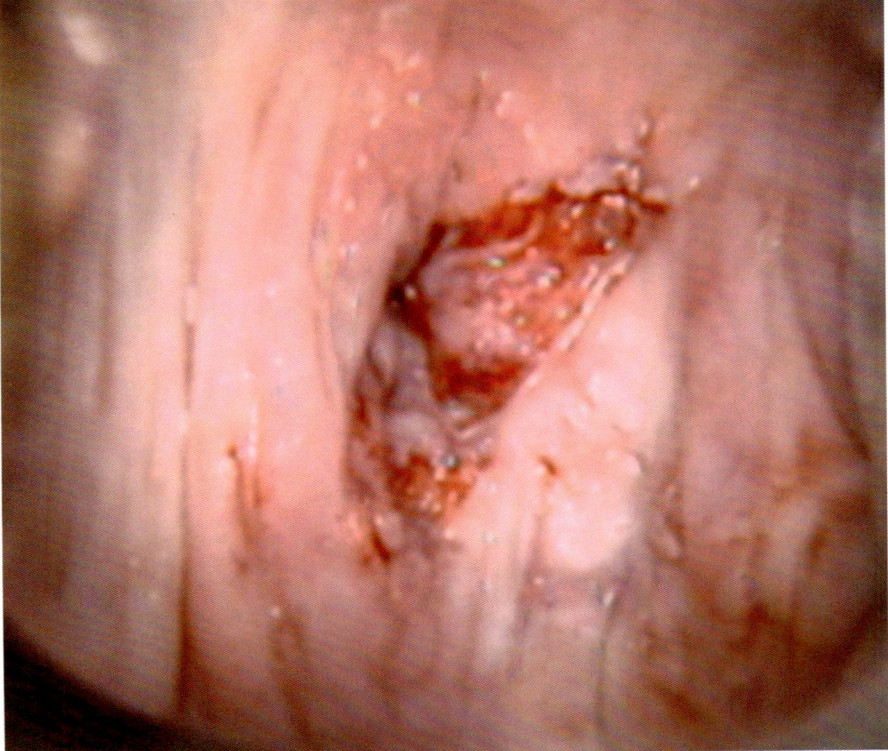

Fig. 11.14: Incomplete visibility of SCJ—cervix after Manchester repair

Missing a Vaginal Lesion

Another significant error is incomplete visualization of the lesion in vagina or missing a sole lesion in vagina. Many a times, the colposcopist's attention is focused so intently on the cervix, that the disease in the vaginal fornices or behind the blades of the vaginal speculum is missed. Screening of disease in the vaginal fornices can be done at the time of application of acetic acid to the cervix by moving the cervix from side to side and up and down by the applicator. After evaluating the cervix, if one is unable to find the source of abnormal Pap test, vagina must be examined more thoroughly before assuming that disease cannot be visualized or cytology is false positive.

False Squamocolumnar Junction

Recognition of SC junction is crucial to identify the upper limit of the lesion. A mistake often made is to take the SC junction as the upper limit of the metaplastic squamous epithehium, while it should be marked by the lower limit of the normal columnar epithelium. A false SC junction may at times be created by abraded epithelium due to trauma (Figs 11.15 and 11.16).

If SC junction is not recognized properly, one may label the colposcopic examination as satisfactory while it is not so. In such a situation, if endocervical curettage is also omitted then abnormal pathology may be missed.

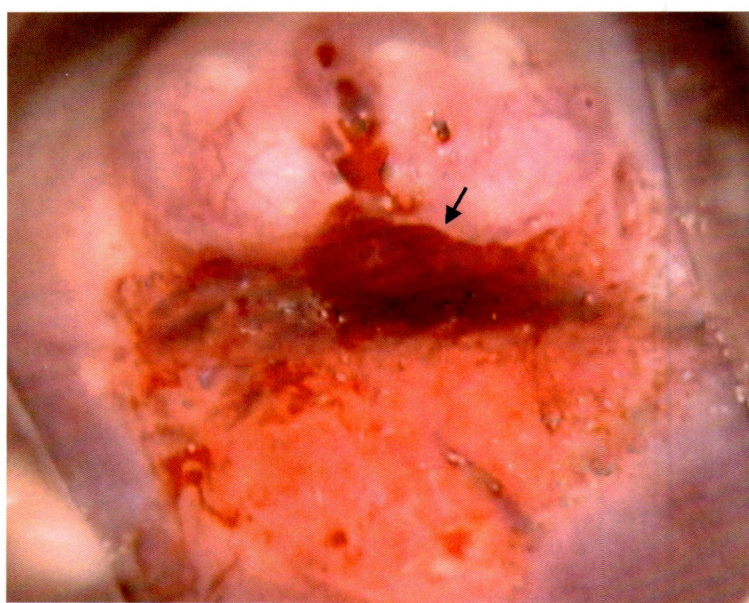

Fig. 11.15: Normal cervix with false SCJ over anterior lip

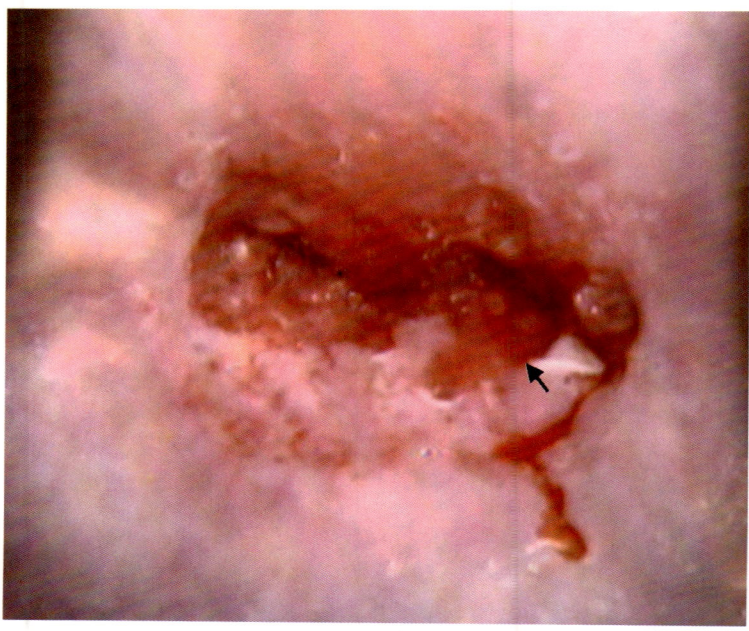

Fig. 11.16: AW epithelium with false SCJ over posterior lip near abraded epithelium

Every attempt should be made to visualize the SCJ in the endocervical canal and see the entire lesion and the entire TZ before reaching to any conclusion. Various methods can be used such as:

a. Timing the colposcopy near ovulation in premenopausal women, when the os is gaping due to effect of estrogens (Fig. 11.17).

b. Cotton tipped applicator or hook to manipulate cervix (Fig. 11.18).

c. Pharmacologic agents like estrogens, misoprostol. Estradiol cream applied intravaginally each evening for 2–3 weeks or Tab conjugated estrogen 0.625 mg given orally for 1 week will convert unsatisfactory colposcopy to satisfactory in 60–70% of cases. However, this therapy has an inherent risk of enhanced coagulation, if patient has to be subjected to surgery. Misoprost 400 mcg tablet used intravaginally 6 hours before the colposcopic procedure can open up the cervix (Figs 11.19A and B) resulting in satisfactory colposcopy in 70–80% cases.

d. Use of endocervical speculum (Fig. 11.20): One has to be judicious in choosing the endocervical speculum. For narrow os, one should use narrow tipped; while for the reproductive os, a broader-tipped speculum can be used. Speculum should be introduced gently because the delicate endocervical epithelium starts bleeding on slight provocation.

e. Osmotic dilators—laminaria tent, lamicel—dilate the cervix with hygroscopic action, but may be difficult to insert in menopausal or stenotic os.

f. Colpomicrohysteroscopy (Fig. 11.21): It enables in vivo evaluation of squamocolumnar junction and endocervix with supravital staining at 20×, 60× and 120× magnifications. This requires special instrument and the expertise.

However, despite using various methods in 20–30% cases, accurate results cannot be obtained.

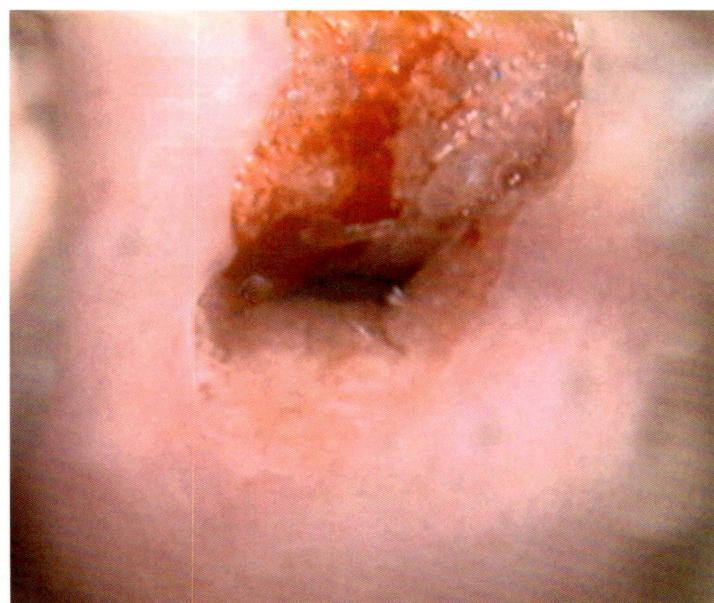

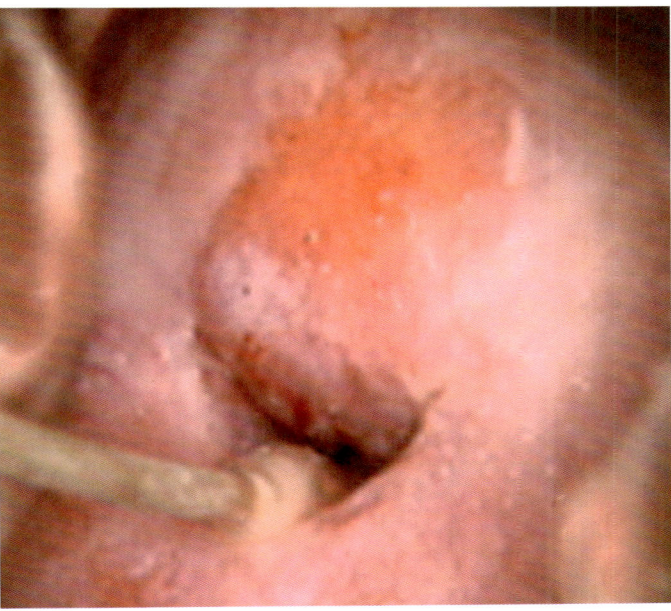

Fig. 11.17: Mid-menstrual gaping os with clear mucus

Fig. 11.18: Manipulation of cervical lips with cotton-tipped applicator

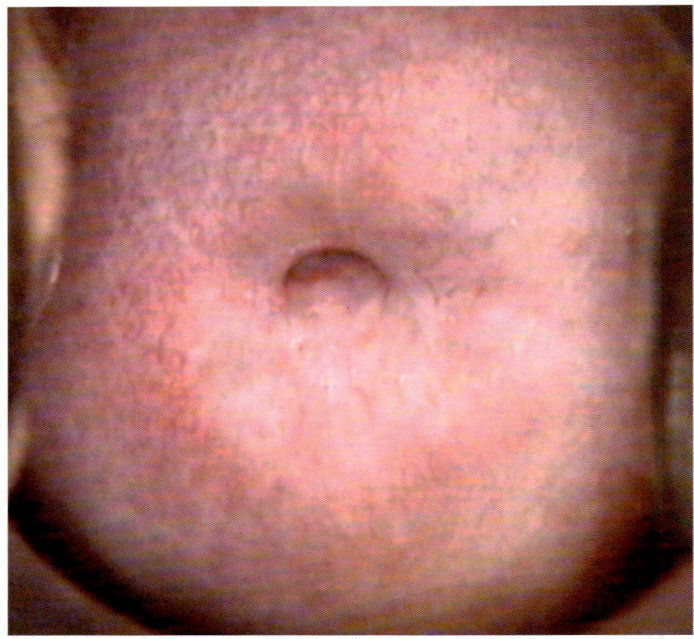
Fig. 11.19A: Incomplete visibility of SCJ

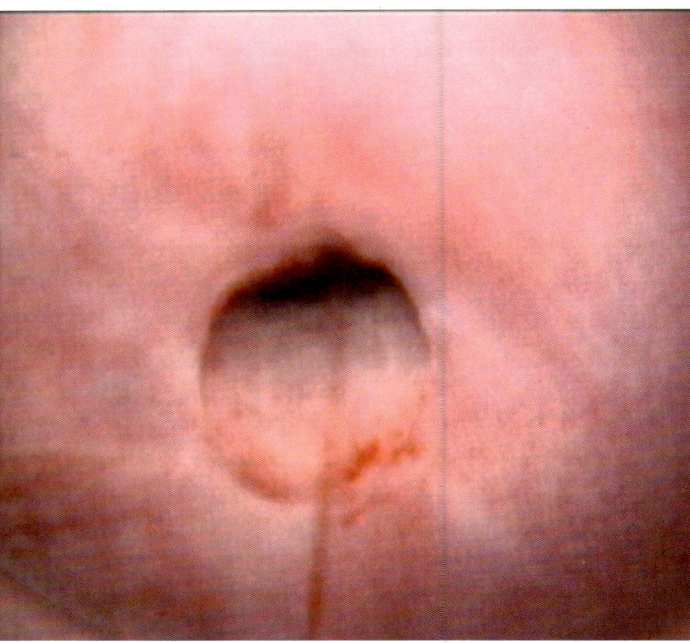
Fig. 11.19B: Cervix after misoprost

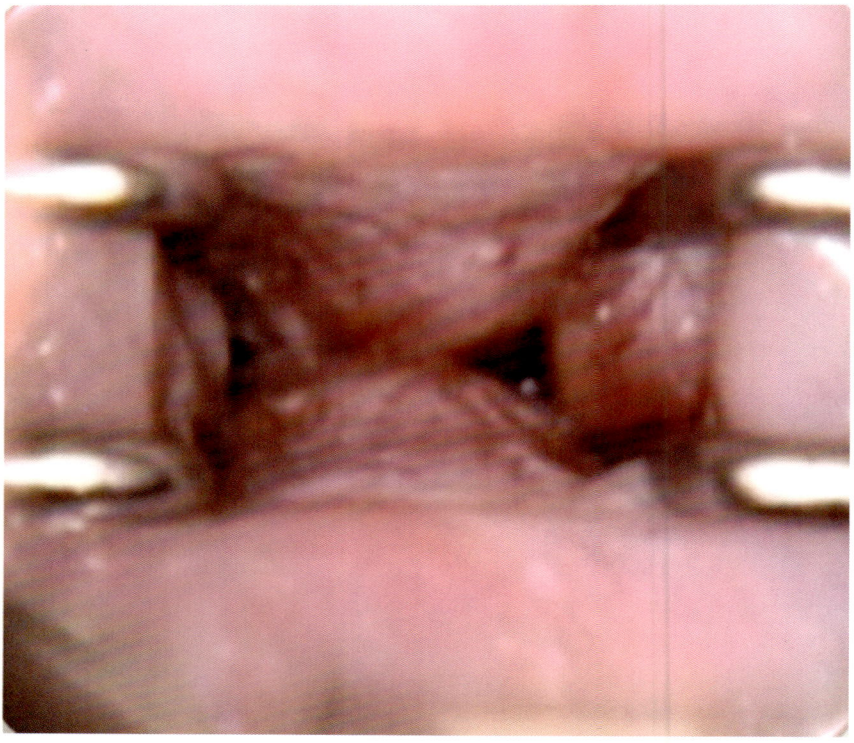

Fig. 11.20: Endocervical canal through endocervical speculum

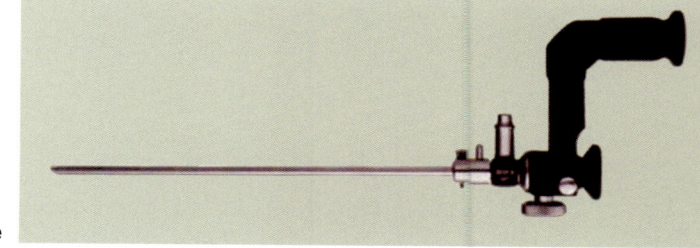

Fig. 11.21: Contact colpomicrohysteroscope

Physiological Conditions Affecting the Colposcopic Pattern

Menopause

The incidence of incomplete visibility of SCJ is much higher (1:4) in women above 40 years of age compared to that in reproductive age (1:40), due to the effect of estrogens.

Colposcopy is tricky and difficult in postmenopausal women because of unsatisfactory colposcopy in 25% of postmenopausal women and because of vaginal atrophy. Moreover, the procedure is painful.

A common problem is that colposcopic findings are normal even though the cytology is showing atypia. The stenotic os and atrophic epithelium in postmenopausal women may result in missing the pathology in the endocervical canal or dysplastic epithelium not taking the whitish hue with acetic acid because of atrophy (Figs 11.22 and 11.23). In such instances, colposcopy is advocated to be carried out after estrogen therapy (conjugated equine estrogen tablet for 1 week or vaginal estrogen cream for 2–3 weeks). Estrogen makes the cervicovaginal epithelium thick enhancing the appearance of dysplastic epithelium which otherwise may not be visible.

Vascular pattern may also be difficult to interpret. Postmenopausal atrophy leads to visualization of larger, deeper, spider-like subepithelial vessels that may be confused with atypical vessels (Fig. 11.24). Branching pattern should be closely scrutinized for differentiation.

Another important point in postmenopausal women is that ASCUS or LGSIL cytology can occur because of estrogen deficiency/senile vaginitis and after treatment with estrogens cytology reverts back to normal.

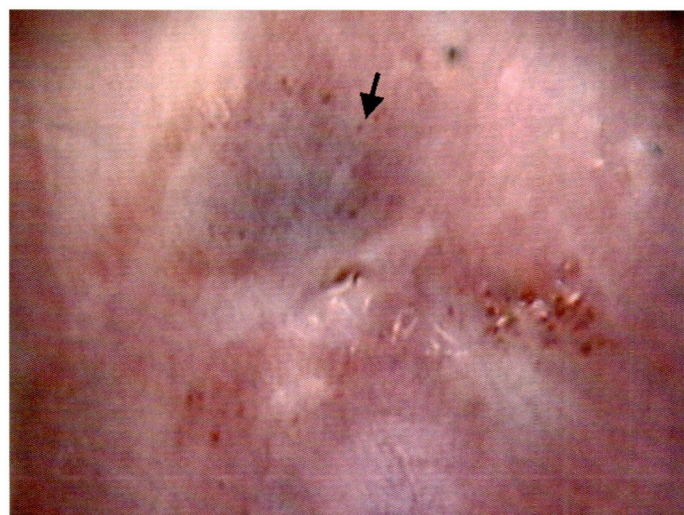

Fig. 11.22: Incomplete visibility of SCJ — squamocolumnar junction is inside the endocervical canal (postmenopausal)

Fig. 11.23: Postmenopausal cervix showing stenotic os and atrophic changes

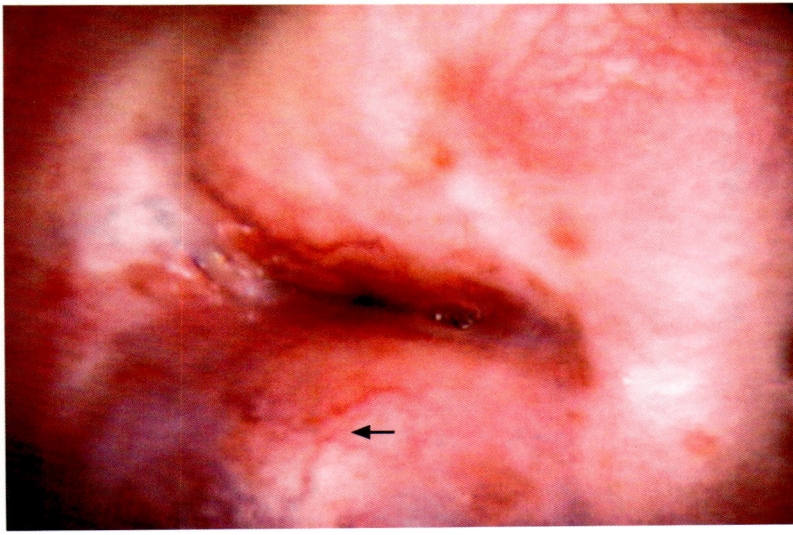

Fig. 11.24: Postmenopausal cervix with deeper spider-like subepithelial vessels

Pregnancy

Errors may occur in association with pregnancy due to physiologic and morphologic changes of pregnancy which may alter the colposcopic image. Vasodilatation and congestion during pregnancy produce accentuated colposcopic patterns with more pronounced mosaic and punctations and enhanced acetic acid effect which may mimic preneoplastic lesions. CIN, if present, may be interpreted as of higher grade than it actually is. In presence of the extensive areas of immature epithelium, it is difficult to exclude low grade CIN lesion.

Pregnancy is a special condition where guidelines to diagnose and manage CIN are different and failure to follow the guidelines is common cause of error. During colposcopy in pregnancy, errors can be minimized by:

a. Use of large speculum covered with condom or lateral vaginal wall retractor (Fig. 11.25).
b. Use of 5% acetic acid for tenacious mucus.
c. Quadrant-wise interpretation of hypertrophied cervix.
d. Remembering that the colposcopic changes in pregnancy are one grade higher than in non pregnant cervix (Figs 11.27A and B).

Deciduosis of cervix can be confused with cervical growth but it will never have atypical vessels.

In first trimester, if colposcopy is unsatisfactory, one may postpone the procedure, because cervical eversion would occur as pregnancy advances. Colposcopic biopsy is safe, if indicated. ECC is contraindicated during pregnancy. However, endocervical brush cytology is safe.

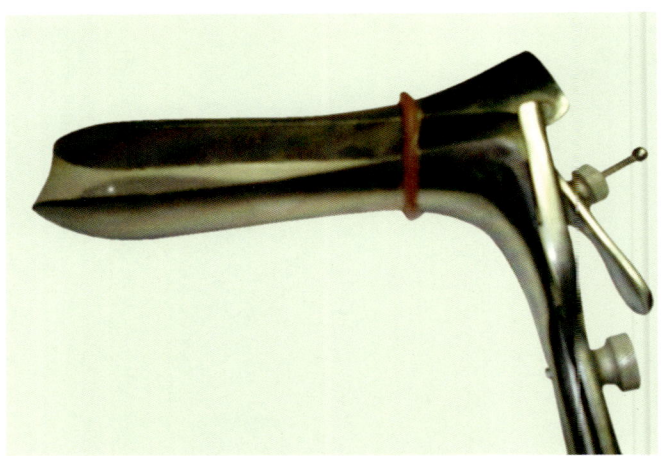
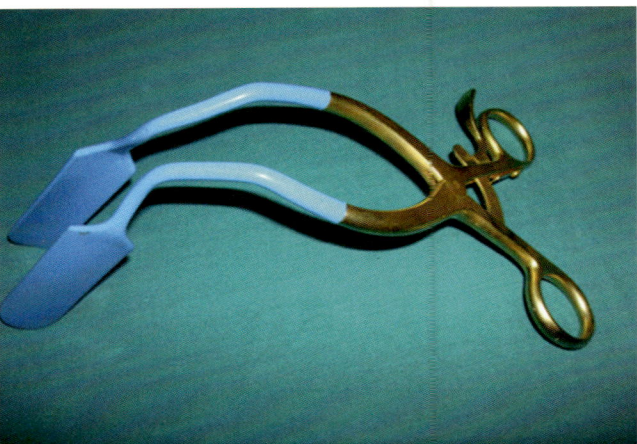

Fig. 11.25: Long-bladed speculum covered with condom and lateral vaginal wall retractor

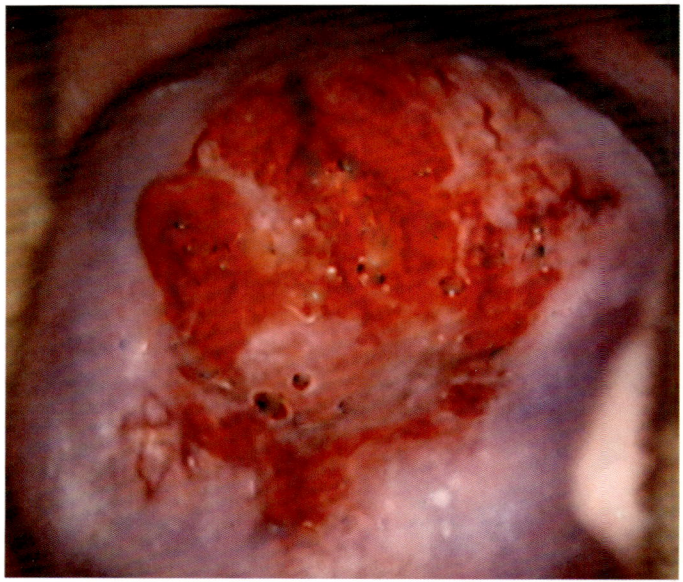
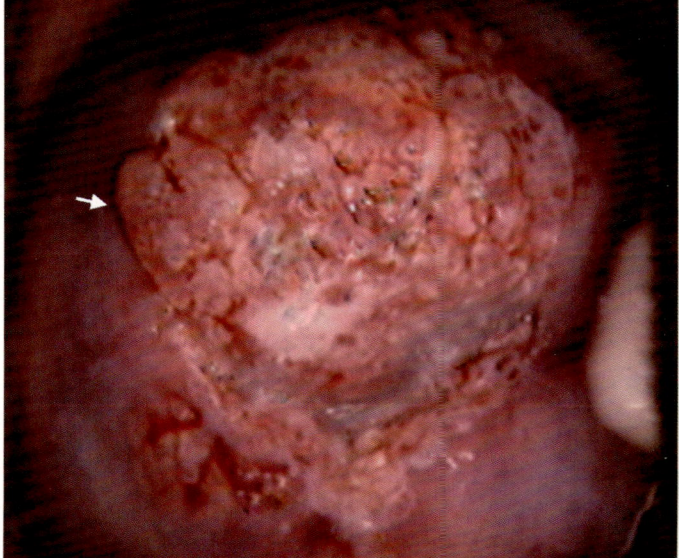

Fig. 11.26A: Hypertrophied and polypoidal cervix with N saline   **Fig. 11.26B:** Hypertrophied and polypoidal cervix after acetic acid

Errors in Biopsy Technique

Atypical transformation zone should be appropriately and adequately biopsied. In atypical TZ, there may be varying degrees of abnormalities and one must take biopsy from the most abnormal area (Figs 11.27 and 11.28). A novice colposcopist may give more importance to minor grades of mosaic or punctations than major grade of acetowhite epithelium or may overlook an area of abnormal vessels leading to biopsy from a wrong area, if only few biopsies are taken. That is why one should take biopsies from multiple sites especially in the beginning and label it accordingly. Biopsy should be colposcopically directed. One must check the site after taking the biopsy to know whether it is from right place or not.

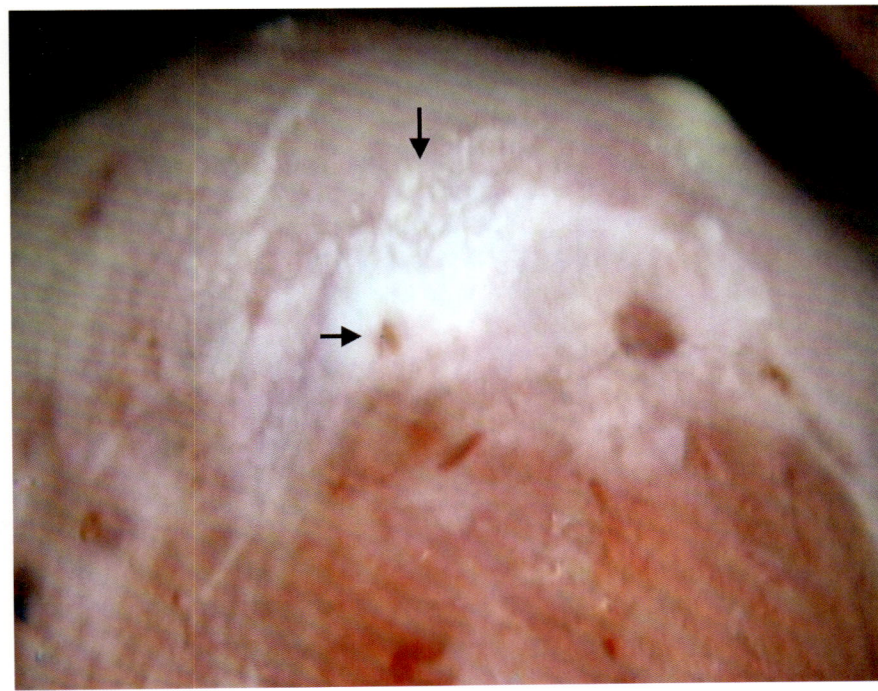

Fig. 11.27: Outer lesion with mosaic is of lower grade compared to adjacent grade 2 AW epithelium

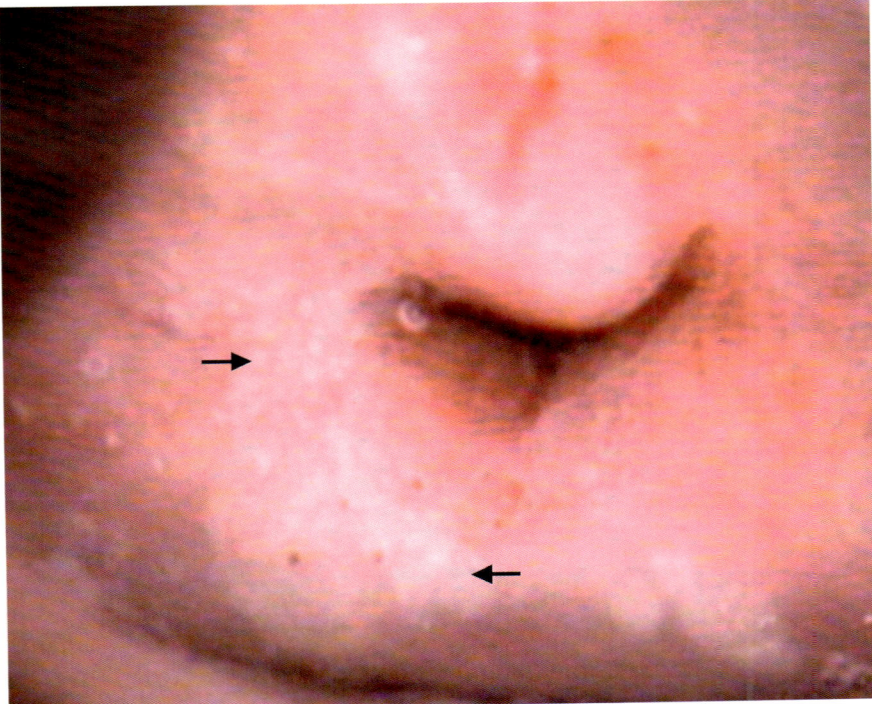

Fig. 11.28: Cervix showing dense AW epithelium at 5–6 O' clock and grade 1 at 7–9 O' clock with mosaic. Cuffed gland openings are also present. Multiple biopsies confirmed higher grade lesion at 5–6 O' clock

Biopsy instrument should be sharp to avoid crushing of tissue. Biopsy forceps should be kept perpendicular to the biopsy site and not tangentially otherwise it may at times give wrong diagnosis on histopathology. Iatrogenic trauma in the form of endocervical curettage (ECC) and cervical biopsy can obscure the lesions. Therefore, there should be a logical progression of events. ECC should always be performed first, followed by posterior cervical lip biopsy, then anterior lip biopsy and vaginal wall biopsy in the end.

Common error is the failure to do endocervical curettage (ECC) in cases of abnormal Pap smear in previously treated patients. Once the TZ is disrupted by cervical therapy, islands of metaplasia or abnormal tissue may be left behind the newly formed squamo-columnar junction. The colposcopy appears satis-factory, and yet there may be disease in the endocervical canal. Other indications of doing ECC are cases of abnormal Pap smear with unsatisfactory colposcopy, with glandular cells on cytology, and before ablative therapy in CIN.

The usual technique of dragging the curette down across the portio of the cervix after curetting the endocervix may dislodge strips of cervical dysplastic epithelium. Therefore, ECC should be performed with the curette remaining in the endocervical canal, and then being gently removed. A cytobrush with a sleeve (straw) has been found to be more sensitive and less painful, resulting in less specimen inadequacy. A cytobrush is rotated 360° briskly 5 times and pulled back into the straw before removing. This technique may prevent contamination of the endocervical sample with ectocervical disease. However, the sample with brush is to be sent in liquid preservative as used in liquid based cytology, which is expensive and not available at every center in India.

Other Sources of Error

Inadequate Training and Experience

Colposcopic competency requires adequate training with an expert colposcopist and enough experience along with an understanding of the pathogenesis and natural history of the disease. An inexperienced colposcopist may find difficulty in colposcopic assessment of various lesions.

ASCCP, RCOG guidelines and study courses on CDs are available on the respective websites and certificates are issued after training and post-evaluation test. At the end of training, delegate should have diagnosed at least 10 high grade lesions under supervision and there should be 80% colposcopic accuracy. Indian Society of Colposcopy and Cervical Pathology (ISCCP) have defined 30 hours of training in their curriculum including the didactic lectures.

Discrepancy among Cytology, Colposcopy and Histology

Another common error is failure to insist on agreement among cytology, colposcopy and histology. There should be close association and good communication between colposcopist and the cytohistopathologist. In case of discrepancy between the three modalities, there should be a review of the reports. Colposcopy demands a multidisciplinary approach.

Improper Documentation

Errors may occur due to improper documentation. To minimize such erros, detailed data documentation should be made regarding:

- Grade of cytological abnormality
- Colposcopic adequacy, visibility of SCJ, type of TZ
- Location of the lesion (inside/outside TZ, by clock position), size and extent of lesion, extension of lesion into endocervical canal or vagina.
- Abnormal colposcopic features should be described location-wise in detail and colposcopic impression should be made in terms of low grade or high grade lesion along with Reid's/Swede colposcopic index score. Histopathological diagnosis should never be made on colposcopy only.

Chapter

12

Screening and Management of Preinvasive Cervical Disease

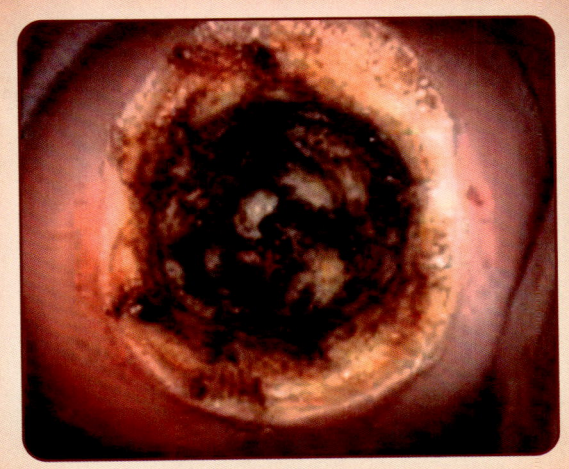

Chapter Outline

Cancer cervix is the second most common cancer globally. India contributes to more than 25% of global disease burden as well as mortality with more than 1.32 lakh new cases diagnosed every year and around 75000 dying from the disease. Magnitude of the problem is more than evident. Only silver lining in the cloud is that cervix is an easily accessible organ; and the cancer is preventable, with well-established etiology, risk factors, and a long latent intraepithelial phase which can be easily detected and treated.

Management requires detection of preinvasive lesions and their treatment, as only detection is insufficient to prevent cancer cervix.

DETECTION

Since preinvasive disease does not have any symptoms, healthy women of target age group have to be screened for detection of the lesions. Organized cervical cytology programs have resulted in a marked reduction of cervical cancer incidence as well as mortality in the developed countries, whereas, the situation has remained largely uncontrolled in developing countries due to ineffective screening programs. Data from different regions of India indicate a slow, but steady, decline in the incidence. However, the rates are still too high and the absolute number of cases is rising due to population growth.

SCREENING PROGRAMS

Organized screening programs seem to offer most efficient screening protection as they ensure regular screening of target women by an invitation, have a published screening policy, a management team responsible for administering the program, with appropriate follow-up of women, proper recording of cancers and an established quality assurance. But such programs involve high cost and are difficult to implement in resource poor countries.

Opportunistic screening: Cervical smears are taken when women visit a doctor for other reasons or make their own appointment. It tends to over-screen some and under-screen other women. Overall reductions in cervical cancer are not as great as with organized programs. Such screening also requires considerable resources.

Camp approach: Most of the times there is limited screening with this approach. It may sensitize the population for screening but can have no impact on incidence/mortality as it is a momentary and limited activity.

Hospital-based screening: It is generally linked to projects restricted to urban centers. It can raise good scientific information but cannot be translated into continuous activity due to lack of resources.

High-risk screening: It is mostly used in gynecology outpatient departments for detection in high-risk individuals or suspicious cervix.

A WHO health survey in 2002 regarding the estimated coverage of cervical cancer screening from 57 countries showed that effective coverage in India was very poor, i.e. the proportion of eligible women who reported having had a pelvic exam and Pap smear in the past three years was < 10%; crude coverage (women have had a pelvic exam but no smear) was around 30% and > 60% women had no coverage, not even a pelvic examination. Even within a country, there are differences in coverage in different age groups, and between rich and poor. Older and poor women, who are at the highest risk of developing cervical cancer, are least likely to be screened. Thus multiple strategies or techniques may need to be pursued within the same country.

SCREENING TOOLS

Available screening tools are based on cytological study of cervical cells, visualization of cervix and detection of HPV DNA.

Cytological Study of Cervical Cells

- **Conventional cytology with Pap smear** involves complex logistics, advanced training, and good program implementation. It is considered to be a very specific test for high-grade precancerous lesions or cancer but its sensitivity is only moderate varying between 30–87% attributed to both sampling and detection errors. The enormous success of cytology based screening program in developed countries is attributed to high screening frequency of 1–5 years, but involves considerable cost and resource implications.

- **Liquid-based cytology (LBC)** and **automated Pap testing** reduce the sampling error and improve the screening accuracy of Pap smears. LBC has the added advantage of "co-testing/reflex testing" for high-risk HPV DNA. Reflex testing means testing for HPV DNA later in the original sample of LBC, in case LBC is reported as ASCUS/LSIL.

- **Clinical down staging:** In developing countries like India, where we still see advanced disease, a simple speculum examination can be good to downstage the disease. Unaided visual inspection of cervix has shown an increase in the detection of early stage disease, however, it may miss majority of precancerous lesions and is not recommended as a screening test.

Visualization of Cervix

- **Colposcopy** also has a limited role as a screening test because of the costly equipment and special training needs.
- **Cervicography** with low cost camera system is also considered inadequate as a stand-alone screening technique, because of loss in visual discrimination inherent in examining an image compared to real time examination. It may have a possible role in combination with cytology or HPV for screening and for triage of women with equivocal cytology.
- **Visual inspection techniques** have been studied extensively in India. Visual inspection with acetic acid (VIA) alone is an inexpensive technique that can be performed easily by all levels of health workers. Results are available immediately and initial treatment can also be provided at the time of the examination. This is an effective screening tool, but has low specificity leading to higher referral rates. Visual inspection technique using a simple magnification device (VIAM) has not shown any advantage over VIA, but visual inspection with Lugol's iodine (VILI) has shown slightly better sensitivity (10% higher) and reproducibility than VIA and is equally specific.

Detection of High-risk HPV DNA

Detection of high-risk HPV DNA in cervical cell specimens can be done by Hybrid capture-2 (HC-2) technique which can detect 13 oncogenic subtypes, or by PCR assay for specific genotyping of HPV 16 and 18 along with detection of other high-risk types. Currently, FDA-approved HPV genotyping test identifies only HPV 16 and 18. Though not FDA approved, but many additional HPV genotyping assays are available now. However, the high cost of these tests restricts their use in low resource settings.

HC-2 has been approved by FDA for primary screening of cancer cervix, as adjunct to Pap smear (co-testing) in women over 30 years age and also for triage of ASC-US smears. For primary screening of women older than 30 yrs of age, HPV testing yields on an average, 10–20% greater sensitivity but 10% lower specificity than cytology, therefore combination of cytology and HPV testing attains very high sensitivity as well as negative predictive value of both approaching 100%, thus allowing extended screening interval of upto 3–5 yrs. When liquid-based cytology (LBC) is used, a reflex HPV DNA test can be performed using the residual liquid from the vial of women with an ASC-US result without the necessity to recall the woman. Nevertheless, HPV reflex testing can also be performed on a separately submitted specimen taken with a brush.

HPV testing could also be added to screening with VIA to increase the specificity of VIA, thereby reducing the referral rates without compromising the sensitivity of the test. A large cluster-randomized trial in a rural setting in India showed that a single round of HPV testing was associated with a significant reduction in the numbers of advanced cervical cancers and deaths from cervical cancer.

Rapid, low-cost oncogenic HPV DNA screening tests are being developed for low-resource countries. The 'care HPV assay' developed by QIAGEN, USA has been evaluated in China. It uses a signal-amplification assay to detect 14 different high risk HPV DNA types; it requires very little work space, does not require electricity or running water, and takes approximately 2.5 hours to perform.

SCREENING RECOMMENDATIONS

Current guideline (Table 12.1) were formulated following a better understanding of the natural history

Table 12.1: ASCCP (2012) guidelines for cervical cancer screening

Population	Recommended method	Comments
< 21 years	No screening	
21–29 years	Cytology alone every 3 years	HPV testing for screening not recommended in this age group
30–65 years	HPV and cytology "Co-testing" every 5 years (preferred)	Screening by HPV testing alone is not recommended
	Cytology alone every 3 years (acceptable)	Routine screening to be continued for 20 years in women with history of ≥ CIN 2 even after the age of 65 years is crossed
>65 years	No screening, if prior screening adequate and negative	
After hysterectomy	No screening in case of total hysterectomy	
Post-HPV vaccination	Recommendations same as for unvaccinated women	

of HPV infection and cervical carcinogenesis and supporting evidence on the performance of different screening tests.

SCREENING AUDIT

Choosing a suitable screening test is only one aspect of a screening program. More fundamental and challenging issue is the organization of the program in its totality, which involves audit as an essential component. The audit would help assess the performance of the program and identify the reason of the failures, which could be due to inadequate coverage, the failure of the screening test, or the failure in follow-up, each indicating the need for a different sort of remedial action.

SCREENING IN POST-VACCINATION ERA

Even post vaccination, screening has to be continued since HPVs 16 and 18 are only responsible for 75% of cervical cancers and also women already infected with high-risk types of HPV will not benefit from these vaccines.

MANAGEMENT OF ABNORMAL PAP SMEAR

Abnormal Pap smear report induces considerable anxiety to the patient and alerts the clinician for further action. Cytology does not give the final diagnosis but only picks up the patients 'at risk', the degree of risk has to be ascertained by further diagnostic procedures. Abnormal Pap smear should be managed at a centre with all facilities for colposcopy as well as treatment.

Abnormal or atypical cytological smear includes a spectrum of conditions ranging from atrophy, trauma and inflammatory to preinvasive and invasive cancers. Clinician must understand the full implication of the abnormal report and whenever in any doubt, it is worthwhile to discuss it with the reporting pathologist.

Presence of abnormal epithelial cells in a Pap smear calls for further evaluation either by repeat cytology, HPV DNA testing for high-risk virus, or by colposcopy depending upon the type of abnormality and the prevalence of associated high grade lesions. The work-up of women with abnormal Pap smear is discussed as per American Society of Cervical Cytology and Pathology (ASCCP) guidelines 2006 which were updated in 2012 (Table 12.1).

Unsatisfactory Cytology

In case of unsatisfactory cytology report, a repeat smear is called for after 2–4 months, following treatment of any underlying factor such as atrophy or inflammation.

Reflex HPV testing is not recommended. However, if the woman is ≥30 years of age and has already been co-tested for HPV and found to be positive, one may do colposcopy immediately; otherwise repeat cytology at 2–4 months is sufficient.

- If repeat cytology continues to be unsatisfactory, colposcopy is recommended.
- If repeat cytology is negative, follow-up can be done with routine screening or co-testing with HPV at one year, if HPV was positive.

Cytology Negative but Absent/Insufficient Endocervical Cells

Absence of endocervical cells on smear suggests that SCJ has not been sampled raising concern for missed disease. However, recent evidence shows a good specificity and negative predictive value of negative cytology despite absent or insufficient endocervical component.

In such a situation, if the woman is ≥ 30 years, it would be preferable to do HPV testing for added margin of safety; however, a follow-up with repeat cytology at 3 years is also acceptable. If HPV testing is done and is negative, women can remain in routine screening. If HPV testing is positive, one could repeat both tests in one year or one could do HPV 16/18 genotyping followed by colposcopy if HPV 16/18 is present and co-testing in 12 months if HPV 16/18 is absent. Women < 30 years can remain in routine screening.

Cytology Negative and HPV Positive Test

For the woman ≥30 years who is cytology negative and HPV positive, there are two options:
- Further triaging with HPV genotyping or mRNA if facility is available
  - If either is positive—immediate colposcopy
  - If negative—co-testing at one year
- Repeat co-testing at one year.
  - If HPV is still positive or cytology is ASC-US or more, colposcopy should be done.
  - If at one year both tests are negative, repeat co-testing at 3/5 years.

ASC-US (Atypical Squamous Cells of Undetermined Significance)

It has been found that prevalence of invasive cancer is low in women with ASC US (0.1–0.2%); hence it can be evaluated by any of the two methods, i.e. repeat cytology after 12 months, immediate high-risk HPV DNA. Both are equally safe and effective. Genotyping is not recommended as its result does not modify the management.

❖ Repeat Pap smear at 12 months:
- If repeat smear shows ASC-US or higher abnormality, further colposcopic examination is recommended.
- If repeat smear is negative, patient can be followed up as in routine screening.

❖ Reflex high risk HPV DNA testing (preferred):
- If HPV DNA is negative, patient can be followed up further by repeat cytology at 12 months or co-testing at 3 years.
- If HPV DNA is positive, colposcopic evaluation is performed.

Patients 21–24 years age need to be managed differently. They are followed by repeat cytology only. HPV DNA testing is not recommended because of high prevalence of HPV in this age group and risk of unnecessary over treatment. Colposcopy is done only if repeat cytology report at 12 months is HSIL/ASC-H or greater or at 24 months ASC US or higher.

In *pregnant women*, management options are same as for non-pregnant women except that colposcopy can be deferred until at least 6 weeks postpartum.

In *women > 65 years* with ASC US but HPV negative, additional surveillance is required after one year, preferably by co-testing but repeat cytology is also acceptable.

ASC-H (Atypical Squamous Cells–High-Grade Lesion cannot be Ruled Out)

Women with ASC–H have a higher prevalence of high grade lesions. Therefore, immediate colposcopy is recommended in all such patients.
- If colposcopy identifies a *high grade lesion* that is proven on biopsy to be CIN 2 or 3, it would be managed accordingly.
- If *high grade lesion is ruled out*, further follow-up is done either by repeat cytology at 6 months interval for 2 years or by HPV DNA at 12 months.

LSIL (Low Grade Squamous Intraepithelial Lesion)

Immediate colposcopy is recommended in LSIL with no prior HPV test or a positive HPV test found on co-testing. Reflex HPV testing is not recommended to triage these women for colposcopy as LSIL has been found to be associated with HPV infection in more than 75% cases.

However, in case co-testing has already been performed, some of LSIL may be found to be HPV negative. In such cases, although colposcopy is acceptable, it is preferable to repeat co-testing at 1 year, as the risk of CIN 3+ in HPV-negative women with LSIL is low. If repeat co-testing at 1 year is ASCUS or worse or the HPV test is positive colposcopy is recommended. If the co-testing result at 1 year is HPV negative and cytology negative, repeat co-testing after an additional 3 years is recommended.

- At the time of colposcopy, If *colposcopy is adequate and a lesion* is identified, directed biopsy is taken and further management is done according to the biopsy report.
- If *no lesion is detected or if the colposcopy is inadequate*, endocervical sampling should also be done. If ECC is negative, patient can be followed up by either repeat cytology at 6 months interval for 2 years or co-testing with HPV DNA at 12 months.

Adolescents with LSIL are followed by repeat cytology only. HPV DNA testing is not recommended because of high prevalence of HPV in this age group and risk of unnecessary over treatment. Colposcopy is recommended only in case of repeat cytology of HSIL/ASC–H or greater at 12 months, or ASC-US or higher at 24 months.

In *pregnant women*, immediate colposcopy may be performed or it can be deferred until at least 6 weeks postpartum, but endocervical curettage should not be done. For pregnant women who have no cytologic, histologic, or colposcopically suspected CIN 2+ at the initial colposcopy, postpartum follow-up is recommended.

HSIL (High-Grade Squamous Intraepithelial Lesion)

HSIL report on cytology carries a high-risk of significant cervical disease with incidence of invasive disease in as many as 2% cases. Immediate colposcopy along with endocervical curettage is recommended in all cases.

- If *colposcopy is satisfactory and a high grade lesion* is identified, directed biopsy is taken and further management is done according to the biopsy report. Instead of directed biopsy, immediate loop electro-surgical excision procedure (LEEP) can also be performed because colposcopy can miss a significant number of CIN 2 and 3 lesions. This is the only clinical situation where role of See and Treat policy is established.
- With *satisfactory colposcopy, if no lesion* is found and ECC is negative, these cases can be closely followed by colposcopy and cytology both at 6 months interval for 1 year. Diagnostic excision is recommended, if HSIL is detected at any of these visits. If both the visits produce negative results, women can return to routine screening.

• If colposcopy is *unsatisfactory or ECC is positive*, diagnostic excisional procedure should be done

In *adolescents* with HSIL cytology, immediate colposcopy should be performed. Immediate *see and treat LEEP is not recommended* in this age group. If no lesion is identified, follow-up is done with cytology and colposcopy both at 6 monthly interval for 24 months. If HSIL report persists with no lesion after 24 months, then diagnostic excision should be done.

In *pregnant women*, immediate colposcopy should be performed. ECC should not be done. Colposcopy directed biopsy can be taken, but diagnostic excision should not be done.

AGC (Atypical Glandular Cells)

Atypical glandular cells could indicate the presence of benign conditions such as reactive changes and polyps or significant neoplastic conditions such as adenocarcinoma in situ (AIS), CIN, and adenocarcinoma of cervix, endometrium, ovaries or fallopian tubes. Significant high grade intraepithelial neoplasia may be seen in up to 40% women and invasive cancer in 3–17% with AGC on cytology.

Cancer risk is lower in women < 35 years of age with AGC, but the risk of CIN 2+ is higher. Therefore, a thorough assessment is required at all ages. Cervical adenocarcinoma is HPV associated and reflex HPV testing can detect them but it does not identify women with endometrial cancer.

All women with atypical glandular cells on cytology should be evaluated by immediate colposcopy, endocervical curettage and regardless of HPV test results. Reflex HPV DNA testing is not recommended. In addition, endometrial sampling should be obtained in those more than 35 years, in those at high risk for endometrial disease even if less than 35 years age or if endometrial cells are present in the smear.

• If initial cytology report is **AGC (NOS)** and no lesions are detected on colposcopy/ECC, patient should be followed up by repeat cytology and HPV testing both at 12 and 24 months, If both the tests are –ve, cotesting is recommended at 3 yrs. If any test is +ve then colposcopy is done.

• If initial cytology report is **AGC favouring neoplasia or AIS**, and no invasive disease has been found on colposcopy/ECC, diagnostic excisional procedure is recommended.

• If endometrial sampling shows any pathology, it is managed accordingly.

• For benign glandular changes: No further evaluation is recommended in premenopausal women, but endometrial assessment is recommended in post-menopausal women.

MANAGEMENT OF HISTOLOGICALLY PROVEN CIN

Definitive management of cervical intraepithelial neoplasia should be based upon the histological proven diagnosis, as the grading of abnormalities on cytology does not always correspond to the histological grading. Appropriate management (neither under nor over-treatment) of these lesions is mandatory for prevention of cervical cancer.

Management of CIN has changed dramatically over past few decades. Various new modalities have evolved. In the past, hysterectomy was the only accepted definitive treatment that is now considered too radical for most of the cases. Now there is a tendency to use conservative modalities as younger patients are being diagnosed with CIN.

Treatment for CIN is based on the philosophy that it is a local disease, where the underlying stroma and lymphatics are not involved. Therefore, conservative treatment by local removal or destruction of pathological tissue is sufficient, provided it is assured that all the abnormal tissues to a depth of 5–7 mm are removed or destroyed. Since whole of the transformation zone (TZ) is at risk, therefore, it is pertinent that entire TZ has to be treated.

TREATMENT MODALITIES

Therapeutic options for conservative management include ablative and excisional modalities (Table 12.2).

Ablative Methods

Aim of ablative therapy is to destroy the full thickness of abnormal epithelium including the glandular crypts up to a depth of 5 to 7 mm as CIN has a tendency to extend into the glandular crypts. Ablation may be performed using cryotherapy, cold coagulation, laser vaporization, or electrocoagulation diathermy. Except electrocoagulation diathermy, all are cost-effective OPD procedures, well acceptable to the patients. The major

Table 12.2: Conservative management options for CIN	
Ablative methods	*Excisional methods*
• Cryotherapy	• LEEP/NETZ/SWETZ
• Cold coagulation	• Cold knife conization
• Laser vaporization	• Laser conization
• Electrocoagulation diathermy	

disadvantage of ablative therapy is that the tissue is not available for histopathological examination. Therefore, success of treatment cannot be judged immediately and a prolong follow-up is required.

Proper patient selection is the key to success of ablative therapy. Patient should be thoroughly evaluated to ensure that all the prerequisites are being met.

Selection criteria
- Lesion should be completely visible along with the entire transformation zone and the squamo-columnar junction—TZ type 1 (Fig. 12.1).
- Pap smear should not contain glandular atypical cells and endocervical curettage should be negative.
- There should be no evidence of invasion or micro-invasion on cytology, colposcopy or biopsy.
- Patient should be compliant as the procedure requires prolong follow-up.

Follow-up facilities of cytology and colposcopy should be available.

Cryotherapy

It destroys the tissue by intracellular crystallization of water. This is the most commonly used ablative method and is an effective treatment for benign and CIN lesions of the cervix in well-selected patients. It is a good technique for small lesions of the cervix. Cryotherapy

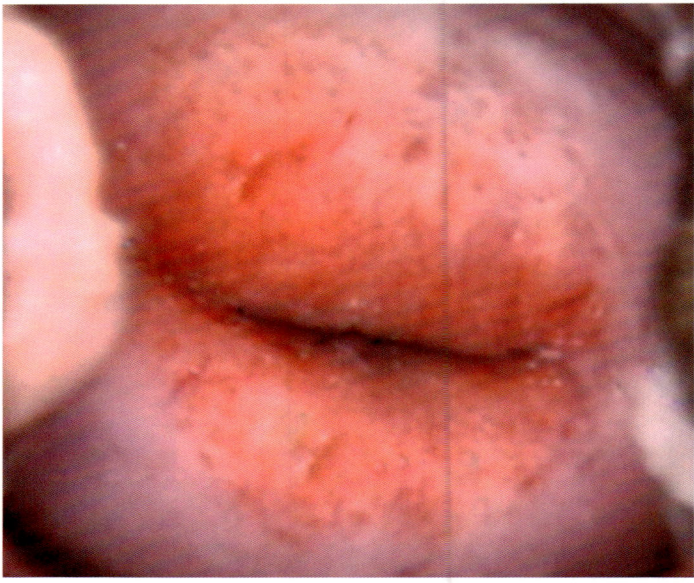

Fig. 12.1: Lesion appropriate for ablation (TZ type 1)

is a poor choice for treatment of lesions extending into endocervical canal (Fig. 12.2) or large lesions extending beyond the probe or in situations where cervical or vaginal anatomy prohibits adequate applications of cryoprobe over the lesions. Procedure is contraindicated in pregnancy, PID or if there is slightest suspicion of malignancy.

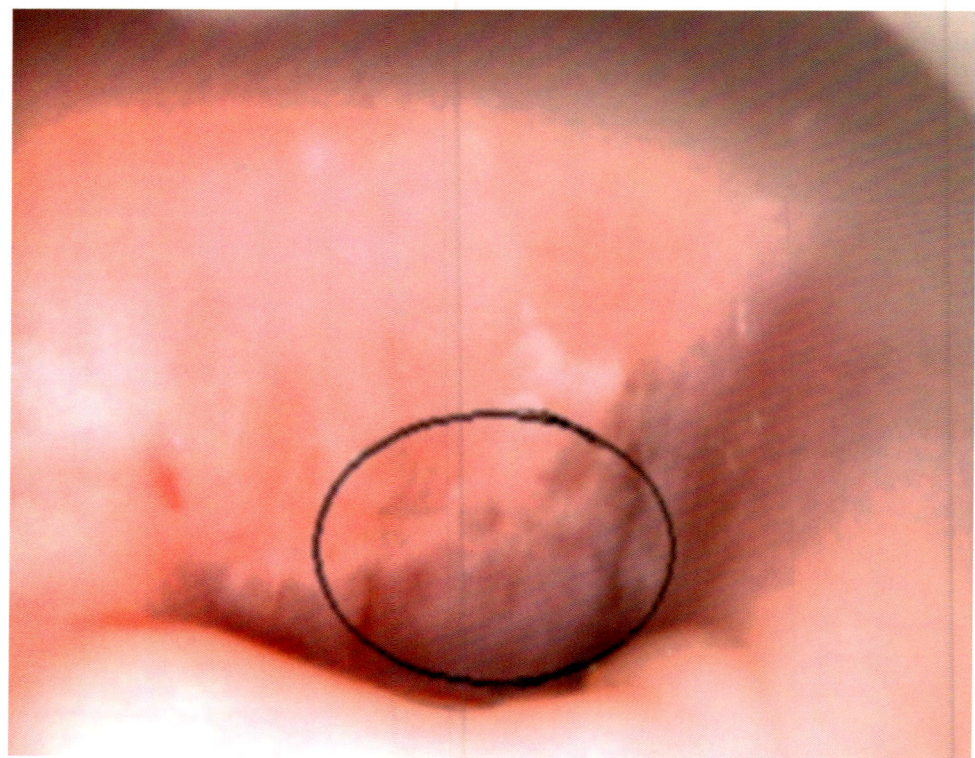

Fig. 12.2: Lesion going into the ECC (TZ type 3)—inappropriate for ablative therapy

It is done with the help of a handheld cryogun with probe using carbon dioxide or nitrous oxide gas as refrigerant. Nitrous oxide (–90°C) is preferred as it is cooler in comparison to carbon dioxide (–60°C). The flow of gas is controlled by a trigger which is used for freezing as well as thawing. Intracellular water gets crystallized destroying the cells under the influence of extremely cold temperature. Adequate tank pressure of more than 40 kg/cm² is necessary for satisfactory results.

Best time for cryotherapy is postmenstrual phase. No anesthesia is required. Premedication is ordered to block unpleasant side effects caused by the release of prostaglandins from dying cells.

After exposing the cervix, topography of abnormal epithelium is rechecked. Probes are available in various size and shapes. Depending upon the size and location of the lesion, appropriate probe that covers the entire lesion but not contact vaginal walls is chosen and placed over the cervix after applying water-soluble lubricant. Thereafter refrigerant is activated. Freezing is continued till an adequate ice ball is formed ideally 7–10 mm beyond the probe edge and not less than 5 mm in any case (Figs 12.3A and B). If the tank pressure of cylinder is good, it usually takes about 3–5 minutes for a good ice ball beyond probe edge to form. Time is not as important as the formation of good ice ball. To

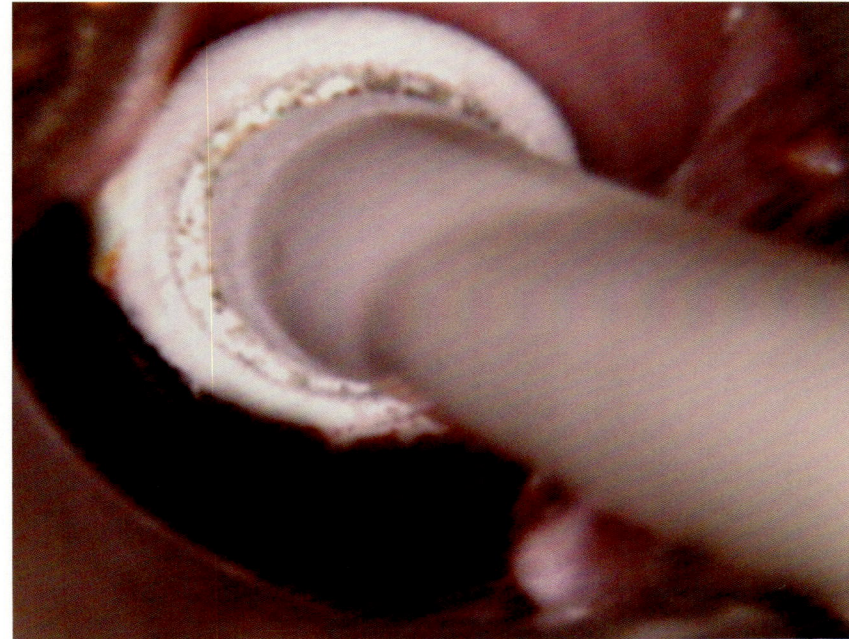

Fig. 12.3A: Ice ball

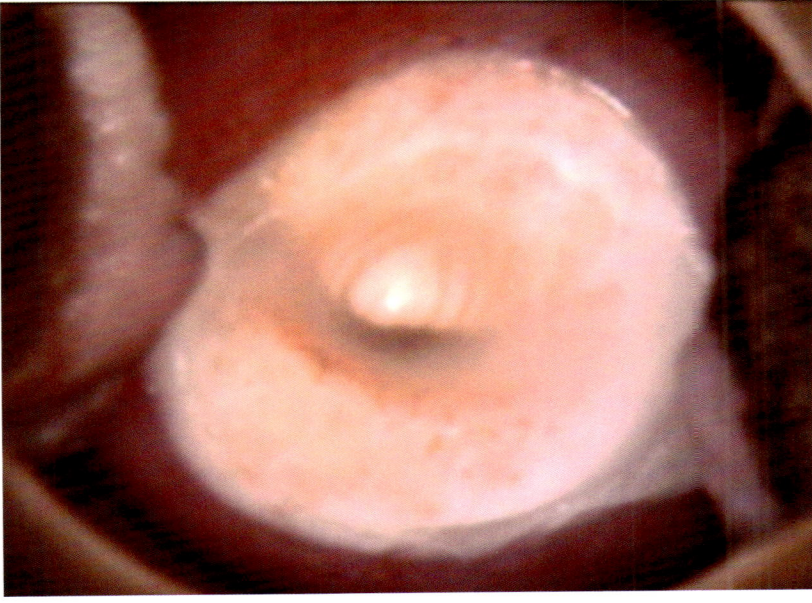

Fig. 12.3B: Cervix after cryo procedure

maximize the cure rate, destruction of all tissues up to a depth of 7 mm should be aimed so that all the involved crypts are destroyed. Effort should be made to include all the metaplastic epithelium. After this, the cryogun is deactivated. Before the second application, cervix should be defrosted first and then the probe is reapplied and the procedure is repeated. This double freeze technique yields better results than single freeze technique.

Side effects are few. There might be slight discomfort at the time of procedure due to release of prostaglandins which is easily relieved by NSAIDs. Some patients may feel flushing or light headedness that is why they should get up slowly after therapy. Later profuse vaginal discharge lasting for 2–3 weeks and scarring of tissue may occur. Bleeding occurs less often. Patient is advised to practice sexual abstinence

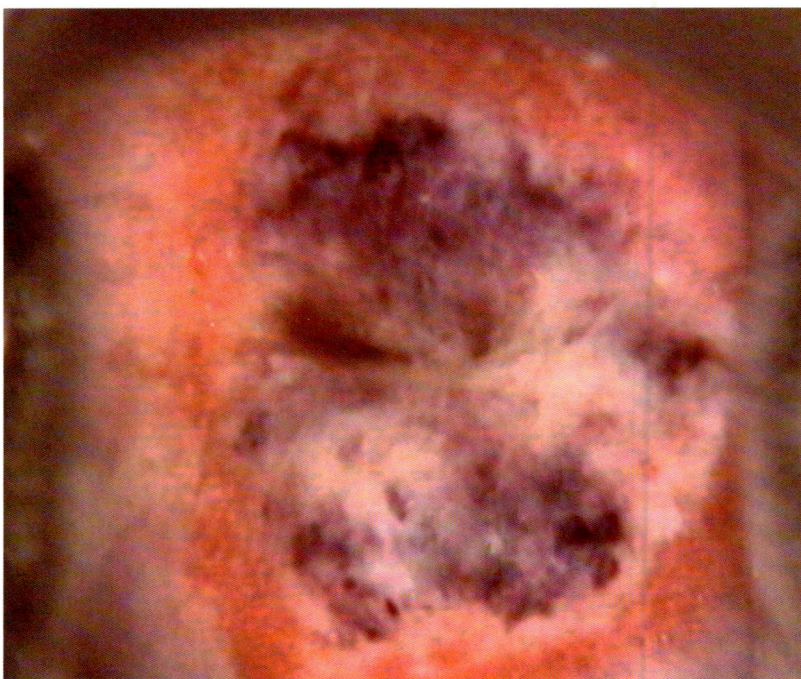

Fig. 12.4A: Cervix 15 days after cryotherapy

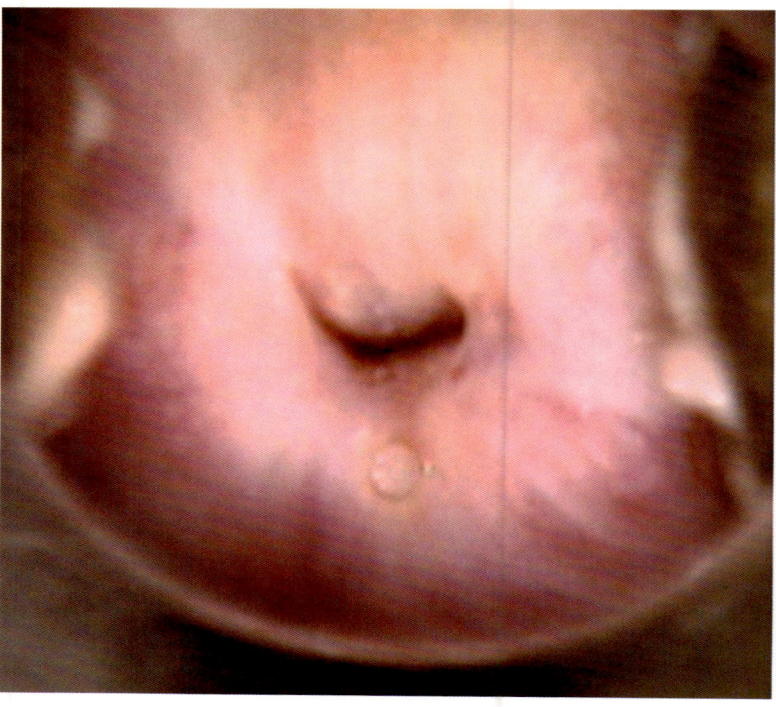

Fig. 12.4B: Cervix 6 months after cryotherapy

for 1 month. Proper rest, local hygiene and institution of antibiotic therapy help in postoperative recovery. There may be sloughing of cervical tissue after freezing that may lead at times to cervical stenosis (Figs 12.4A and B).

After healing, the squamocolumnar junction may recede inside the endocervical canal. Follow-up is performed 6 months after the procedure using cytobrush for Pap smear. If cytology remains abnormal after six months, it is considered as treatment failure and conization should be considered as the next therapeutic procedure as a possibility of co-existing invasive cancer may be one of the reasons of failure. In properly selected cases, cure rate of cryotherapy has been reported as high as 96%.

It is generally preferred to have the diagnosis of CIN firmly established before deciding the management plan and offering the type of treatment. However, there are exceptions to this rule. To maximize treatment coverage especially in developing countries, women may be offered treatment at their first visit to the clinic during colposcopy/ VIA. Otherwise patients who are lost to follow up would not receive any treatment for the lesions and may progress to invasive lesions. This approach may be used by expert colposcopist to maximize treatment coverage while at the same time minimizing the number of clinic visits. In case single visit treatment is decided, directed biopsy must be taken before cryotherapy to confirm the histological nature of the lesion which has been treated because ablative treatment does not provide any tissue specimen for histological examination.

Cold Coagulation

Semm's cold coagulator (Fig. 12.5) coagulates tissue at a temperature of 100°C. Thermo sound probe is applied to the cervix for at least 20 seconds in 4 to 5 overlapping areas to destroy whole transformation zone. Local cold coagulation offers the advantage of easy portability, no gas requirements and requires a far shorter treatment time compared to cryotherapy. It is electrically operated, and it incorporates automatic self-sterilization analgesia is recommended for large lesions. Mild degree of pain, discharge or infection may occur. Cure rate up to 94% is reported.

Electrocoagulation Radical Diathermy

In electrocoagulation diathermy (Fig. 12.6), the whole transformation zone is destroyed by combination of fulguration and coagulation using needle and ball electrodes. For adequate destruction (7–10 mm), general anesthesia has to be used as the procedure is very painful. Lesion is identified under colposcopic view and cervix is dilated up to (7 mm). First the whole area is fulgurated with needle electrode at 2 mm apart points followed by coagulation of intervening tissue with ball electrode. It can be used for large lesions, occupying more than 75% of the ectocervix or extending to the vaginal wall, where cryotherapy or cold coagulation cannot be used.

Bleeding and discharge are common among late complications. Cervical stenosis is common. SC junction is usually visible and cytological follow-up is easily performed. Up to 99% success rate has been reported with this technique.

Radical diathermy is different from diathermo-coagulation in which heat is used to destroy cervical epithelium only to a depth of 2–3 mm that is too superficial to be recommended for the treatment of CIN.

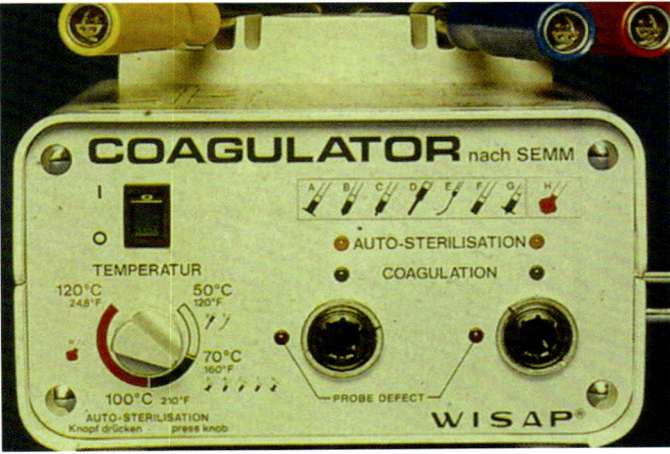

Fig. 12.5: Semm cold coagulator

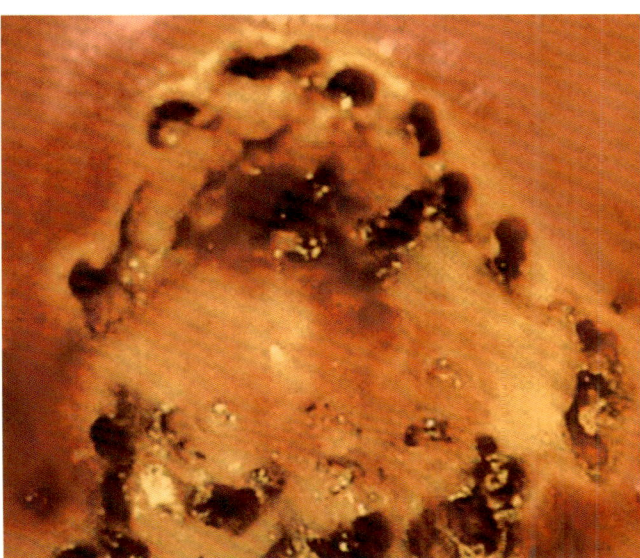

Fig. 12.6: Cervix after electrocoagulation diathermy

Laser Ablation

This treatment modality has been extensively used with success rate equal to that of cryotherapy. Laser allows more precise tissue destruction, leaves less necrotic tissue, heals faster and squamocolumnar junction usually does not recede inside the canal. It can also be used for large intraepithelial lesions particularly those involving vaginal cuff or lateral fornices.

Local anesthesia with paracervical block is given underneath cervical mucosa and cervix is stained with 50% Lugol's iodine. The peripheral margins are outlined with CO_2 laser and the whole transformation zone is ablated up to 7 mm depth. Central button is destroyed along the axis of cervical canal up to 12 mm. Immediate complications are few. Delayed bleeding and mild pain have been reported. It results in minimal structural cervical deformity and does not affect future fertility. Scarring and stenosis of cervical os are rare. However, the equipment is very costly, requires extensive training, and is not available in many centers.

Excisional Methods

With ablative methods, clinician takes a calculated risk, as even in best hands, cytology and colposcopy both carry a definite inter- and intra-observer error. Various studies report 0.1 to 1% incidence of missed invasive cancer at the time of ablation. Such cases have medical, financial and legal implications. This problem is overcome by excisional methods.

The aim of an excisional treatment is to remove the lesion/transformation zone in its entirety and submit it for histopathology. Excisional methods are being preferred in modern practice as these are diagnostic as well as therapeutic. Completeness of excision can be assessed and invasion can be ruled out with confidence, if performed under colposcopic guidance.

Excision Treatment Types

Excision can be carried out by any of the accepted methods, electrosurgical loop/needle, and straight wire excision of TZ, laser, or cold knife. Whichever method is used, whole of the transformation zone should be excised. Size and shape of the excision should be decided by the colposcopic findings and should correspond to the type of TZ described by IFCPC (Figs 4.33A to C). IFCPC (2011) has recommended to avoid the terms: "conization," "cone biopsy," "big loop excision," and "small loop excision" as each of these may mean different things to different health care providers. Each of the excision types is associated with a different technique as well as with altered risk of incomplete excision and subsequent morbidity.

Type 3 excision is indicated for resection of a type 3 TZ, glandular disease, suspected microinvasion, large CIN 3 lesion to rule out invasion, and for repeat treatment.

Type 3 excision is associated with greater difficulty and risk of long-term morbidity as well as a high risk of incomplete excision and residual disease. In such cases, one may consider alternatives to LLETZ such as SWETZ/NETZ, cold knife or laser excision.

When the lesion is extending inside the endocervical canal, microcolpohysteroscopy, if available, may be used to map the upper limit of the lesion and tailor the size of the cone as complication rate is directly related to the size of the cone removed.

Shape of the cone should be truncated (Fig. 12.7) as with a conical cone, gland crypts at the apex may be transected leaving behind the residual disease (Fig. 12.8). Properly planned, colposcopically-guided excision has fewer complications.

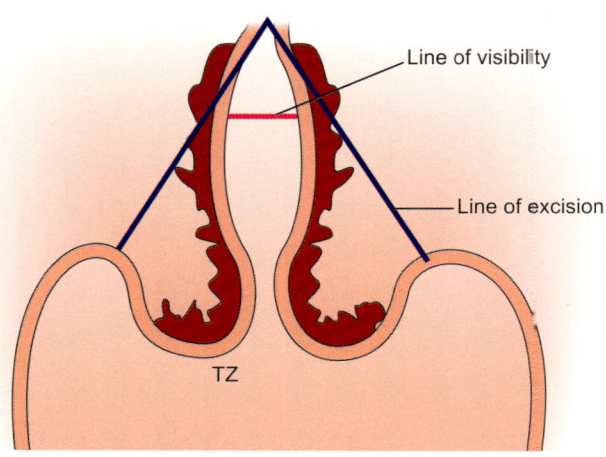

Fig. 12.7: Cylindrical cone

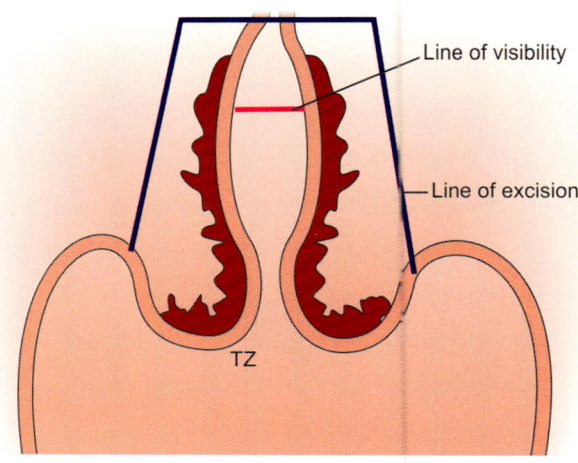

Fig. 12.8: Ideal truncated shape

Excisional Techniques

Techniques used for excision include loop electrosurgical excision procedure (LEEP) also called large loop excision of transformation zone (LLETZ), its variations are: Needle excision of transformation zone (NETZ) or straight wire excision of transformation zone (SWETZ), cold knife conization (CKC), and laser conization.

Loop Electrosurgical Excision Procedure (LEEP) or Large Loop Excision of Transformation Zone (LLETZ)

This procedure is fast gaining popularity in modern treatment of CIN. Excision is performed with a diathermy loop made of a very thin steel/tungsten wire (0.2 mm diameter) with insulated shaft is used along with a monopolar electrosurgical generator wattage set at 25–50 using blend current. Loops are available in various dimensions of width and depth. Loop is selected according to site and size of the lesion. Less than 2 cm diameter loop is recommended to minimize the tissue damage, as larger loops use more power.

The procedure should be done in postmenstrual phase. Any cervicitis or vaginitis, if present, should be treated beforehand as any infection may give rise to secondary hemorrhage. The procedure is done under local intracervical anesthesia. Insulated speculum should be used along with smoke evacuator. Loop is advanced into cervix just lateral to transformation zone or 5 mm lateral to the lesion until required depth of 1 cm is reached (Figs 12.9A and B).

SWETZ and NETZ refer to the same technique in which the TZ is excised with a straight diathermy wire instead of a loop. The point of the wire is employed like a knife and the size and shape of excised tissue is determined by the configuration of coloposcopic abnormality rather than by predetermined shape of the instrument. Also the deep cutting edge is not obscured during an NETZ procedure. NETZ is more likely to produce a specimen in one piece and with clear margins as compared to LLETZ. However, it takes too longer to perform and is difficult to learn.

To get a clean cut, loop is moved slowly and not pushed across the cervix and is withdrawn just beyond the contralateral margin of the transformation zone. If there are any bleeding points at the base of the excisional tissue (Fig. 12.9C), they can be treated with ball electrode.

A special device such as **Cone biopsy excisor** (Fig. 12.10A) can also be used. It has a linear rigid wire with central fully insulated shaft to protect endocervix. It removes accurate cone, requires less wattage, hence less thermal artifacts. Its design permits precise positioning (Fig. 12.10B) and good hand control. It can be used as OPD procedure under local anesthesia.

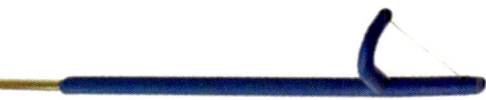

Fig. 12.10A: Cone biopsy excisor

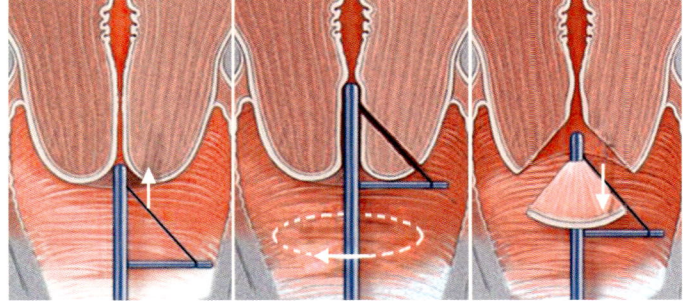

Fig 12.10B: Conization procedure using cone biopsy excisor

When LEEP is performed for type 3 excision, it has to be done in two parts. A large loop is used to remove the broader ectocervical portion, and upper endocervical portion is removed with a smaller in a top hat manner (Fig. 12.11). Excision of the TZ in multiple fragments can complicate the histopathological assessment. In type 2 and 3 excisions, endocervical sampling can be considered after the excision.

Advantages: LEEP can be done on an outpatient basis and tissue is available for histopathology which reduces

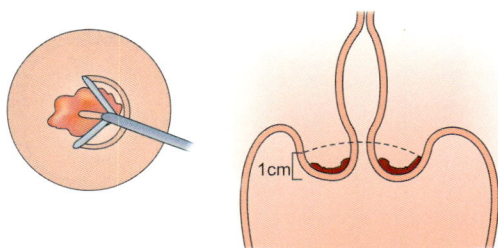

Fig. 12.9A: LEEP procedure—diagrammatic

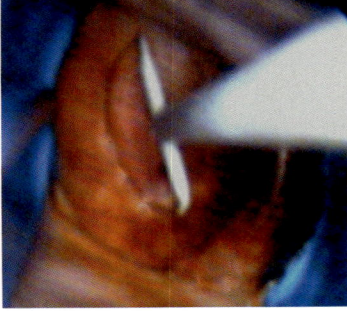

Fig. 12.9B: LEEP in progress

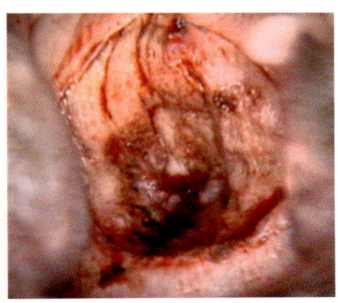

Fig. 12.9C: Base of the cervix after LEEP excision

the anxiety of the patient. Postoperative discomfort is minimal and healing is rapid. It can be diagnostic as well as curative during a single visit. If no invasion is reported and margins of the tissue removed are free, no further treatment is required. It also offers a valuable safeguard as the removal of entire transformation zone can pick up any area of unsuspected invasion which could otherwise have been missed.

Complications including pelvic infection, bleeding and stenosis of os are much lower as compared to that with cold knife conization. In comparison to Laser conization, it is cost-effective, requires no special equipment and can be done easily with the usual operation theatre equipment. Its success rate is 90%. This technique has found high acceptability in developing countries because of low cost of the equipment and treatment.

Side effects are few. Patient may experience blood-stained discharge for 2–3 weeks. If at any time after therapy there is purulent discharge, pain in abdomen or bleeding, patient must report immediately. Infection can be controlled by local and systemic antibiotics. Bleeding can usually be controlled by packing, fulguration, Monsel's paste or silver nitrate stick. Rarely a stitch may be required. Incidence of cervical stenosis is extremely low.

See and treat policy: Since LEEP is a simple procedure which can be diagnostic as well as curative. Its use has been recommended as a single clinic visit treatment termed "See and Treat" policy. It is highly beneficial and provides the opportunity to treat patients with significant lesions where follow-up visit is a problem and patient may not return for therapy, and may get lost for follow-up. However, at times, it may lead to unnecessary excision because many low grade lesions like regenerative or metaplastic epithelium may mimic CIN. Hence, this "See and Treat policy" is now recommended only for definite high grade lesions only.

Cold Knife Conization (CKC)

Cold knife conization is performed with help of scalpel under general anesthesia (Fig. 12.12). In the past, cold knife conization was the only excisional method available. It has well recognized short- and long-term morbidity, major complication being intraoperative and postoperative hemorrhage that can be minimized by injecting the cervix preoperatively with adrenaline 1 in 200,000. Despite the high rate of complications, cold knife conization still has an important place in the treatment. Moreover, facilities for LEEP or Laser are not available in many centers.

CKC has clear advantage over LEEP and Laser as it gives excisional margins that are not affected by thermal artifact.

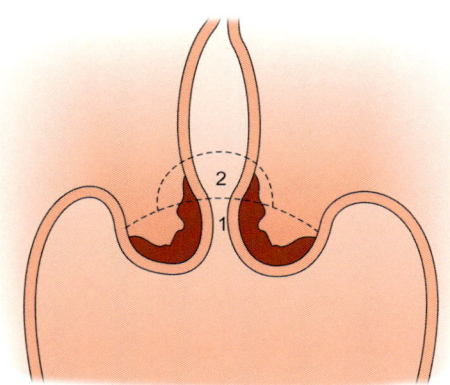

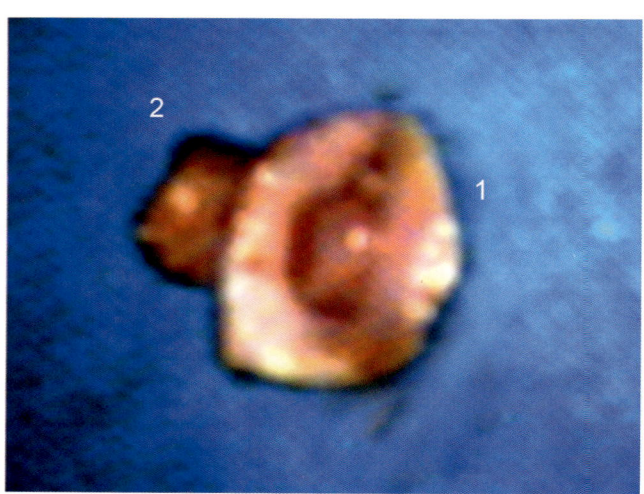

1-lower part, 2-upper part

Fig. 12.11: Type 3 excision by LEEP

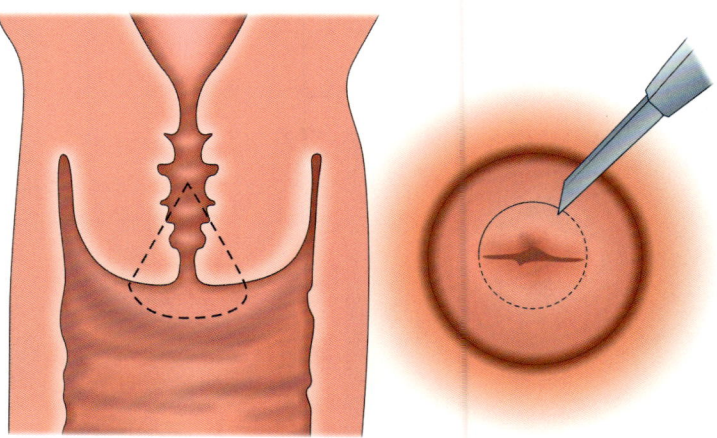

Fig. 12.12: Cold knife conization—diagrammatic

Laser Conization

When conization is indicated, laser (Fig. 12.13A) is an ideal method of treating CIN lesions. But instead of cone, a cylinder of tissue should be removed. The sides of cylinder should be as flat as possible. For this procedure, cutting mode of laser should be used. Spot size of laser is reduced to minimum but higher power available is used for cutting.

After colposcopic evaluation of cervix and applications of Schiller's iodine, area to be cut must be marked out with laser leaving 3 mm of healthy tissue around. Then cutting is done vertically into the cervix and incision goes up to 1 cm depth. To avoid the thermal damage and to facilitate cutting, the central portion of cervix is drawn away from the beam using fine surgical hooks. While cutting, the capillaries retract and there is hardly any bleeding (Fig. 12.13B). Side effects are similar to those of ablation. Fertility is not affected.

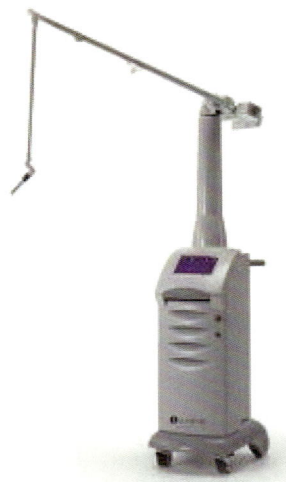

Fig. 12.13A: Laser equipment

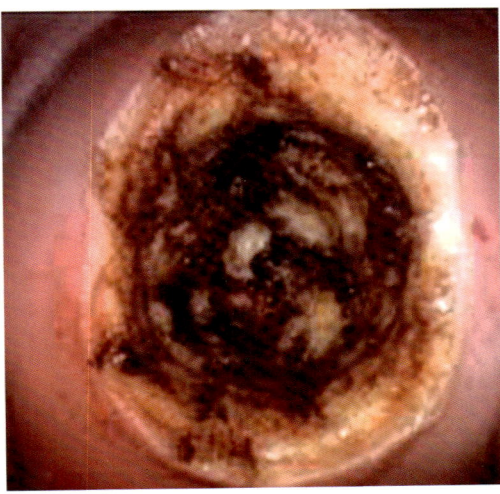

Fig. 12.13B: Crater after laser conization

Before sending the specimen to the histopathologist, its dimensions should be noted (Fig. 12.14) as follows:
- Length is the distance from the distal or external margin to the proximal or internal margin of the excised specimen.
- Thickness is the distance from the stromal margin to the surface of the excised specimen.
- Circumference (optional) is the distance surrounding the perimeter of the excised specimen.

When excised specimen is removed in multiple pieces, each piece specimen should be measured separately.

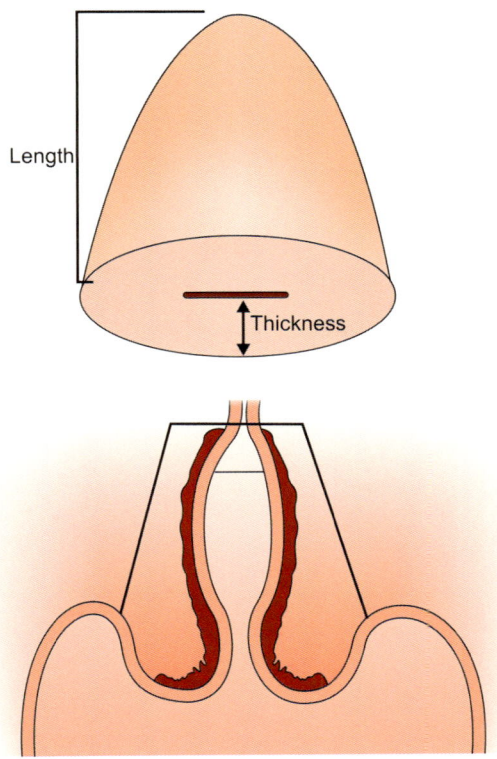

Fig. 12.14: Dimensions of the excised specimen

Hysterectomy

In general, hysterectomy is not required for treatment of CIN except for the following indications:
1. Associated uterine or ovarian pathology.
2. Elderly patients with recurrent disease despite multiple attempts at conservative therapy.
3. Lesions extending extensively into vaginal fornices.
4. Rarely cancer phobia.

Vaginal hysterectomy or laparoscopic assisted vaginal hysterectomy (LAVH) is preferred as removal of vaginal mucosa over portio vaginalis of cervix is better removed. Follow-up of patients is required for detection of vaginal intraepithelial neoplasia which may develop later in 1% of cases.

Follow-up after excision: Margin status of the excised specimen should be noted. Although positive margins increase the risk of recurrence, a negative status does not rule out residual disease, so the patient should remain under follow-up. If on histology report, the margins of the LEEP are found to be positive, one should not immediately decide for retreatment but wait and watch.

All the patients are advised to come after 4 months for repeat Pap smear and colposcopy, if required.

A post-LEEP button may be seen at follow-up visit (Fig. 12.15). This is a regenerative change and has no significance in the absence of any other abnormality.

Role of HPV testing in follow-up after treatment: It has been established that HPV testing post-treatment can more quickly and efficiently detect a treatment failure and predict residual/recurrent CIN with significantly higher sensitivity and not significantly lower specificity than follow-up cytology. HPV DNA testing has also been found to be more sensitive than histology of the section margins.

Treatment of residual and recurrent lesions: The presence of residual disease warrants excision of the TZ. Such cases are generally not suitable for ablation as the post-treatment recurrence frequently occurs in the endocervical canal where it is not colposcopically detectable.

RECOMMENDED TREATMENT GUIDELINES

Though cervical squamous intraepithelial neoplasia (CIN) is graded into 3 grades, but for the purpose of management, two-tier grading into low grade (CIN 1) and high grade (CIN 2, 3) is used based on the risk of progression to invasive cancer, which has been reported to be only 1% in CIN 1 but 5% and 12% for CIN 2 and 3, respectively.

Treatment is individualized depending upon age of the patient, desire for fertility, size and grade of lesion, prior cytology report, treatment history, operators experience, co-existent pathology, and resources available.

CIN 1

Management of CIN 1 (low grade lesions) poses a difficult challenge for the clinician, as majority of the lesions will undergo spontaneous regression. Risk of occult CIN 3+ is more when CIN 1 is preceded by HSIL, ASC-H or AGC (approximately 15%) than when preceded by ASC-US or LSIL on cytology report (approximately 4%). That is why now the recommended management is based on the preceding cytology report:

- **CIN 1 preceded by "lesser abnormalities":** Lesser abnormalities includes ASC-US/LSIL on cytology, positive HPV 16/18, and persistent HPV positive. Observation and immediate treatment are both accepted policies for such patients.

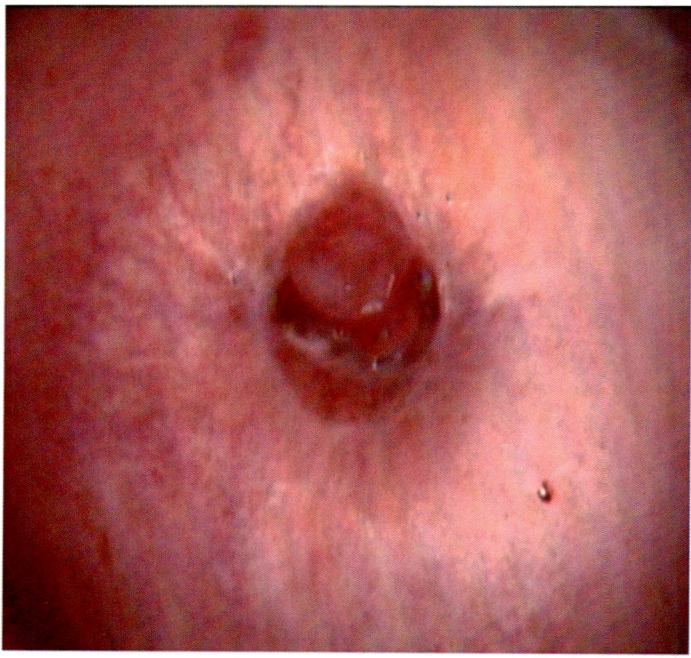
After saline application

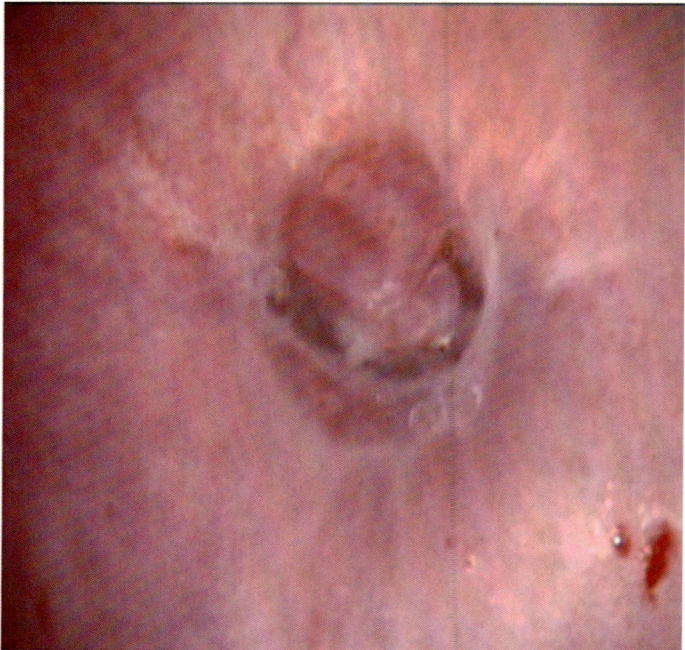
After acetic acid application

Fig. 12.15: Cervix 6 months after LEEP showing post-LEEP button

– Immediate treatment is recommended when the lesion is extensive or the patient is not reliable for follow-up.

– Majority of the patients can be kept under observation by repeat cytology at 6 months interval for 2 years or co-testing with HPV at 12 months. If both are negative, co-testing is repeated after 3 years. If repeat cytology at any time is ASC-US or higher or if the HPV is positive then colposcopy is done.

If the lesion persists for more than 2 years:

o Patient can be treated with either ablative or excisional methods, if the colposcopy is satisfactory.

o Excisional method should be chosen, if colposcopy is unsatisfactory, endocervical sampling is positive, or if the CIN 1 has been persisting after previous treatment.

- **CIN 1 preceded by ASC–H, HSIL or AGC NOS:** Management depends on the colposcopy and endocervical sampling findings.

  – Excisional method should be chosen, if colposcopy is unsatisfactory, or endocervical sampling is positive.

  – Patients with satisfactory colposcopy and negative endocervical sampling can be kept under observation with co-testing (both cytology and HPV) at 12 and 24 months.

    o If reports are negative at both visits, age-specific routine screening to be performed after 3 years.

    o If at any time, cytology is reported as HSIL, diagnostic excision should be done.

    o If HPV is positive or cytology is abnormal but less than HSIL, then colposcopy is performed.

- **CIN 1 (special population):**

  – *Young adults (21–24 years)* with CIN 1 are followed by repeat cytology only. Colposcopy is recommended only in case of repeat cytology of HSIL or greater at 12 months or ASC–US or higher at 24 months. HPV DNA testing is not recommended because of high prevalence of HPV in this age group and risk of unnecessary over treatment.

  – *Young adults* with CIN 1 preceded by ASC–H, HSIL or AGC NOS, observation for up to 24 months using both colposcopy and cytology at 6 month intervals is recommended, provided the colposcopic examination is adequate and endocervical assessment is negative.

  – *Pregnant* women with CIN 1 are followed up without treatment.

CIN 2, 3

Due to high rate of progression and persistence of these lesions, it is recommended that all women with CIN 2, 3 should be treated immediately. Patients are not kept under observation alone except in special population (*young adults* and *pregnant*).

– Either excisional or ablative methods can be used, if colposcopy is satisfactory and the lesion size is small

– Only excisional methods are recommended in

  o Inadequate colposcopy

  o Large CIN 2, 3 lesions

  o Recurrent CIN 2, 3 lesions

– If CIN 2, 3 is detected at the margins of excisional cone or in the endocervical sample obtained immediately after the procedure, follow-up is done with cytology and endocervical sampling at 4–6 months after treatment. Alternately a repeat diagnostic excision can also be performed. In case repeat excision is not feasible or there is persistent or recurrent CIN 2/3, hysterectomy can be performed.

Special population:

– *Adolescents* with CIN 2 with satisfactory colposcopy and negative endocervical sampling can be followed by repeat cytology and colposcopy both at 6 months interval for 24 months, whereafter treatment is recommended, if CIN 3 develops subsequently or if CIN 2 persists. In case of unsatisfactory colposcopy and specified CIN 3 lesions, immediate treatment is recommended even in this age group.

– *Pregnant* women with CIN 2, 3 should be followed up by colposcopy and cytology both at interval of 3 months and at 6 weeks postpartum. Repeat biopsy or diagnostic excisional procedure is indicated only if invasive cancer is suspected on cytology and colposcopy. Unless invasive cancer develops, treatment is not recommended during pregnancy.

Follow-up: Apart from treatment, a strict follow-up protocol is mandatory for these cases.

Follow-up should be done by co-testing (both cytology and HPV) at 12 and 24 months.

- If reports are negative at both visits, age-specific routine screening to be performed after 3 years.

- If any test is abnormal then colposcopy with endocervical sampling is performed.

Despite treatment, the risk of carcinoma is much higher in this category. These cases require routine surveillance up to 20 years even if this period extends beyond 65 years of age.

Adenocarcinoma in situ (AIS)

Management of women with AIS is quite challenging due to its multifocal nature, skip lesions and lesions extending into the endocervical canal. Hence, it is difficult to determine the extent of disease and completeness of excision by conservative methods.

- Hysterectomy is preferred, if patient has completed her family.
- Excisional conization is done, only if future fertility is required as it carries a high failure rate. If margins and endocervical sampling show CIN or AIS, repeat excision can be tried to increase the likelihood of completeness of excision. Follow-up is done at 6 months using combination of co-testing (cytology and HPV), colposcopy and endocervical sampling. Hysterectomy is done as soon as the patient completes her family. Prolong follow-up is required if the patient is not willing for hysterectomy.

Cold knife conization is preferred for the treatment of AIS, with the whole specimen taken out in a single piece for proper interpretation of margin status which is very important for further planning and management.

NEWER TECHNOLOGIES FOR CERVICAL CANCER SCREENING

Current technologies are relatively inefficient at identifying individuals at risk for disease and require longitudinal testing over a woman's lifetime which is not feasible in low-resource settings. Several new approaches are currently being developed in three broad areas.

Screening Methods Utilizing HPV Diagnostics

No reliable methods exist to identify those lesions that are likely to regress or progress. New screening strategies focus on identification of oncogenic HPV infection and viral activity.

HPV integration is a key molecular event in the transition from an innocuous HPV infection to one that has oncogenic potential and results in increased expression of the viral E6 and E7 proteins. Increased expression of these proteins results in the disruption of host cell proteins, p53 and pRb and cell cycle regulation, resulting in cell cycle progression. In the normal cell, cell cycle progression is activated by CDK 4/6 and in part regulated by p16. Increased expression of p16 in cells driven by viral oncogene-mediated cell-cycle dysregulation can be detected through cellular immunostaining. Tests that detect the integration of HPV into the host cell may provide a useful way of screening women at risk for cervical cancer.

Detection of p16 (INK4a) correlates closely with viral integration. Detectable p16 expression has been found to be associated with increasing severity of dysplasia. Data are promising but current usage of the p16 biomarker is limited due to variability depending on the stains used.

High-risk HPV messenger RNA (mRNA) is another biomarker. Quantification of high-risk HPV mRNA would provide indirect functional information about the transcriptional activity of the virus by evaluating the activity of E6 and E7. It shows great promise to stratify the risk of progression to high-grade dysplasia in women with abnormal cytology.

The E6 strip test is also a biomarker that indicates viral integration. The test detects the HPV-E6 oncoprotein of HPV types 16, 18 and 45, in cytologic samples positive for oncogenic HPV DNA. Results are available in one hour and show good histologic correlation.

Strategies Identifying Epigenetic Changes

Methylation biomarkers: Aberrant methylation of tumor suppressor genes is a known cause of cell cycle dysregulation. Many genes are currently being evaluated as potential methylation biomarkers for cervical cancer and may have future clinical utility in low resource settings.

Telomerase RNA component (TERC) identification: Another area of biomarker research is in the use of telomerase RNA component (TERC) identification by fluorescence in situ hybridization. Many studies indicate that TERC identification may become a useful screening tool for cervical cancer.

Screening Methods Utilizing Proliferation Markers

Other biomarkers under evaluation for cervical cancer screening include CDC6 and MCM5. These proteins are present in normal cells only during the activation of the cell. Dysplastic cells have unregulated cell cycles and as a result, CDC6 and MCM5 reflect cell proliferation. MCM5 appears to be a biomarker that is expressed independent of high-risk HPV infection and may in the future serve as a useful marker for both HPV- dependent and HPV-independent cervical dysplasia.

NEW ADVANCEMENT IN THE TREATMENT OF CIN

Terameprocol

Terameprocol is a novel transcription inhibitor with potential antiviral, antiangiogenic, and antineoplastic activities. Phase I/II clinical trials with Terameprocol vaginal ointment (1%, 2%) in HPV-linked cervical intraepithelial neoplasia have shown an excellent safety profile, with only mild self-limiting treatment-related adverse events, but no serious adverse events and no detectable absorption of Terameprocol.

Vaginal and Vulval Lesions

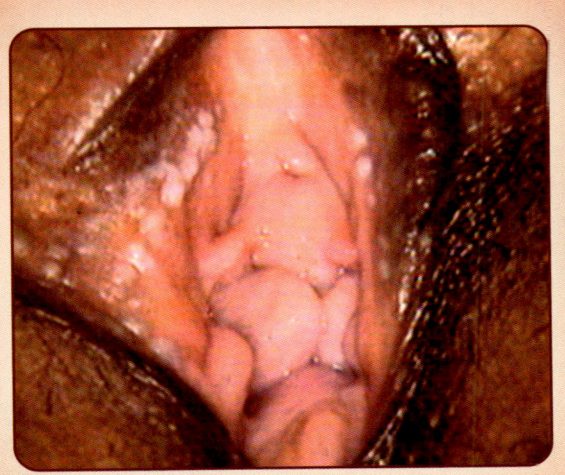

Chapter Outline

VAGINAL LESIONS

Colposcopic terminology used for describing vaginal lesions is almost same as for cervix and has been defined for the first time by IFCPC in 2011 (Table 13.1). Though at times transformation zone may be seen in the vagina also, where islands of columnar epithelium are found within the squamous epithelium (adenosis), the cervical transformation zone types are irrelevant in the vagina.

NORMAL FINDINGS

Vagina is lined by glycogenated, stratified squamous epithelium. In comparison to cervix, connective tissue of vagina is loose, more abundant and vascular. Hence normal vaginal epithelium is seen as mature, pink and smooth surface with numerous rugae (Fig. 13.1).

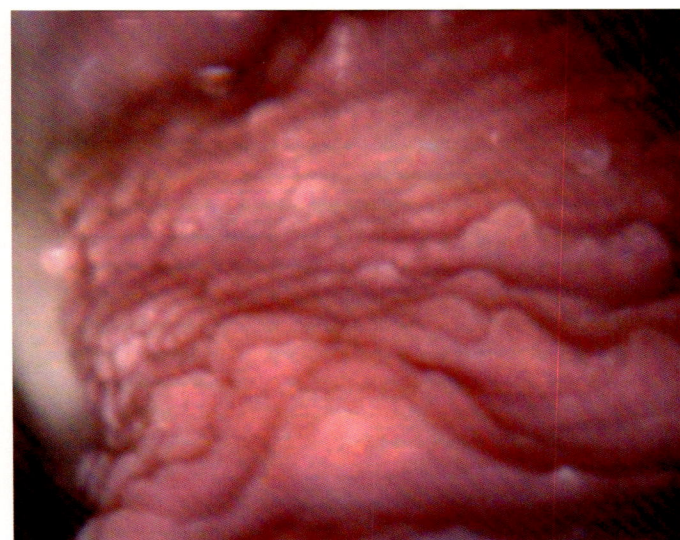

Changes in surface contour are more pronounced in vagina because of loose vaginal texture. At higher magnification, terminal capillary network may be seen. The color and blood vessel distribution of both normal and atypical findings is same as that of cervical epithelium. But, in comparison to the cervix, vagina shows higher colposcopic grade for the same degree of histological abnormality.

MISCELLANEOUS FINDINGS

Congenital Transformation Zone

It is a physiological condition seen in about 4% of normal females, wherein the normal transformation zone may be seen extending to the vaginal fornices. This transformation zone arises from metaplasia occurring during intrauterine life which reaches full maturation into glycogenated squamous epithelium. It is frequently found on the outer side of the adult transformation zone. It contains usual gland openings and retention cysts and is indistinguishable from the typical transformation zone of the adulthood. Unlike cervical transformation zone, it is not at risk of attaining neoplastic potential.

Fig. 13.1: Normal vagina — pink smooth surface with numerous rugae

Table 13.1: IFCPC nomenclature of vagina		
General assessment	Adequate/inadequate for the reason (i.e. inflammation, bleeding, scar)	
Normal colposcopic findings	Squamous epithelium Mature Immature	
Abnormal colposcopic findings	General principles	Upper one-third/lower two-thirds, anterior/posterior/lateral (right or left)
	Grade 1 (minor)	Thin acetowhite epithelium Fine punctation Fine mosaic
	Grade 2 (major)	Dense acetowhite epithelium Coarse punctation Coarse mosaic
	Suspicious for invasion	Atypical vessels **Additional signs:** Fragile vessels, irregular surface, exophytic lesion, necrosis, ulceration (necrotic), tumor/gross neoplasm
	Non-specific	Columnar epithelium (adenosis) lesion staining by Lugol's solution (Schiller's test): Stained/non-stained, leukoplakia
Miscellaneous findings	Erosion (traumatic), condyloma, polyp, cyst, endometriosis, inflammation, vaginal stenosis, congenital transformation zone	

Occasionally, this epithelium remains immature, non-glycogenated and is seen extending to vagina as mild acetowhite area (Fig. 13.2). At times, it may show fine regular punctations (Figs 13.3A and B) or mosaic and even patchy keratosis, confusing it with an abnormal lesion. However, histology is confirmatory which generally shows normal mature or minimally altered metaplastic squamous epithelium.

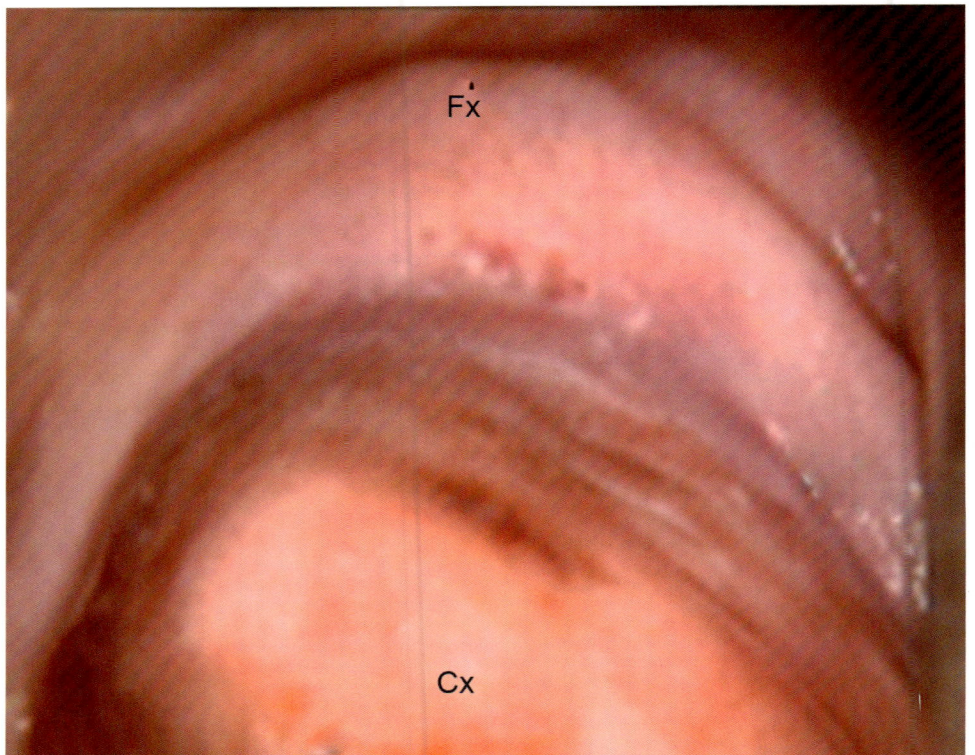

Fig. 13.2: Metaplastic epithelium seen as gr 1 AW epithelium extending into anterior fornix

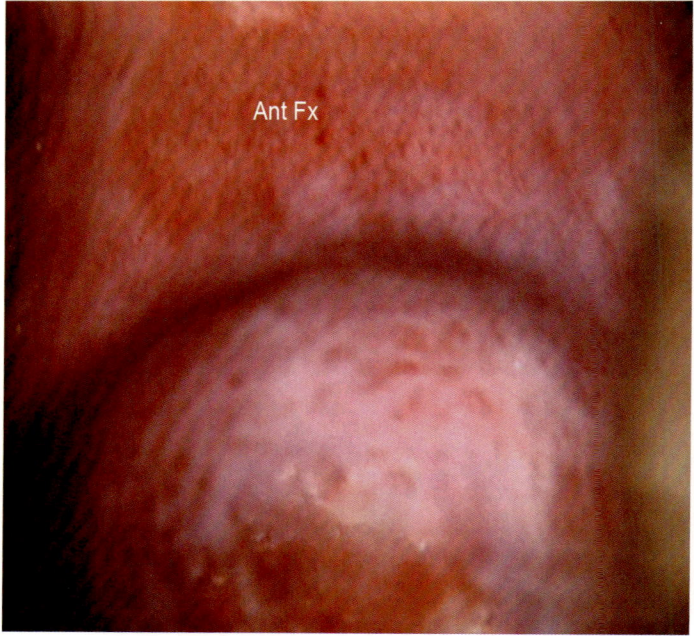

Fig. 13.3A: Immature metaplastic epithelium with fine punctations extending up to vaginal fornix

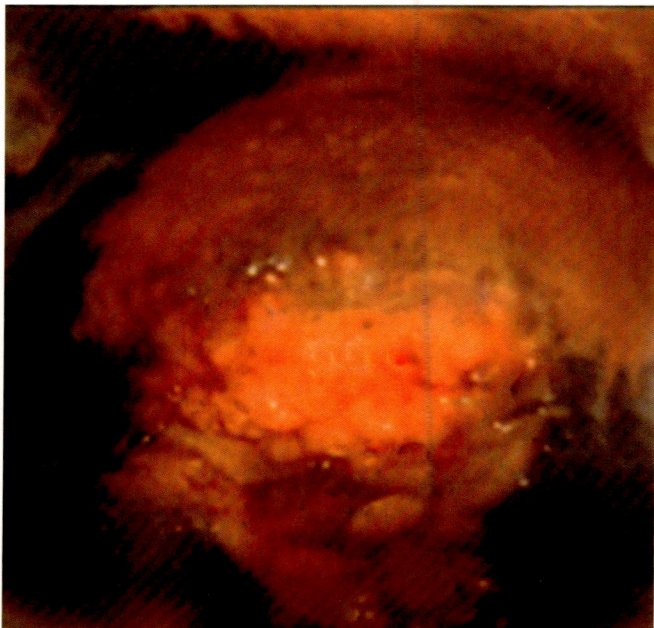

Fig. 13.3B: Same cervix after Lugol's iodine application showing non-glycogenated epithelium over cervix and upper vagina

ABNORMAL FINDINGS

Non-specific

Vaginal Adenosis

Persistence of columnar epithelium over vagina after birth is termed as "adenosis". It is a benign condition, seen occasionally in women less than 20 years of age. In about 90%, this is attributed to diethylstilbesterol (DES) exposure *in utero*.

Columnar epithelium covers the cervix as well as the upper vagina. Mostly this whole area undergoes metaplasia and is eventually converted into mature metaplastic epithelium, but in some females findings may persist.

Colposcopy: Transformation zone is very wide. Vaginal fornices may show varied appearances. Columnar epithelium is very rarely seen. Most common presentation is large areas of immature metaplastic epithelium which is acetowhite (Fig. 13.4). Fine punctations or mosaic may also be seen at times. Transformation zone may show usual islands of columnar epithelium, gland openings and nabothian cysts. Findings may be confused with intraepithelial neoplasia, however, histology is confirmatory which shows metaplastic epithelium.

Exact significance of this atypical appearance is not known. Incidence of CIN is reported high in such cases. VAIN may also be present. Most serious complication is development of clear cell adenocarcinoma in young females, risk being 1.4 per 130 females exposed to DES *in utero*.

Leukoplakia

White patches which are often multifocal, can be found in vagina in certain conditions like HPV infection (Fig. 13.5) and following the use of diaphragm, pessary or estrogen cream (Fig. 13.6).

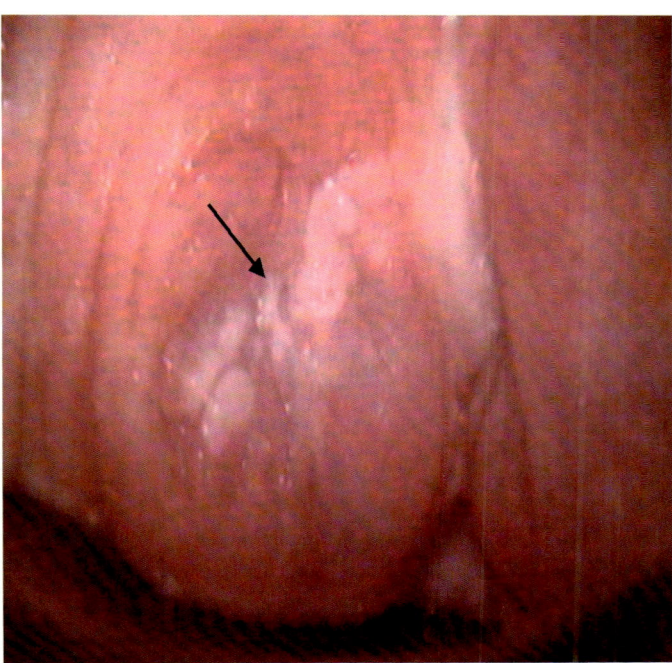

Fig.13.5: Leukoplakic patches seen at vault (1 year after hysterectomy) suggestive of HPV infection

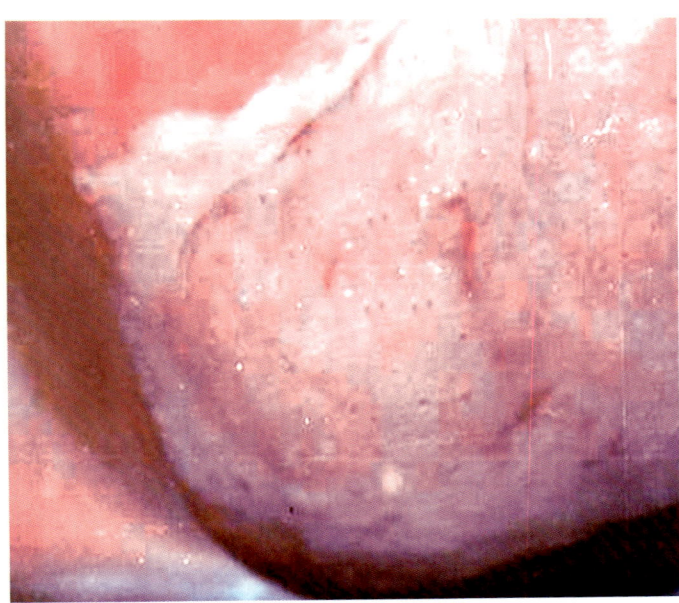

Fig. 13.4: Acetowhite epithelium reaching in posterior fornix along with multiple gland openings

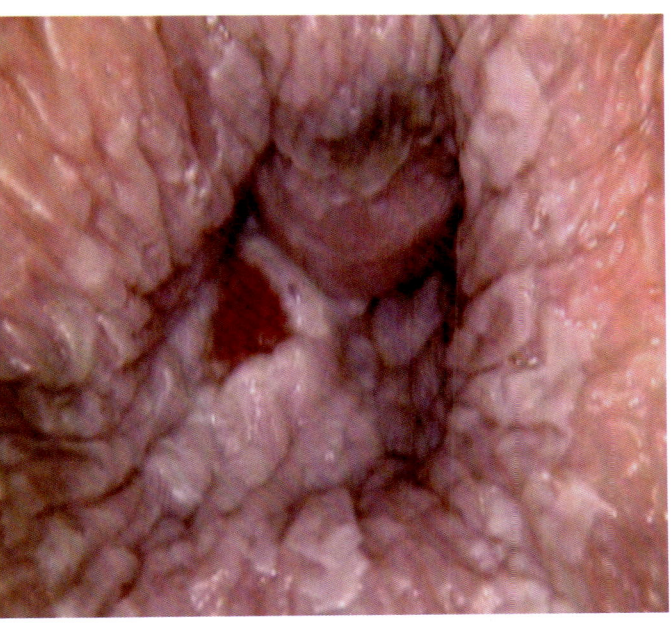

Fig. 13.6: Keratosis with vaginal wall prolapse

Infections

Trichomonas vaginalis

Vagina shows strawberry spots and leopard appearance, similar to *Trichomonas* infection of cervix (Figs 13.7A and B).

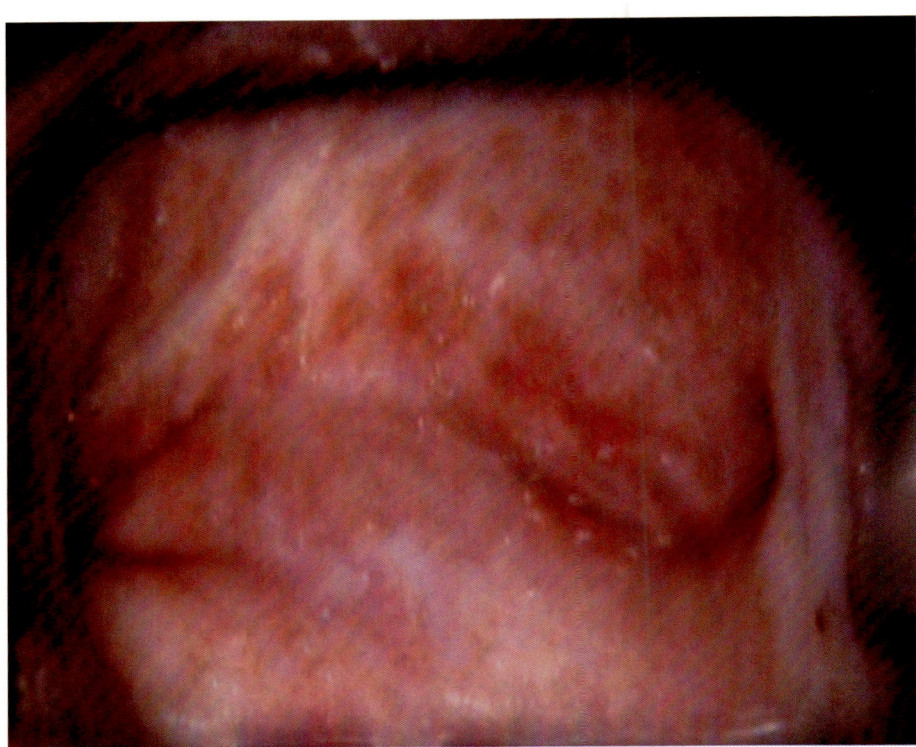

Fig. 13.7A: *Trichomonas* infection vault—strawberry spots

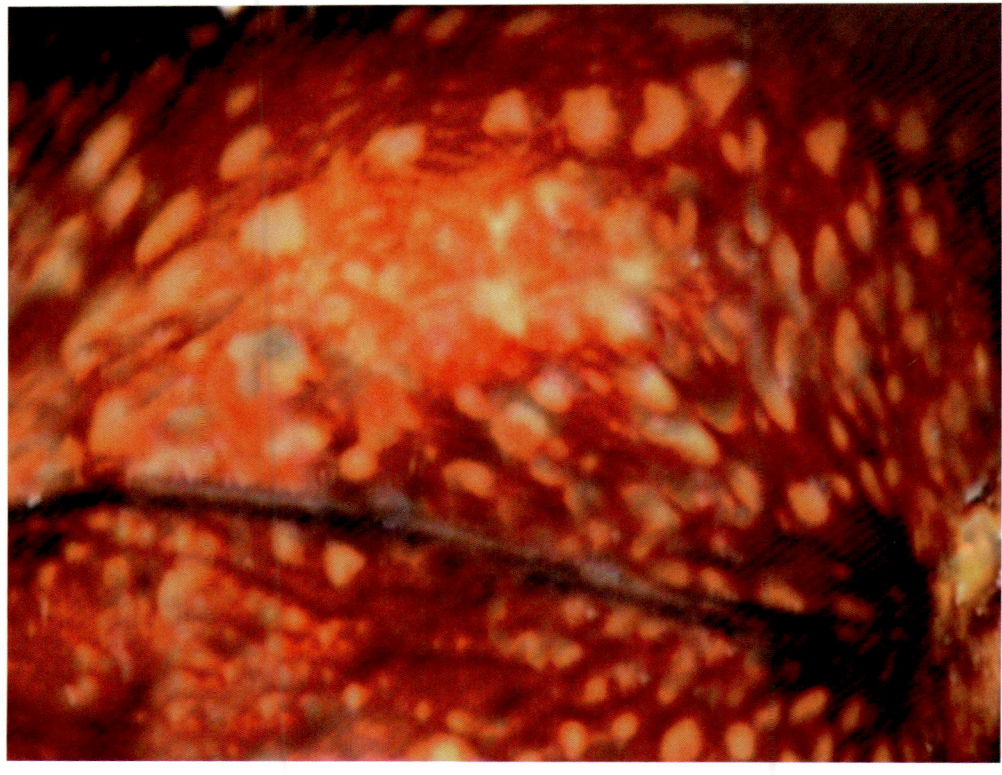

Fig. 13.7B: Vault after Iodine application—leopard appearance

Human Papillomavirus Infection

These lesions are often found in association to that of cervix and vulva. Like elsewhere, HPV infection in vagina also may produce microscopic or macroscopic lesions. Findings are same as in the cervix.

Subclinical papilloma viral infection (SPI) can be found as leukoplakic patches (Fig. 13.5), micropapillary projections with or without central vessel (Figs 13.8A to C).

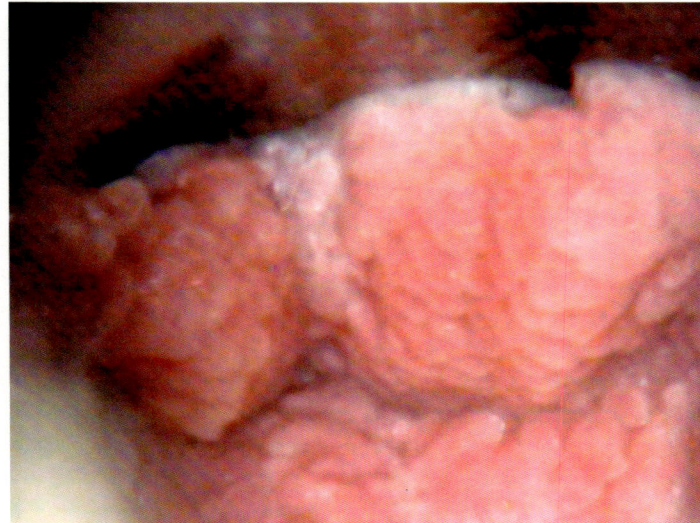

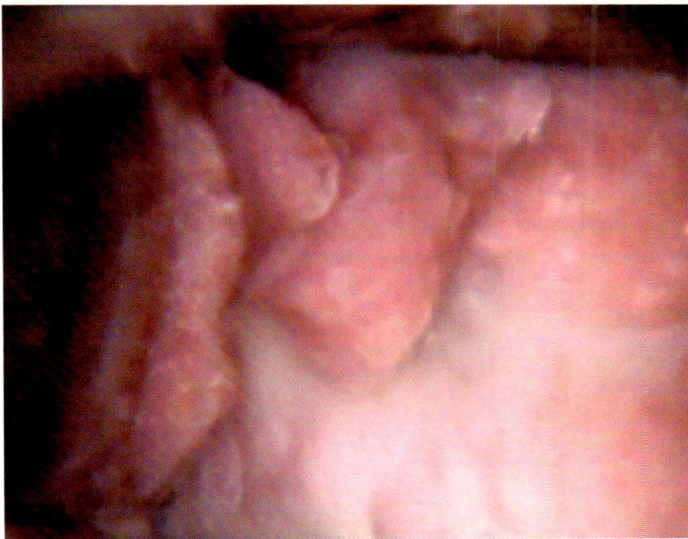

Fig. 13.8A: Micropapillary lesion vagina

Fig. 13.8B: Micropapillary lesion vagina

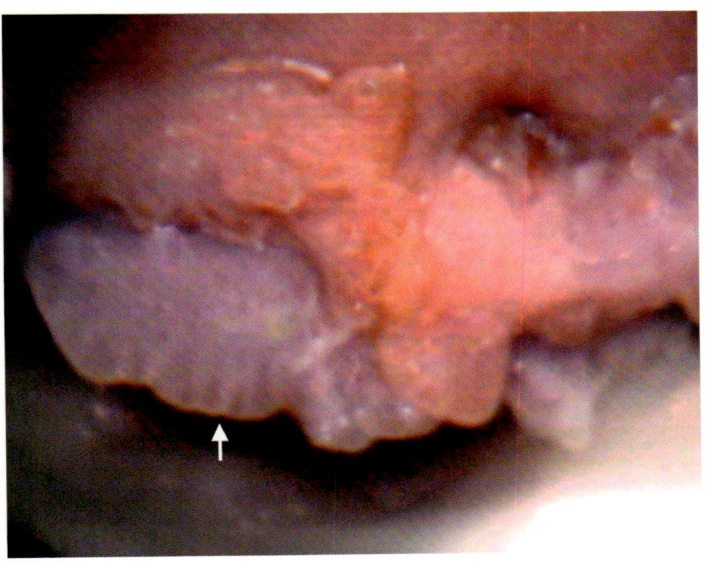

Fig. 13.8C: Micropapillary lesion vagina with central vessels

Subclinical papilloma viral infection can also present as acetowhite specks known as asperities (Fig. 13.9).

SPI may occasionally be confused with exaggerated vaginal rugosities of papillary type but they do not turn white after acetic acid application.

Like anywhere else, macroscopic lesions are visible to naked eye in form of condyloma (Figs 13.10 and 13.11).

Intraepithelial neoplasia may coexist with SPI, and colposcopically differentiation may be difficult. Histology is confirmatory.

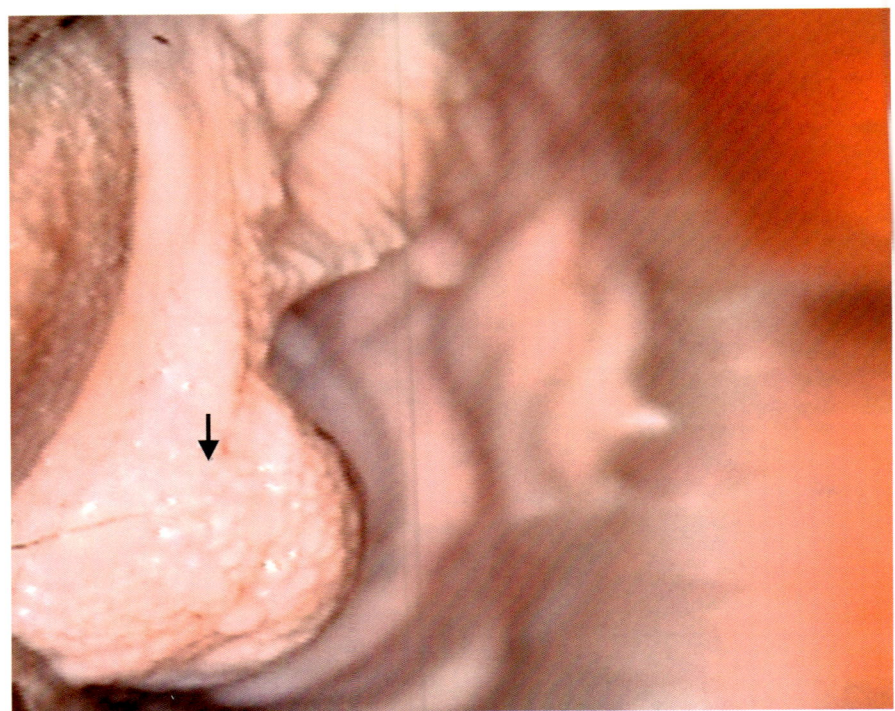

Fig. 13.9: Asperities in lower vagina

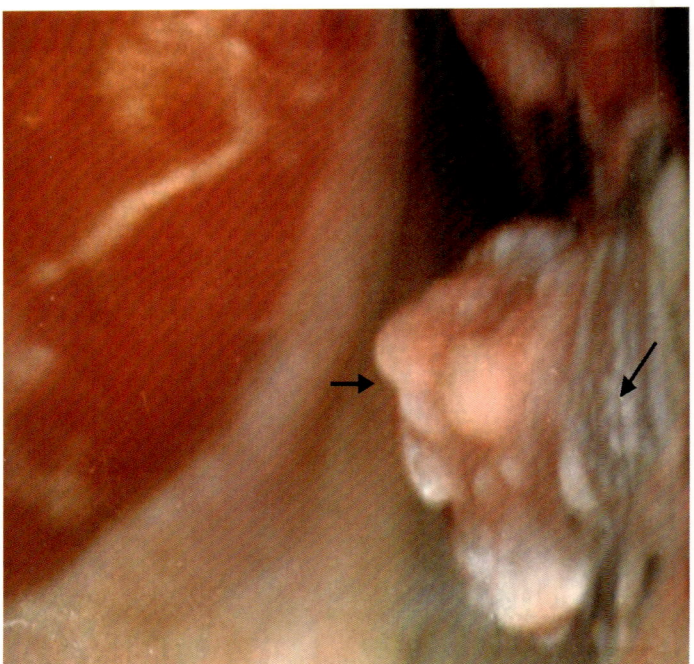

Fig. 13.10: Exophytic condyloma with asperities in upper vagina

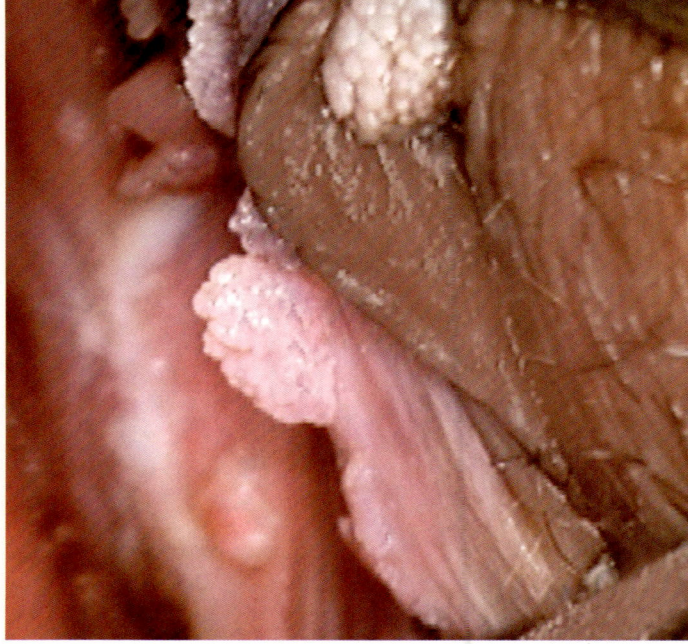

Fig. 13.11: Multiple exophytic condylomas in vagina and vulva

Vaginal Intraepithelial Neoplasia (VAIN)

Approximately 50% of these lesions are multifocal. One must look for these lesions in cases of cervical and vulval neoplasia as well as condyloma, after pelvic irradiation, and in presence of abnormal smear in post-hysterectomy cases done for CIN or invasive disease.

90% of lesions are located in upper vagina. Like its cervical counterpart, VAIN is graded as VAIN I, II and III depending upon the degree of undifferentiated cells in the epithelium.

Colposcopy: Vaginal epithelium may get traumatized and detached by minor trauma because of decreased intercellular cohesion in the dysplastic epithelium. Unprepared epithelium may show slightly raised areas of pinkish color (Fig. 13.12). Leukoplakic patches with sharp borders may also be seen usually in the fornices. Coarse and irregular punctations may be seen according to the degree of underlying pathology (Fig. 13.13).

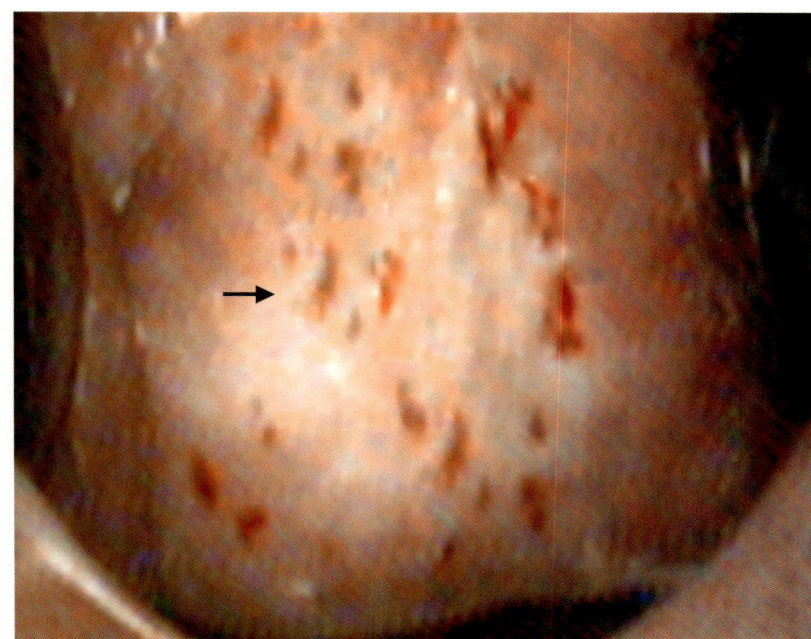

Fig. 13.12: Raised hyperemic spots and minute ulcerations in fornix

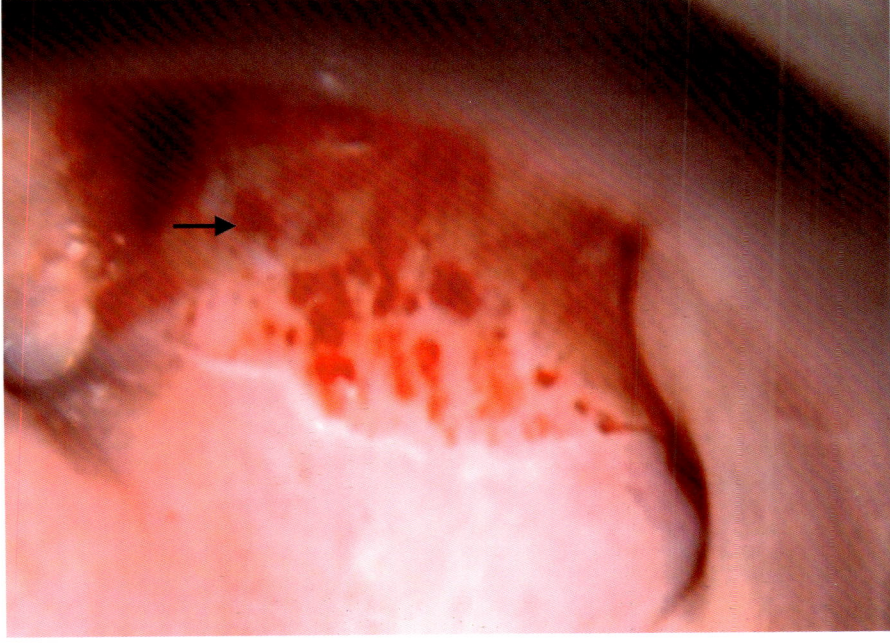

Fig. 13.13: Coarse punctations at vault along with AW epithelium

After application of acetic acid, lesions become acetowhite, degree of whiteness being dependent on the grade of the lesion (Figs 13.14, 13.15A and B).

Lugol's iodine does not stain the lesions as they are non-glycogenated.

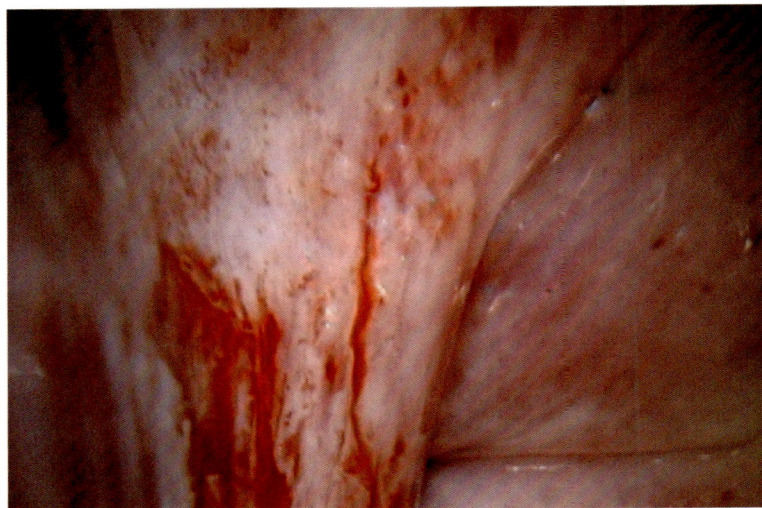

Fig. 13.14: Acetowhite epithelium with coarse punctations in upper vagina

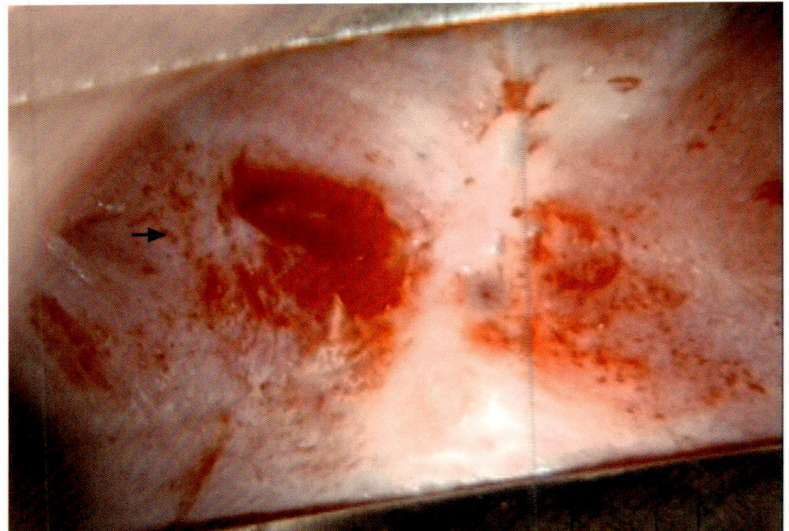

Fig. 13.15A: Acetowhite epithelium with coarse punctations over vault

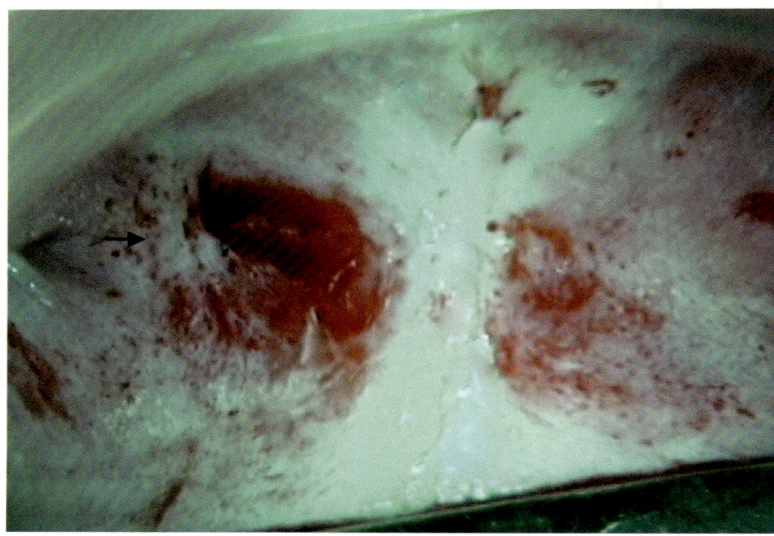

Fig. 13.15B: Same vault under green filter

Suspicious of Invasion/Invasive Carcinoma

Primary vaginal carcinoma is very rare (Fig. 13.16A). Colposcopic appearance is same as that of cervical carcinoma. Early invasion shows acetowhite epithelium with irregular contour and atypical blood vessels (Fig. 13.16B).

Usually invasive lesions are extension from squamous carcinoma of cervix (Fig. 13.17).

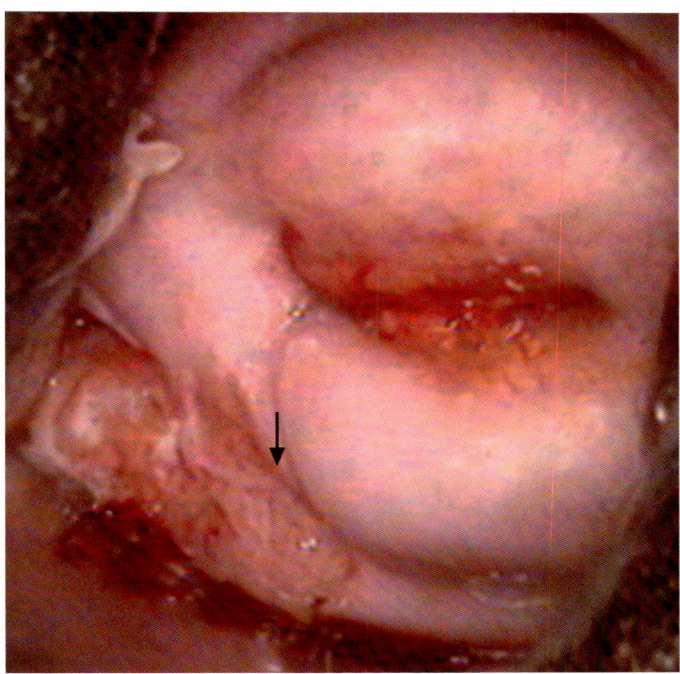

Fig. 13.16A: Lesion with irregular contour seen in right fornix away from normal TZ

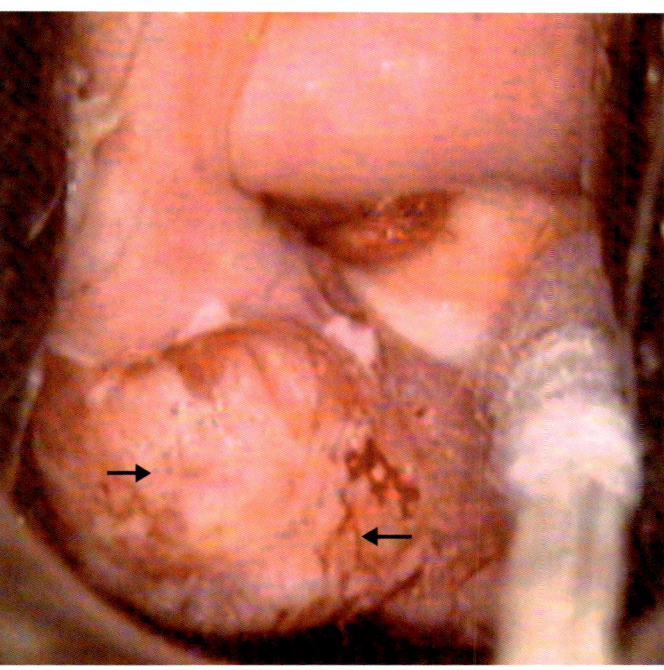

Fig. 13.16B: Same lesion under higher magnification with thick AW epithelium and atypical vessels

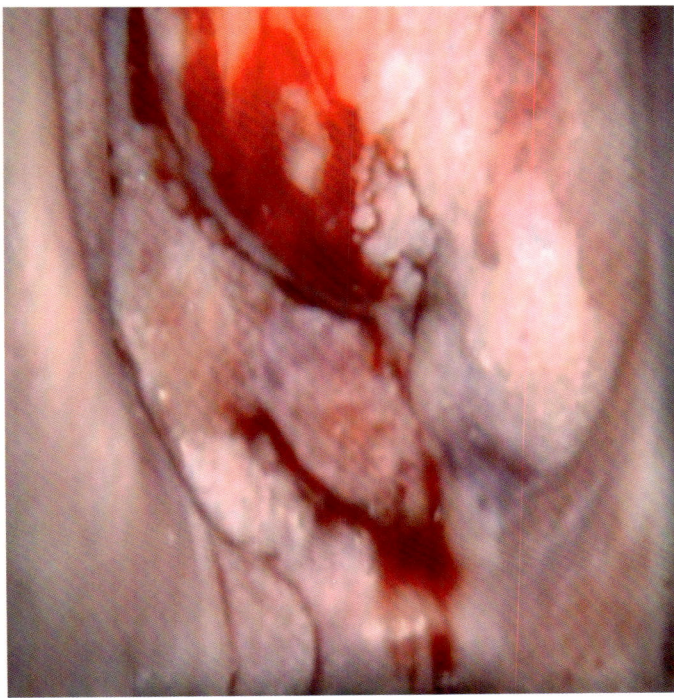

Fig. 13.17A: Vaginal extension from cancer cervix

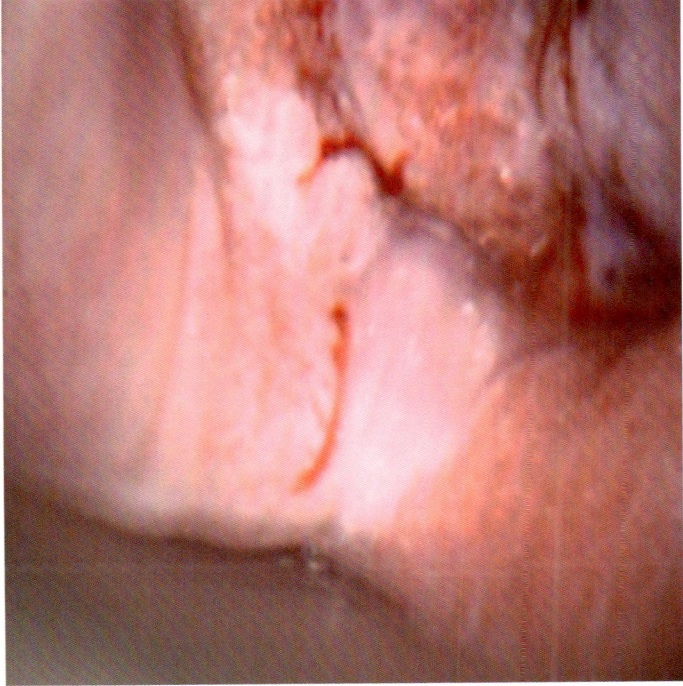

Fig. 13.17B: Same lesion under high magnification

VULVA

Diagnosis of vulvar disease presents an enigma to the clinicians and many women affected by vulval symptoms are referred to the colposcopy clinic, though the role of colposcope in the management of vulvar disease is limited.

Vulva is the part of the female genital tract located between the genitocrural folds laterally, the mons pubis anteriorly, and the anus posteriorly. It is divided into hairy and non-hairy areas. Hairy area includes the labia majora composed of folds of adipose and fibrous tissues, which form the lateral boundaries of the vulva, and fuse anteriorly into the mons pubis. Posteriorly, they terminate 3–4 cm anterior to the anus where they are united by the posterior commissure or fourchette. Non-hairy areas are clitoris, labia minora, inner surface of labia majora, vestibule, posterior fourchette and immediate perianal mucosa. The vestibule is the area between the hymen and Hart's line. Structures found in the vestibule include the urethra, periurethral (Skene's) glands, major vestibular (Bartholin's) glands, and the minor vestibular glands.

NOMENCLATURE OF VULVA

The International Federation of Cervical Pathology and Colposcopy has introduced the clinical/colposcopic terminology of vulva (Table 13.2) which can be used by the gynecologists and the colposcopists for appropriate diagnosis and treatment as well as consistent reporting of vulvar lesions. It includes the "basic definitions", "normal findings" as well as "abnormal findings" of vulva.

Various structures of the vulva and anus and whether they are composed of skin (hairy/non-hairy portions) or mucosa are described in the basic definitions section. It is important to know this as the conditions involving non-hairy regions may be treated by CO_2 laser vaporization whereas those affecting hairy portions would require excisional treatment.

The nomenclature also emphasizes that conditions like micropapillomatosis, sebaceous glands (Fordyce spots) are normal findings and may be mistakenly diagnosed as genital condylomata acuminata and treated by CO_2 laser vaporization. Similarly, vestibular redness alone is a normal finding and not a sign of dermatitis or inflammation.

Table 13.2: The IFCPC (2011) terminology of vulva (including anus)

Section	Pattern		
Basic definitions	*Various structures*		
	Urethra, Skene duct openings, clitoris, prepuce, frenulum, pubis, labia majora, labia minora, interlabial sulci, vestibule, vestibular duct openings, Bartholin duct openings, hymen, fourchette, perineum, anus, anal squamocolumnar junction (dentate line)		
	Composition		
	Squamous epithelium, hairy/non-hairy, mucosa		
Normal findings	Micropapillomatosis, sebaceous glands (Fordyce spots), vestibular redness		
Abnormal findings	General principles: Size in centimeters, location		
	Lesion type:	*Lesion color:*	*Secondary morphology*
	Macule	Skin-colored	Eczema
	Patch	Red	Lichenification
	Papule	White	Excoriation
	Plaque	Dark	Purpura
	Nodule		Scarring
	Cyst		Ulcer
	Vesicle		Erosion
	Bulla		Fissure
	Pustule		Wart
Miscellaneous findings	Trauma		
	Malformation		
Suspicion of malignancy	Gross neoplasm, ulceration, necrosis, bleeding, exophytic lesion, hyperkeratosis with or without white, gray, red, or brown discoloration		
Abnormal colposcopic/other magnification findings	Acetowhite epithelium, punctation, atypical vessels, surface irregularities. Abnormal anal SC junction (note location about the dentate line)		

Source: Bornstein J, Sideri M, Tatti S, et al. 2011 Terminology of the Vulva of the International Federation for Cervical Pathology and Colposcopy. J Lower Genital Tract Dis 2012;16(3):292.

Rest of the table includes nomenclature for recognizing the pattern of the lesion/s for further evaluation and differential diagnosis. This can be done using a magnifying lens or by colposcopic examination.

Abnormal findings are defined by the size, location, type, and color of the lesion, and secondary morphology, if present. The characteristics of the type of lesions and the secondary morphology are further defined in detail (Tables 13.3 and 13.4).

The findings suspicious of malignancy and abnormal colposcopy findings suggestive of intraepithelial neoplasia are also defined. and such lesions should always be biopsied. Colposcopy of vulva following acetic acid application, though not advised in routine,

would help to delineate the lesion and choose the biopsy site in such cases.

Colposcopic Findings

Colposcopy of vulva is very different from that of the cervix as they differ in their anatomic structure. Technique of colposcopic examination of vulva, referred to as vulvoscopy has been described in Chapter 3.

Colposcopic pattern depends upon thickness of the skin as it affects the opacity. Thickness varies from person to person in different areas of vulva and different lesions. Hairy part of the vulva is thicker than non-hairy part. Degree of hyperkeratosis, acanthosis, or papillomatosis affects the colposcopic pattern. Vascularization can be visualized in the non-hairy part only.

Table 13.3: Definitions of primary lesion types

Term	Definition
Macule	Small (<1.5 cm) area of color change; no elevation and no substance on palpation
Patch	Large (>1.5 cm) area of color change; no elevation and no substance on palpation
Papule	Small (<1.5 cm) elevated and palpable lesion
Plaque	Large (>1.5 cm) elevated, palpable, and flat-topped lesion
Nodule	A large papule (>1.5 cm); often hemispherical or poorly marginated; may be located on the surface, within, or below the skin; nodules may be cystic or solid
Vesicle	Small (<0.5 cm) fluid-filled blister; the fluid is clear (blister: A compartmentalized, fluid-filled elevation of the skin or mucosa)
Bulla	A large (>0.5 cm) fluid-filled blister; the fluid is clear
Pustule	Pus-filled blister, the fluid is white or yellow

Source: Bornstein J, Sideri M, Tatti S, et al. 2011 Terminology of the Vulva of the International Federation for Cervical Pathology and Colposcopy J Lower Genital Tract Dis 2012;16(3):292.

Table 13.4: 2011 IFCPC terminology of the vulva definitions of secondary morphology presentation

Term	Definition
Eczema	A group of inflammatory diseases that are characterized by the presence of itchy, poorly marginated red plaques with minor evidence of microvesiculation and/or subsequent surface disruption
Lichenification	Thickening of the tissue and increased prominence of skin markings. Scale may or may not be detectable in vulvar lichenification. Lichenification may be bright-red, dusky-red, white, or skin-colored in appearance
Excoriation	Surface disruption (notably excoriations) occurring as a result of the "itch-scratch cycle"
Erosion	A shallow defect in the skin surface; absence of some, or all, of the epidermis down to the basement membrane; the dermis is intact
Fissure	A thin, linear erosion of the skin surface
Ulcer	Deeper defect; absence of the epidermis and some, or all, of the dermis

Source: Bornstein J, Sideri M, Tatti S, et al. 2011 Terminology of the Vulva of the International Federation for Cervical Pathology and Colposcopy. J Lower Genital Tract Dis 2012;16(3):292.

Normal Findings

Normally introital epithelium is smooth in childhood whereas extensive or localized papillary or villiform pattern is seen in reproductive age group. It is not seen in old age. These vestibular papillae (micropapillomatosis) are mildly acetowhite, located on the inner aspect of labia minora, and generally have a single base for each projection (Fig. 13.18). These may be mistaken as HPV-induced lesions (Fig. 13.19).

Fordyce's spots are small, painless, raised, pale, white spots or bumps 1–3 mm in diameter, may be seen on vulvar mucosa in women of all ages. These are a form of ectopic sebaceous glands. They are a normal finding and are not associated with any disease or infection.

After acetic acid application, a mild acetowhite area of few millimeters may be visualized just lateral to vulvo-vaginal line on the medial aspect of labia minora but not extending to fourchette. This is a normal finding (Fig. 13.20). Any other discrete acetowhite area or whiter in grade is taken as abnormal.

Iodine application has no role in vulvoscopy as vulva is non-glycogenated (Fig. 13.21).

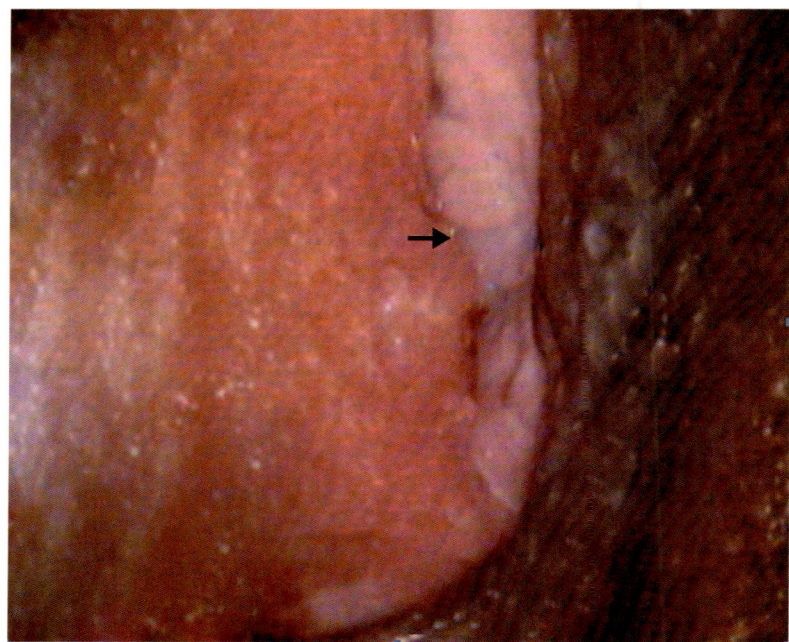

Fig. 13.18: Vulva showing normal finding of vestibular papillae

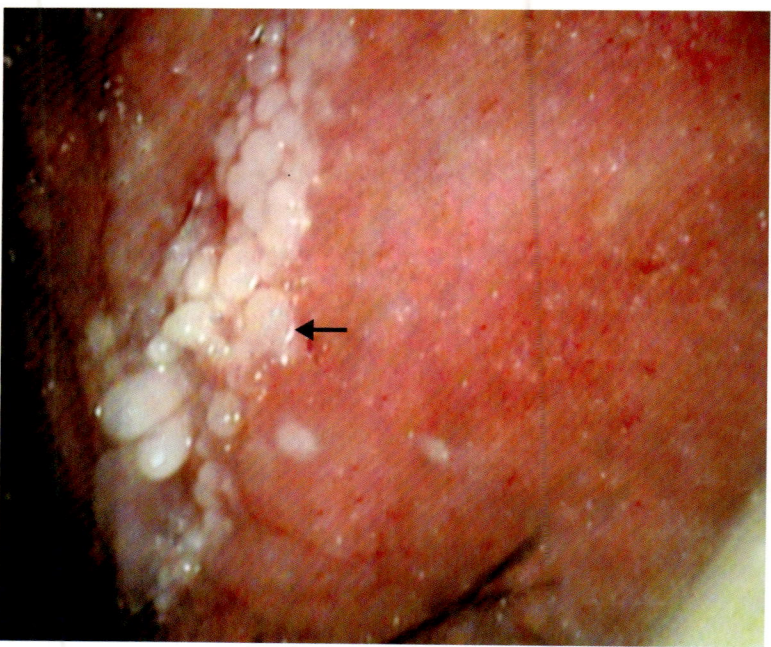

Fig. 13.19: Introitus showing big vestibular papillae that may be confused with HPV-induced lesion

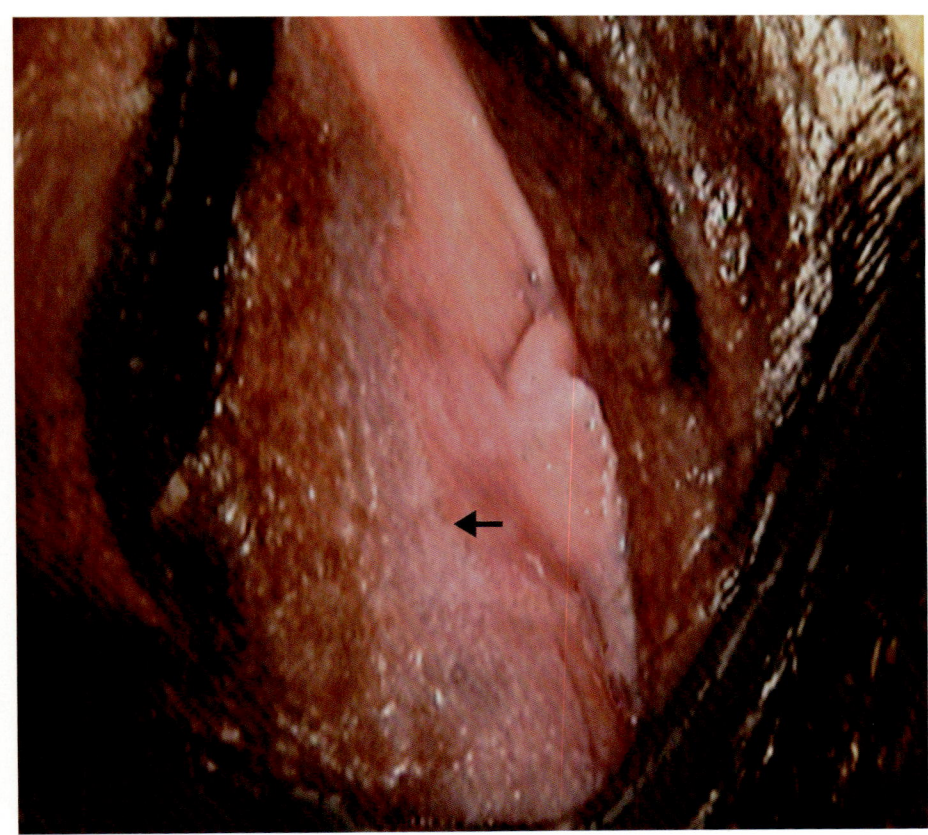

Fig. 13.20: Medial aspect of right labia minora showing wavy line of mild acetowhiteness

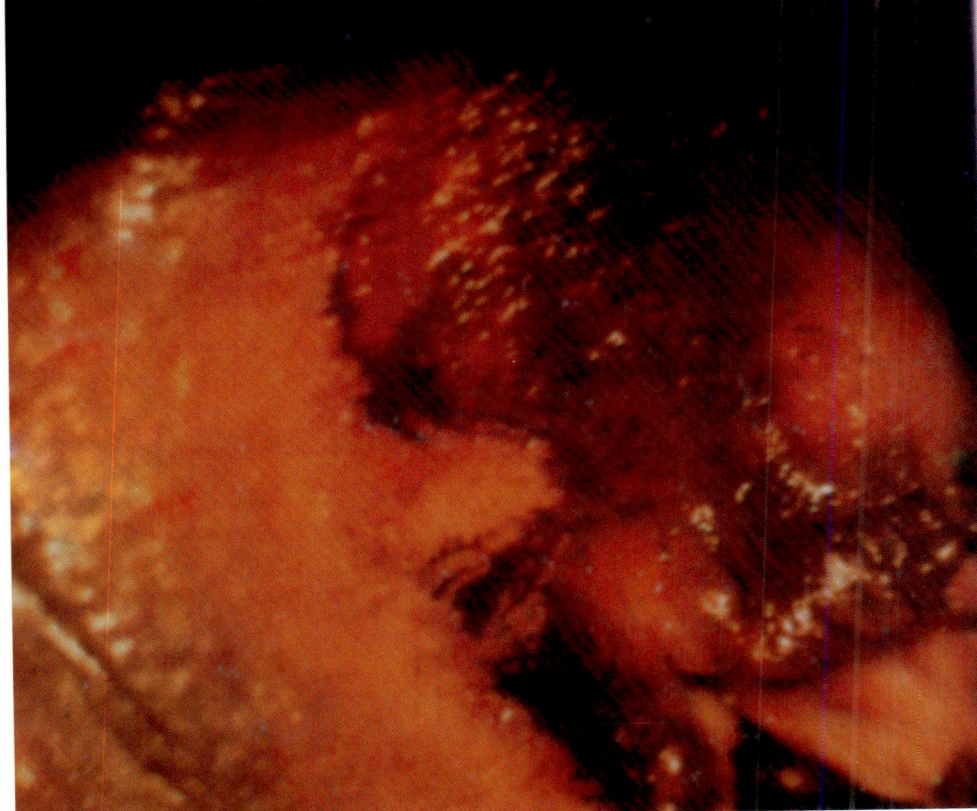

Fig. 13.21: Vulvovaginal line demarcating iodine positive vaginal epithelium from non-glycogenated keratinized vulval skin

Vulvar Dermatosis and Vulvar Intraepithelial Neoplasia (VIN)

Various terms have been used to define the precursors of vulvar squamous cell carcinoma. Bowen first reported on these squamous intraepithelial lesions in 1912, which were commonly referred to as Bowen's disease; since then, a myriad of confusing clinical and histopathological terms such as leukoplakia, Bowenoid papulosis, erythropsia of Queyrat, squamous cell carcinoma in situ, hyperplastic dystrophy, etc. have been employed to describe these vulvar precancerous lesions.

The International Society for the Study of Vulvar Disease (ISSVD) in 1987 simplified the terminology and adopted the single term of VIN, graded as VIN 1, 2, and 3 depending upon the extent of cellular abnormalities within the epithelium, in the same way as for cervical intraepithelial neoplasia (CIN).

However, the natural history of vulvar lesions did not provide any evidence that the morphologic spectrums of VIN 1, 2, and 3 reflected a biologic continuum, nor that VIN 1 was a cancer precursor. Atypical cells in the lower one/third of epithelium can be seen in a variety of chronic dermatological conditions, most of which have no relation to vulvar squamous cell neoplasia (Table 13.5). Hence, ISSVD (2004) decided to abolish the term VIN 1 and use the term vulvar dermatosis for these lesions.

On the keratinized portion of vulva, these lesions may present (Figs 13.22 to 13.28) as white, lichenified or hyperkeratotic and sometimes hyperpigmented area. In non-hairy portion, lesion may be erythematous or gray. They may also present as warty lesions.

Based on the characteristics of lesions, ISSVD introduced a clinical classification of vulval dermatological disorders in 2011 (Table 13.6) which was also taken into consideration by the IFCPC nomenclature committee while formulating 2012 terminology.

Colposcopy does not have much role in these clinically evident lesions except for directing the biopsy site and mapping the limits of the lesion at the time of excision.

Table 13.5: Vulvar dermatosis (previously referred as VIN 1)
Keratosis
Psoriasis
Seborrheic keratosis
Candidiasis
Lichen planus
Lichen sclerosus
Lichen simplex chronicus
Squamous epithelial hyperplasia
Hyperplastic dystrophy with atypia
Vulvar vestibulitis
Micropapillomatosis labialis
Flat/papular condyloma
Condyloma accuminata

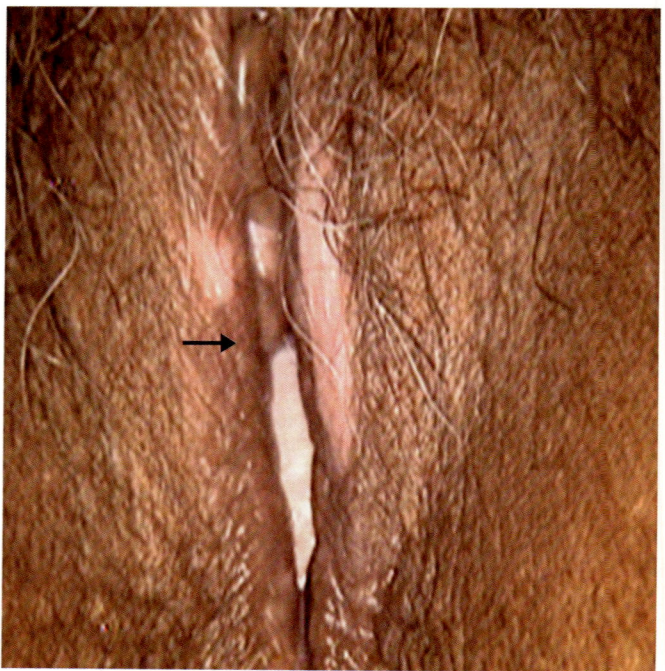

Fig. 13.22: Vulvar dermatosis—abnormal finding of white plaques over both labia minora

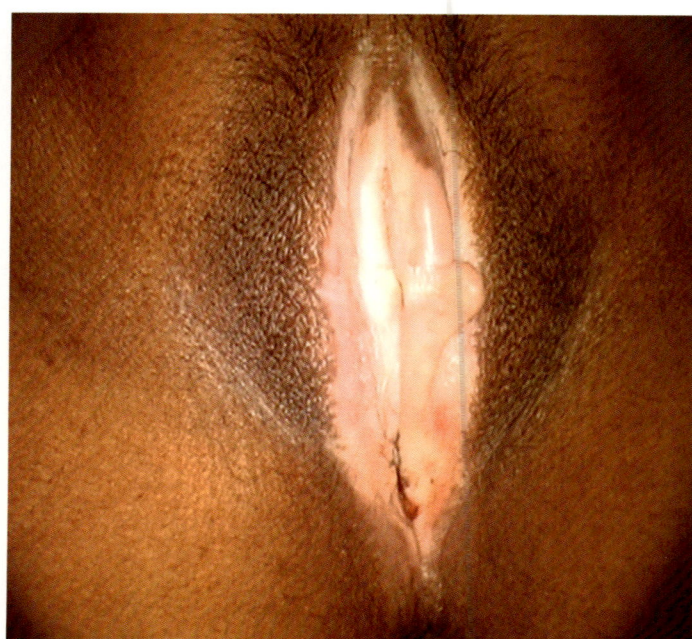

Fig. 13.23: Vulvar dermatosis—white lesion involving both labia minora and part of majora

Table 13.6: ISSVD (2011) clinical classification of vulvar dermatological disorders

Lesion characteristics	Example
Skin-colored lesions	
Papules and nodules	Molluscum, warts, cysts
Plaques	LSC, VIN
Red lesions	
Eczematous and lichenified	LSC, contact dermatitis
Patches and plaques	Candidiasis, psoriasis, VIN
Red lesions	
Papules	Angiokeratoma, H. suppurativa
Nodules	Furuncles, VIN
White lesions	
Papules and nodules	Fordyce spots, molluscum contagiosum, wart, scar, VIN, squamous cell carcinoma, milium, epidermal cyst, Hailey-Hailey disease
Patches and plaques	Vitiligo, lichen sclerosus, post-inflammatory hypopigmentation, lichenified diseases (when the surface is moist), lichen planus, VIN, squamous cell carcinoma
Dark lesions (brown, blue, gray, black)	
Patches	Melanocytic nevus, vulvar melanosis, lichen planus, post-inflammatory hyperpigmentation, acanthosis nigricans, melanomainsitu
Papules and nodules	Melanocytic nevus , warts (HPV), VIN, seborrheic keratosis, angiokeratoma, mammary-like gland adenoma (hidradenoma papilliferum), melanoma
Blisters	
Vesicles, bullae	Herpes virus infections (simplex, zoster), acute eczema, bullous lichen sclerosus, lymphangioma circumscriptum, immune blistering disorders
Pustules	Candidiasis, folliculitis
Erosions and ulcers	
Erosions	Erosive lichen planus, candidiasis, LSC, psoriasis, Crohn's disease, VIN eroded variant, ruptured vesicles/ bullae, extramammary Paget's disease
Ulcers	Excoriations (related to eczema, LSC), aphthous ulcers (idiopathic or secondary to Crohn's, Behçet's, viral infections), herpes virus infection, ulcerated squamous cell carcinoma, primary syphilis chancre
Edema	
Skin-colored	Crohn's disease, post-radiation and post-surgical lymphatic obstruction, idiopathic lymphatic abnormality, post-infectious or post-inflammatory
Pink or red edema	Venous obstruction, cellulitis, inflamed Bartholin duct cyst/abscess, Crohn's disease, mild vulvar edema with inflammatory vulvar disease

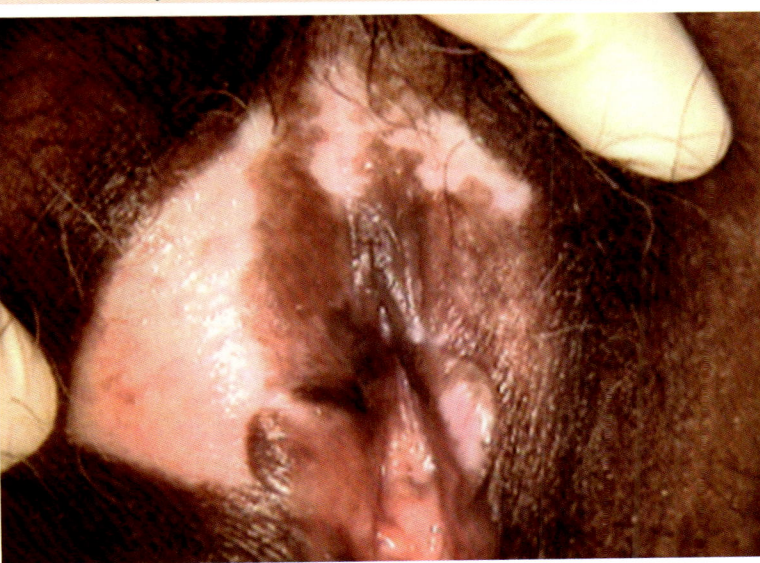

Fig. 13.24: Vulvar dermatosis—white patches involving labia minora and majora with hyperpigmentation in paraclitoral area

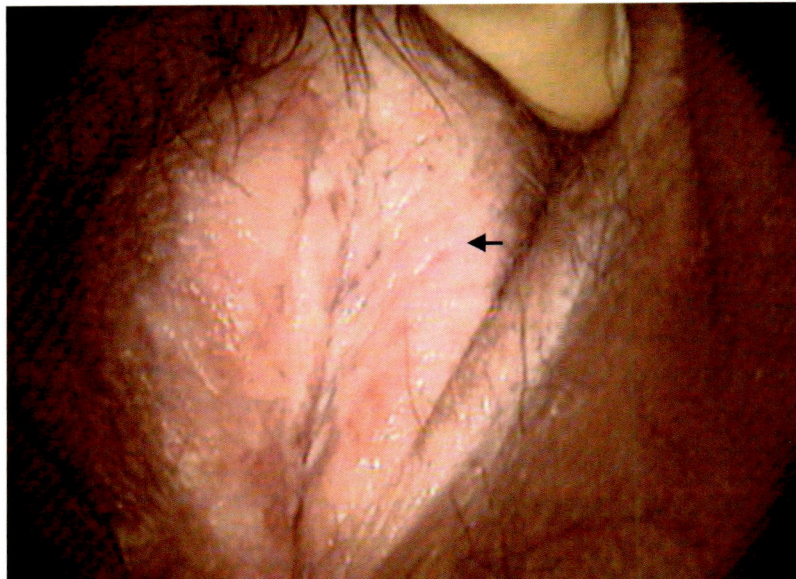

Fig. 13.25: Vulvar dermatosis—white raised lesion with lichenification and AW epithelium over left side

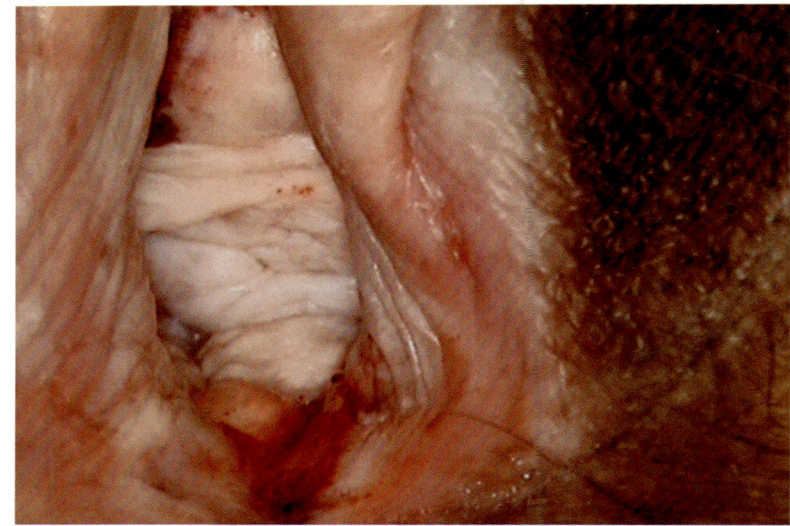

Fig. 13.26: Vulvar dermatosis—white patchy lesion with fissures involving labia minora and fourchette with loss of labia minora

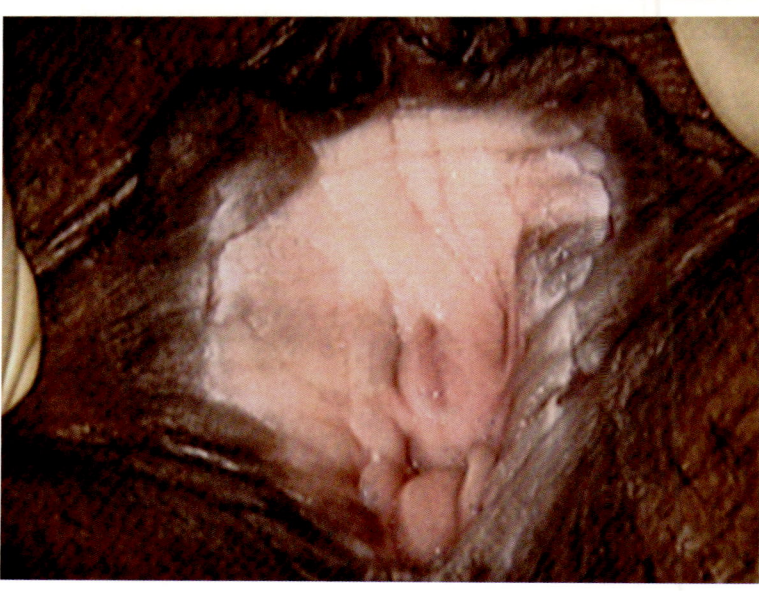

Fig. 13.27: Vulvar dermatosis—flat papular, pigmented and non-pigmented lesions with partial loss of labia minora

Human Papillomavirus Infection

Papillomaviruses are known to cause genital warts that were called "acuminate" as these lesions taper gradually to a sharp point, resembling the tips of leaves of the olive tree. These spiked growths tend to fuse with individual contiguous lesions to produce a cauliflower shaped or "Fig. shape" (condylomatous) lesion (Fig. 13.28).

Condylomata acuminata are small, usually multifocal lesions, involving the external genitalia, perineum and epithelium of lower genital tract. HPV lesions may be microscopic (Fig. 13.29) or macroscopic (Fig. 13.30) like all the other sites.

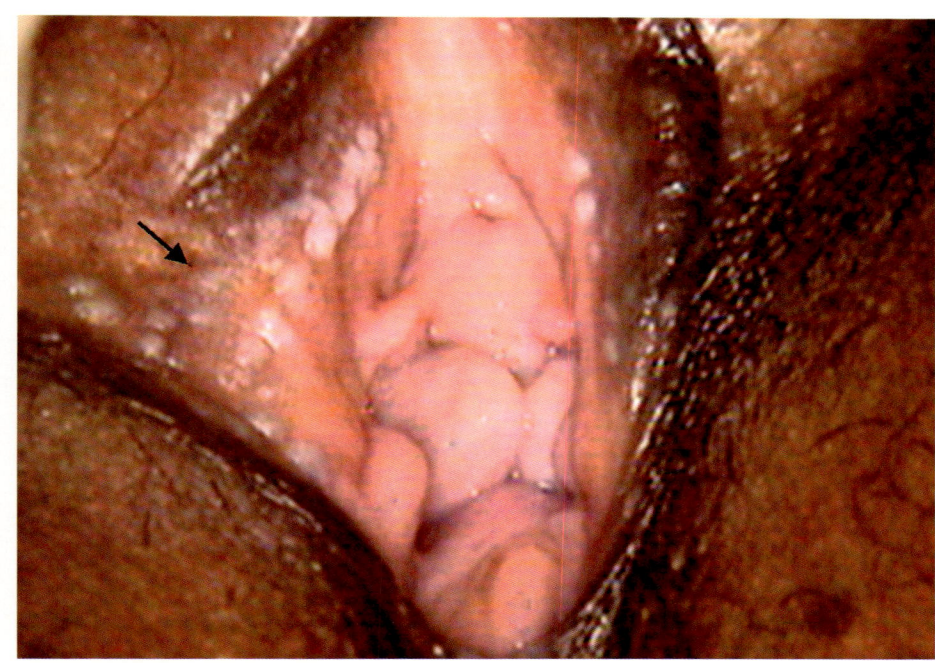

Fig. 13.28: Multiple raised AW papules over medial aspect of labia minora suggestive of condylomas

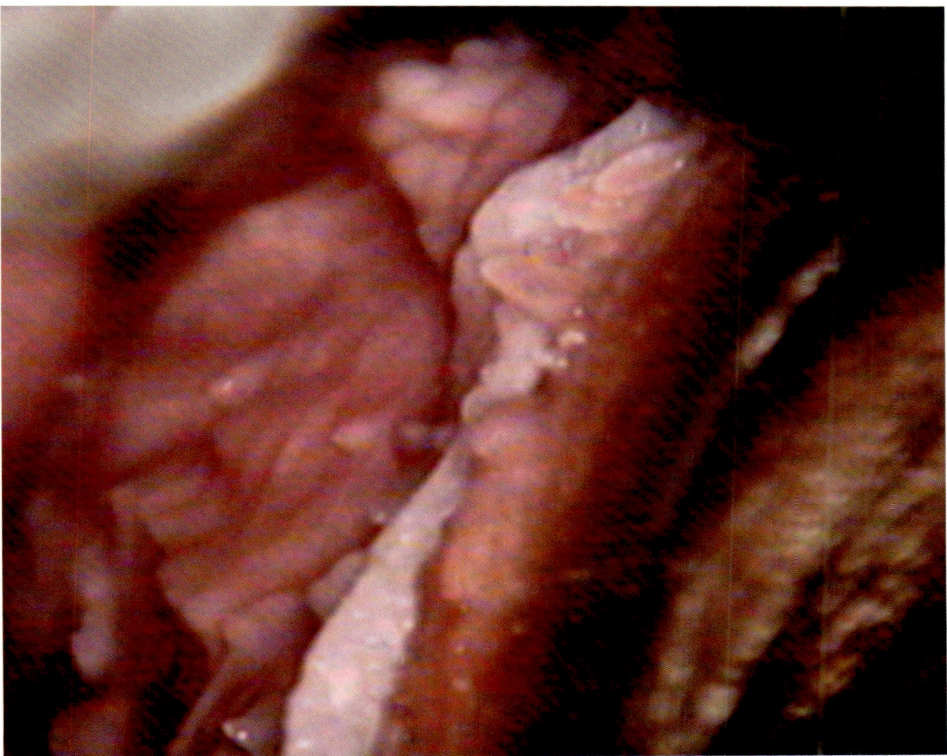

Fig. 13.29: AW lesion with micropapillary surface

Initially, warts may be reddish brown because of parakeratosis (Fig. 13.31). However, with time and exposure to local trauma, they become gray or white (Fig. 13.32) because of hyperkeratosis and generalized keratin disturbance associated with viral infection.

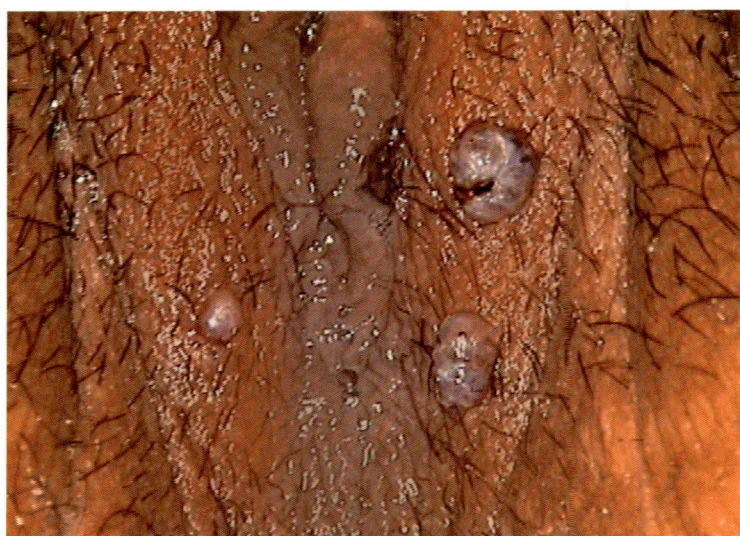

Fig. 13.30: Grayish dark nodular lesions with irregular surface

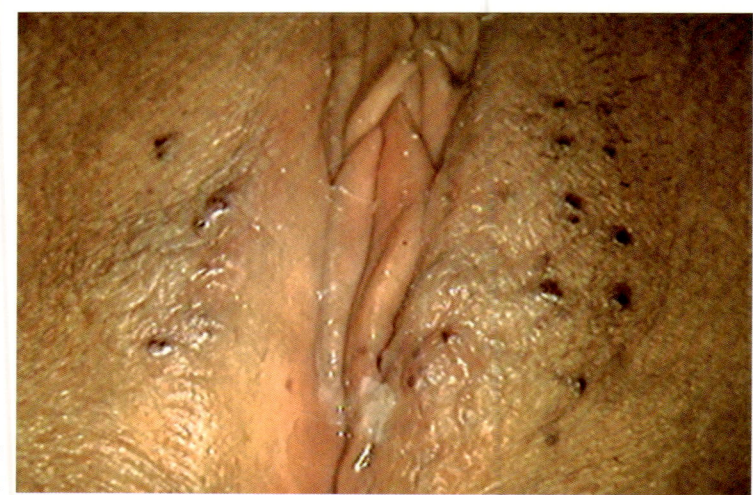

Fig. 13.31: Reddish brown nodules suggestive of condyloma

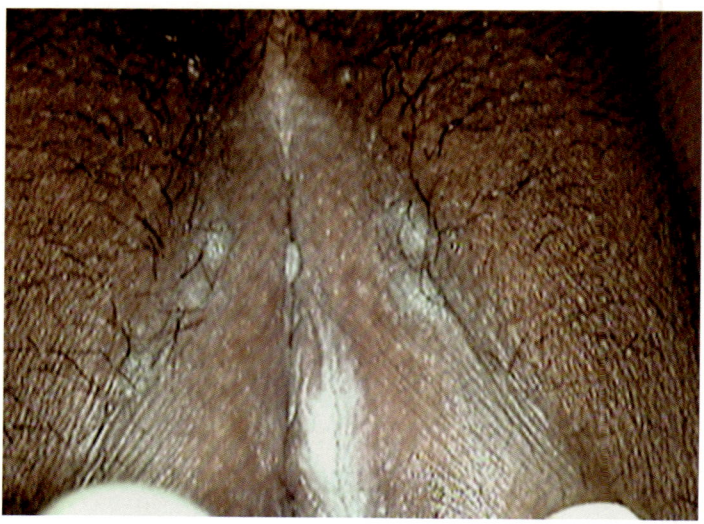

Fig. 13.32: Grayish white nodular warts with rough surface

More common subclinical papillomavirus infection (SPI) may be visualized as acetowhite epithelium either with a flat or micropapillary surface (Figs 13.33 and 13.34).

Discrete acetowhite spots or micropapillae may be seen in paraclitoral, introital or perianal area (Fig. 13.35).

Diagnosis of subclinical genital HPV lesions may at times be confused with normal vestibular papillae (micropapillomatosis). However, the papillations in micropapillomatosis generally have a single base for each projection, whereas HPV lesion typically has multiple projections coming off a single base (Fig. 13.36).

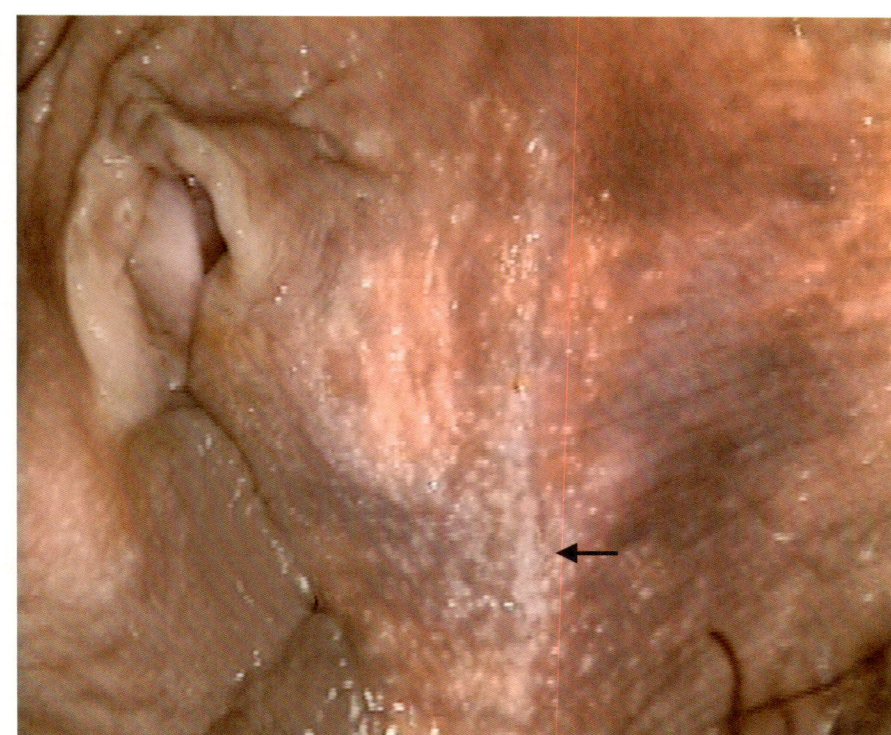

Fig. 13.33: White specks or asperities over labia minora

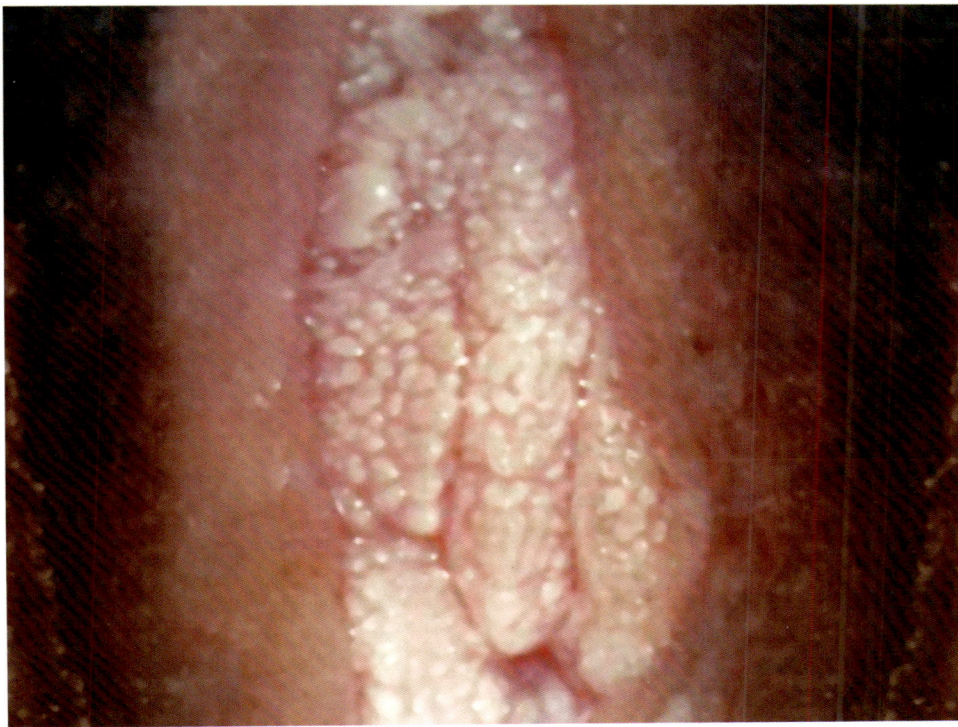

Fig. 13.34: Acetowhite lesion with micropapillary surface in non-hairy portion of vulva

Papillomavirus lesions are at times indistinguishable from VIN, which may also be found associated in 7–13% of cases (Fig. 13.37). VIN associated with HPV is more frequent in younger women, less likely to be invasive, and more often multifocal.

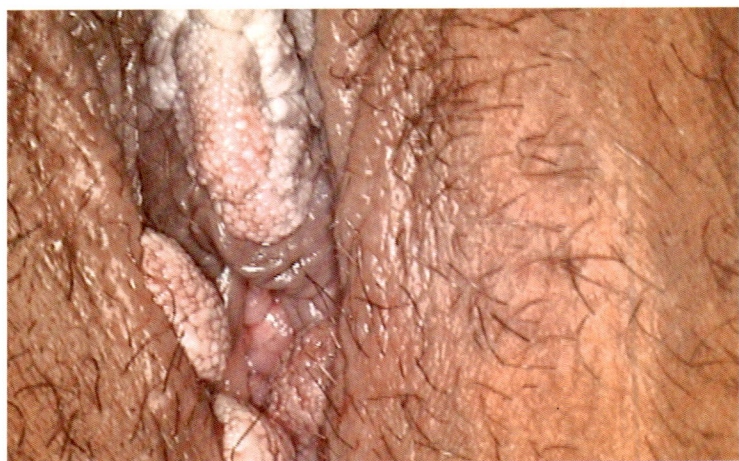

Fig. 13.35: AW micropapillary warty lesion

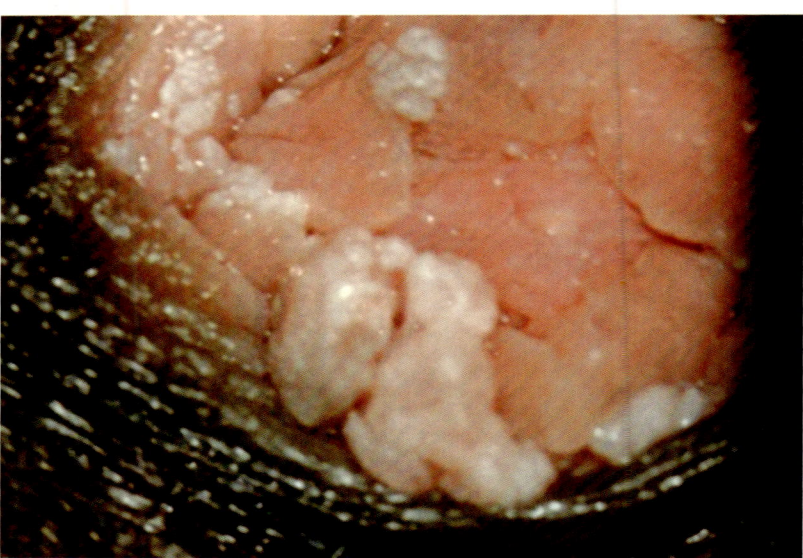

Fig. 13.36: Multiple AW projections with irregular surface at introitus suggestive of condylomatous lesions

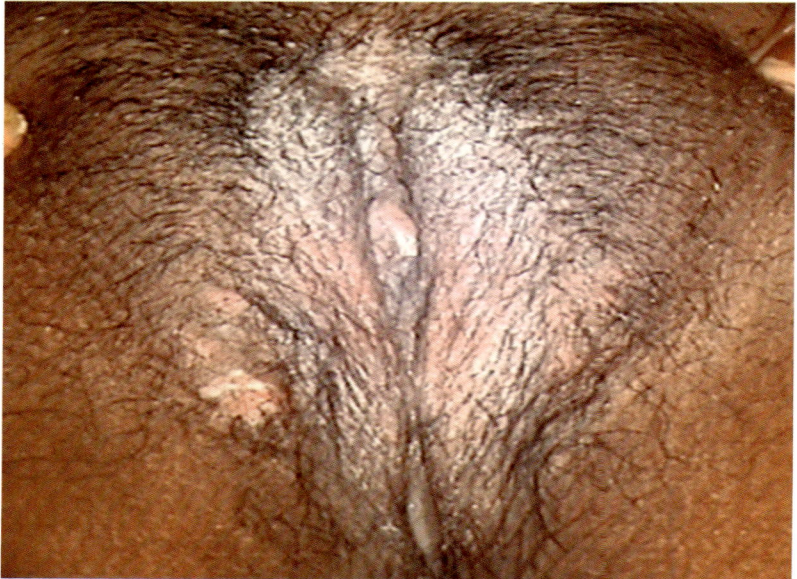

Fig. 13.37: Thickened raised reddish brown epithelium along with warty lesion (VIN-u, mixed warty basaloid)

Vulvar Intraepithelial Neoplasia (VIN)

VIN is part of a syndrome of multifocal epithelial changes of the anogenital tract. The key to diagnosis of VIN is a high index of suspicion. However, definitive diagnosis is made by colposcopic evaluation followed by biopsy.

Colposcopy is particularly helpful in the diagnosis of VIN and invasive cancer. White, red, and hyper-pigmented lesions are associated with VIN and vulvar cancer. Biopsy is required for definitive diagnosis.

Biopsy and histological confirmation should be considered in the following situations:
- Lesions surrounded by either thickened skin or color changes.
- Raised, red or pigmented lesions
- Presumed genital warts that fail to respond to two or three office treatments.
- Vulvar changes such as squamous cell hyperplasia and lichen sclerosus that do not respond to medical therapy.
- Suspicion of neoplasia

Table 13.7 depicts the different classifications given for VIN.

Histologically, the terms warty, basaloid, and differentiated (simplex) are used. The World Health Organization (WHO) classified VIN according to the 3-grade system for both the warty/basaloid types and the simplex type.

Table 13.7: Classification of vulvar intraepithelial neoplasia (VIN)

- WHO (2003)
  - VIN 1,2,3 (warty type/basaloid type)
  - VIN 1,2,3 (simplex type)
- ISSVD (2004)*
  - VIN, usual type (VIN 2, 3)
    - o Warty type
    - o Basaloid type
    - o Mixed warty-basaloid type
  - VIN 3, differentiated type
- Bethesda-like system (2005)
  - Low-grade VIL (condyloma VIN 1)
  - High-grade VIL (VIN 2/VIN 3)

*VIN 1: abolished terminology

In 2004, ISSVD modified their VIN terminology, using a 2-tier classification into VIN usual type and VIN differentiated type. The term VIN is now applied only to the histologically high-grade squamous lesions that were the former VIN 2 and VIN 3 or differentiated VIN.

A Bethesda-like grading system of low-grade vulvar intraepithelial lesions and high grade vulvar intraepithelial lesions has also been proposed in 2005. Condyloma acuminatum and discrete raised lesions with minimal atypia and lacking the features of dermatosis (VIN 1) were categorized into low-grade VIL.

Thus, two distinct pathways have been demonstrated (Fig. 13.38) for carcinogenesis from normal epithelium through precursor lesions (VIN) into keratinizing and warty/ basaloid types of vulvar SCC.

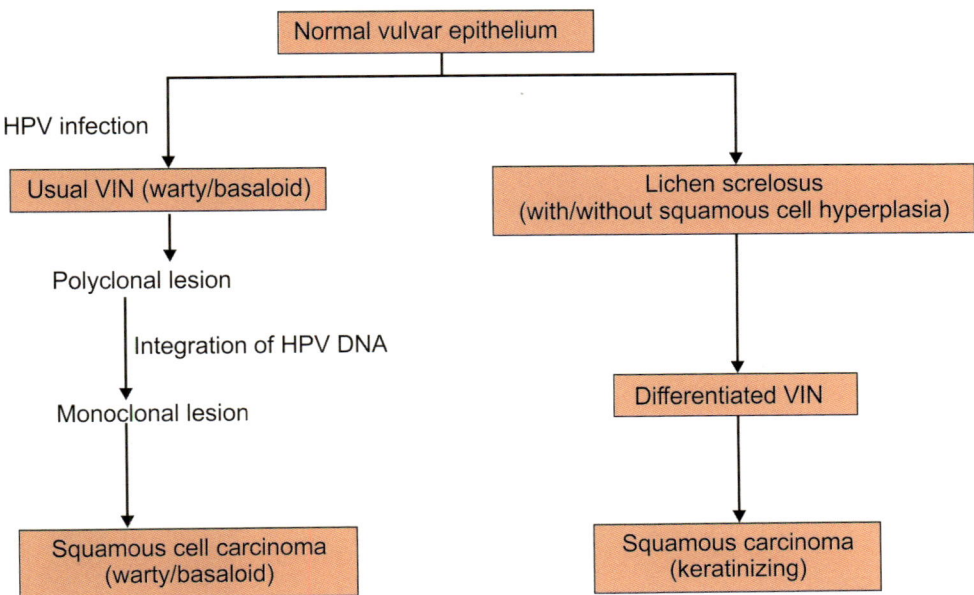

Fig. 13.38: Pathogenesis of VIN and squamous cell carcinoma of the vulva

Clinically, two distinct clinicopathologic subtypes of VIN exist: Usual VIN (VIN-u) and differentiated VIN (VIN-d). In terms of presentation, HPV-related VIN (VIN usual) tends to be asymptomatic and is often discovered at the time of evaluation for an abnormal Pap smear or genital warts.

Because multicentric disease is commonly encountered, particularly in younger women, a complete exam should include the cervix and vagina. Up to 50% of women with VIN will have antecedent or concomitant lower genital tract neoplasia, usually cervical or vaginal intraepithelial neoplasia. Vulvoscopy (colposcopy of the vulva) can be of help to magnify diseased areas. Vascular changes seen on cervical colposcopy are often not seen on the vulva. Biopsy of any suspicious areas should be liberally undertaken.

VIN lesions may occur anywhere on the vulva, including the periurethral and perianal areas, and are often multifocal. Lesions are usually elevated and have a rough surface, although flat lesions can also be seen. The color can be brown, white, gray or red (Figs 13.39 to 13.45).

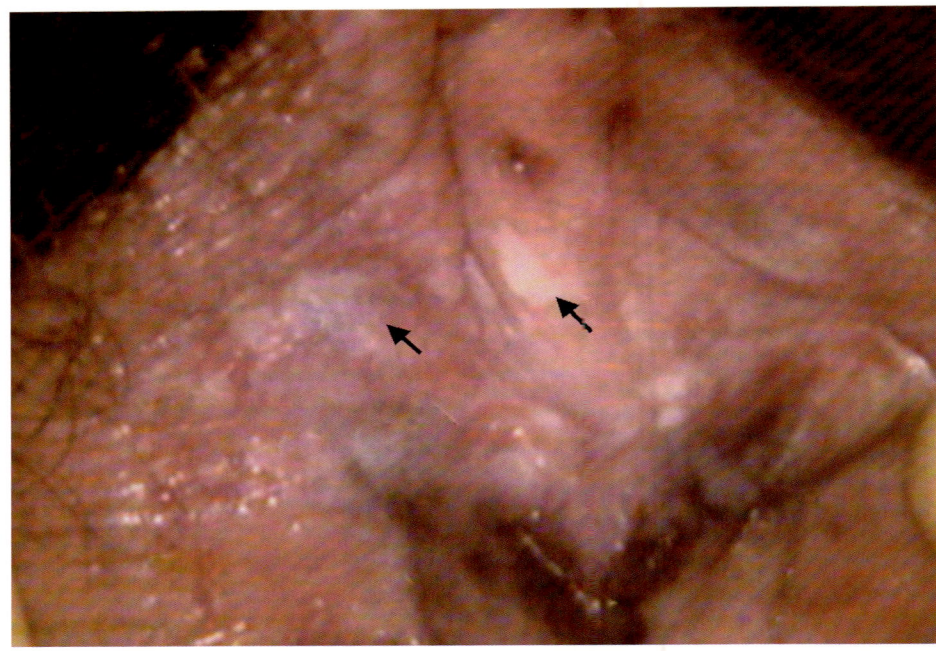

Fig. 13.39: AW epithelium over labia minora and in periurethral area (VIN-d)

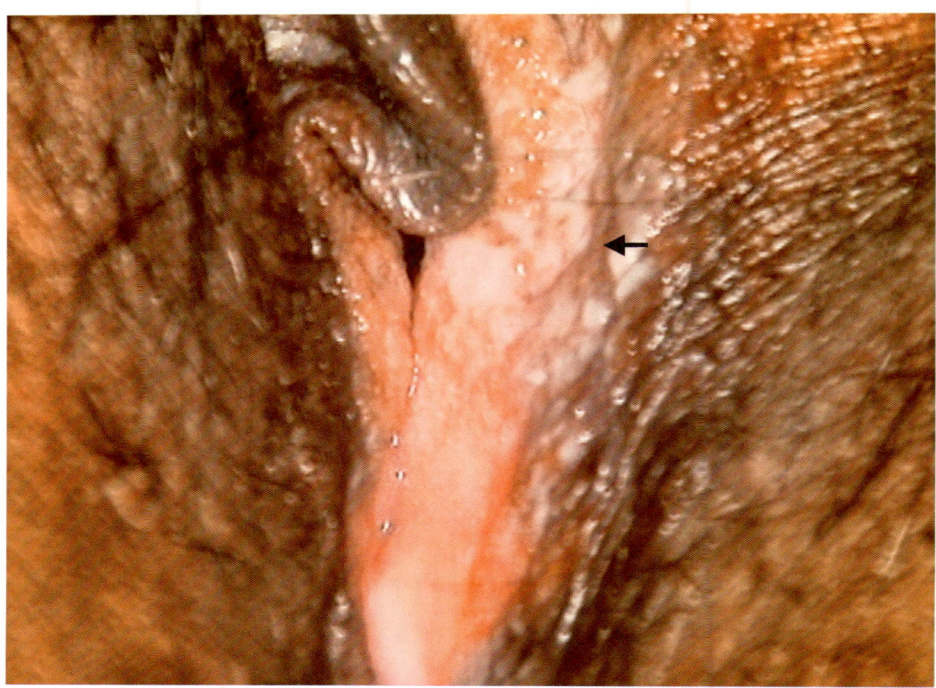

Fig. 13.40: Thick raised white patches with irregular surface at places and acetowhitening (VIN-d)

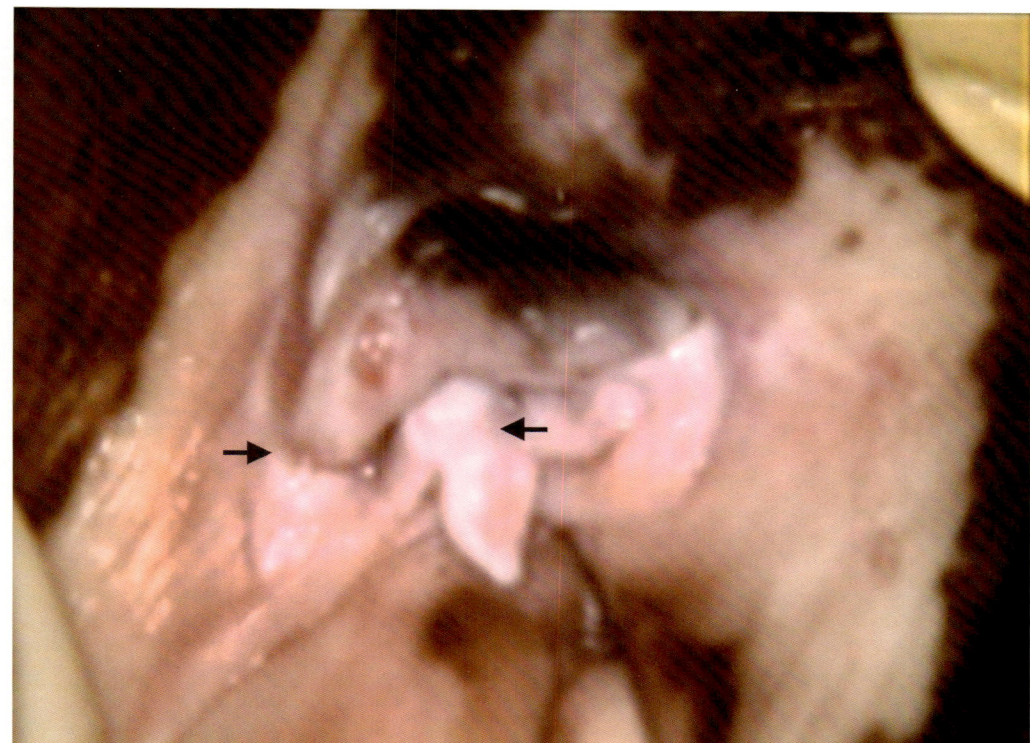

Fig. 13.41: Smooth acetowhite lesion in clitoral area along with white patches over both labia minora (VIN-d)

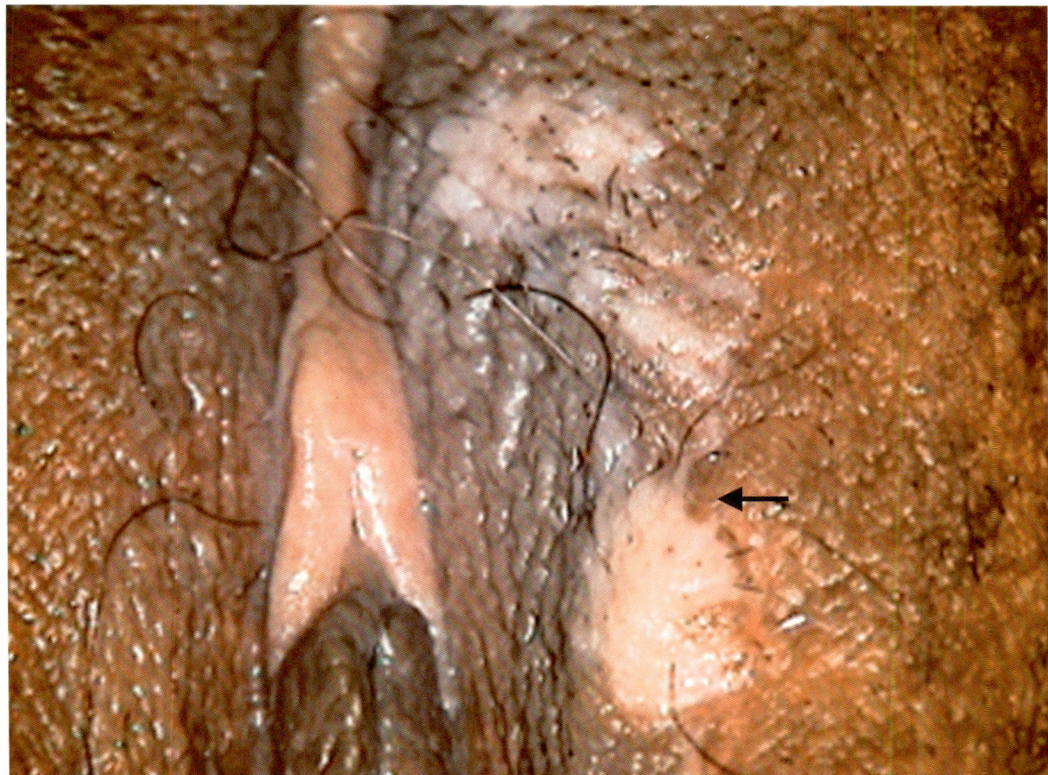

Fig. 13.42: AW lesion over labia minora, with white gray color changes and irregular borders (VIN-u)

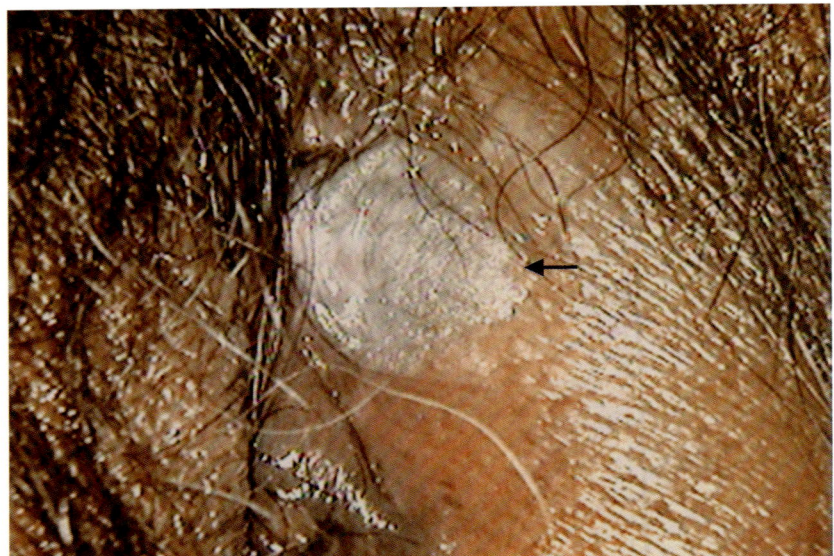

Fig. 13.43: Rough keratotic lesion in paraclitoral area (VIN differentiated)

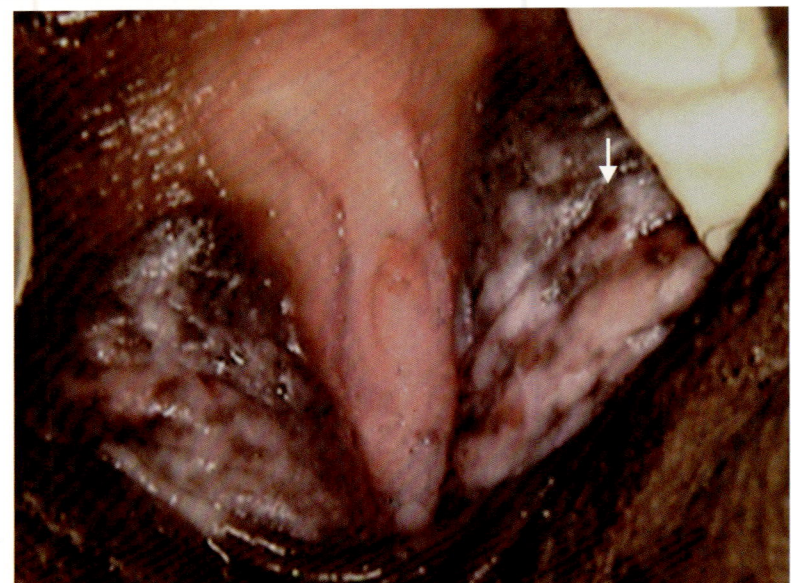

Fig. 13.44: Thick raised white patches with irregular surface at places and acetowhitening (VIN-u)

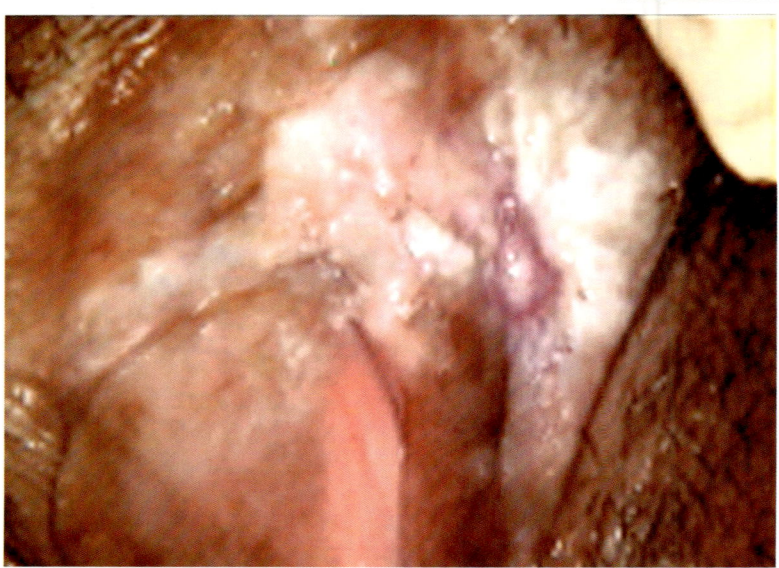

Fig. 13.45: Thick raised white patches along with AW epithelium and ulcer involving clitoris and paraclitoral area (VIN-d)

Differentiated VIN, in contrast, occurs in older women, often in the setting of other non-neoplastic epithelial disorders such as lichen sclerosus, lichen simplex chronicus, or lichen planus. Patients are usually symptomatic, with a long history of pruritus and burning. As compared to VIN usual, differentiated VIN is associated with a higher risk (> 95%) of progression to invasive squamous cell carcinoma of the vulva.

Carcinoma Vulva

Corresponding to two distinct types of VIN, two types of vulvar carcinoma are seen, the characteristics of which are described in Table 13.8. As opposed to the typical keratinizing vulvar squamous carcinomas seen in older women (in which oncogenic HPV infection ranges from 2–23%), HPV-related basaloid and warty carcinomas (75–100% of which harbor HPV) tend to arise in younger women. As a result, the risk factors typically associated with HPV-related disease (number of sexual partners, early age at first coitus, and abnormal Pap smears) while applicable to women with

Table 13.8: Characteristics of two types of squamous cell carcinoma of the vulva

Characteristics	Warty or basaloid type	Keratinizing type
Frequency	20–35%	65–80%
Age	Younger	Older
	55 (35–65)	77 (55–85)
Precursor	Warty or basaloid VIN	Lichen sclerosus differentiated VIN
Association with HPV	Associated with HPV high-risk types	No relation to HPV
Prognosis	Better	Worse

HPV-associated vulvar cancers, do not hold for those with keratinizing carcinomas.

The presentation of early invasive vulvar cancer is similar to those of symptomatic VIN. As invasion proceeds, a distinct tumor is likely to be recognized. The most common signs are red, pink, or white bumps, often with rough or eroded surfaces. A persistent, non-healing ulcer is also another presenting sign (Figs 13.46A and B).

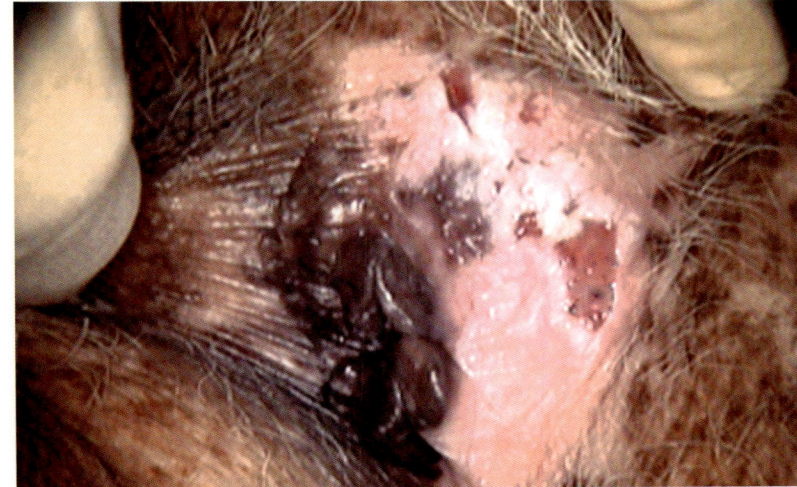

Fig. 13.46A: Non-healing ulcer along with dense, raised AW lesion over widespread white lesion in paraclitoral area

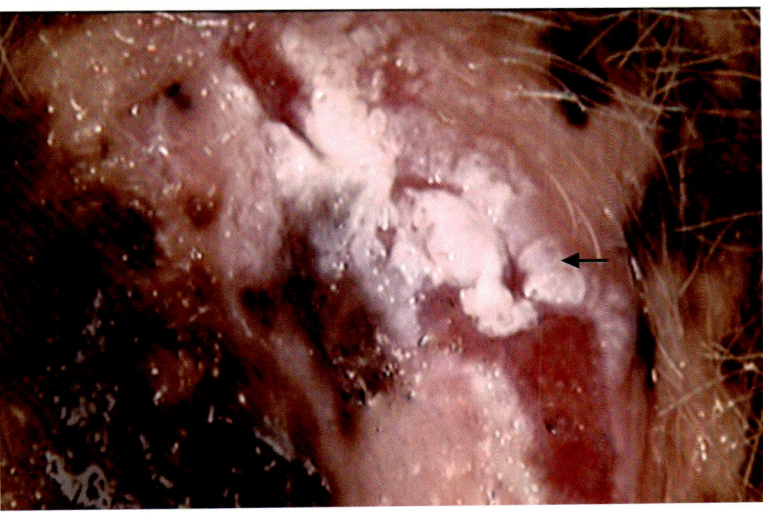

Fig. 13.46B: Same lesion with atypical vessels under higher magnification

About 25% cases are asymptomatic and lesions are subclinical which are difficult to be picked up on naked eye examination. Colposcopically, these lesions can be seen as slightly raised/micropapillary area or leukoplakia. After acetic acid application, lesions may assume marked whiteness with sharp borders (Fig. 13.47A) or may be diffuse in appearance. Punctations or rarely mosaic may be seen on the medial aspect of labia minora. Presence of atypical vessels suggests invasion (Fig. 13.47B). Definitive diagnosis can be achieved by biopsy only.

Verrucous carcinoma, the other subtype of invasive squamous cell vulvar cancer, appears with cauliflower-like growths similar to genital warts (Fig. 13.48).

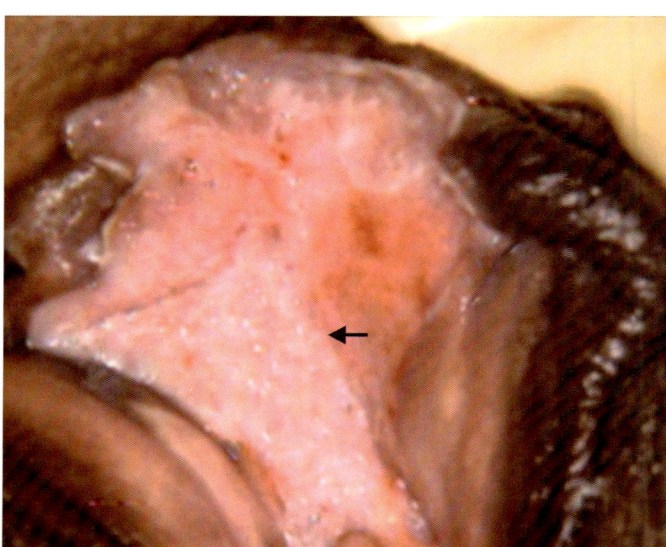

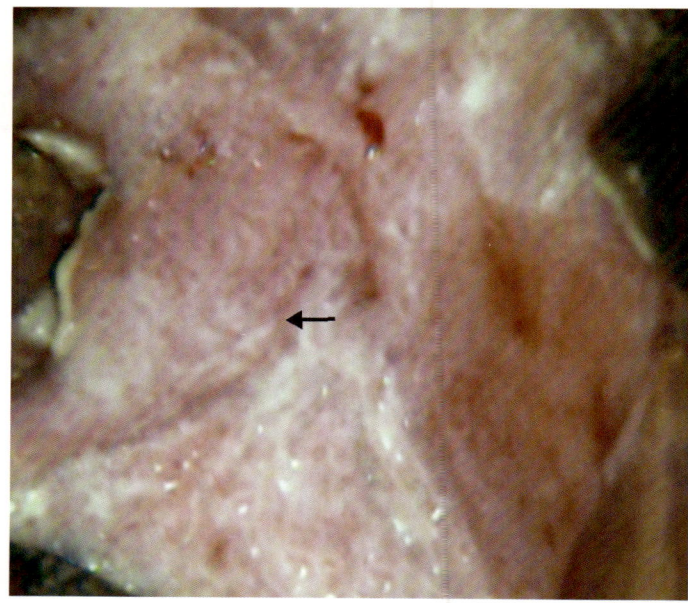

Fig. 13.47A: AW epithelium with slightly irregular, raised surface over labia minora

Fig. 13.47B: Same lesion under higher magnification—atypical vessels and punctations are visible

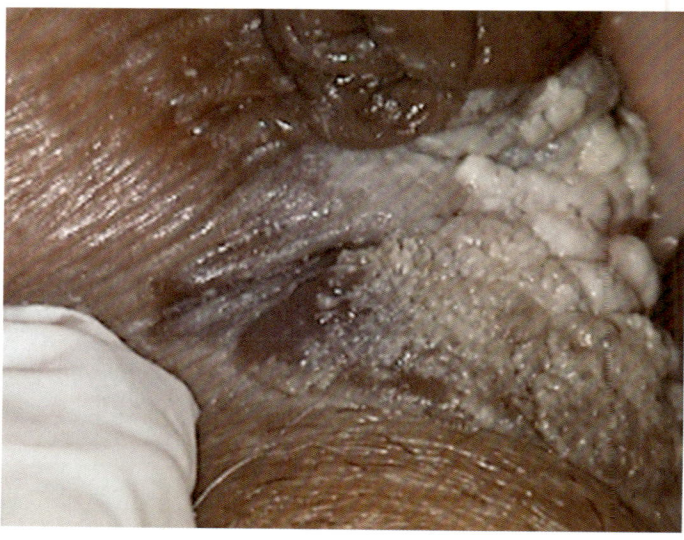

Fig. 13.48: Cauliflower keratotic growth over vulva

Chapter

14

Treatment of Vulvovaginal Diseases

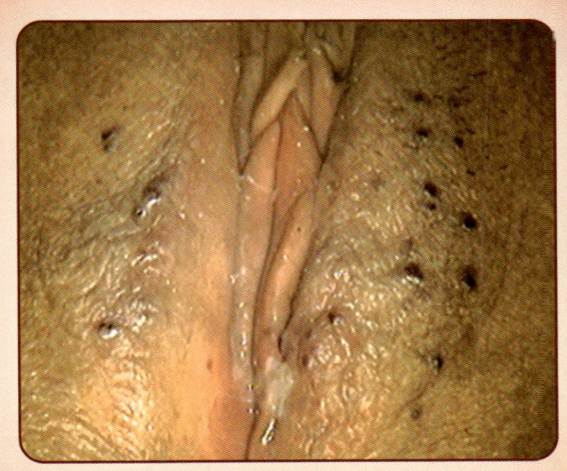

Chapter Outline

VULVAL LESIONS

Vulval symptoms are common in women and cause considerable distress. They are also often chronic and can substantially interfere with sexual function. Community based surveys indicate that about one-fifth of women have significant vulval symptoms lasting over three months at some time in their lives. Correct diagnosis and treatment reduces morbidity.

Vulvar pruritus and pain are common presenting symptoms. Among vulval dermatosis, contact dermatitis, lichen sclerosus, lichen planus and vulvar intraepithelial neoplasia are the ones that are often associated with both pruritus and pain. Itch or pain may be caused by dermatitis, recurrent candidiasis and the recently recognised pain syndromes—vulvar vestibular syndrome and dysesthetic vulvodynia.

Though diagnosis is usually apparent after a thorough history and examination, conditions commonly co-exist and are complicated by prior treatment. An early, accurate diagnosis should enhance management of vulval conditions, particularly pain syndromes.

The etiology of these vulvar skin conditions is multifactorial. Therefore, patient education, behavior modification, and regular follow-up are essential to ensure effective control of symptoms and management of the skin conditions. A pragmatic approach to management of chronic vulval symptoms is outlined.

History and Examination

Thorough history should be obtained regarding itching with or without pain, intermittent or constant, if worse before or during menses and any precipitating factors. History of sexual dysfunction or unrecognized depression should also be sought.

A thorough examination with adequate light is essential, as changes can be subtle. Examination may be normal or clear lesions may be present. Cotton bud can be used to elicit pain in the vestibular area in women with a history S/O vulvar vestibular syndrome.

Investigations

A vaginal or vulval swab is required to rule out infection as this can cause secondary dermatitis. Candidiasis can often coexist with other conditions. If fissures or ulcers are present, PCR should be done for HSV.

Biopsy is required for any abnormal examination finding that persists for more than six weeks without a clear diagnosis.

Treatment

Counseling is important as vulval conditions commonly respond slowly to the treatment, usually over weeks to months. The aim of therapy is to control symptoms rather than to cure the condition.

Principles of good vulval skin care should be part of the treatment of all conditions. Any irritants identified should be avoided, such as tight-fitting clothing, detergents, soaps, etc. that may irritate vulvar skin. Specific treatment for different vulval conditions is outlined below.

CONDITIONS WITH MINIMAL CLINICAL FINDINGS

Vulvar Vestibular Syndrome

Vulvar vestibular syndrome (VVS) is also known as vestibulitis, vestibulodynia, vestibular pain syndrome and localized vulval dysesthesia. Its exact prevalence is difficult to estimate, but studies suggest it may be more common than is recognized. A history of knife-like or excessive pain on contact to the genital area would be consistent with the syndrome.

Altered pain perception is the major feature of this syndrome. The typical patient is a nulliparous woman in her 20s or early 30s who often develops symptoms suddenly. The pain is characterized by extreme tenderness to pressure within the vulvar vestibule. Pain with attempted vaginal entry is the most common complaint. In the absence of localized pressure, women are symptom-free. It may follow a precipitating inflammatory condition or occur spontaneously. With time, this sensitivity to pressure or stretch may preclude intercourse or the insertion of tampoons. Pain characteristically may improve after initial penetration. Many women have associated urinary symptoms of frequency and bladder irritability in the absence of infection.

Physical signs are restricted to exquisite tenderness in the region of the posterior (less commonly the anterior) vestibule. Gentle pressure with a cotton swab commonly elicits pain.

Management is often difficult and prolonged and involves both behavioral and medical interventions. Coexisting disease (such as Candidiasis) should be excluded and irritants should be avoided. Sympathy and strong positive reassurance are required and sexual counseling should be offered. A number of treatments have been tried, including xylocaine gel 30 minutes before intercourse and pelvic floor retraining with biofeedback, as vaginismus is common. Low-dose tricyclic antidepressants, such as amitriptyline 10–75 mg at night, may be helpful in some patients and newer agents for neuropathic pain show promise. Cases that do not respond to medical treatment, may be offered surgery in the form of vestibulectomy.

Dysesthetic Vulvodynia

Dysesthetic vulvodynia (also known as essential vulvodynia and generalized vulval dysesthesia) occurs mainly in older patients. The predominant symptom is chronic, poorly localized vulval burning or pain. No abnormalities are found on examination, but there may be diffuse and variable hypersensitivity and altered perception to light touch. The exact etiology is unclear, but the condition shares some features with neuropathic pain syndromes (e.g. poor localization, persistence after removal of the noxious stimulus, little response to routine analgesia, and often a burning quality). Referred pain from the back or pelvis and recurrent herpes simplex should be excluded. If the description of the pain is bizarre or inconsistent, psychogenic pain should be considered but is rare.

Low-dose tricyclic antidepressant (e.g. amitriptyline, 10–75 mg at night) is the standard treatment for dysesthetic vulvodynia. Gabapentin, desipramine, and imipramine have also been reported as beneficial.

CONDITIONS WITH ABNORMALITIES ON EXAMINATION

Dermatitis

Dermatitis is common condition in women presenting with chronic vulval symptoms. Subtypes include atopic, seborrheic, irritant, allergic and corticosteroid-induced dermatitis and lichen simplex chronicus. It is more common in individuals with atopy, whose skin is less able to tolerate environmental insults. Contact allergens have been identified in many women diagnosed with vulval dermatitis, commonly medications. Itch is a common presenting symptom, although burning can occur, if the mucosa is involved. Clinical signs may be subtle and include poorly defined erythema, scale, fissures, lichenification and excoriation.

Common causes of irritation should be carefully sought and avoided. Therapy should begin with a potent topical corticosteroid (e.g. methylprednisolone aceponate) until symptoms have resolved. At this point, a weaker corticosteroid, such as 1% hydrocortisone, can be continued for a further two to three months. This cycle can be repeated, if disease activity flares. Drugs with antihistamine and sedative properties, at night, can be helpful in controlling nocturnal scratching.

Recurrent Vulvovaginal Candidiasis

Vulvovaginal candidiasis is considered recurrent when at least four discrete documented episodes occur in one year, or at least three in one year that are not related to antibiotic therapy. The condition is common. The pathophysiology of recurrent infection is unclear, but appears to involve an abnormality in the host–microorganism relationship.

Recurrent vulvovaginal candidiasis presents primarily with itch, but burning, especially after intercourse, is also common. It is characteristic for these symptoms to flare in the week before menses and to improve with the onset of menstruation. Clinical appearance is often not helpful in making the diagnosis. Vulval erythema, subtle swelling and occasionally longitudinal fissures may be seen. It is uncommon to find vaginal discharge of acute candidiasis. Low vaginal swabs for hyphae may be negative in up to 50% of women with culture-positive symptomatic vulvovaginal candidiasis. Most cases are caused by C. albicans, but other species may also be responsible which may be relatively resistant to treatment.

About 90% of uncomplicated cases of vulvovaginal candidiasis respond to oral or topical antifungals, although a secondary irritant contact dermatitis from topical imidazoles may occur. Longer treatment for 14 days is required for recurrent vulvovaginal candidiasis, followed by a maintenance regimen for six months. Some recommended maintenance regimens include clotrimazole (500 mg vaginal suppositories weekly), oral ketoconazole (100 mg daily), oral fluconazole (100–150 mg weekly) and oral itraconazole (400 mg monthly or 100 mg daily). Compliance is better with oral therapy. One in 10 000–15 000 persons exposed to ketoconazole may develop hepatotoxicity.

If there is a significant dermatitic reaction, 1% hydrocortisone ointment is useful, at least in the early stages. About 70% of women with other non-albicans species respond to intravaginal boric acid (600 mg daily in a gelatin capsule for 14 days). Topical flucytosine (4%) has also been used.

Combined pills can be continued as long as the estrogen dose is low (20–30 µg ethinylestradiol), or may occasionally be replaced with progesterone—only contraception. Asymptomatic male sexual partners should also be treated.

White Lesion—Lichen Sclerosus

It is an idiopathic inflammatory skin disease that has a predilection for the genital skin. It has been linked to several autoimmune diseases. It is a chronic, progressive, lifelong condition.

Lichen sclerosus most commonly presents with pronounced itch, although burning and dyspareunia can also occur. It may occur anywhere over the vulval, perineal or perianal skin and is uncommon at extra genital sites. The vagina is not involved. Typically, it presents with well-defined white plaques and an atrophic, wrinkled surface. There may also be purpura, hyperpigmentation, erosions, fissures and edema. Long-standing disease may result in labial shrinking, obliteration of the clitoral hood and occasionally restriction of the introitus, resulting in difficult and painful intercourse.

The diagnosis should be confirmed by skin biopsy. Patient should be explained about chronicity of the disease and lifelong treatment. Treatment should aim to control symptoms, minimize scarring and detect malignant change early. Potent topical corticosteroids are symptomatically effective in over 90% of women, providing rapid symptomatic relief and variable objective improvement. Betamethasone dipropionate ointment (0.05%) or clobetasol propionate 0.05% is used initially twice daily for a month, then daily for two months and gradually tapered.

2% testosterone or 2% progesterone has also been used but topical clobetasol is the most effective drug in relieving symptoms and improving objective and histopathologic findings. Whereas the long-term use of high potency steroids are reported to result in adverse changes on the vulva, such as atrophy and striae, the long-term use of clobetasol in patients with lichen sclerosus rarely has any adverse effect.

After the completion of the above routine, the patient is re-examined and advised to use the clobetasol once or twice a week. Commonly, when women complain of a sudden recurrence of vulvar pruritus, this may be associated with another cause for pruritus such as a candidal infection.

In patients who have persistent debilitating pruritus despite the above therapy, there are two other approaches.

1. Triamcinolone suspension (5 mg) diluted in 2 ml of normal saline injected subcutaneously beneath the skin of both labia majora. The suspension is slowly injected as the needle is withdrawn, then tissues are massaged to aid distribution of the suspension. This often results in relief of the pruritus, following which the patient stops scratching the vulvar tissue. By the time the effects of the injections have abated, the symptom of pruritus remains quite mild and is even absent and can usually be controlled by topical medication.

2. Intramuscular triamcinolone is injected into the thigh or gluteus muscle (1 mg/kg). No more than 80 mg should be given at a time. This can be repeated in 6–8 weeks.

Annual follow-up is recommended, as longitudinal studies suggest that the lifetime risk of squamous cell carcinoma within the affected area is about 2–5% compared to <0.01% without lichen sclerosus. It has been found that women with squamous cell hyperplasia occurring in a background of lichen sclerosus constitute a distinct group at higher risk of developing invasive cancer.

Psoriasis

Psoriasis is less common than lichen sclerosus. It can be easily mistaken for atopic dermatitis, but clues include a family history of psoriasis and evidence of psoriatic lesions elsewhere on the skin (scalp, natal cleft or nails). Clinically, psoriasis on the vulva may lack scale, but it tends to be more symmetrical, erythematous and well defined than dermatitis.

Psoriasis often requires more aggressive and prolonged treatment than dermatitis. Weaker-potency corticosteroids, such as 1% hydrocortisone, are often insufficient for maintenance, and a stronger corticosteroid, such as betamethasone valerate (0.02% twice daily), is often needed.

Atrophic Vaginitis

Estrogen deficiency causes the vaginal epithelium to become thin, pale and dry. Symptoms include superficial dyspareunia, minor vaginal bleeding and pain from splitting caused by friction. Topical vaginal estrogen creams are beneficial. Estriol cream or pessaries are used daily for three weeks and then once or twice a week for maintenance.

Human Papillomavirus Infection of External Genitalia

Spontaneous regression of genital warts can occur in up to 30% of affected patients. Regression, however, does not necessarily lead to viral clearance, as viral genomes can be detected in normal epithelium for months to years following clearing of visible disease. However, in immunocompetent women, the cell-mediated immunity that results in lesion regression most likely controls latent HPV infection. Therefore, disease recurrence is less likely. Immunosuppressed women are at increased risk of developing HPV-related manifestations. They include those receiving long-term corticosteroid therapy or chronic immunosuppressive treatment, as well as immunosuppressed women with HIV infection.

The goal of therapy in general is physical destruction or removal of visible disease, not eradication of HPV infection.

Multiple treatment options are available for genital warts of the lower genital tract. The choice of treatment or observation is determined by the extent of the genital HPV lesions, clinical symptoms, presence of any suspicious area for malignant transformation, and by clinician and patient preference. Risk assessment including age and immune status is also an important part of planning therapy.

The following options for treatment of vulvar and perianal lesions are available.

Patient applied treatments include
- Imiquimod 5% cream
- Podophyllotoxin 0.5% solution or gel
- Sinecatechins 15% ointment

Provider-administered therapies include
- Trichloroacetic or bichloroacetic acid 80–90%
- Podophyllin 10–25%
- Cytodestructive treatment
- Surgical removal

Such therapies have been the mainstay of treatment. Local irritation (e.g. pain, burning and soreness), erythema, edema and at times, ulceration can result from the use of any of the medications. Careless or excessive use can result in extensive burning of the epithelium, with resultant scar formation.

Surgical excision or laser vaporization should be reserved for patients with extensive disease. Alternative regimens include intralesional interferon, photodynamic therapy, and topical cidofovir.

Topical Chemodestructive Agents

Patient applied

Imiquimod
Imiquimod is expensive. It is an immune response modulator. Although the exact mechanism of action is not definitely known, it induces cytokines locally, including alpha-interferon, various interleukins, and tumor necrosis factor. More recently, imiquimod has been shown to influence toll receptors. Studies demonstrate reduced recurrence of genital warts post-treatment.

The cream works better in females than in males with an overall complete clearance rate of 72% reported compared to 33% in males when applied 3 times a week for up to 16 weeks. It is not recommended for treatment of urethral, vaginal or cervical warts and in pregnancy. It should be applied sparingly to each wart 3 times per week alternate days for up to 15 weeks. The treatment area should be washed with a mild soap 6 to 10 hours after application. A major advantage of imiquimod over other patient-applied treatments is that the cream can be used even on areas that are difficult to see as its application does not have to be limited exactly to the HPV lesion.

Patient should be evaluated by a clinician approximately once a month to determine the effectiveness of treatment and whether treatment needs to be continued. Use of imiquimod does not preclude treatment by the clinician with other modalities such as TCA, cryotherapy, etc. as the combination may result in much quicker clearance than treatment with any one treatment used alone. Healing occurs within 2–3 weeks leaving hardly any scarring.

Side effects: Local skin reactions such as redness, erosions, itching, flaking and swelling are common but usually mild. If such reactions are severe, cream should not be applied until the reaction has subsided.

Podophyllotoxin 0.5% solution and gel
This is a purified podophyllin. Purified podophyllotoxin is a much better product than podophyllin because the toxic components present in podophyllin have been eliminated standardizing the amount of beneficial podophyllin in the medicine so there is no variability in this product.

It is available in a solution or gel form which is usually self-applied by patients initially twice daily for three days followed by four days without therapy. The cycle may be repeated up to four times.

The total wart area treated should not exceed 10 cm², and the total volume should be limited to 0.5 ml per day. It is not recommended in children and pregnancy.

Although approximately 80% will have better than 50% reduction in wart volume within 2–4 weeks of beginning treatment, reported total clearance is 37% at 4 weeks and 44% at 8 weeks. Remaining latent virus results in a decreased real cure rate.

Side effects: Virtually non-toxic. Irritation to skin may occur.

Sinecatechins 15% ointment
It is the latest agent for the treatment of warts. Sinecatechin 15% cream is a botanical drug product extracted from green tea leaves. It is a mix of catechins and other components. Catechins are bioflavonoids, polyphenols and powerful antioxidants shown to

enhance immune system function and to fight tumors. 0.5 cm strand of ointment is applied in a thin layer using a finger over all external warts three times a day for up to 16 weeks only. It is not to be washed off afterwards. It is not recommended in pregnancy. 53.6% complete clearance is reported with a 16 week median time to complete clearance.

Side effects: Erythema, pruritus, burning, pain/discomfort, erosion/ulceration, edema, induration and vesicular rash may occur.

Clinician Administered Therapies

Tri- or bichloroacetic acid (TCA or BCA)

It is the most commonly used office treatment. Most effective strength is 80–85% and is well tolerated, although significant burning occurs in the treated area for 2 to 5 minutes.

It may cause burns, if spilled, hence should be applied by clinician weekly or fortnightly. Before application, surrounding normal epithelium should be coated with a protective substance, as 5% lidocaine gel, and then solution is applied with help of a small cotton-tipped applicator to the wart. It is allowed to dry first before patient sits or stands. If excess acid has been used, treated area should be powdered with talc, sodium bicarbonate or liquid soap preparations. It may be repeated weekly.

It can be used in pregnancy, children, in the vagina, perianally and urethral meatus.

It is effective in 50 to 85%, if used weekly until warts are gone.

It is totally non-toxic, may cause shallow skin ulcerations at times that heal quickly.

Podophyllin

It is an extract of the May apple plant and the oldest treatment for genital warts. It works by binding to cellular microtubules, thereby stopping cell division.

It is carefully applied to the wart and then washed off by the patient between one and four hours after application. It may be repeated weekly, if needed. To avoid toxicity, one application should be limited to < 0.5 ml podophyllin or an area of < 10 cm² warts treated per session and no open lesions or wounds should be present in treatment area. It should be washed off 4 to 6 hours after application. It often results in pain at the site of application in 1 to 3 days.

It should not be used inpregnancy, children, or in the vagina, inside the anal canal, or on thin, ulcerated skin.

Reported response is 32 to 79% after 3 to 6 months of regular weekly application. There is a significant problem with variability of strength of podophyllum preparations, which makes response rates very variable and also increases the risk of side effects.

Podophyllin in 10–25% benzoin is rarely used now as severe side effects have been reported with this drug. Neurotoxicity and bone marrow depression may occur, if applied over too large an area. Fetal death is reported when applied during pregnancy.

Cytodestructive Treatment

These methods are used, if all above treatments fail, or in combination with chemodestructive agents.

Cryotherapy

Cryotherapy is a common office treatment for external genital HPV lesions. It destroys the lesions by freezing. It can be used in many ways, can be applied in the form of liquid nitrogen through soaked cotton-tipped applicators or through cryoprobe or by spraying liquid nitrogen on each wart. Procedure is easy with low cost. Healing takes approximately 2–4 weeks.

It can be used in pregnancy, on the cervix and perianally. Response rate is 63–88%. It is usually done once a week until clear.

Side effects: There are very few side effects. Each freeze stings during the freeze but generally no pain is felt afterwards. There is very little scarring.

Electrocautery

It burns each wart using monopolar current. It used to be the mainstay of therapy 15 to 25 years ago and still continues to be an effective option. It is still a good form of treatment, especially in those who have failed treatment with other methods. Generally, works faster than topical agents but requires local anesthesia. It is difficult to use with extensive warts unless done under general anesthesia, or with several separate treatments of smaller sections done under local anesthesia. It may be used in pregnancy, on the vulva and may also be used carefully on small warts in the vagina and perianal region. Its response rate is 70–90%.

Side effects: May cause scarring because there is far less control over damage to surrounding tissues than with other cytodestructive treatments such as cryotherapy or laser.

Laser

Laser uses a high intensity light beam to burn warts. It is very effective but the high cost and expertise is the main drawback that has greatly reduced its use. Laser is rarely used as the first-line of therapy except to treat multifocal high-grade precancerous changes throughout the lower genital tract, massive warts or thick keratotic or extremely extensive lesions not responsive to local therapy.

It requires general anesthesia for large areas to be treated, or local anesthesia for small areas. It may be used safely in pregnancy, in the vagina, cervix, urethra and the perianal areas. It may be very painful during the healing phase of 1 to 3 weeks depending upon the size of the area treated.

Surgical Removal

Surgical removal is indicated in case of extensive warts.

Adjunctive Agents

5% 5-FU and 1% 5-FU

These creams were used extensively in the 1980s but are used less often today due to side effects.

It is cytotoxic, inhibits production of both RNA and DNA in the cell that has an antiproliferative effect. It gives rise to hypersensitivity reaction that stimulates the immune system. It is applied sparingly to each wart one to three times per week.

Success of treatment partly depends upon the amount of inflammatory reaction, as are the complications. For external warts, 5-FU is not as successful as when it is used for treatment of vaginal warts. 5-FU is rarely used today. When used, it is probably best used as an adjuvant post-treatment along with other methods to prevent recurrence as over the margins.

Side effects: It is very irritating to external skin, may cause deep ulcerations which are very painful and difficult to heal. Chronic dyspareunia may result when used on the vestibule.

Long-term follow-up care and prevention

Self-examination supplemented by periodic check ups by health care providers is recommended to assess for recurrence of HPV disease on external areas.

If a patient does not respond to a given product by the fourth week, she should be switched to another form of therapy and a biopsy should be taken to exclude cancer or precancer.

Pregnant patients with external HPV lesions

Spontaneous resolution of warts occurs in most of the patients following delivery and recovery from pregnancy-induced immunosuppression. Therefore,

most of the lesions should be left for observation and not treated.

TCA, liquid nitrogen, or electrocautery all can be used to treat external genital HPV lesions at any time during pregnancy.

Imiquimod and sinecatechins are not approved for use in pregnancy.

Podophyllin and podophilox, 1% and 5% 5-FU are contraindicated in pregnancy.

Laser is best reserved for persistent lower genital tract lesions at 30 to 32 weeks gestation.

Cesarean section vs vaginal delivery

Some clinicians advocate cesarean section to prevent laryngeal papillomatosis due to perinatal transmission. Reported rate of this occurrence is low 1–4/100,000 births. No controlled studies has suggested that cesarean section prevents this condition as laryngeal papillomatosis has been reported in children born even by cesarean section, therefore cesarean section is not recommended only to prevent papillomatosis. The one clinical indication for cesarean section that involves HPV is the presence of extensive vaginal and/or introital warts blocking the birth canal.

Vulval Intraepithelial Neoplasic (VIN)

Current treatments for VIN, have largely resulted in suboptimal outcomes. Response rates have been poor and relapse rates high. Recurrence rates following many medical or surgical therapies range from 39% following local excision and 70% after laser ablation to 90% in some studies of 5-fluorouracil.

Agents that enhance or induce strong cell-mediated immune responses are likely to hold the greatest promise not only for control of HPV-related disease but also for reduction of future recurrences. Imiquimod's efficacy in the treatment of genital warts is well-established, and its use has been shown to be associated with encouraging results in the treatment of VIN 2 and VIN 3 with a greater than 90% response rate.

Treatment of VIN in pregnancy is deferred until completion of the pregnancy. In some cases, regression of such lesions may occur.

Treatment of VIN must be individualized depending upon patient age, symptoms, distribution and size of lesions, malignant potential, psychological issues, and recurrence rates. All modalities for treatment of VIN have high recurrence rates.

The principal therapies for the treatment of VIN are local excision and local destruction.

Treatment options

- Observation (VIN 1 and, perhaps VIN 2, only).
- Excisional:
  - o Wide local excision
  - o Skinning vulvectomy
  - o Simple vulvectomy with adequate surgical margins of 1 cm around the lesion.
- Destruction: Can be done by laser vaporization, cryocautery, 5-fluorouracil (5-FU) and imiquimod.

VIN 1 and 2

Now VIN 1 is considered as chronic dermatological condition. Most women with VIN under the age of 40 have HPV as the cause and the lesions undergo spontaneous regression in majority of cases; hence such lesions may be kept under close observation. Persistent lesions require therapy.

Alternatively small lesions may be treated by cyto-destruction (electrocautery, laser, freezing, tri- or bichloroacetic acid) or immunomodulation with imiquimod.

Avoiding aggressive treatment is particularly important in pregnancy, as most of them spontaneously resolve in postpartum period.

Immunocompromised or immunosuppressed patients such as diabetics and HIV-seropositive have a much higher incidence of HPV infections and VIN as compared to general population, and spontaneous regression is unlikely in such cases.

Women who smoke should be encouraged to quit, since spontaneous regression is rare in smokers and recurrence rates are very high in smokers after treatment.

VIN 3

VIN 3, at any age, should be treated, and it is essential that the patient be informed of the requirement for long-term follow-up.

High-grade (VIN 3) which is at risk for invasion is most commonly a solitary lesion that is larger than the more "acute" multifocal papules or may cover large areas of the external genitalia with thickened, flat, often multicolored (red, white and pigmented) epithelium. Such large areas of involvement require either multiple biopsies to rule out invasion prior to laser ablation or should be excised in their entirety.

Treatment options

- Wide local excision of individual lesions by a scalpel. Recurrence rates as high as 32% are reported.
- Laser vaporization may be used on either single lesions or widespread disease. Approximately 75–85% of VIN lesions are found in non-hairy areas. It is a good treatment when extensive multifocal disease occurs in young individuals. Depth of destruction must be tailored with 2.5 mm depth in hairy and perianal areas and lesser depths (1–2 mm) in areas such as the labia minora, clitoris where the skin thickness is less than 3 mm. Deeper ablation may result in scarring and dyspareunia.
  Recurrence rates of 5 to 40% have been reported.
- Cryocautery is rarely used to treat high-grade VIN due to the inability to accurately measure the depth of tissue destruction. However, small focal papules (previously termed Bowenoid papulosis) can usually be safely destroyed by this method.
- Electrocautery of such lesions is also likely to be acceptable treatment due to the low malignant potential of these lesions.
- 5-FU has been used to treat VIN but causes severe pain and has recurrence rates as high as 75%. It may be most helpful as an adjunct to laser, applied post-treatment to healing laser margins to reduce the potential for recurrence.
- Increasing evidence supports the use of topical imiquimod for VIN 3 also.

Currently radical treatments like skinning vulvectomy, or simple vulvectomy are not advocated in most of the cases, due to the gross disfigurement that often occurs following such surgery. However, when risk of invasion is high, or extensive symptomatic disease cannot be treated by any other manner, then this approach may be justified.

Follow-up

Lifetime follow-up is required for patients with VIN. They have to be followed every 3 months initially. For the multifocal and immunocompromised patient, multiple recurrences of VIN are common, occurring in at least one-third of cases.

VAGINAL LESIONS

The natural history of vaginal HPV lesions including vaginal intraepithelial neoplasia [VAIN] is not well understood. Host immunity produces spontaneous resolution of low-grade lesions in most cases. Therefore, it is best not to over aggressively diagnose and treat these low-grade lesions. However, these lesions may serve as a significant viral reservoir, until regression occurs. All high-grade VAIN 2, 3 should be treated.

Treatment of VAIN 1 and Vaginal Warts

Many clinicians choose not to treat vaginal warts or VAIN 1 in expectation of spontaneous resolution in most of the lesions. However, all these patients require follow-up to evaluate progression or regression.

Lesions must be treated in:

- Non-compliant patient for follow-up.
- Concern about occult higher grade disease.
- Cosmetic and/or concerns about sexual transmission of HPV.

Treatment options for low-grade vaginal HPV lesions are limited:

- *Cryotherapy with liquid nitrogen.* The use of a cryo-probe in the vagina is not recommended because of the risk for vaginal perforation and fistula formation.
- *Tri- or bichloroacetic acid (TCA or BCA).* It works well on small individual lesions. It should be applied colposcopically with the wooden end of cotton-tipped applicator.
- *Imiquimod:* Imiquimod is not FDA-approved for intravaginal use. Though several reports in the literature show favorable results.

Imiquimod can be clinician applied directly to individual vaginal HPV lesions under colposcopic guidance, as with TCA, but this requires at least a once-a-week application. Reports where patients have self-applied imiquimod to the vagina have often lead to excessive introital pain and irritation.

Treatment of VAIN 2, 3

VAIN 2 in a young woman may reasonably be treated similar to VAIN 1. **VAIN 3** should always be treated.

Options for treatment of VAIN 2, 3 include:

- *Laser,* which requires special expertise, particularly when used in the vagina.

- *Local excision, loop excision, and partial vaginectomy* are all options depending on extent of the VAIN and concern for invasion. Risks of injury to bladder, rectum, ureters, and blood vessels require special expertise and are, therefore, best managed by a specialist with expertise in these techniques.

If VAIN involves the vaginal cuff post-hysterectomy for CIN, it is best excised to rule out invasive cancer.

Problem-Based Management

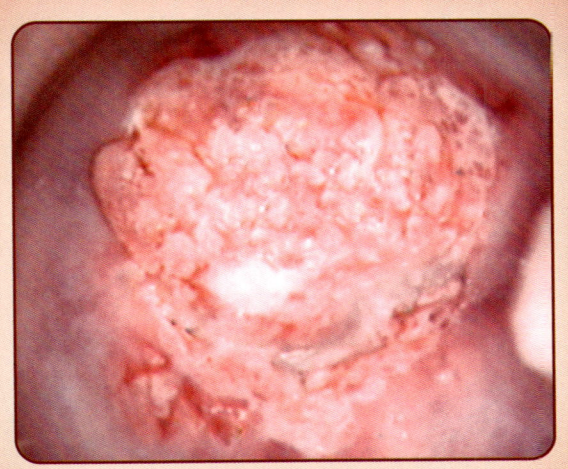

Chapter outline

CASE 1

A healthy, 25-year-old, P1 L1, went for cervical cancer screening, where her Pap smear and HPV DNA testing was done. Cytology was reported as ASC–US and HPV DNA was found to be positive for high risk virus.

Q.1. What is your advice to this patient who is very anxious and worried?

Ans.: The woman should be counseled that HPV infection is very prevalent at young age, majority of infections are transient and clear on their own within 1–2 years; most of the women with minor cytological abnormalities do not have or develop high grade lesions over time. So there is no cause for anxiety.

However, regular followup is essential. If the patient is too anxious, she can be advised immediate colposcopy or further triaging with E6/7 mRNA depending upon the facilities available.

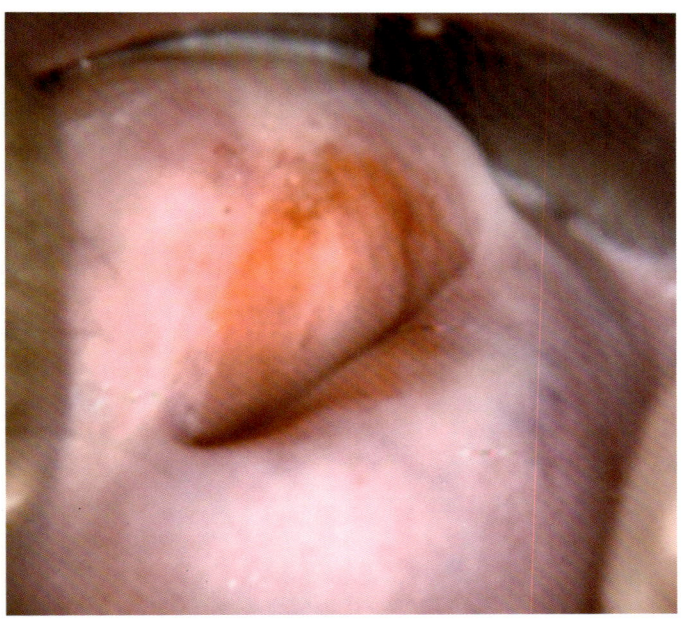

After saline application

Q.2. Colposcopy images are shown. Describe the findings.

Ans.: It is an adequate colposcopy with SCJ entirely visible. Lower endocervical canal can be seen due to ectropion. Transformation zone is type 1 and does not show any abnormality.

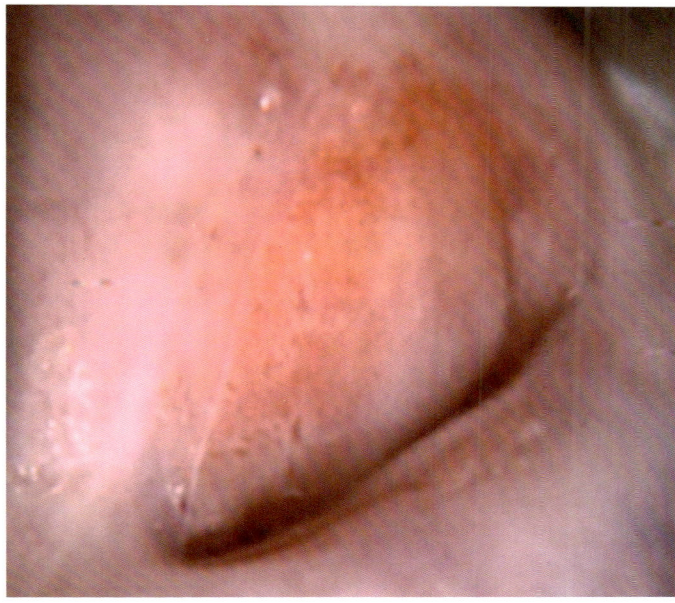

After application of acetic acid

Q.3. What is the further management plan?

Ans.: Patient would be called for followup after 12 months for repeat Pap smear. If repeat cytology is ASC–US or more, further colposcopy is recommended. If cytology remains negative for 24 months then patient is kept on routine surveillance.

Comments

1. The prevalence of invasive cancer is very low (0.1–0.2%) in women with ASC–US and is induced only by persistent infection with HR-HPV types.

2. Cancer screening in women less than 30 years age is done by Pap smear only. HPV DNA testing is not recommended because of its high prevalence in this age group as it may lead to unnecessary anxiety.

3. In presence of +ve HPV DNA test, vulva and vagina should also be examined carefully, if cervix does not show any lesion.

CASE 2

A 32-year-old, P3L3, presented with excessive vaginal discharge and postcoital bleeding. Per speculum examination showed non-specific discharge from cervix and cervical ectopy, bleeding on touch.

Q.1. What would be the plan of management?

Ans.: Examination of vaginal and cervical discharge for sexually transmitted infections followed by Pap smear after treatment of infection.

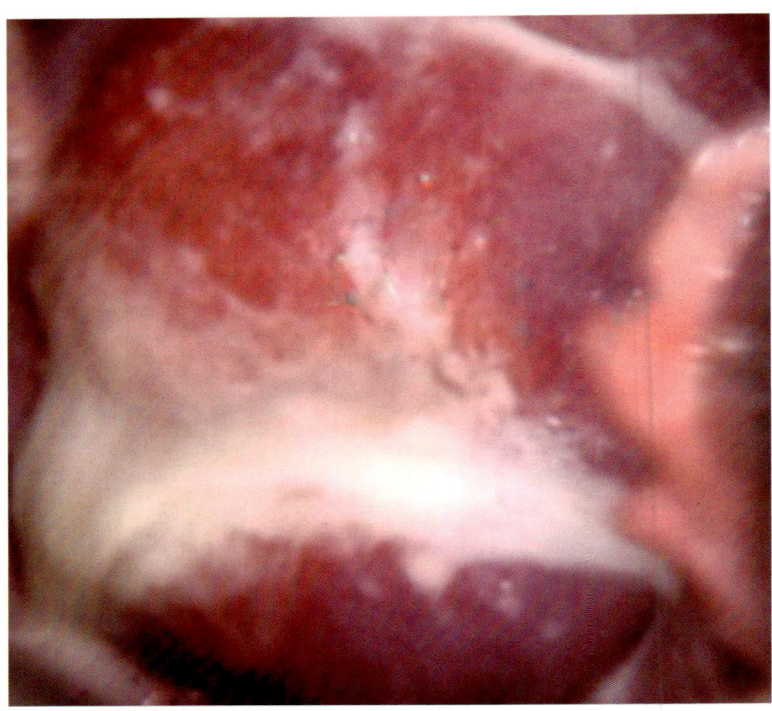

Cervix in unprepared state

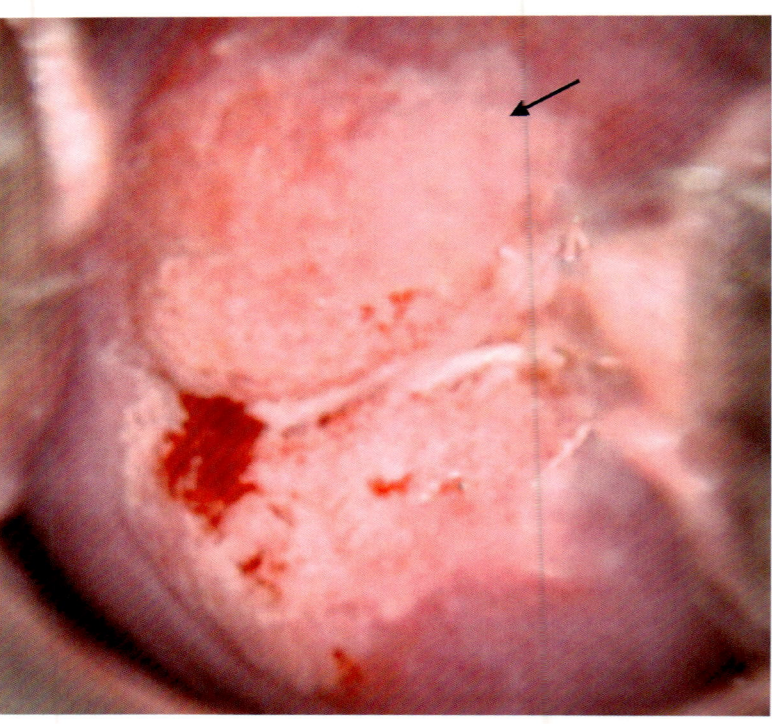

After acetic acid application

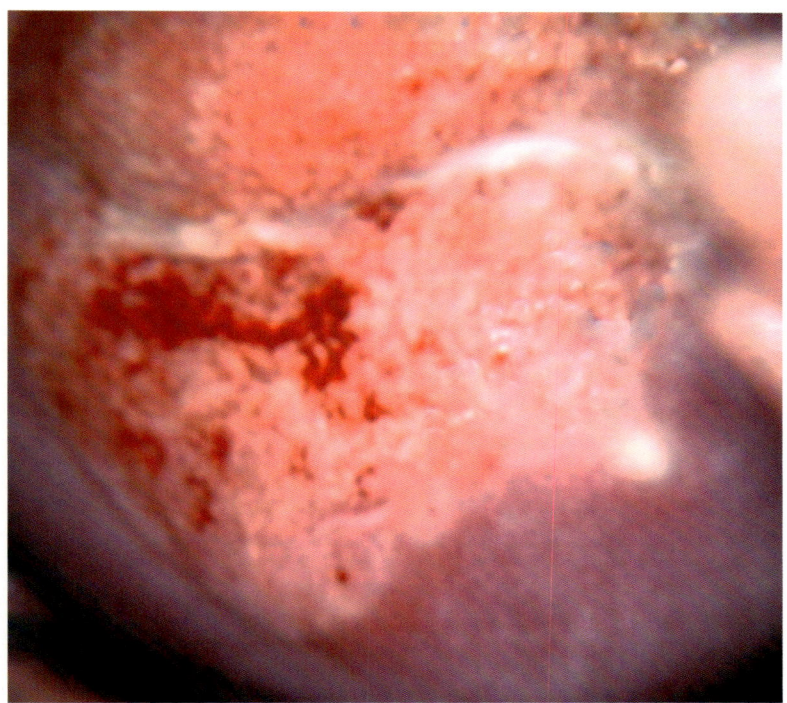

Same cervix—magnified view

Q.2. Pap smear was reported as LSIL. Colposcopy images are shown. Describe the findings?

Ans.: Colposcopy is adequate and shows ectopy. SCJ is completely visible. Type 1 transformation zone shows minor (Gr 1) abnormal finding. Thin, flat, AW lesion with irregular geographic border is seen at 1 O' clock position, inside the TZ. It is seen in its entirety. Posterior lip shows immature metaplastic epithelium.

Q.3. Directed biopsy from 1 O' clock was reported as HPV-related changes with CIN 1. How would you manage this patient?

Ans.: Patient would be kept under observation and followed up with cytology at 6 and 12 months or HPV DNA after 1 year.

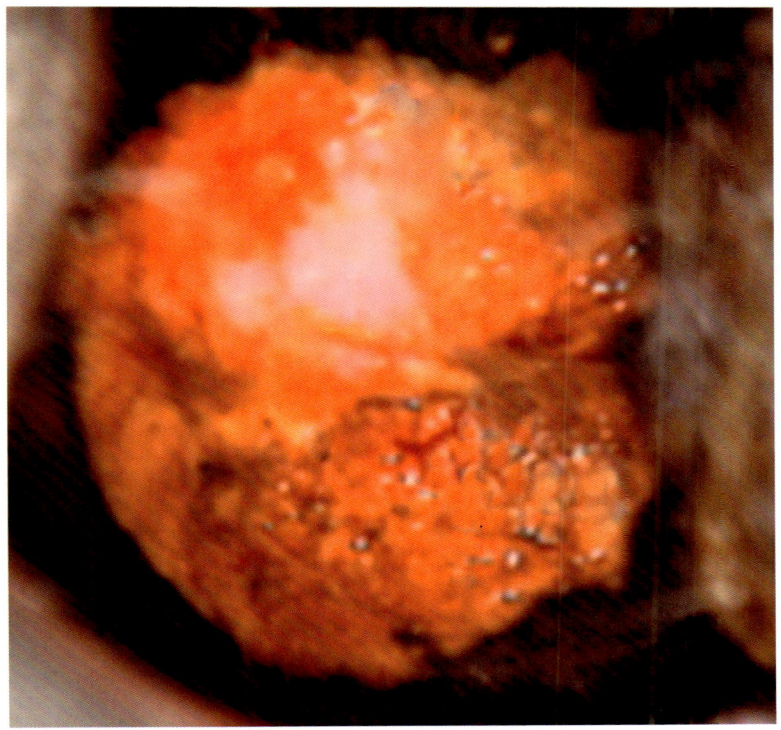

After Lugol's iodine application

Comment

Compliant patient of CIN 1 preceded by LSIL cytology and satisfactory colposcopy need not be treated immediately and can be kept under observation with regular follow-up for 2 years. In such cases, there is very small risk of unrecognized high grade lesion but risk of occult or unrecognized cancer is nil. If CIN 1 persists after 2 years or is found to be progressing at anytime, it can be treated by ablation or excision accordingly.

CASE 3

A 34-year-old, P1L1with cervical cytology report of HSIL, was referred for colposcopy.

Q.1. Describe the colposcopic findings.

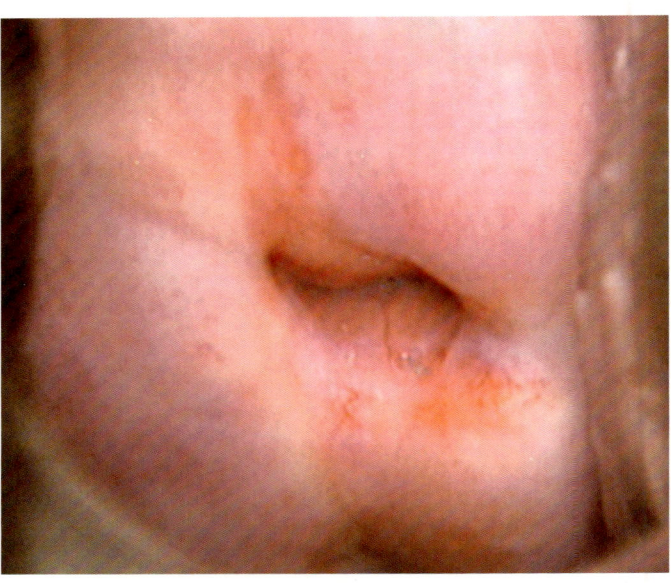

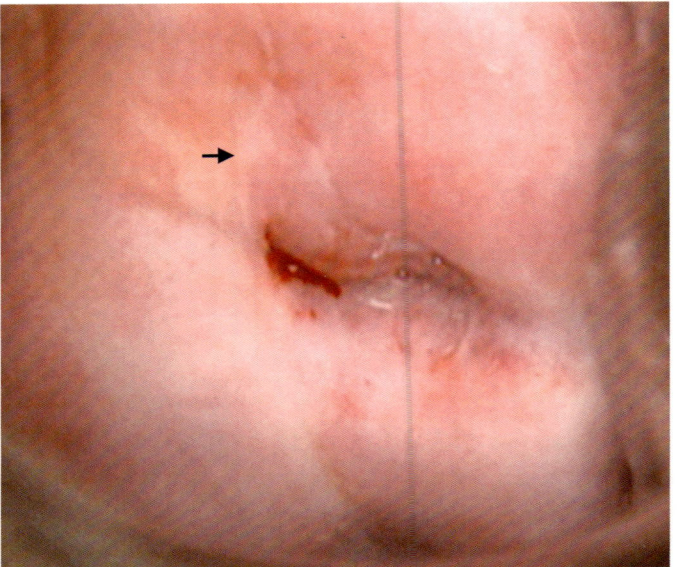

After acetic acid application

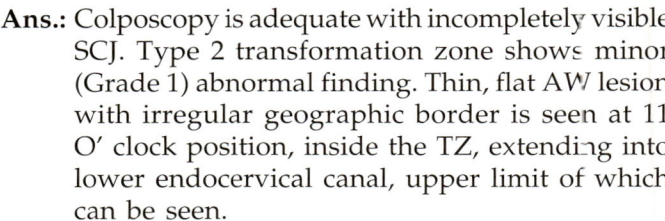

After saline application

Ans.: Colposcopy is adequate with incompletely visible SCJ. Type 2 transformation zone shows minor (Grade 1) abnormal finding. Thin, flat AW lesion with irregular geographic border is seen at 11 O' clock position, inside the TZ, extending into lower endocervical canal, upper limit of which can be seen.

Q.2. What else would you like to do at this time?
Ans.: Biopsy from 11 O' clock with endocervical sampling in view of HSIL cytology.

Q.3. Biopsy was reported as koilocytosis with CIN 1 and endocervical sampling was negative. What would be further line of management?

Ans: In view of discordance between cytology and histopathology reports, Pap smear would be repeated. If repeat Pap smear also shows HSIL only, it would need immediate treatment by excisional method.

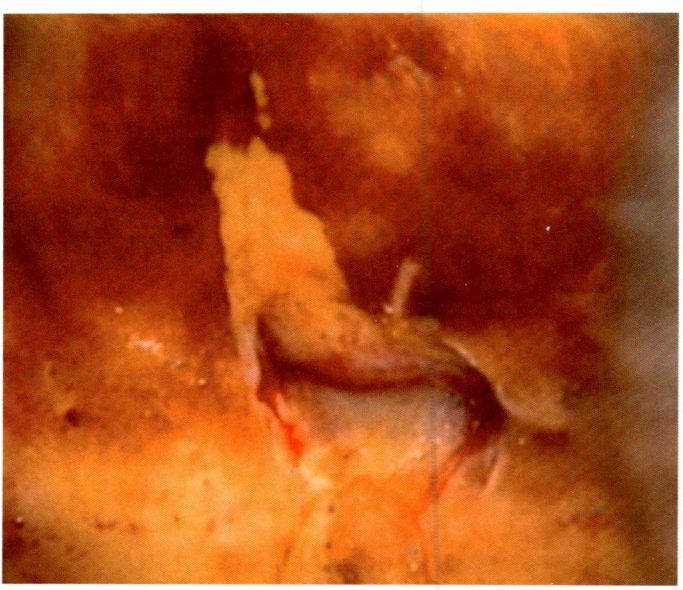

After Lugol's iodine application

Comment

Because of high specificity of Pap smear, persistent HSIL on Pap smear with discordant findings on colposcopy calls for diagnostic excision. However, if CIN 1 preceded by HSIL has satisfactory colposcopy and negative endocervical sampling, she could be just kept under observation with 6 monthly follow-up by both colposcopy and cytology. After one year follow-up, women with 2 consecutive negative reports of cytology as well as colposcopy can return to routine screening program.

CASE 4

A 35-year-old, P0L0, presented with intermenstrual bleeding P/V for 1 year, referred for colposcopy with cytology report of HSIL.

Q.1. Colposcopy pictures are shown. Describe the colposcopic findings.

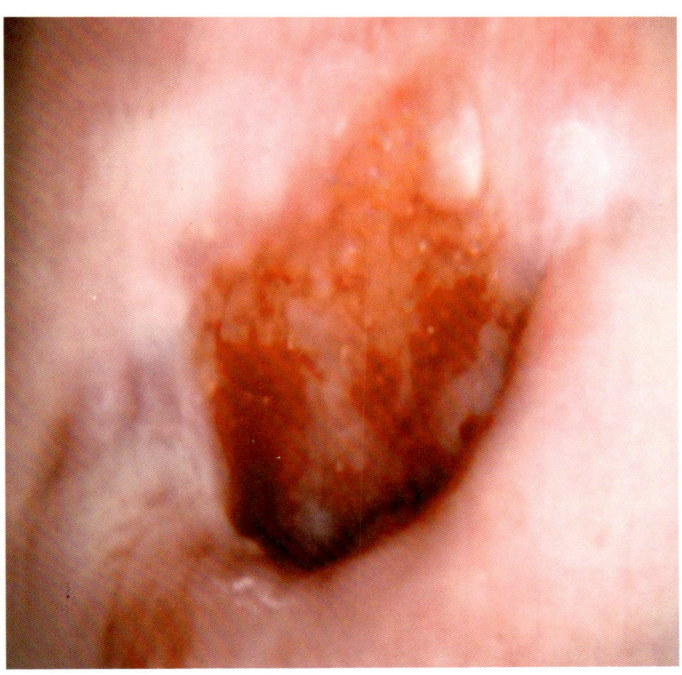

After saline application

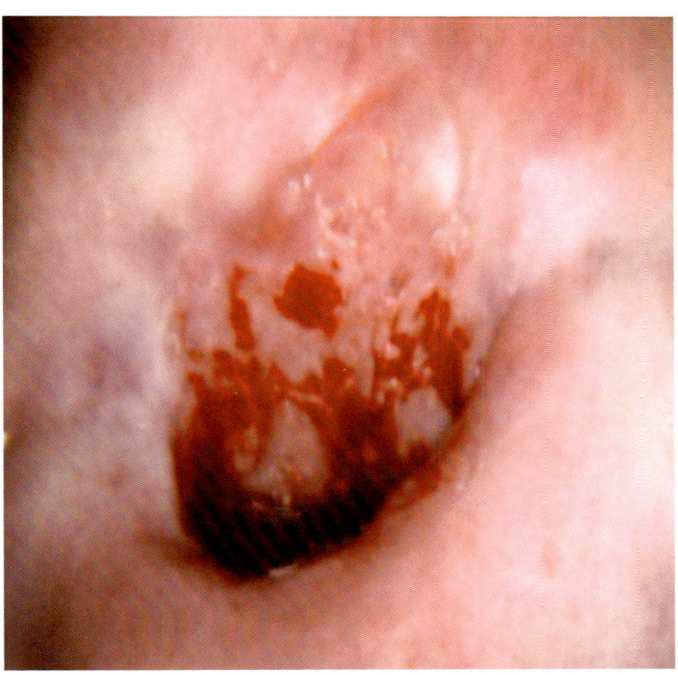

After acetic acid application

Ans.: Colposcopy is adequate, SCJ not visible.

Type 3 TZ shows major (grade 3) abnormal findings, with raised AW lesion and friable vessels on the anterior lip between 9 and 3 O' clock, reaching inside the endocervix. Upper limit is not visible.

Few coarse punctations are seen. No atypical vessels are seen.

Q.2. Biopsy was reported as microinvasion up to a depth of 1 mm only. What should be the plan of management?

Ans.: Cold knife excision (type 3) should be done to rule out invasion.

Q.3. Excision specimen did not show any other focus of microinvasion or invasion, and no lymph vascular space invasion, margins as well as endocervical curettings were negative. What would be the further advice?

Ans.: No further treatment is required. Patient should be closely monitored with cytology, colposcopy and endocervical curettage.

Comment

In a nulliparous patient, conization is sufficient treatment for cancer cervix stage 1A1 (invasion < 3 mm) provided accurate evaluation of conization specimen has been done as per prescribed norms (12 sections in stepwise fashion).

With no LVSI, negative endocervical curettings and sufficient, negative clear margin, patient can be left for close follow-up, since incidence of lymph node involvement without LVSI is extremely low in this stage (only 0.8%). It requires close and prolong monitoring, every 3 monthly for 2 years and then 6 monthly for 3 years.

CASE 5

A 35-year-old, P5L3, presenting with history of postcoital bleeding and cryocautery 1 year back was referred for colposcopy with a cytology report of HSIL.

Q.1. Describe the colposcopy findings?

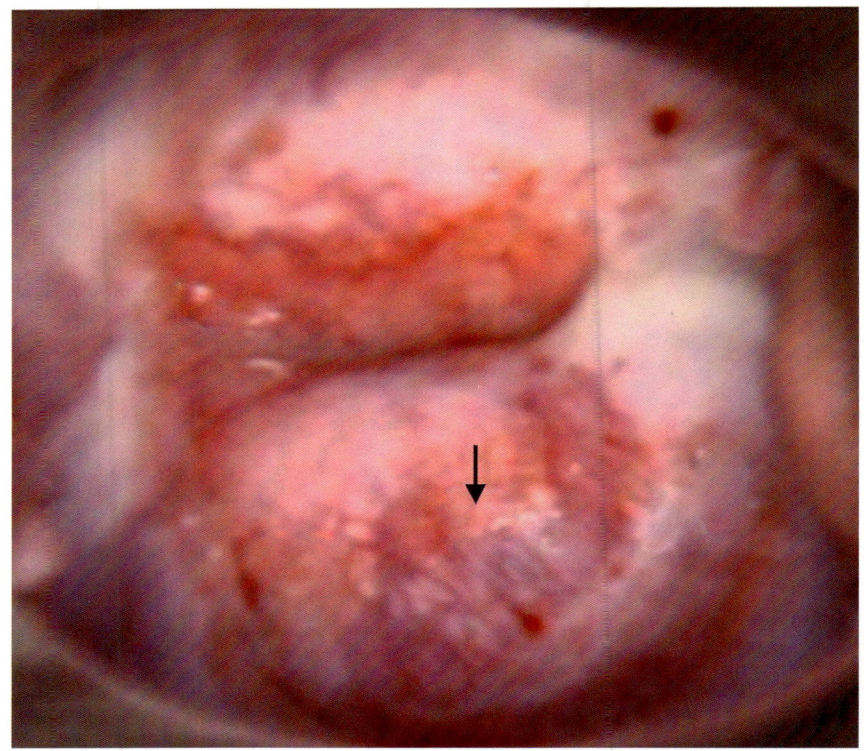

After saline application

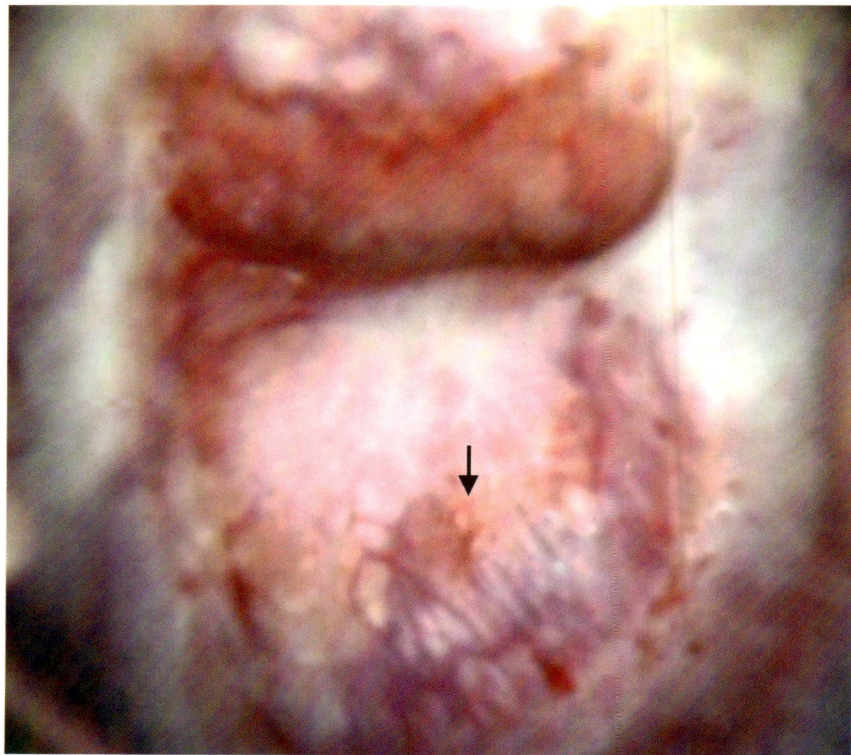

Under green filter

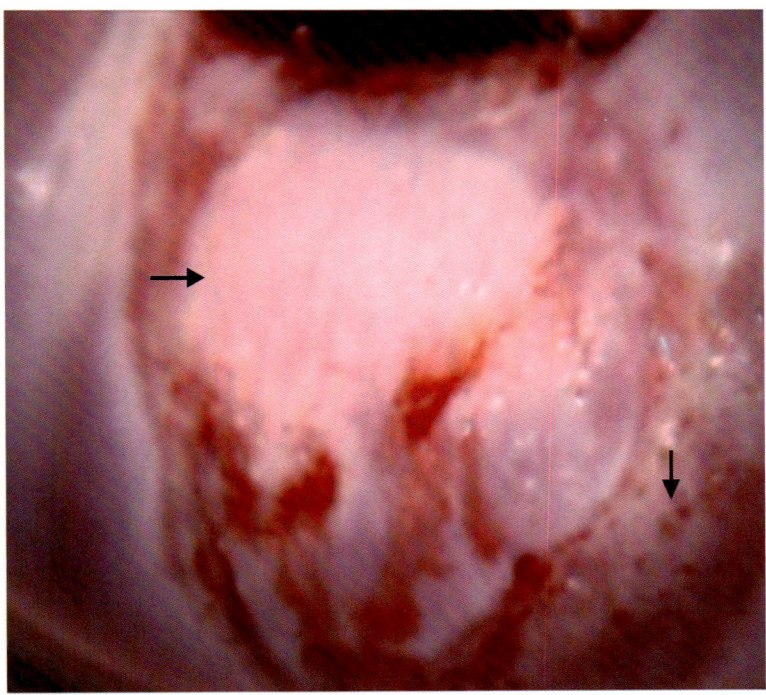

After acetic acid application

Ans: Colposcopy is adequate with partially visible SCJ. Type 2 transformation zone shows major (grade 2) abnormal finding. Dense, AW lesion with raised suface, sharp border along with inner border sign, coarse mosaic in the center and coarse punctations between 4 to 7 O'clock is seen on posterior lip, inside the TZ, extending into lower endocervical canal, upper limit of which can be seen. No atypical vessels are seen.

Q.2. Biopsy taken from posterior lip at 6 O' clock was reported as CIN 3. What would be the plan of management?

Ans.: Excision of TZ (type 2) and ECC to assess extent of the lesion and rule out invasion.

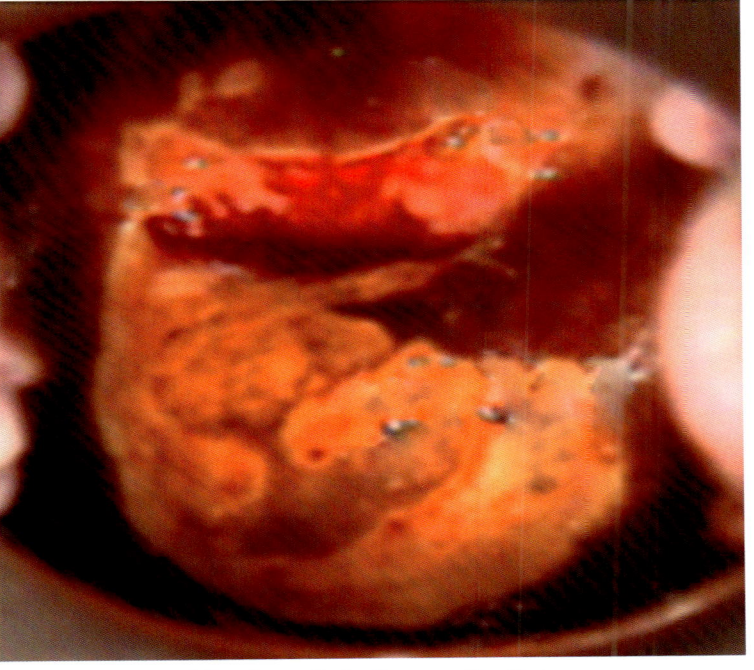

After Lugol's iodine application

Comment

A large high grade lesion would need immediate treatment with excisional method. If there is no invasion in the excised specimen, patient can be kept under follow-up with repeat cytology and endocervical sampling at 6 months after treatment. If CIN 2/3 is detected at the margins of excisional cone or in the endocervical sample obtained immediately after the procedure and repeat cytology/ endocervical sampling at 4–6 months reveals the same, then repeat excision or hysterectomy should be recommended.

CASE 6

A 35-year-old, P0A2, presented with excessive vaginal discharge. Wet smear showed pus cells +++, negative for TV and Candida. Vaginal culture is sterile. Pap smear showed severe inflammation.

Q.1. What would be plan of management?

Ans.: She should be treated with a course of doxy-cycline for 14 days. Repeat cytology would be taken after 6 weeks.

Q.2. Pap smear was reported as moderate inflammation. Colposcopy was performed. Describe the colposcopy findings.

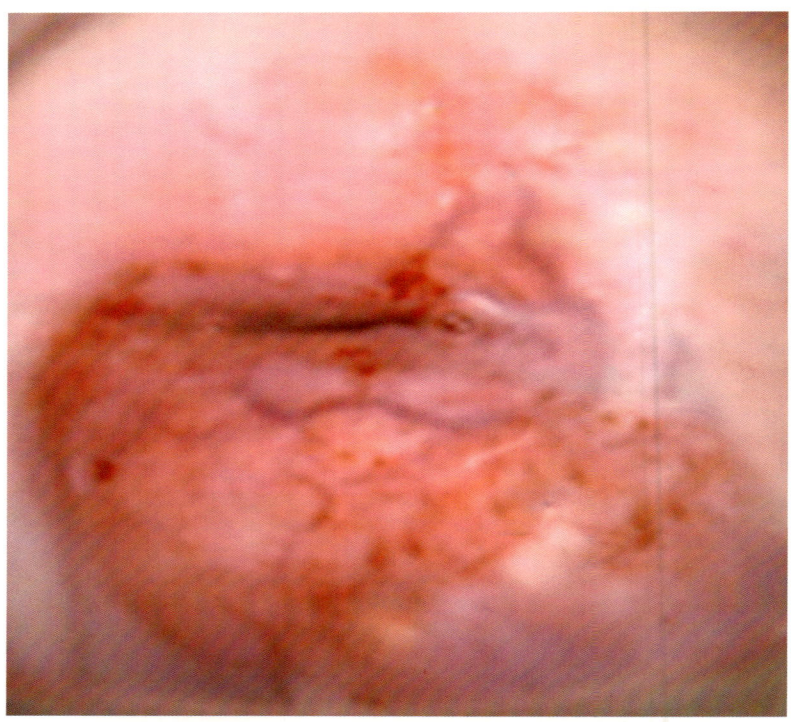

After saline application

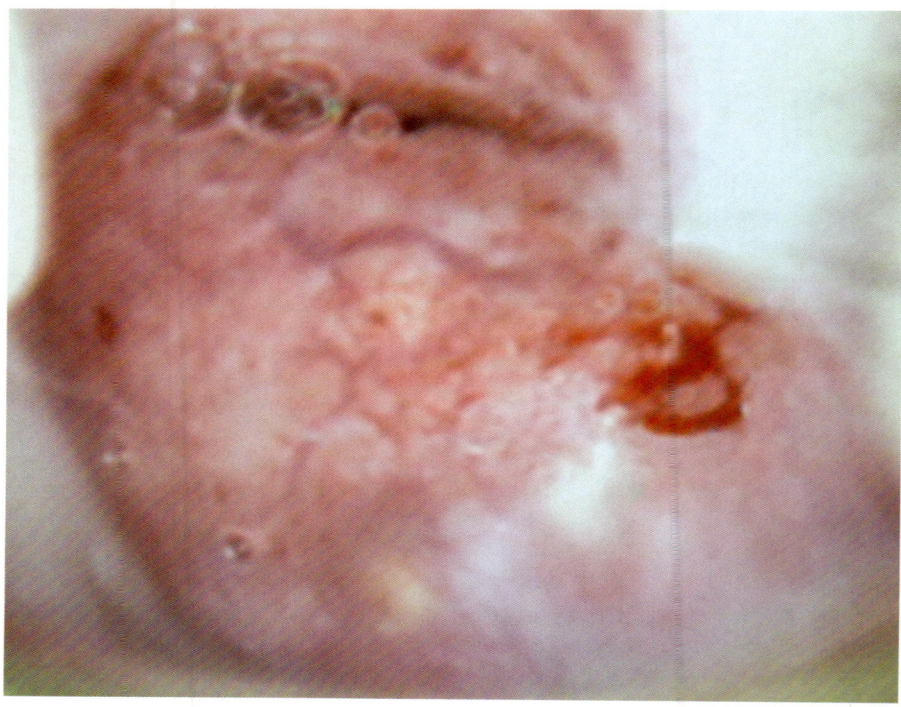

Under green filter

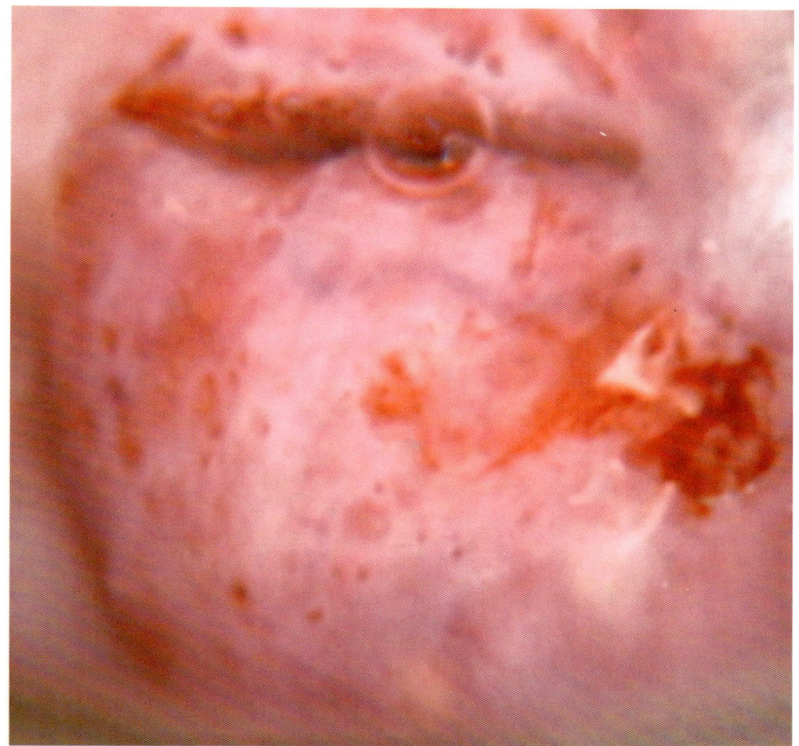

After acetic acid application

Ans.: Colposcopy adequate, SCJ completely visible. TZ type 1. Generalized aceto-whitening of TZ mainly over posterior lip. Vascularity increased but no abnormal vessels are seen. Iodine uptake is patchy. Findings are suggestive of inflammation.

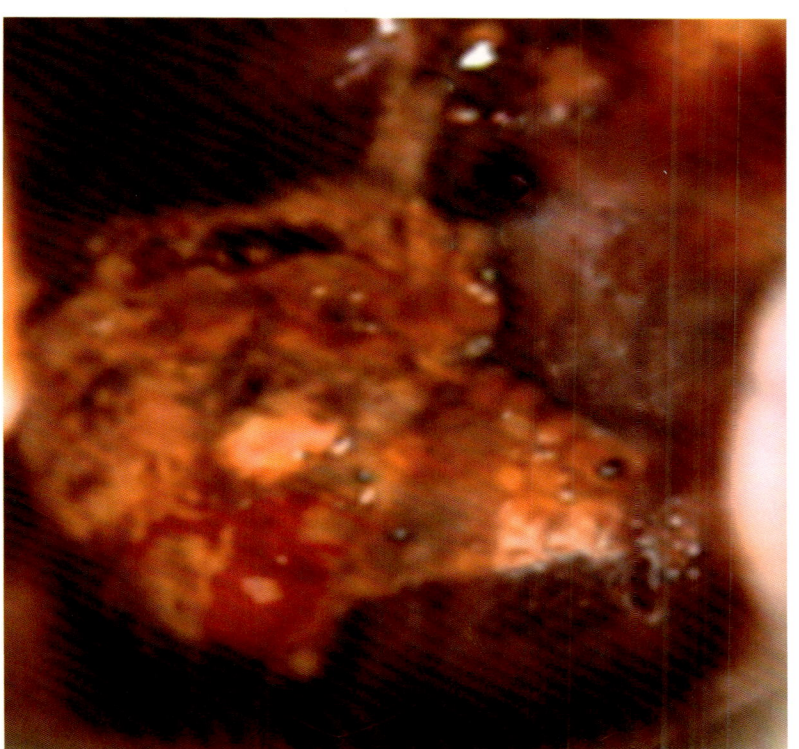

After Lugol's iodine application

Comment

Inflammation increases the false negative rate of cytology. Therefore, in case of persistent inflammatory smear despite antibiotic treatment, colposcopy must be done especially in woman at high-risk for cancer cervix.

CASE 7

A 32-year-old, P3L3, with an ASC–US report on routine screening underwent colposcopy.

Q.1. Describe the colposcopy findings?

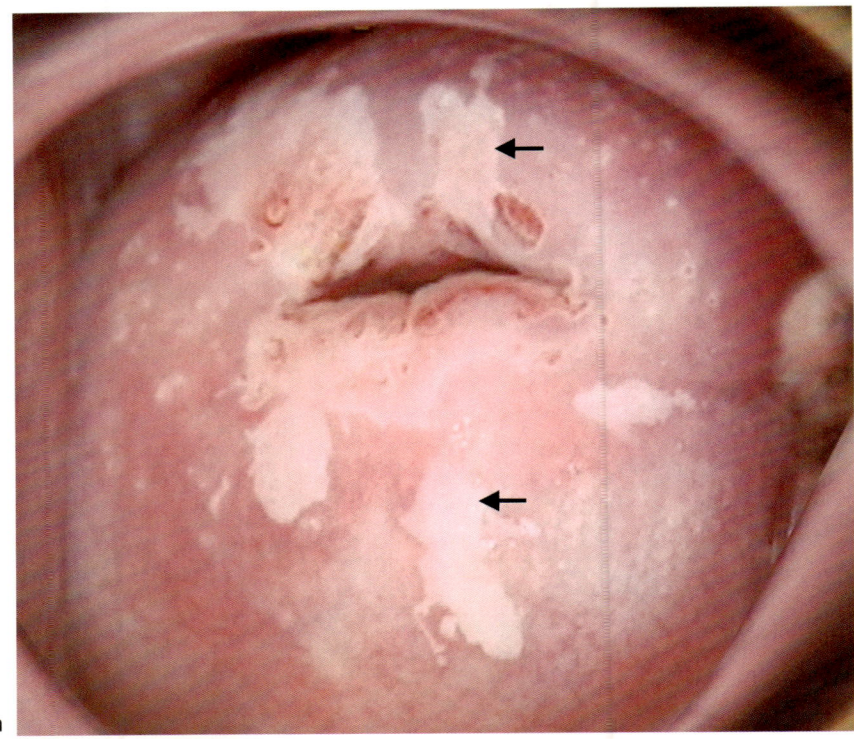

Cervix after acetic acid application

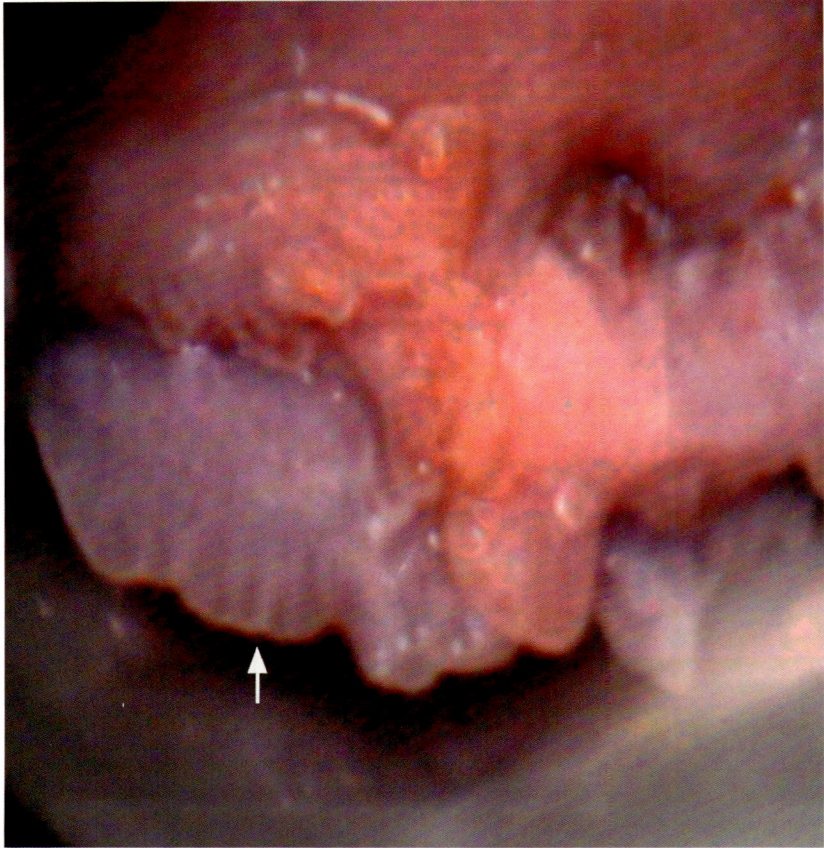

Anterior wall of vagina

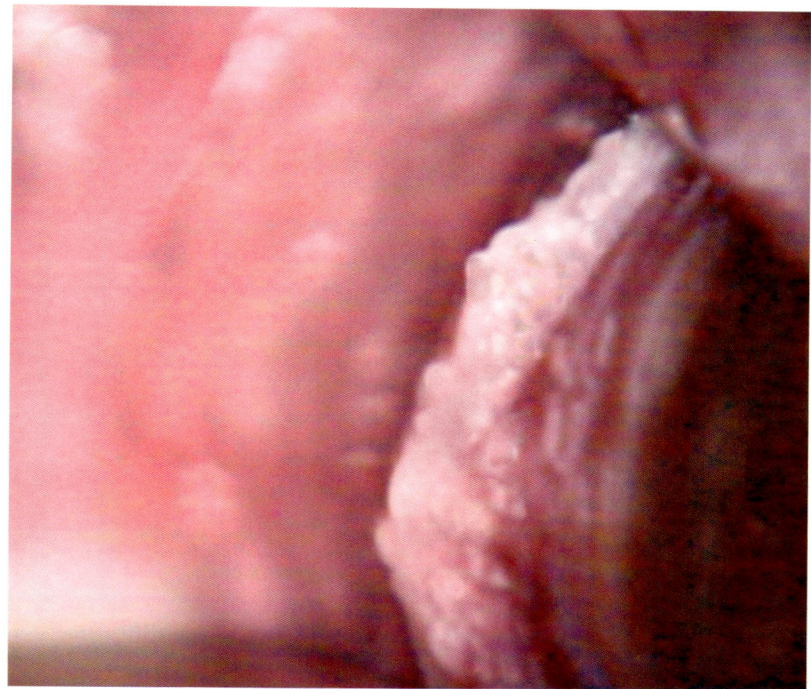

Vulva—introitus

Ans.: Colposcopy is adequate. SCJ is completely visible. TZ is type 1 showing minor abnormal findings. Many tongues of AW epithelium with ill-defined margins and flat surface are seen extending beyond TZ. No vascular abnormalities are seen. Anterior vaginal wall reveals warty lesion, asperities are seen at introitus and small warts are seen in the paraclitoral area.

Q.2. What should be the further plan of management?

Ans.: Since HPV-related changes are seen involving vulva, vagina and also cervix. HPV DNA testing for high-risk types should be done. If positive, cervical biopsy would be done to rule out co-existing CIN.

Q.3. Biopsy shows only HPV-related changes. Should any treatment be advised for vulval and vaginal lesions?

Ans.: No treatment is required for vulval and vaginal lesions. However, if the patient is too anxious, vulval warts can be treated with local therapy.

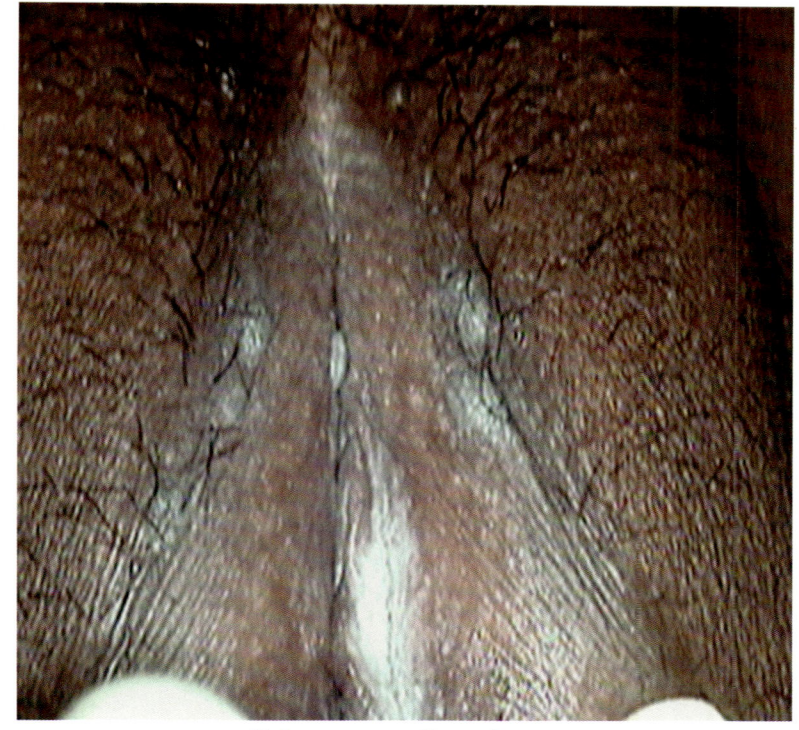

Vulva — paraclitoreal area

Comment

Women with HPV infection need to remain under long-term follow-up and get their partner(s) also examined for HPV infection.

CASE 8

A 32-year-old, G2P1L1, with 12 weeks pregnancy, complained of excessive vaginal discharge. Per speculum examination revealed unhealthy cervix. Pap smear was reported as LSIL. She was referred for colposcopy.

Q.1. Colposcopy picture is shown. Describe the findings.

Ans.: Colposcopy adequate, SCJ not visible. TZ is type 2 showing ectopy with hypertropic polypoidal epithelium and grade 1 acetowhitening probably due to deciduosis of pregnancy. Within this TZ, there is another small denser AW lesion with ill-defined margins at 11–12 O' clock near the SCJ. No abnormal vessels are seen.

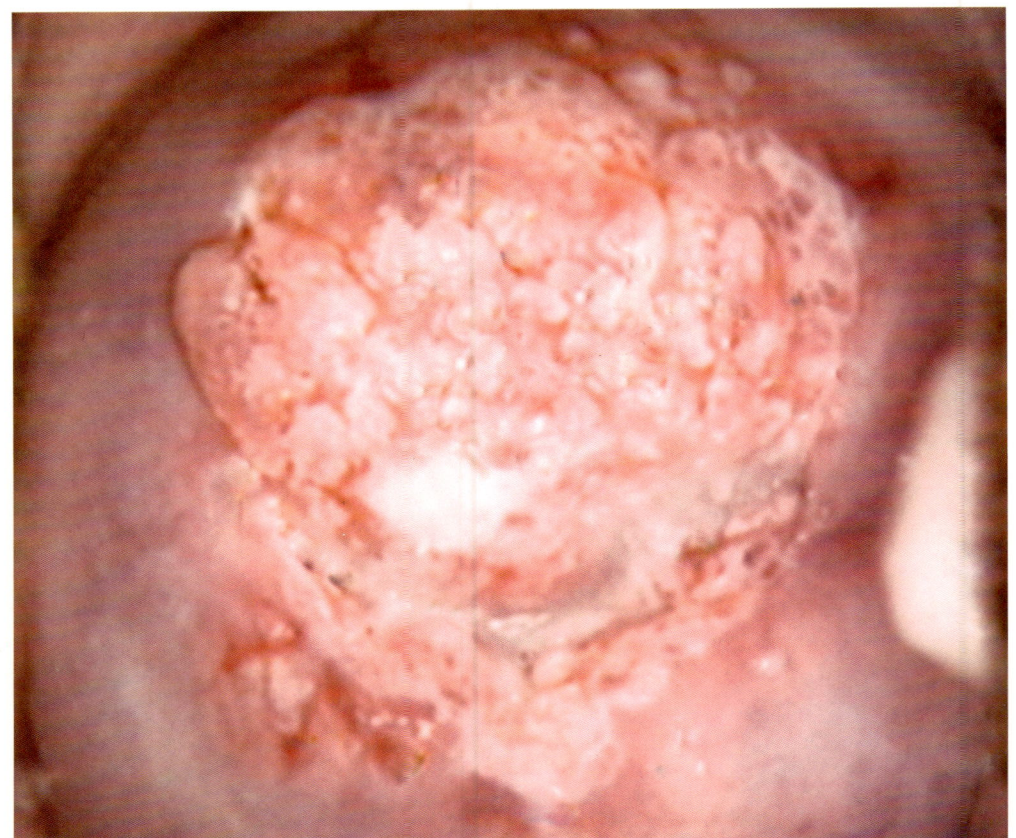

After acetic acid application

Q.2. What is your plan of management?

Ans.: Colposcopy and cytology would be repeated after three months. If higher grade is reported, then biopsy would be done. If grade remains the same, then patient would be just followed up till 6 weeks after postpartum.

Comment

Due to hormonal changes in pregnancy, colposcopic findings are one grade higher than the non-pregnant cervix for a given pathology. Therefore, caution should be observed in interpretation.

CASE 9

A 53 years asymptomatic postmenopausal woman is referred with Pap smear report of LSIL. On per speculum examination, cervix and vagina are normal in appearance. Colposcopy showed menopausal cervix, and the squamo-columnar junction could not be visualized.

Q.1. How will you manage?

Ans.: First of all Pap smear should either be reviewed, or repeated after a short course of estrogen either oral for one week or vaginal application for 2–3 weeks. Estrogen helps in converting unsatisfactory colposcopy into satisfactory one in 30% of cases.

Q.2. Review smear is LSIL, colposcopy was repeated. Describe the findings.

Ans.: Colposcopy is adequate, thin, flat, AW epithelium present over anterior lip, reaching inside endocervix. Upper limit of the lesion is not visible.

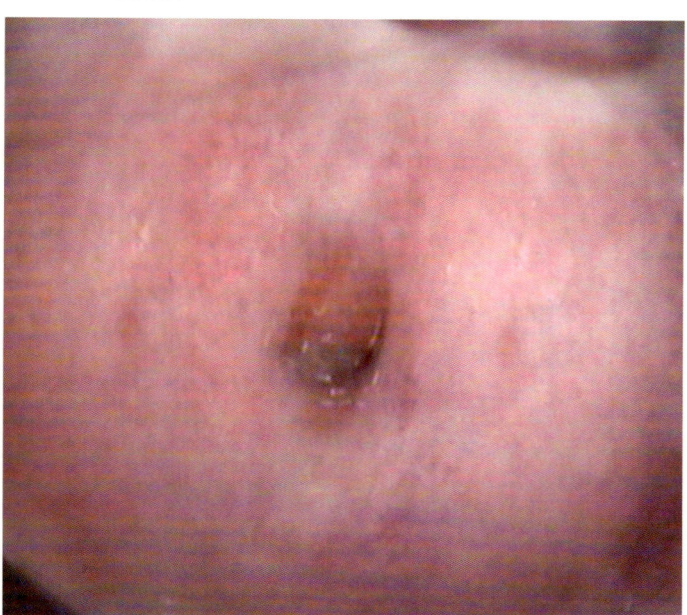

After saline application

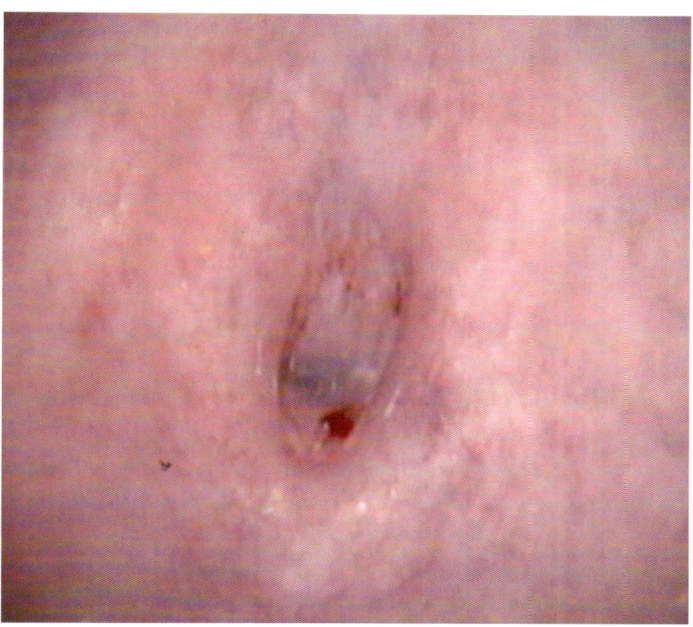

After acetic acid application

Q.3. In case of transformation zone is abnormal with unsatisfactory colposcopy, will you wait for 2–3 weeks for the estrogen effect?

Ans.: Intravaginal misoprost 400 mcg can be given 4–6 hours prior to the colposcopy. This might open the os and convert unsatisfactory colposcopy into satisfactory. If colposcopy remains unsatisfactory despite everything, biopsy can be taken from the abnormal area along with ECC. Alternatively even diagnostic conization can be considered.

Comment

In postmenopausal women, cytology and colposcopy both can be very tricky. Because of atrophic changes, cytology may be reported as abnormal, SCJ recedes inside endocervix and acetowhite change may not be evident on colposcopy because of decreased thickness of the epithelium. In this age group, cytology as well as colposcopy should always be performed after estrogen supplementation. A short course of estrogen is innocuous and produces no harm.

CASE 10

A 33-year-old, P0L0, with history of postcoital bleeding was referred for colposcopy with cytology report of atypical glandular cells

Q.1. Describe the colposcopic findings.

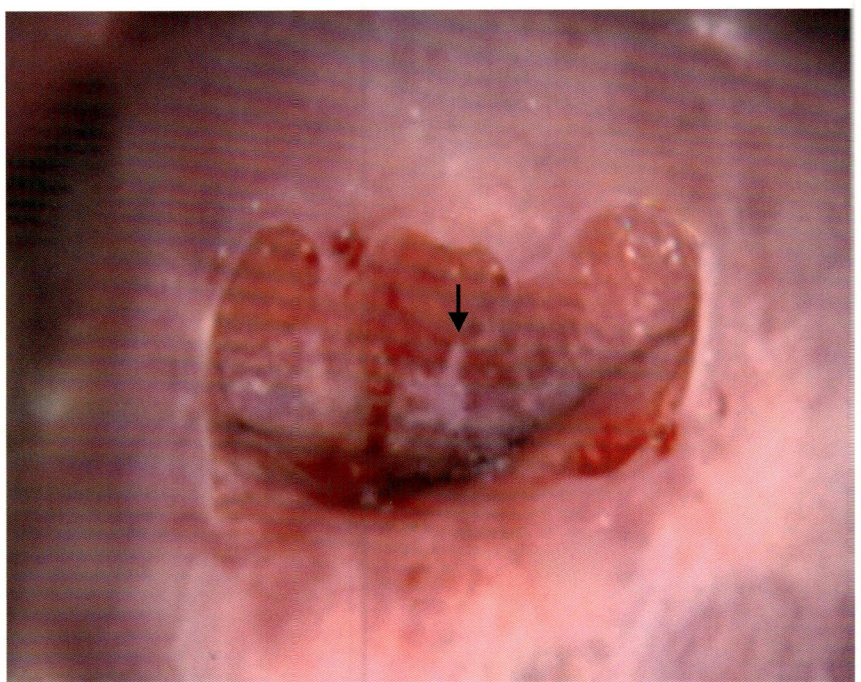

After acetic acid application

Ans.: Colposcopy is adequate, SCJ partially visible. TZ type 2 with an isolated small elevated acetowhite lesion over columnar epithelium not contiguous with SCJ.

Q.2. What would be the further plan of management?

Ans.: In view of the above colposcopic findings and atypical glandular cells on cytology, type 3 excision of TZ would be done with endocervical curettage after excision.

Q.3. Excision specimen showed AIS on histopathology with clear margins and negative ECC. What is your advice?

Ans.: Close follow-up every 6 months using combination of cytology, HPV DNA testing, colposcopy and endocervical sampling till she completes her family when hysterectomy should be undertaken. However, if margins/endocervical sampling were positive, repeat excision could have been tried to ensure completeness of excision.

Q.4. Would you do endometrial biopsy in this case?

Ans.: Endometrial sampling is generally not required in women with atypical glandular cells who are < 35 years of age. However, if endometrial cells are present in the smear or the woman is at high risk for endometrial malignancy, then endometrial sampling is required.

Comment

Management of women with AIS is quite challenging due to its multifocal nature, skip lesions, difficulty in determining the extent of disease and inability to ensure the completeness of excision by conservative methods. Hysterectomy is recommended, if patient has completed her family because of high failure rate of excision.

Cytology for the Gynecologists

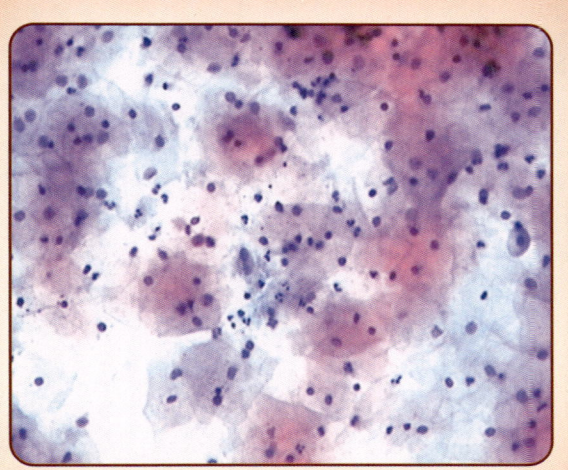

Chapter Outline

Cervical cytology is the standard screening test for cervical cancer and premalignant cervical lesions. The present chapter highlights the practical points for the gynecologists who are the ones mainly responsible for cervical cancer screening in our country where there is no well-organized national cervical cancer screening program. It emphasizes the practical aspects of specimen procurement and fixation, the reporting formats, along with interpretation of cytology findings in cervical preneoplasitc and neoplastic lesions, vaginal lesions and cervicovaginal infections.

An understanding of basic cytology and histology of cervix is essential for the gynecologist to have a close co-ordination with the cytopathologists, to ensure delivery of quality health care. Cervical cancer screening strategies and techniques, as well as the follow-up of abnormal cytology results are discussed separately.

SAMPLE COLLECTION

It is essential to obtain a quality sample to ensure test reliability and minimize false negative rates. Most pre-malignant and malignant lesions of the cervix arise at the squamocolumnar junction/in the transformation zone (TZ). Thus one must take care that the whole circumference of the transformation zone has been sampled and sufficient well-preserved cells are collected.

Time of Sample Collection

Ideal time for taking Pap smear is around mid-cycle, although in case of opportunistic screening, it can be taken at any point in the cycle as the woman may never come back again. One should avoid taking a smear during menstruation as the presence of blood will obscure the findings. Sample taken during late secretory phase may be unsatisfactory because of marked cytolysis due to large numbers of Doderlein bacilli, which are the normal vaginal flora at this time of the cycle. Patient should not use vaginal douche, pessary or any type of lubricant 24 hours before smear is taken.

Exposing the Cervix

With the woman in lithotomy position, a bivalve retaining speculum of the appropriate size is inserted in vagina. The cervix is visualized under adequate directed light with the speculum in situ. A lubricant should not be used for insertion of the speculum as it may result in unsatisfactory smear due to contamination with the lubricant jelly. Bimanual examination should not be carried before sampling to prevent lubricant contamination, trauma or dislodgement of diagnostic cells.

Collection Device

The collection device is important for ensuring sample adequacy. A variety of devices are available for obtaining conventional cervical samples such as wooden/plastic spatula, "broom-type" samplers and endocervical brushes that may be used depending upon the clinical situation. The use of cotton-tipped swab is not recommended.

A single sample obtained with either a spatula or "broom-type" brush should be adequate if the transformation zone is visible. However, if the TZ is not visualized as in postmenopausal woman or following previous cervical treatment, endocervical brush should be used to obtain endocervical sample in addition to the ectocervical. In pregnant woman, an endocervical brush should be avoided.

Collection Technique (for Conventional Pap Smear)
Obtaining Cellular Sample

When using a spatula/Combi brush to collect sample, the long thin end is inserted in the endocervical canal and the broad arm of spatula is rotated 360° over ectocervix in clockwise or anticlockwise direction 4–5 times (Fig. 16.1). It should be applied with some degree

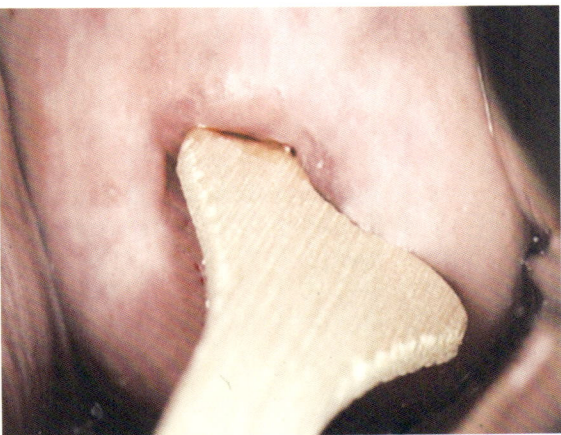
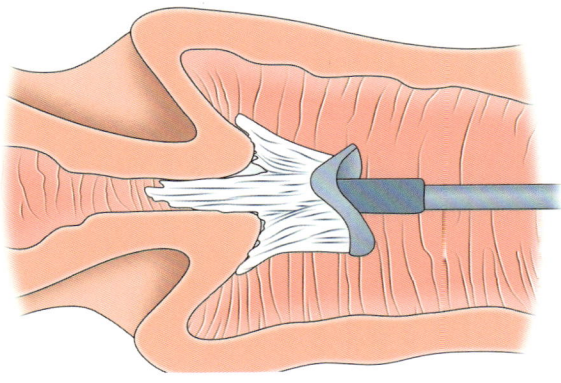

Fig. 16.1: Long arm of Ayre's spatula or Combi brush is inserted and rotated gently in clockwise direction

of firmness and rotated around the full circumference of the cervix. For "broom-type" sampler, it should be rotated 5 times in a clockwise direction with the central longer bristles in the canal. Slight bleeding is to be expected and will not interfere with interpretation. However, forceful scraping may lead to trauma and excessive bleeding and blood will interfere with interpretation. Particular care should be taken in young women with cervical erosion as they tend to bleed easily. Similarly, a small amount of mucus does not affect interpretation. However, if a large plug of mucus obscures the external os, it can be removed gently with a swab prior to sample collection.

If spatula alone is used for endocervix and an endocervical brush sample is taken separately, this should follow the spatula sample as it may cause slight bleeding. The brush is gently inserted into the endocervix and rotated gently one-half to one full turn.

Smear Preparation

The spatula with the sample should be rapidly but lightly stroked, evenly across the surface of the precleaned prelabeled glass slide without any delay, so that all the material obtained is transferred forming a thin and uniform smear (Fig. 16.2). If material is more, spread on multiple slides. Cells obtained with the endocervical brush are placed on the glass slide by a rolling action and with the "broom-type" sampler a firm paint stroke motion is used across the slide. The broom is then turned over and the paint stroke motion is repeated over the same area. In case where two applicators have been used, both the spatula/"broom-type" and endocervical brush samples may be placed on one slide. Slides that have been stored for long period should not be used as there may be fungal overgrowth that can result in interpretation errors.

Smear Fixation

Utmost care should be taken to immediately fix the wet slides by immersion in 95% alcohol or spraying with fixative to prevent air-drying artifact which can occur within seconds, particularly the smears from post-menopausal patients and blood-stained smears dry very rapidly. Prefixation air-drying can result in interpretation errors due to degenerative changes with loss of cellular features.

For wet fixation with alcohol, the volume of the alcohol must be sufficient to cover the slide and alcohol should be changed regularly to maintain the efficacy of fixation. The smears are immersed immediately in prelabeled coplin jars or wide mouth bottles filled with 95% ethanol. Ideally separate containers of fixatives should be used for each patient but in practice a wide mouth bottle or coplin jar is used for 8–10 smears. Proper labeling of slides is imperative. Care must be taken to note down the ID no. of the patient on the slide to prevent mixing of cases. The smears should be taken out from the container and kept in slide mailer plastic boxes or wrapped in soft tissue paper for transportation to the laboratory along with properly filled requisition form.

Spray fixation with an aerosol fixative is a good alternative, protects the smears from drying and is generally considered more convenient. Spray fixatives are made of water-soluble polymers and various fixatives are available commercially. When applying spray fixative, one should follow the manufacturer's instructions and take due precautions to prevent cell loss and to ensure proper fixation. Spray should be applied immediately on wet smear in smooth and steady manner. Distance between nozzle of spray can and smear should ideally be 10–12 inches (25–30 cm). If nozzle is too near to the smear, there can be dislodgement of cells; cell may freeze and get damaged causing distortion artifacts like perinuclear halo. If too far, sufficient fixation may not take place. Following fixation, the smear should be left on a level surface (not at an angle) and allowed to dry. The fixative beyond expiry date should not be used. Good brand of hair sprays can also be used in case of non-availability of cytosprays, but are better avoided.

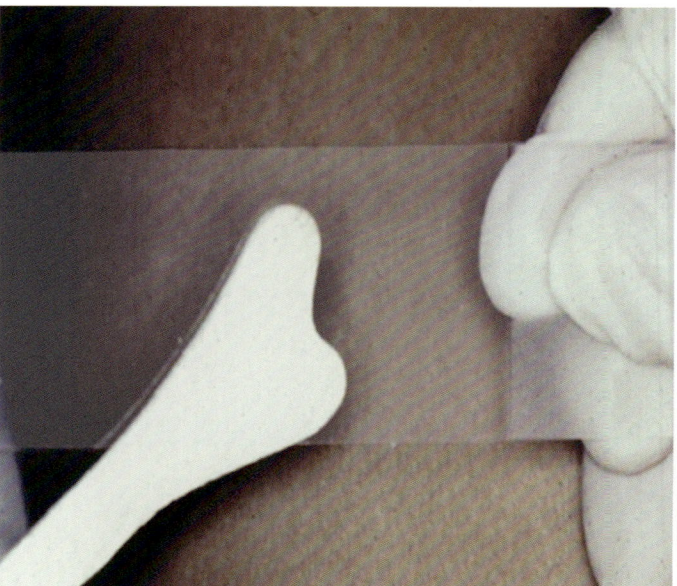

Fig. 16.2: Material from spatula is transferred to the smear to prepare thin evenly spread smear

Collection Technique (for Liquid-Based Preparation)

Under this concept, a broom-type sampler is used to sample the transformation zone of the cervix following the manufacturer's instructions. The broom is pushed gently into the endocervical canal until it reaches deep enough for the shorter bristles to contact the ectocervix. It is then rotated in a clockwise direction 5 times to obtain the sample. Back and forth rotation is avoided. After removing from the cervix, the sampling device with the collected cells is immersed in the liquid in the sample vial and is rinsed well to ensure transfer of 100% cells homogneously into preservative fluid which has mucolytic agents and chemicals to lyse red cells (Fig. 16.3). In *thin prep*, the sampler is pushed into the bottom of the vial forcing the bristles to spread apart for about 10 times, is swirled vigorously to further release material into the preservative solution, the broom is discarded and the vial capped. In *autocyte prep*, the entire detachable head of the broom is removed from the handle of the sampler and placed into the appropriate vial which is then capped, labeled and sent to the laboratory for processing.

Fluid is processed either through automated machines or manually to prepare thin small monolayer smears. Smears are free of mucus, red cells and other contaminating particles and have reduced number of neutrophils. Only part of fluid with homogeneous cell suspension is used to prepare smears for examination. Remainder of the cellular material is used for ancillary

studies like immunocytochemistry, HPV detection and molecular genetics. The preservative fluid is ethanol/methanol based and has shelf-life of sample cells for four weeks at room temperature and 6 months under refrigeration. Shelf-life of the fluid is 36 months from the date of manufacture without cell sample.

Conventional Pap Smear vs. Liquid-Based Cytology

Conventional Pap smear has a relatively low sensitivity (about 60%) due to potential errors during sampling or interpretation. Sampling errors may be caused by loss of cells during transfer from the sampling device on to the slide (Fig. 16.4). There may be interpretation errors where in the abnormal cells on the slides are not identified. Reasons could be unequal distribution of cells on the slide, thick and thin areas and variable cell fixation, difficulty in recognizing abnormal cells in thick areas and cells enmeshed in mucus, red blood cells and heavy neutrophilic exudates (Fig. 16.5). Moreover, large

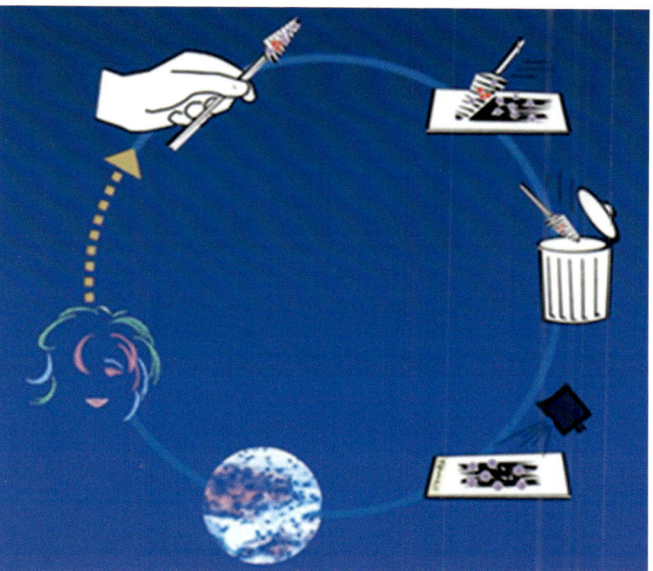

Fig. 16.4: Atypical cells represented by red dot on the sampling device sometimes gets discarded in the dustbin while taking conventional Pap smear

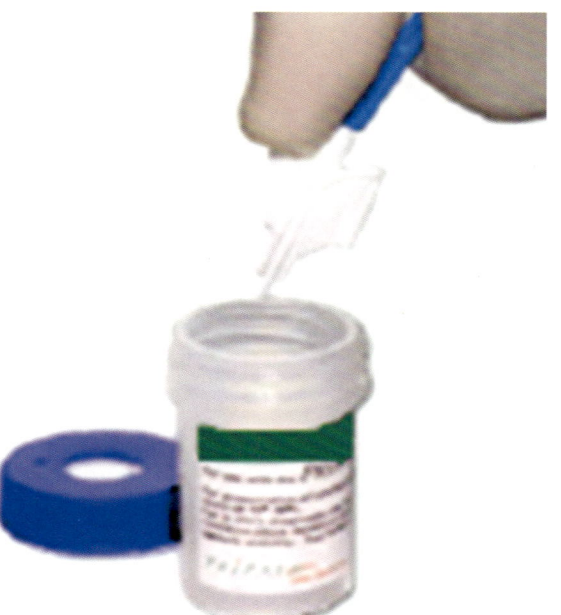

Fig. 16.3: In liquid-based cytology, material collected on the sampling device is immersed into the preservative solution and rinsed well to obtain a homogeneous suspension of cells

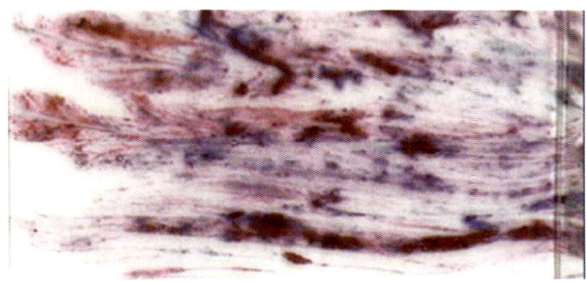

Fig. 16.5: Conventional Pap smear is spread over large area of the slide and may have uneven thickness

areas of smear are to be examined and sometimes multiple smears are prepared. Examination is time consuming and tiring which may lead to missing of abnormal cells due to fatigue.

Liquid-based cytology has the advantages of reduction in the smear screening time, uniform spread of cells (Fig. 16.6), with reported increase in detection of HSIL in LBC smears as compared to conventional Pap smears, and the facility of conducting ancillary studies on the same sample. However, some pathologists feel there may be interpretation errors due to alteration in cellular cytology caused by suspension of cells in the liquid medium; absence of intercellular relationship and absence of mucus deprives the screener with vital clues for interpretation. Moreover, it is expensive as compared to conventional Pap smear and preparation of smears is more time consuming.

SAMPLE SUBMISSION

The glass slide/specimen vial must be labeled with patient's name and identification no. and packaged carefully to prevent breakage or leakage and transported to the laboratory for processing. All specimens should be submitted to the laboratory accompanied with completed laboratory requisition forms. Laboratory requisition form should include the following clinical details written clearly or typed

- Patient's Name, Age, Address, Identification No., Telephone No.

- Date of procedure, referring Doctor with contact details
- Source and site of origin of specimen with identifying symbols
- Method of collection
- Clinical symptoms and signs
- Date of Last Menstrual Period
- Special situations-pregnancy, postmenopausal, oral contraceptive/other hormonal use
- Provisional clinical diagnosis
- Prior abnormal cytology/histology report
- Prior treatment if any.

Causes for rejection of specimen or limited reports:
- Incomplete and/or improper labeling
- Insufficient pertinent clinical history
- Specimen not fixed on slide immediately
- Obscuring inflammation, debris, or excessive air drying
- A broken slide will be rejected and discarded as a biohazard.

Schedule for repeat smears

In general, all repeats should not be performed within 6–8 weeks. It is because the scraped surface may not have re-epithelialized and the chance of a false negative result is increased. If colposcopic investigation is performed within this period upon a report of possible or definite abnormality, a concurrent cytology sample is not recommended.

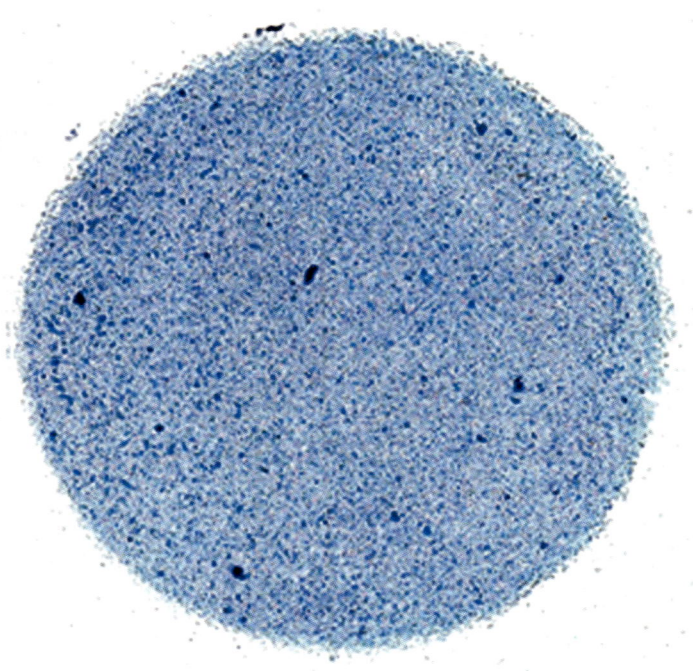

Fig. 16.6: Smear prepared in LBC is a small circle of 1–1.5 cm diameter and cells are spread uniformly

TYPES OF CELLS SEEN ON CERVICAL CYTOLOGY

Normal Findings

Basal Cells

Basal cells are small (10 µ) in size and possess blue cytoplasm. Nuclei are large about 8 µ in size. N:C ratio is high. Basal cells generally do not shed, but may be seen in smears obtained from vigorous endocervical brushing and present as sheets of small endocervical cells with uniform dense nuclei. Basal cell hyperplasia may occur in early metaplasia

Parabasal Cells

Parabasal cells are round cells, 10–15 µ in size and show cyanophilic cytoplasm (Fig. 16.7), with centrally located vesicular nuclei. Cytoplasm is more abundant than basal cells.

Intermediate Cells

Intermediate cells are large (15–40 µ), polyhedral in shape, and possess abundant cytoplasm and central vesicular nuclei. Cytoplasm is amphophilic to light basophilic in color (Fig. 16.8).

Navicular Cells

Navicular cells are a variant of intermediate cells. Cells become oval or boat-shaped and show folding of cytoplasm (Fig. 16.9). Glycogen deposits stain yellow. These are seen is pregnancy and early menopause, however, are not diagnostic of pregnancy. Thus it is importance to mention the age of the woman and clinical history of amenorrhoea, if present.

Superficial Cells

Superficial cells are large (40–60 µ), polyhedral cells with abundant eosinophilic cytoplasm and small dense pyknotic nuclei, with small perinuclear halo in many cells (Fig. 16.10). In abnormal conditions, these cells are keratinized and are seen as anucleate, polygonal, pink, transparent cells.

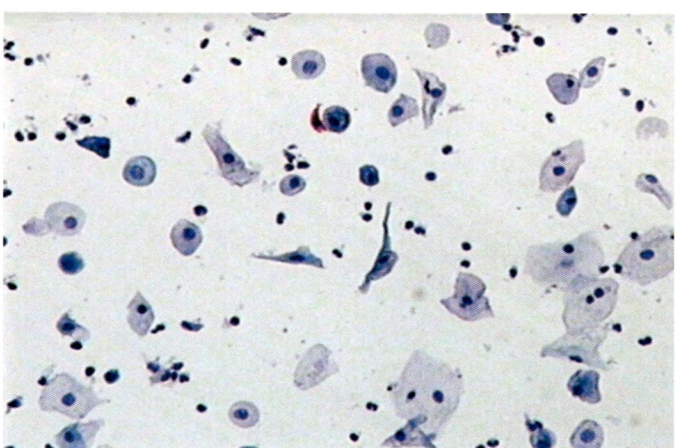

Fig. 16.7: Parabasal cells

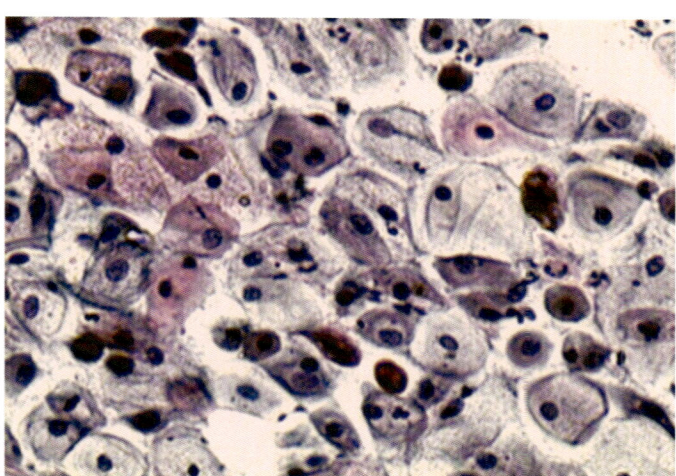

Fig. 16.9: Navicular cells

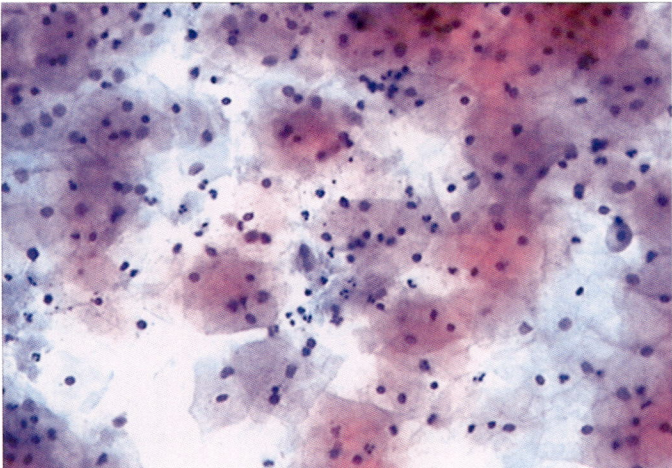

Fig. 16.8: Intermediate cells

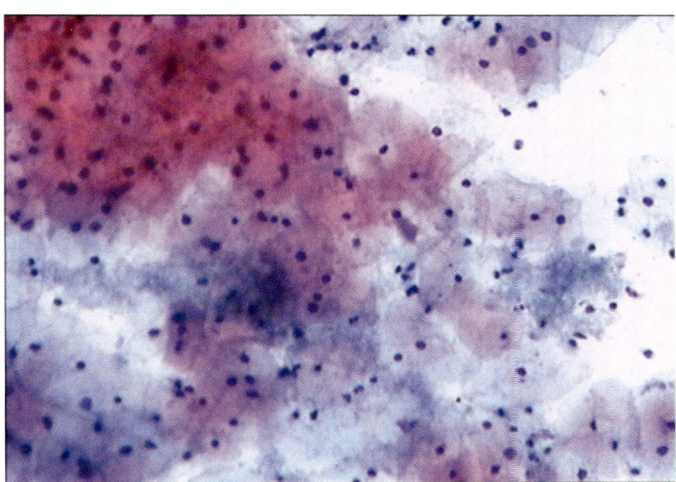

Fig. 16.10: Superficial cells

Endocervical Cells

Endocervical columnar cells measure 20 µ in length and 10 µ in width and possess light blue, opaque or clear cytoplasm. Nuclei are vesicular, 8 mm – 15 µ in size located at the basal side of cell away from lumen giving appearance of "picket cells" in longitudinal view (Fig. 16.11A) and "honeycomb" appearance on end-on view (Figs 16.11B and C).

Squamous Metaplasia

Polygonal parabasal cells and endocervical cells are seen together. Cells of immature metaplasia are identified as parabasal metaplastic cells arranged in sheets and having clearly visible sharp cells borders, angulation, cytoplasmic processes and spikes. Cytoplasm is basophilic or eosinophilic (Fig. 16.12).

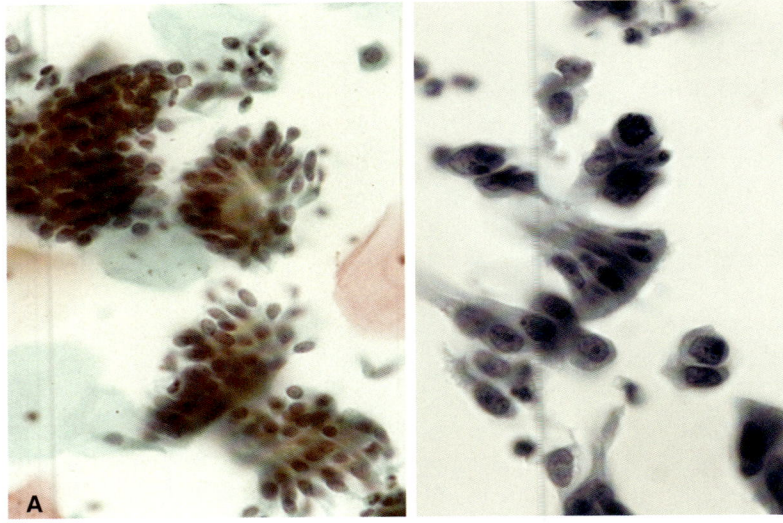

Fig. 16.11A: Clusters of columnar endocervical cells showing "picket fence" arrangement of cells in the right side picture

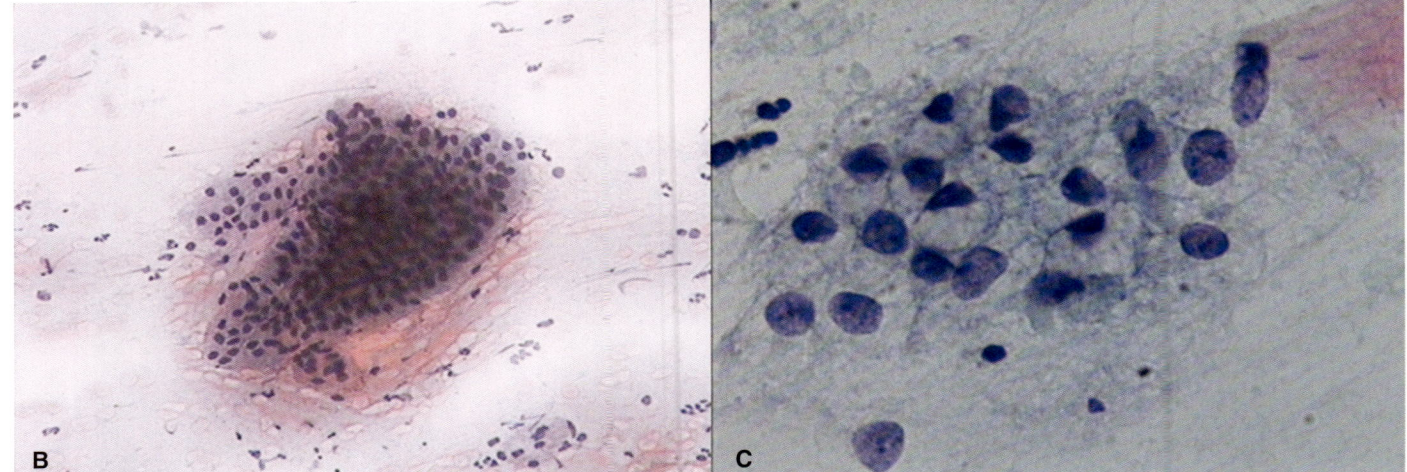

Figs 16.11B and C: Endocervical cells showing honeycomb appearance on end-on view

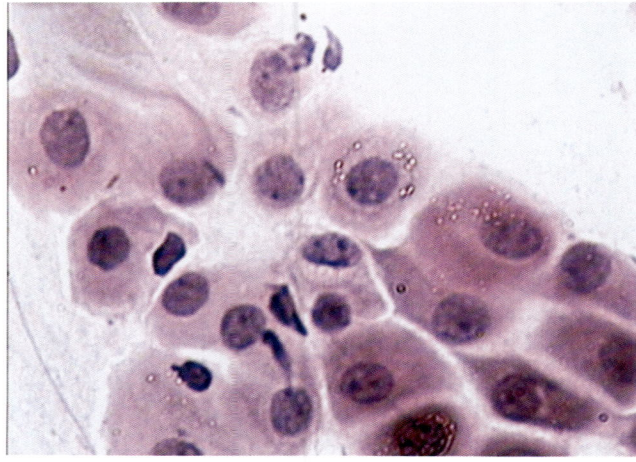

Fig. 16.12: Metaplastic parabasal cells show sharp angulated borders and cytoplasmic spikes

Normal Pap Smear

In child bearing age, predominantly superficial cells and intermediate cells are seen (Fig. 16.13). Parabasal cells are seen only occasionally in normal smears but are seen in certain situations which will be described later. Basal cells are seen rarely. Endocervical cells form an important constituent of the Pap smear. Neutrophils may be present.

In menopausal women, cytology findings are affected by withdrawal of estrogenic activity. In early menopause, estrogen deficiency is mild. There is reduction in the number of superficial and predominance of intermediate cells and some large parabasal cells (Fig. 16.14). As estrogen deficiency increases, thick crowded and large clusters of intermediate large parabasal cells are seen. Some cells may resemble navicular cells. In advanced stage of menopause, estrogen levels are markedly low. Yield of cellular material is poor due to dryness of genital tract. Dominant cell is parabasal type; there is enhanced eosinophilia of the cytoplasm and pyknosis of nuclei, nuclear breakup and marked variation in cell size. Sometimes there is enlargement of nuclei of parabasal cells and such cells may be mistaken for dysplastic cells. Occasionally sheets of spindle cells may be seen which may be mistaken for malignant cells. Endocervical cells are few or absent.

It is now almost established that carcinoma cervix is preceded by cellular abnormality of surface epithelium. Most high grade lesions start de novo though some low grade lesions may develop into cancer. Transformation zone is the site of initiation in most cases.

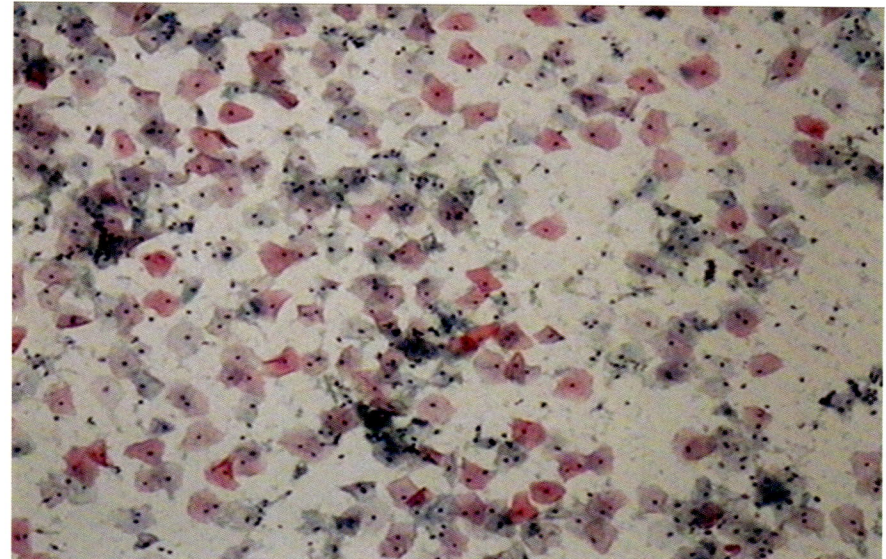

Fig.16.13: Normal Pap smear with mixture of superficial and intermediate cells. Endocervical cells are not seen in this field

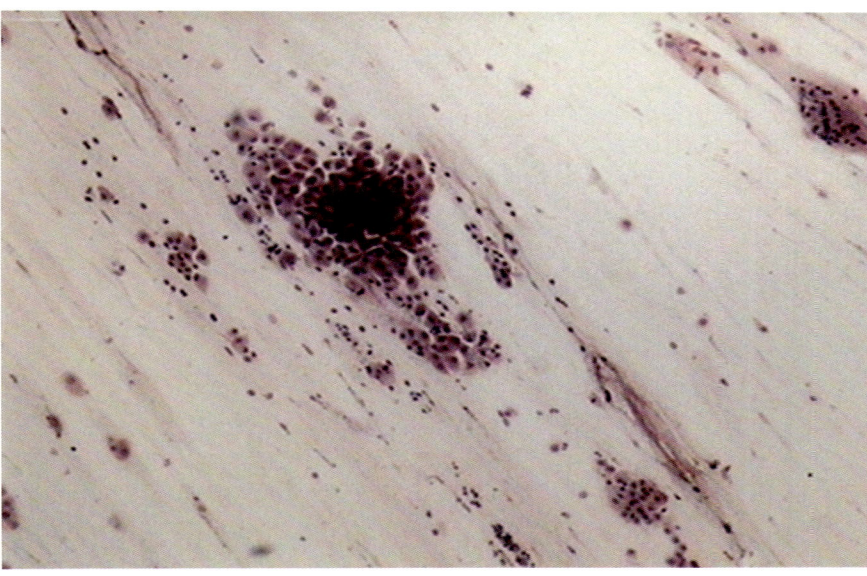

Fig. 16.14: Smear from postmenopausal woman shows crowding of parabasal cells

Abnormal Findings

The term "dyskaryosis" meaning 'abnormal nucleus' is used to describe cells with nuclear abnormalities and maturity of cytoplasm and is still used in UK. The term "dysplasia" is also used to describe the same, mainly in USA. Both these terms can be used interchangeably.

Dysplastic (Dyskaryotic) Cells

Dysplastic (dyskaryotic) cells show slight to moderate nuclear abnormalities (enlargement and hyperchromasia) in well differentiated squamous or glandular lesions. More advanced lesions show nuclear enlargement, hyperchromasia, along with high N:C ratio, coarse chromatin and thickened nuclear membrane.

Dysplastic squamous cells are of 3 types:

1. Intermediate dysplastic cells seen in LGSIL.
2. Parabasal dysplastic cells resemble closely parabasal or metaplastic cells in size and shape but have atypical nuclei. Cells lie singly or in clusters or strings or files. These cells are seen in HGSIL or cancer.
3. Small parabasal and basal dysplastic cells. These cells indicate more aggressive lesion. Cells lie scattered loose or in loose clusters or in syncitia.

Dysplastic Endocervical Cells

Dysplastic endocervical cells are uncommon and difficult to recognize. They may be seen in HGSIL or early adenocarcinoma, and are seen as columnar cells with enlarged hyperchromatic or pale nuclei and large nucleoli.

Koilocytes

Koilocytes are mature squamous cells of intermediate type with abnormal enlarged hyperchromatic nuclei that are smudged, homogenous, and are surrounded by sharply demarcated perinuclear halo. Sometimes binucleation/multinucleation may be seen. Koilocytes are characteristic of HPV infection and are seen with both low-risk and high-risk types of HPV infection and form the criteria for the diagnosis of LGSIL.

Leukoplakia

White discoloration or abnormal keratinization of cervical surface is called leukoplakia. This is because of keratinization of superficial cells which are seen as anucleate, polygonal, transparent cells with pink or yellow cytoplasm. Brown cytoplasmic granules may be present and ghost nuclei are seen.

Parakeratosis/Pseudoparakeratosis

Also presents as white patch clinically. Small nucleated squmaous cells present in sheets Cause is not known. But such cells can be seen in HPV infection, low grade and high-grade squamous lesions.

CERVICAL CYTOLOGY REPORTING

Terminologies/Classifications

Papanicolaou, the founder of contemporary diagnostic cytology, proposed a classification in 1943 (Table 16.1), but it did not reflect current understanding of cervical neoplasia, classes had no equivalents in histopathologic terminology, and did not reliably communicate clinically relevant information. Over the years, different systems and terminologies evolved to overcome the deficiencies of the previous ones. WHO and CIN classifications had the drawbacks of lack of reproducibility in assigning lesions to different categories and the biological behavior of the lesions did not correspond with the cytological categories. Terminology for reporting cervicovaginal smears was further standardized by The Bethesda System (TBS) in 1988. Since the goal of any screening program is to detect the precursor lesions and treat them early in order to halt their progress to frank cancer, it is of utmost importance for the clinicians and the pathologists to be familiar with the terminology, morphology and management protocols of the precancerous lesions.

Table 16.1: Evolution of reporting system precancerous lesions of cervix

Papanicolaou's classification

Class I:	Absence of atypical or abnormal cells
Class II:	Atypical cytology but no evidence of malignancy
Class III:	Cytology suggestive of but not conclusive for malignancy
Class IV:	Cytology strongly suggestive of malignancy
Class V:	Cytology conclusive for malignancy

WHO classification proposed by Reagen and Patten in 1962:
- Mild dysplasia
- Moderate dysplasia
- Severe dysplasia
- Carcinoma in situ

CIN classification: Proposed by Richart in 1967 to further improve upon the concept of disease continuum.
- CIN I
- CIN II
- CIN III

The Bethesda system: Standardized in 1988, revised twice there after current system developed in 2001

BETHESDA SYSTEM (2011) FOR REPORTING CERVICAL CYTOLOGIC DIAGNOSIS

Bethesda system (Table 16.2) considered cervico-vaginal smear as a medical consultation and stressed it to be reported in clear, unambiguous language so as to establish an effective communication with the referring consultant and facilitate cyto-histologic correlation.

Table 16.2: The 2001 Bethesda system for reporting cervical cytologic diagnosis

I. Specimen type

Indicate conventional smear (Pap smear) vs. liquid-based

II. Specimen adequacy

Satisfactory for evaluation

(presence/absence of endocervical/transformation zone component and any other quality indicators, e.g. partially obscuring blood and inflammation)

Unsatisfactory for evaluation ... (specify reason)

- Specimen rejected/not processed (specify reason)
- Specimen processed and examined, but unsatisfactory for evaluation of epithelial abnormality (specify reason)

III. General categorization (optional)

Negative for intraepithelial lesion or malignancy—*see* interpretation/result

Epithelial cell abnormality (specify 'squamous'/ 'glandular')—*see* interpretation/result

Other (e.g. endometrial cells in a woman > 40 years of age)—*see* interpretation/result

IV. Interpretation/result

Negative for intraepithelial lesion or malignancy

(State whether or not there are organisms or other non-neoplastic findings)

Organisms:

- *Trichomonas vaginalis*
- Fungal organisms morphologically consistent with *Candida* spp
- Shift in flora suggestive of bacterial vaginosis
- Bacteria morphologically consistent with *Actinomyces* spp.
- Cellular changes consistent with herpes simplex virus

Other non-neoplastic findings (optional to report):

- Reactive cellular changes associated with inflammation (includes typical repair) radiation intrauterine contraceptive device (IUD)
- Glandular cells status post-hysterectomy
- Atrophy

Epithelial cell abnormalities

Squamous cell

Atypical squamous cells (ASC):
- ASC of undetermined significance (ASC–US)
- ASC—cannot exclude HSIL (ASC–H)

Low grade squamous intraepithelial lesion (LGSIL)

Encompassing: HPV, mild dysplasia, and CIN 1

High grade squamous intraepithelial lesion (HGSIL)

Encompassing: Moderate and severe dysplasia, CIS, CIN 2, and CIN 3

Squamous cell carcinoma

Glandular cell

Atypical glandular cells (AGC)

Specify endocervical, endometrial, or gladular cells not otherwise specified

Atypical glandular cells, favor neoplastic

Specify endocervical cell or not otherwise specified

Endocervical adenocarcinoma in situ (AIS)

Adenocarcinoma

Other:

Endometrial cells (in a woman > 40 years of age—specify if 'negative for squamous intraepithelial lesion')

Automated review and ancillary testing (include if appropriate)

Educational notes and suggestions (optional)

Specimen Adequacy

Satisfactory for evaluation

Cervicovaginal smear should be representative of epithelia of ectocervix, endocervix and should include transformation zone as aim of cervical smear examination is detection of abnormal cells which generally arise in the transformation zone. Therefore, ideally the smear should contain squamous cells, metaplastic cells (TZ) and/or endocervical cells, and should not be obscured by the presence of blood/inflammation, etc. However, since the absence of endocervical cells/presence of partially obscuring factors have not shown to increase the risk of a false negative report; TBS 2001 considers such specimens to be reported as "satisfactory for evaluation". but the comments about the TZ components/partially obscuring factors are placed in the narrative report which should be read carefully by the clinician to note that the transformation zone was not sampled and to improve the specimen adequacy henceforth.

In conventional Pap smears, cervical mucus itself is evidence of smear adequacy in absence of endocervical cells. However, in liquid-based preparations, this valuable resource is lost. Since only a part of sample aliquot is used in smear preparation, 5000 well preserved squamous cells per smear and 10 endocervical cells form the basis of adequacy. In older women, TZ may be situated within endocervix canal and is much more difficult to sample and presence of endocervical cells or mucus is not necessary for adequacy.

Any smear containing abnormal cells is considered satisfactory for evaluation irrespective of the number of cells present.

Unsatisfactory for evaluation

When the smear does not contain adequate cellular material for reliable interpretation, it is reported as "unsatisfactory for evaluation". The report would specify, whether the specimen was rejected and not processed (with reason); or whether it was processed and examined, but found unsatisfactory for evaluation of epithelial abnormalities. The causes of unsatisfactory smears could be:

1. Heavy inflammation obscuring cells (Fig. 16.14)
2. Air drying artifact (Fig. 16.15)
3. Excessive cytolysis (Fig. 16.16)
4. Bloody smear with only few cells
5. Uniformly thick smear
6. Scanty cellular material
7. Lubricant contaminant
8. Inadequate fixation
9. Unrepresentative material
10. Menstrual cells

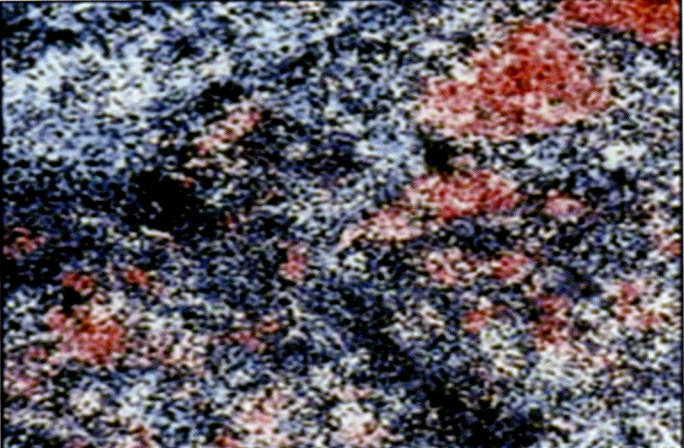

Fig. 16.14: Pap smear shows heavy infiltrate of neutrophils masking epithelial cells

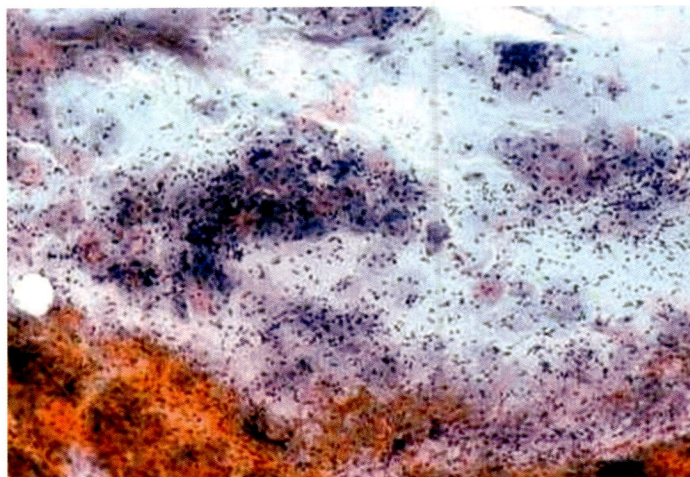

Fig. 16.15: Air drying effect due to lack of immediate fixation shows polychromasia and smudgy morphology of cells

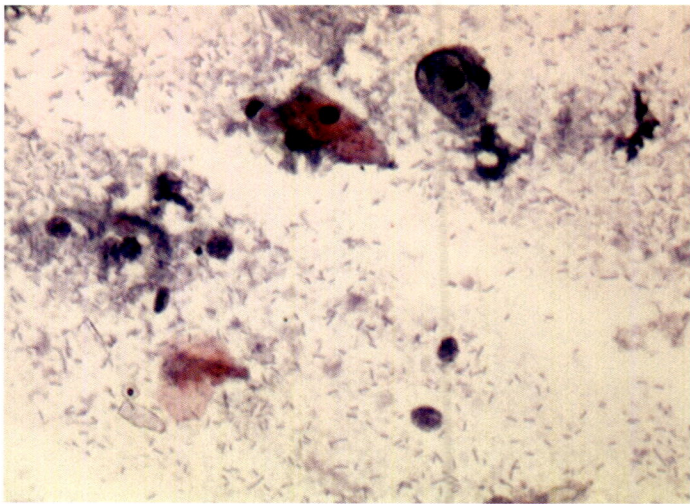

Fig. 16.16: Heavy presence of Doderlein bacilli and fragmentation and cytolysis of cell cytoplasm due to excess of progesterone effect

Interpretation/Result

Negative for Intraepithelial Lesion/Malignancy

In TBS 2001, cervical cytologic specimens that contain no epithelial abnormalities are listed under the category "negative for intraepithelial lesion or malignancy." This includes the previous categories of "within normal limits" and "benign cellular changes". The presence of organisms and other non-neoplastic findings are included as a comment in this "negative" category.

Organisms

Trichomonas vaginalis

Organism appears as gray-green round or elliptical in shape, 8–20 μ in size. Nucleus is situated eccentrically (Fig. 16.17). Sometimes flagella may be seen at one pole. Leptothrix infection (long curving organisms) may be associated in some cases.

Smear background is dirty due to cell necrosis. Squamous cells show marked eosinophila of the cytoplasm, perinuclear halo and pallor or apoptosis of nuclei. Florid squamous metaplsia may be seen.

Candida albicans (Synonym: Monilia)

Candida appears in yeast form and pseudohyphae. Yeast form appears as small round or oval, 8–10 μ in size, encapsulated or budding organisms. Pseudohyphae are seen as thin filaments (Fig. 16.18) of bamboo with spores. Cellular abnormalities are not significant.

Gardnerella vaginalis (Synonyms: Corynebacteria vaginalis, Haemophilus vaginalis):

These appear as short rods on Pap stain. These adhere to surface of squamous epithelial cells. Such cells are called "clue cells" (Figs 16.19A and B). Bacilli are present in the background also. *Gardnerella vaginalis* are the main cause of bacterial vaginosis. These should not be

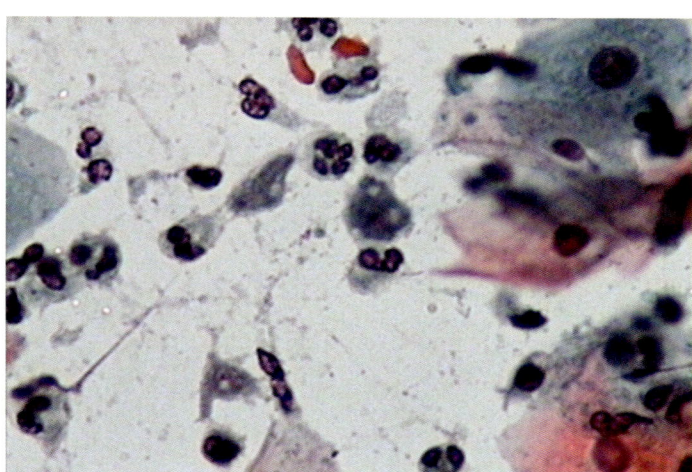

Fig. 16.17: Pear-shaped Trichomonads seen in the center of the field with blue gray cytoplasm and indistinct thin nuclei

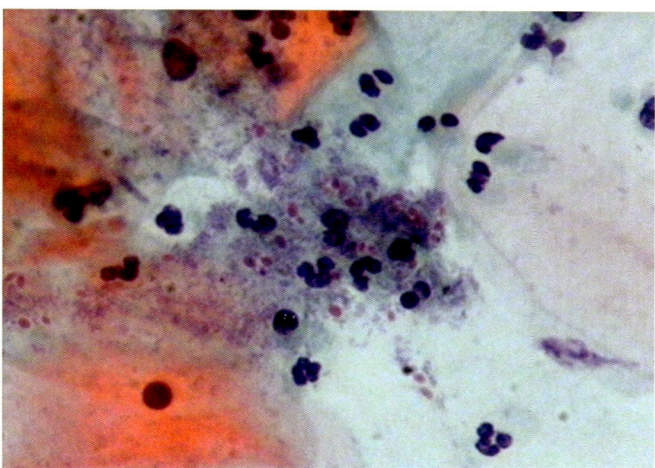

Fig. 16.18: Budding red-colored yeasts seen in Candida infection

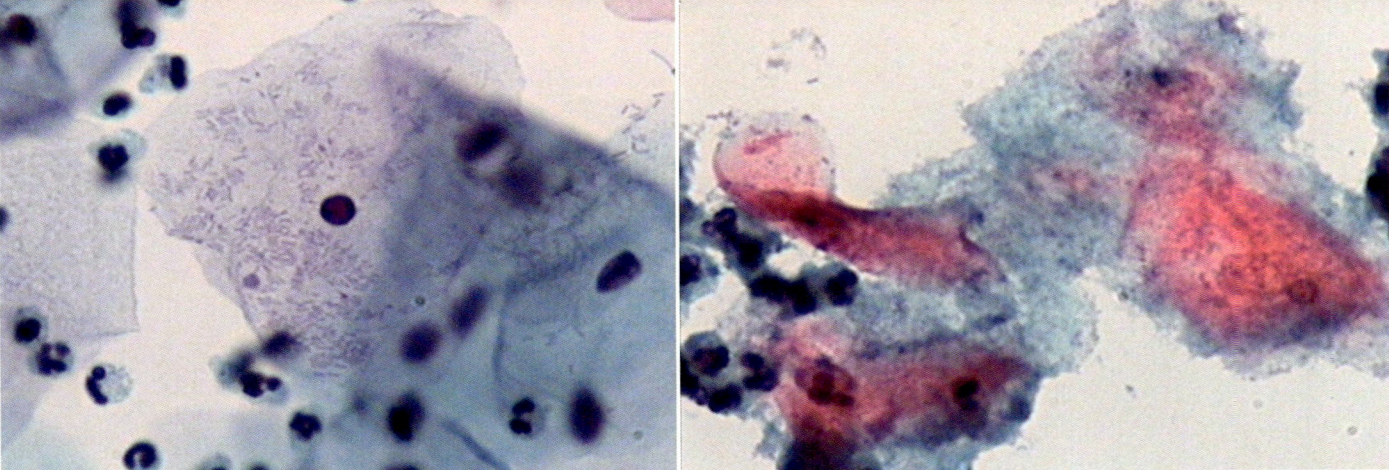

Figs 16.19A and B: "Clue cell" with small organisms adherent to the cytoplasm of squamous cells

mistaken for lactobacilli which cause cytclysis of intermediate cells and may adhere to the surface of cells. Lactobacilli form the normal flora of vagina and are increased in pregnancy and postmenopausal women (Fig. 16.20). In bacterial vaginosis, there is a change of bacterial flora from lactobacilli to mixed organisms. Smears show dirty background due to organisms and presence of clue cells.

Actinomyces

Actinomyces are gram-positive filamentous organisms and are seen as balls or colonies of basophilic filaments in smear. Colonies may be surrounded by neutrophils. Actinomyces infection is mostly seen in IUD wearers (Fig. 16.21).

Genital herpes

In early stage, there is marked cell enlargement. Nuclei become opaque and basophilic, show ground glass appearance and peripheral condensation of chromatin.

Nuclear vacuoles due to viral inclusions may appear (Fig. 16.22).

In late stage, nuclear crowding, molding of nuclei and multinucleation appear. Large eosinophilic inclusion surrounded by clear area may be present. Nuclear fusion may lead to hyperchromatic nuclear masses and be mistaken for malignant cells (Fig. 16.23).

Other Non-neoplastic Findings

Reactive cellular changes associated with

Acute inflammation: Smear has dirty appearance due to presence of neutrophils, necrotic cells, cell debris and bacteria (Fig. 16.24). Cell cytoplasm has deeper eosinophilia particularly in trichomonal infection. There is increase in the number of parabasal cells due to loss of superficial cell layers. Metaplastic cells may be present.

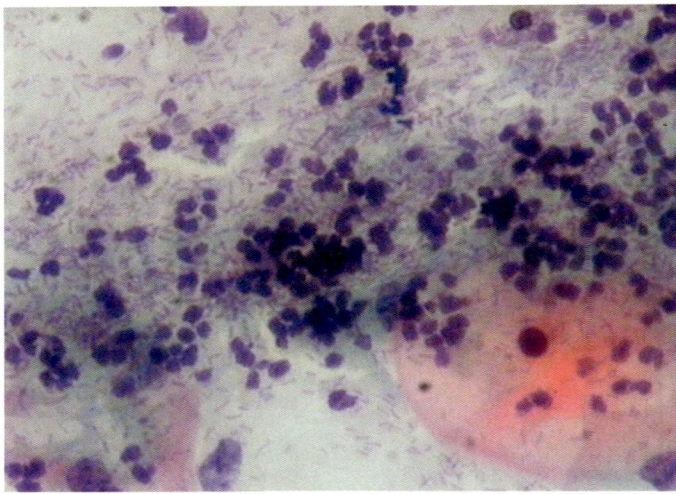

Fig. 16.20: Large number of Doderlein bacilli are seen with neutrophils

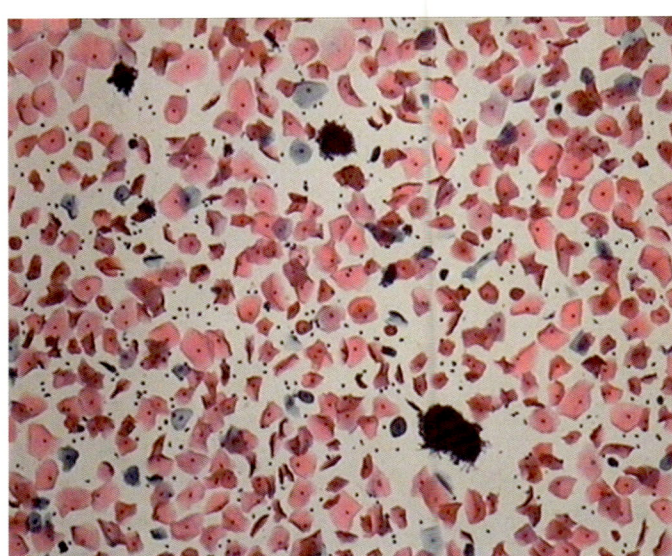

Fig. 16.21: Colonies of Actinomyces organisms

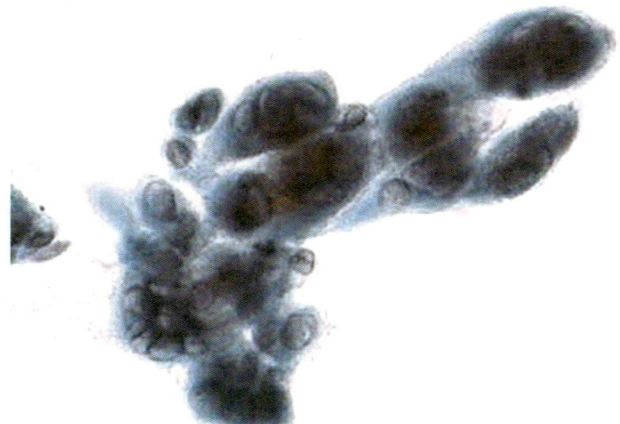

Fig. 16.22: Large multinucleated cells with clear nucleoplasm in herpetic infection

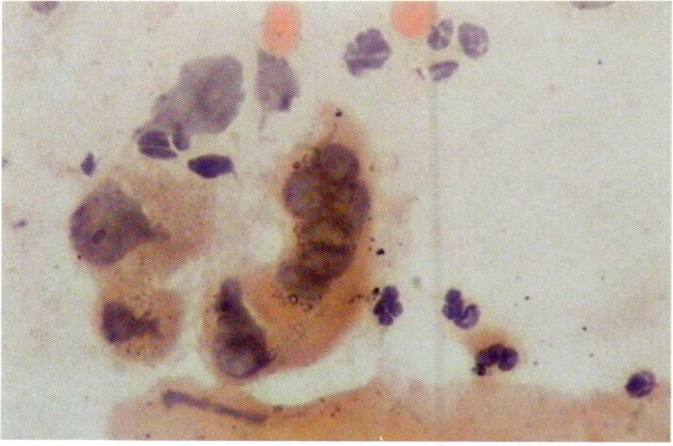

Fig. 16.23: Multinucleation and nuclear molding is evident

Nuclei are homogeneous and show mild enlargement, perinuclear halo, binucleation, small nucleoli may be seen. Bare nuclei of multinucleated cells may be present. Cytoplasmic vacuoles may contain neutrophils. Mitosis may sometimes be seen.

Infection in postmenopausal women: Inflammation may cause increased cell maturation, increase in cell necrosis, cell debris, pyknosis of nuclei or nuclear enlargement along with neutrophilic exudate (Fig. 16.25).

Chronic inflammation: Smear shows lymphocytes, macrophages and plasma cells. Multinucleated macrophages can be seen in granulomatous conditions like tuberculosis.

Repair, regeneration: Repair of cervix after surgical procedures or infections or radiotherapy may show

cellular changes which may resemble florid squamous metaplasia (Fig. 16.26).

Effect of intrauterine devices: IUDs may lead to florid squamous metaplasia or repair reaction. Presence of bacteria and actinomyces or other organisms and presence of calcified amorphous debris or calcified spherical bodies in the smears are noted.

Human papillomavirus infection: Human papillomavirus (HPV) is now recognized as causative agent for carcinoma cervix. Smears show marked koilocytoatypia. Cells show perinuclear halo, nuclear atypia, binucleation and thickening of peripheral cytoplasm of intermediate cells (Fig. 16.27).

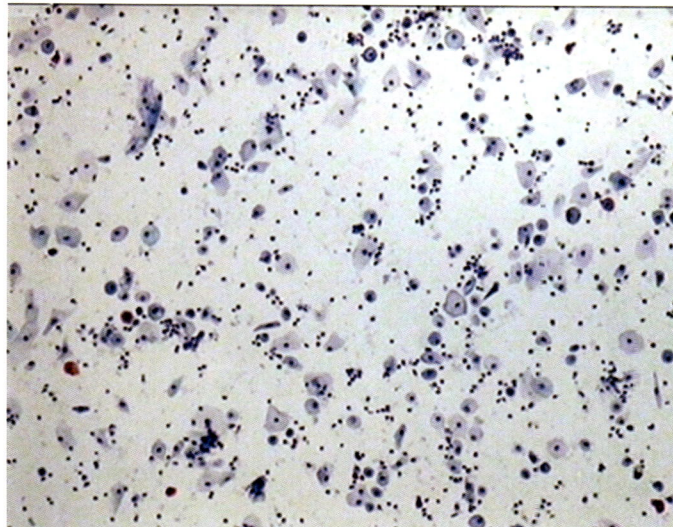

Fig. 16.25: Postmenopausal smear showing acute inflammatory cells and a few intermediate and superficial cells. Nuclear enlargement is not observed in this case

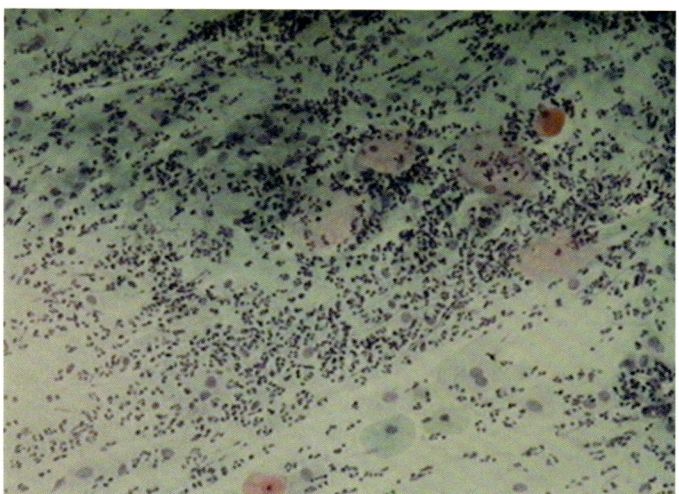

Fig. 16.24: Acute inflammatory exudates

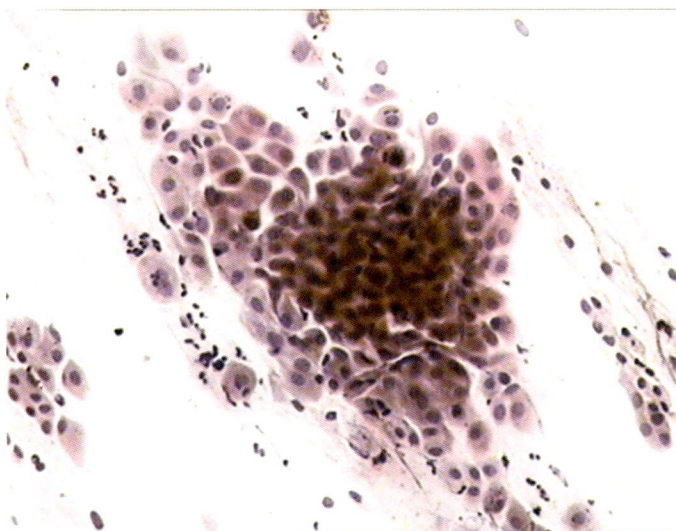

Fig. 16.26: Large sheets of metaplastic squamous cells

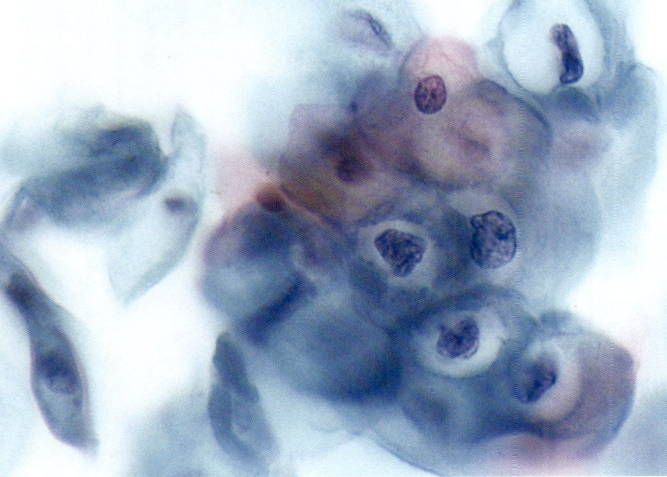

Fig. 16.27: Koilocytes in HPV infection showing perinuclear vacuole, condensation of peripheral cytoplasm and crenation of nuclei

Epithelial Cell Abnormalities and Squamous

Atypical Squamous Cells of Uncertain Significance (ASC–US)

A new terminology "atypical squamous cells of undetermined significance (ASC–US)" was introduced in 1988. Bethesda classification to encompass equivocal cytological abnormalities which show more than inflammatory atypia but fall short of definitive criteria to be labeled as SIL. Outcome of ASC–US in different clinical settings varied from mostly benign lesions to potentially ominous lesions in some cases because of their differing management protocols. Thus in 1991, Bethesda Committee recommended to qualify ASC–US lesions into 3 categories: ASC–US-favor reactive, ASC–US, not otherwise specified (ASC–US–NOS), and ASC–US-favor neoplastic outcome. However, there was tremendous over-usage of ASC–US diagnosis, without significant pick up of lesions on follow-up, resulting in unnecessary biopsies and workload. In Bethesda 2001 system, the term ASC–US was replaced by 'ASC' (atypical squamous cells) which was assigned dichotomous qualifiers:

1. **ASC–US:** To denote cytological changes suggestive of SIL but are quantitatively insufficient for definitive interpretation. The term "undetermined significance" emphasizes that a specific diagnosis cannot be made and that further triage may be appropriate ASC–US will include most cytology results previously categorized as ASC–US–NOS or ASC–US, favor SIL. It excludes cytology suggestive of HSIL.

   The cells show nuclear enlargement 2½–3 times a normal intermediate squamous cell nucleus, slightly increased N/C ratio, minimal hyperchromasia, evenly distributed chromatin with a smooth and regular nuclear membrane (Fig. 16.28).

2. **ASC–H:** It includes cytological changes suggestive of HSIL but lack criteria for definitive interpretation. In ASC–H, the cytological changes are suggestive of HSIL but lack criteria of definitive interpretation.

   ASC–H has high predictive value for CIN 2/3 outcome on follow-up.

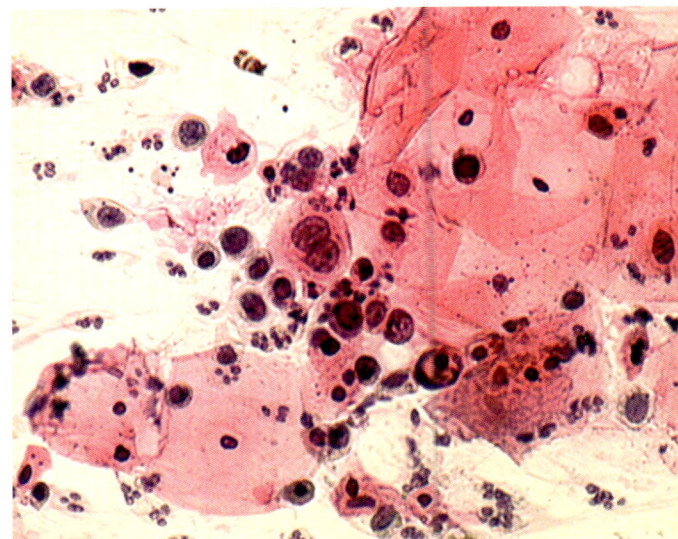

Fig. 16.28: ASC–US: There is nuclear enlargement and mild hyperchromasia

Low Grade Squamous Intraepithelial Lesions (LGSIL)

The category of LSIL includes the following categories: human papillomavirus (HPV), mild dysplasia, and CIN 1. Cytological features of dyskaryotic intermediate and superficial cells are seen in Figs 16.29A and B.

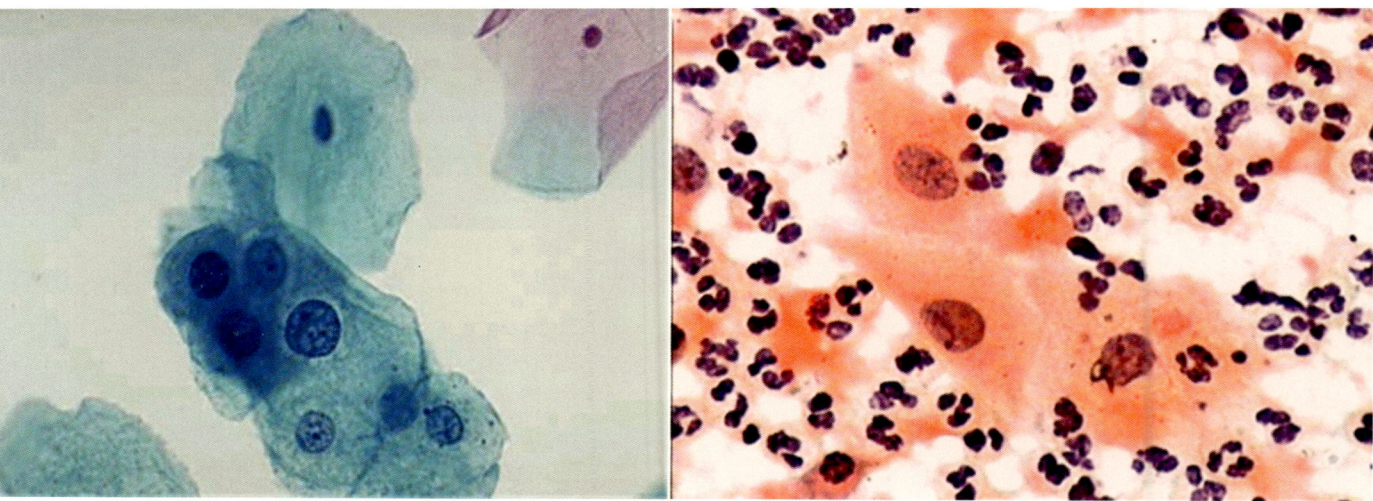

Figs 16.29A and B: Nuclear enlargement and mild hyperchromasia on intermediate cells

Koilocytes, if present, signify LGSIL. A few dyskaryotic parabasal cells may be seen. Background is generally clear, and there is no inflammation.

High Grade Intraepithelial Lesion (HGSIL)

The category of HSIL includes moderate dysplasia, severe dysplasia, and carcinoma in situ, or CIN 2, 3. HSIL lesions are characterized by the presence of marked nuclear abnormalities. Cells may lie as streaks-trapped in mucus (Fig. 16.30). Abnormal shapes like cancer cells may be present. Atypical endocervical cells may be seen. Background shows inflammation. Differentiation from invasive cancer may be impossible.

Squamous Cell Carcinoma Cervix

Smear shows necrotic material, blood, and debris in the background which forms tumor diathesis. Inflammation and necrotic material may obscure cancer cells. Marked pleomorphism and abnormalities of squamous cells are seen (Fig. 16.31). Apoptotic or necrotic cells and abnormal mitotic figures may be seen. Large sheets of tumor cells or tumor fragments may be present.

In keratinizing squamous cell carcinoma, keratinized cancer cells, anucleate squamous cells, intermediate type of undifferentiated malignant cells or small cancer cells, naked nuclei and abnormal shapes, tadpole or spindle cells are present in the smear. There is marked variation in size and shape of cells. Cells possess thick dense orange or yellow cytoplasm and highly abnormal nuclei varying in size. Multi-nucleated cells and mitotic figures may or may not be present (Figs 16.32A to D).

Spindle-shaped cells and abnormal shapes like tadpole cells suggest invasion (Fig. 16.33).

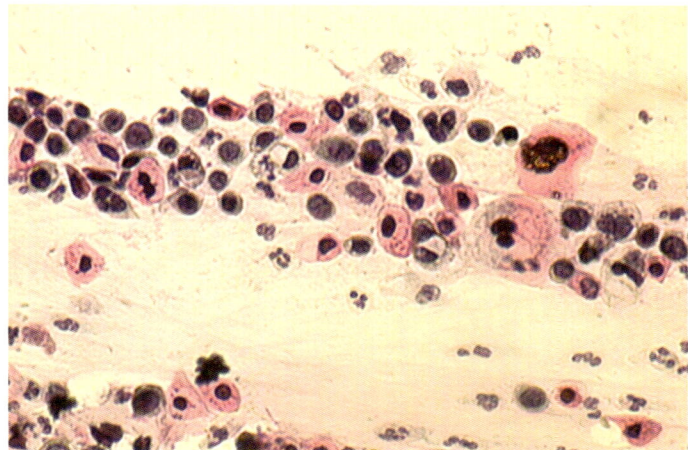

Fig. 16.30: Large number of parabasal cells showing nuclear enlargement and hyperchromasia

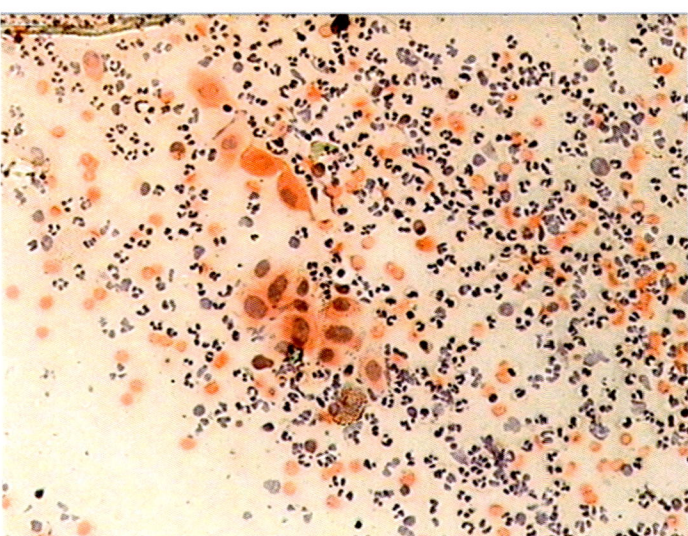

Fig. 16.31: Squamous cell carcinoma cervix showing large highly atypical keratinized cells with abundant deeply eosinophilic cytoplasm

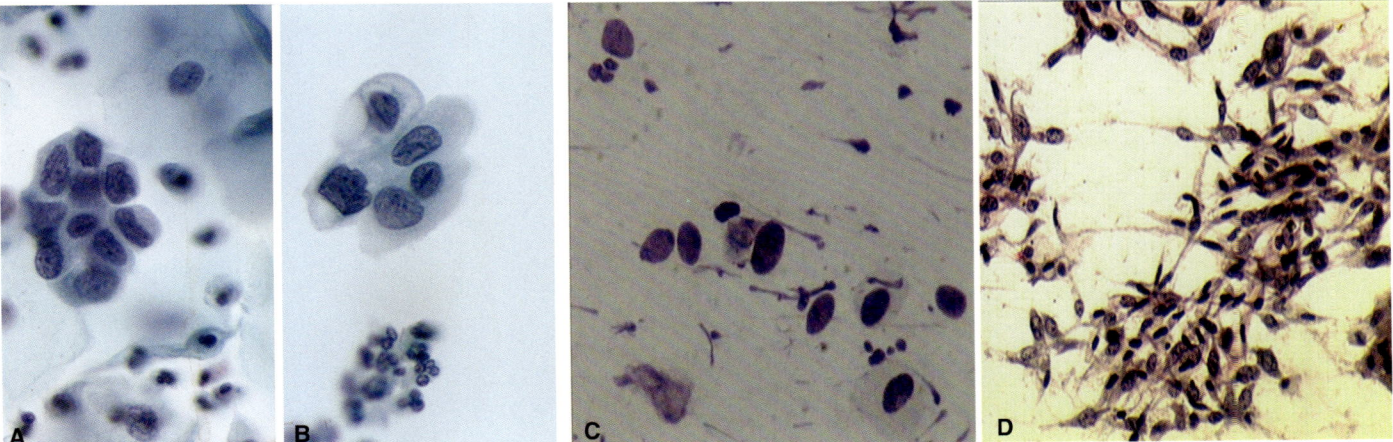

Figs 16.32A to D: Spindling of malignant epithelial cells

Squamous pearls with concentric arrangement of malignant cells, if present, indicate invasive cancer but may be seen in HGSIL (Fig. 16.34).

In invasive small cell carcinoma, undifferentiated cancer cells are seen. Cytoplasm is variable but scanty and basaophilic (Fig. 16.35). Cells are oval or round but shapes may vary. Highly abnormal nuclei are present. Mitosis is present. Cytoplasm is fragile and degenerates easily. Tumor diathesis is present.

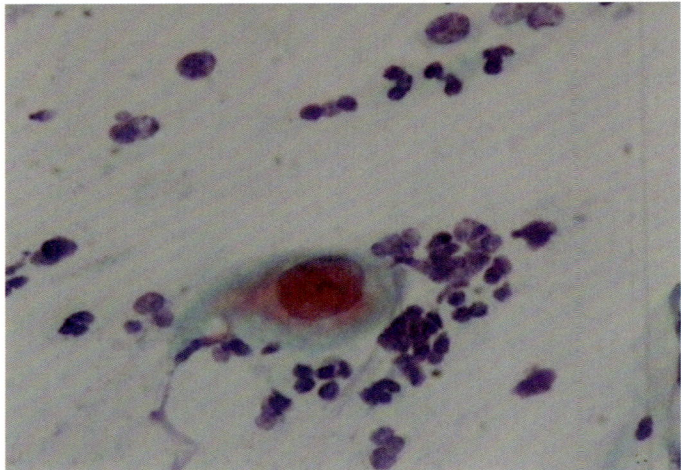

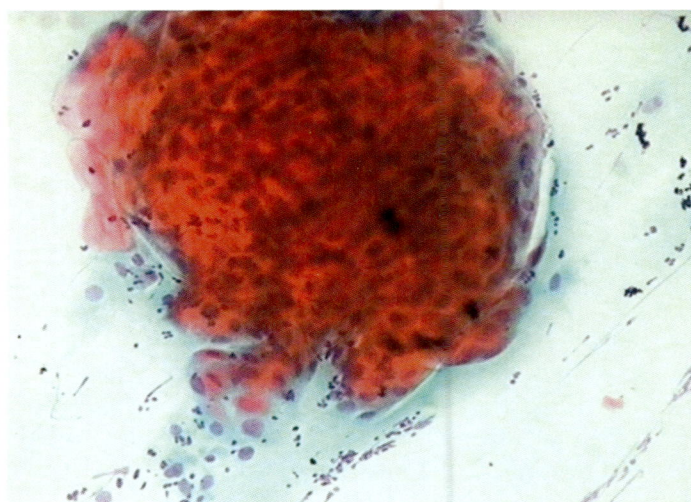

Fig. 16.33: Tadpole cell in squamous cell carcinoma

Fig. 16.34: Keratin pearl in squamous cell carcinoma

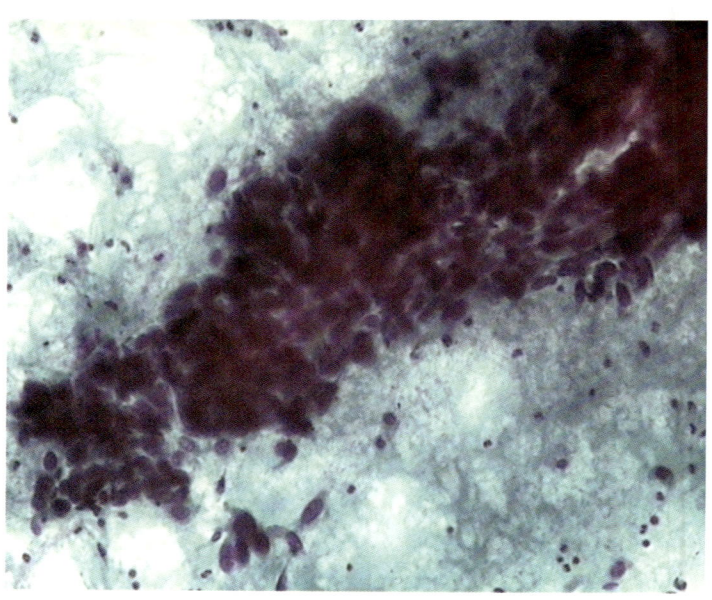

Fig. 16.35: Necrotic background representing tumor diathesis in carcinoma

Epithelial Cell Abnormalities, Glandular

TBS 1988 used the term "atypical glandular cells of undetermined significance" (AGUS) to describe "cells showing either endometrial or endocervical differentiation displaying nuclear atypia that exceeds obvious reactive or reparative changes but lack unequivocal features of invasive adenocarcinoma." The terms such as "favor reactive" and "favor neoplastic" could be used to describe the spectrum of AGUS that ranged from benign appearing reparative findings to adenocarcinoma in situ.

There were several problems associated with the use of the term AGUS. One could get confused between AGUS and ASC–US, with the potential risk of under management, as the finding of AGUS could be a marker for significant glandular or squamous pathology. Thus, in TBS 2013, the term AGUS is replaced with "atypical glandular cell" (AGC) and the term "favor reactive" is eliminated; the laboratory will try to indicate origin of the AGC as endocervical, endometrial, or unqualified (not otherwise specified). The terms "AGC, favor neoplastic" and "adenocarcinoma in situ (AIS)" are listed as separate categories.

AGC (favor neoplastic)

Sheets of tightly packed glandular cells are seen with pseudostratification, crowding, nuclear hyperchromasia, pallisading and rosette formation. Stripped off nuclei reveal frayed/feathered appearance (Fig. 16.36). Chromatin is fine to coarsely granular. Nucleoli may or may not be present.

Adenocarcinoma in situ (AIS)

Nuclear and cellular changes are more marked (Fig. 16.37). It is difficult to differentiation between AIS and adenocarcinoma.

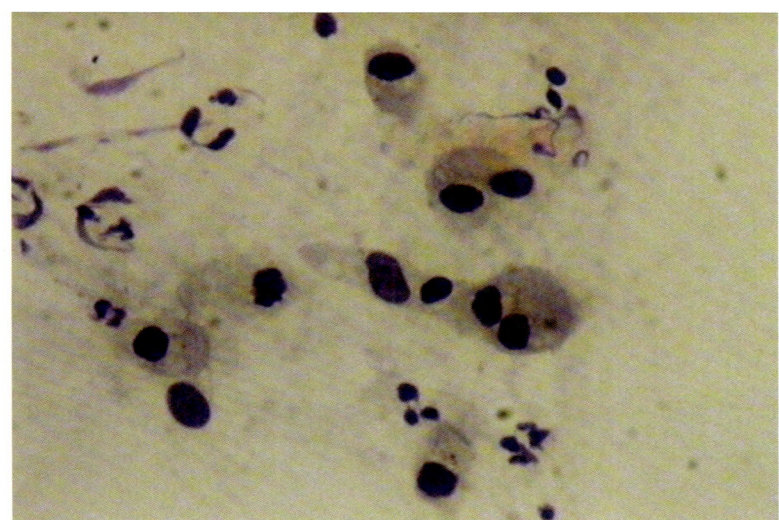

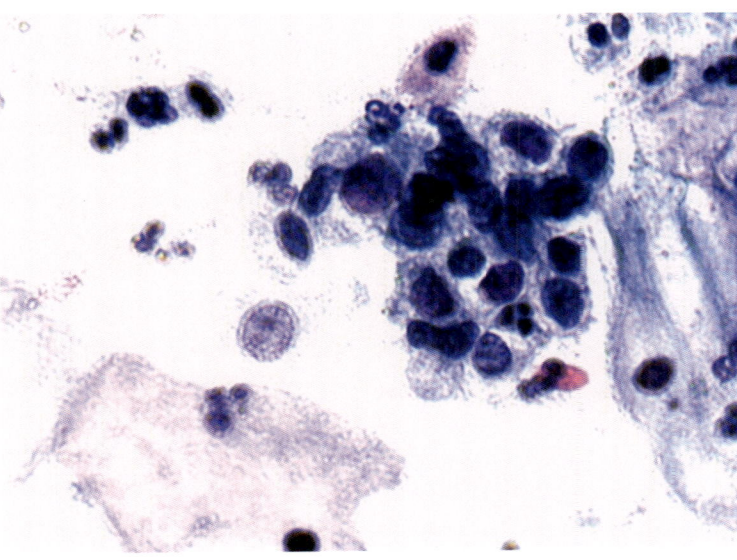

Fig. 16.36: AGC favoring neoplasia with columnar cells showing nuclear enlargement and hyperchromasia

Fig. 16.37: AIS showing tightly packed cells with marked cellular and nuclear atypia. Cytoplasmic fraying is evident

Invasive endocervical adenocarcinoma

Columnar cells possess cytoplasmic vacuoles, nuclear enlargement, eccentric nuclei, large eosinophilic nucleoli, multiple nucleoli and papillary spherical clusters. There is overlapping of nuclei and clusters may have a lumen (rosette or glands). Such cells are seen in adenocarcinoma, squamous cell carcinoma and HGSIL. It is difficult to differentiate between dysplastic and malignant endocervical cells. However, in adenocarcinoma, smear shows necrotic and bloody background.

Signet ring cells may be present. Mitotic figures and apoptotic nuclei are present. A few dysplastic squamous cells may be seen (Fig. 16.38).

Other

This category is created for reporting normal or abnormal endometrial cells in women who are 40 years or older, as the presence of even benign-appearing endometrial cells on cervical cytology in women who are at least 45 years of age is more often associated with endometrial adenocarcinoma and endometrial hyperplasia than with benign endometrium. However, since cervical cytology is primarily a screening test for squamous epithelial lesions and squamous cancer, it is not reliable for detection of endometrial lesions.

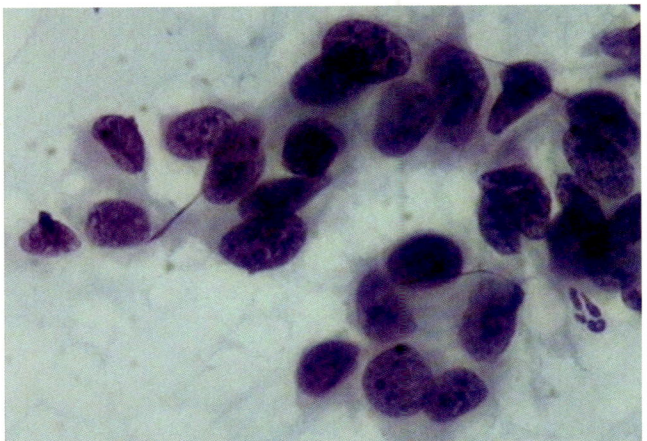

Fig. 16.38: Large round cells with extremely large hyperchromatic nuclei forming rossete or gland in adenocarcinoma

Ancillary Testing and Educational Notes

If slides are scanned by automated computer systems, the type of system used should be reported with the result. Ancillary testing such as HPV DNA is performed, if appropriate, and reported with the cytology results.

Written comments regarding the interpretation of a cytologic specimen are optional and may be conveyed to the clinician by the pathologist as a means of clarification and information.

Appendix-1

COLPOSCOPY REPORT FORM

Name of patient: Date of Visit:

Age of patient:

Hospital identification no.:

Address and Phone no.:

Last menstrual period:

Pap smear report:

HPV DNA report:

Reason for colposcopy referral:

Report

- Colposcopy adequate/inadequate (specify reason)
- SCJ visible entirely/partially/not visible
- TZ type 1/2/3
- **Cervix:** Normal/Abnormal

    Normal – OSE: Mature/Atrophic, CE: Ectopy/Metaplsia/NC/GO

    Abnormal findings if present

    – Location of lesion: Inside TZ/Outside TZ, at .... O'clock

    – Size of lesion: Occupying .... quadrants, ... % of cervix

    – Minor/Major/Suspicious for Invasion/Non-specific/Miscellaneous

    – Scoring system used with score of findings

- **Vagina**: Normal/Abnormal
- **Vulva**: Normal/Abnormal

Biopsy taken/not taken: If taken specify site and location ....

Endocervical sample (ECC) taken/not taken:

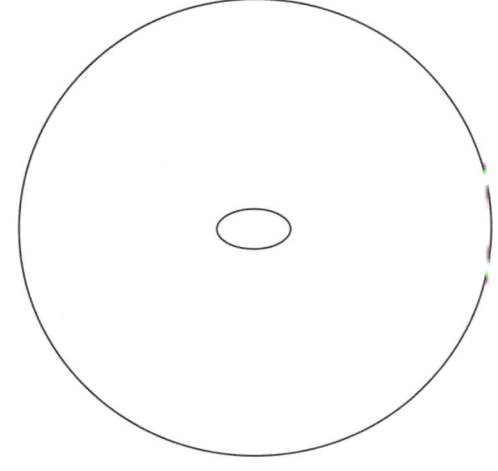

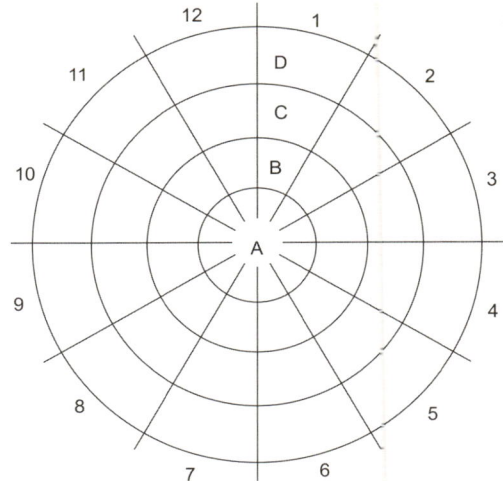

Cervix

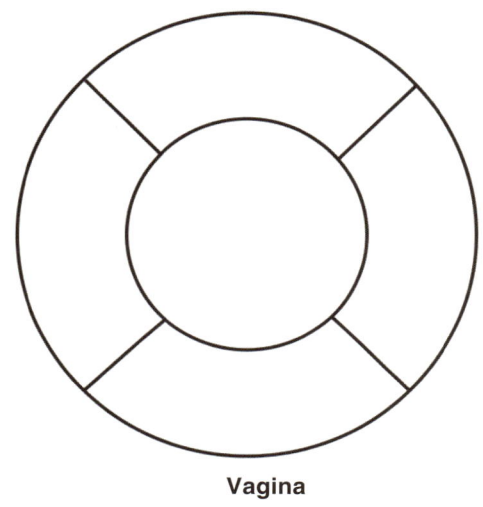

Vagina

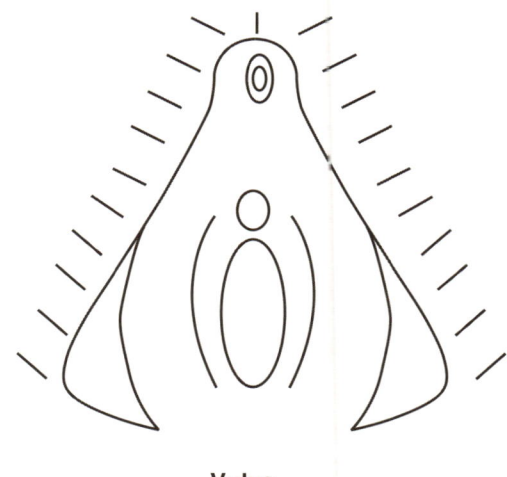

Vulva

Final Impression

Cervix/vagina/vulva:

Normal/Inflammation/Low grade/High grade lesion/Suspicious of invasion

Recommendation

Repeat Pap smear

HPV DNA— high-risk

Cryocautery

LEEP/Conisation

Routine surveillance

Follow-up

Biopsy Report:

Signature
Name of Colposcopist

Appendix-2

PREPARATION OF CHEMICAL REAGENTS USED IN COLPOSCOPY

Acetic Acid

Acetic acid is always used freshly prepared. Unused solution should be discarded at the end of the day.

1 % (for collin's test): Glacial acetic acid 1 ml + 99 ml of distilled water

3 % (examination of cervix): Glacial acetic acid 3 ml + 97 ml of distilled water

5 % (examination of vulva): Glacial acetic acid 5 ml + 95 ml of distilled water

The requisite amount of glacial acetic acid should be added carefully to distilled water and mixed thoroughly.

- Use of undiluted acetic acid can cause severe chemical burn.
- Glacial acetic acid bottle should remain tightly closed.

Lugol's Iodine

Required ingredients:

Potassium Iodide (KI): 10 g

Iodine crystals (I2): 5 g

Distilled water: 100 ml

First potassium iodide is dissolved in water. After it is completely dissolved, iodine crystals are added slowly while shaking the solution. The whole solution is filtered and stored in a tightly capped brown bottle. Shelf-life of this solution is 1 month. The 'Use by' date should be specified on the bottle label.

Monsel's Paste

Required ingredients:

Ferric sulfate base: 15 g

Ferrous sulfate powder a few grains only

Glycerol starch: 12 g

Sterile water: 10 ml

Glycerol starch is prepared separately. Ingredients required are Starch: 30 gm, Glycerin: 390 gm and sterile water: 30 ml. Starch is dissolved in sterile water in a China crucible, followed by addition of glycerin and shaking it well. The crucible and its contents are heated over a burner, mixing constantly with a spatula until it takes a thick consistency. It should not be overheated or it will turn yellow. Prepared glycerol starch can be stored in a cool place for one year.

Preparation of Monsel's paste: While preparing Monsel's paste one should be careful as it emits heat. A few grains of ferrous sulfate powder are added to 10 ml of sterile water in a glass beaker and shaken. Ferric sulfate base is dissolved in this solution by stirring with a glass stick till it becomes crystal clear. This ferric sulfate solution is added slowly to 12 gm of already prepared glycerol starch, mixing constantly till a homogeneous mixture is made.

This paste is stored in small brown color bottle. Paste should be used after approximately 2–3 wks. After 2–3 wks of evaporation paste looks like mustard. If too thick, sterile water can be used to make it thin. Shelf-life of Monsel's paste is 6 months. The 'Use by' date should be specified on the bottle label with the instruction to shake well before use.

Bibliography

1. Anderson MC, Jordan JA, Morse AR, Sharp F. Integrated Colposcopy: For colposcopists histopathologists and cytologists. 2nd ed. London and NewYork: Chapman and Hall Medical 1996.

2. Apgar BS, Brotzman GL, Spitzer M eds. Colposcopy: Principles and Practice; an integrated textbook and atlas. Philadelphia. WB Saunders Company 2002.

3. Bornstein J, Bentley J, Bösze P, Girardi F, Haefner H, Menton M, Perrotta M, Prendiville W, Russell P, Sideri M, Strander B, Tatti S, Torne A, Walker P. 2011 colposcopic terminology of the international Federation for Cervical Pathology and Colposcopy. Obstet Gynecol. 2012 Jul;120(1):166–72.

4. Bornstein J, Sideri M, Tatti S, Walker P, Prendiville W, Haefner HK; Nomenclature Committee of International Federation for Cervical Pathology and Colposcopy. 2011 terminology of the vulva of the International Federation for Cervical Pathology and Colposcopy. J Low Genit Tract Dis. 2012 Jul; 16(3):290–5.

5. Brown AJ and Trimble CL. New Technologies for Cervical Cancer Screening. Best Pract Res Clin Obstet Gynaecol. 2012 April; 26(2): 233–242.

6. Burghardt E, Pickel H, Girardi F. Colposcopy-Cervical Pathology Textbook and Atlas, 3rd edn, New York (NY): Thieme, 1998.

7. Cartier R. Practical Colposcopy. S Karger AG (Switzerland) 1977.

8. Das SK, Nigam S, Batra A, Chandra M. An Atlas of colposcopy, cytology and histopathology of lower female genital tract. Delhi: CBS publishers 1995.

9. Giuntoli RL, Atkinson BF. Atkinson's Correlative Atlas of Colposcopy, Cytology & Histopathology. Lippincott; 1997.

10. Khanna N, Dalby R, Tan M, Arnold S, Stern J, Frazer N. Phase I/II clinical safety studies of terameprocol vaginal ointment. Gynecol. Oncol. (2007) Dec; 107(3):554-62.

11. Kohli M, Lawrence D, Haig J, Anonychk A, and Demarteau N. Modeling the impact of the difference in crossprotection data between a human papillomavirus (HPV)-16/18 AS04-adjuvanted vaccine and a human papillomavirus (HPV)-6/11/16/18 vaccine in Canada BMC Public Health 2012, 12:872

12. Kolstad P, Stafl A. Atlas of Colposcopy. Baltimore: University Park Press, 1972.

13. Massad LS, Einstein MH, Huh WK, Katki HA, Kinney WK, Schiffman M, Solomon D, Wentzensen N, Lawson HW. 2012 ASCCP Consensus Guidelines Conference. 2012 updated consensus guidelines for the management of abnormal cervical cancer screening tests and cancer precursors. Obstet Gynecol. 2013 Apr; 121(4):829–46.

14. Nazeer S, Shafi MI. Objective perspective in colposcopy. Best Pract Res Clin Obstet Gynaecol. 2011 Oct; 25(5):631–40.

15. Prendiville W, Ritter J, Tatti S, Twiggs LB. Colposcopy: Management Options. Philedelphia. WB Saunders; 2003.

16. Saslow D, Solomon D, Lawson HW, Killackey M, Kulasingam SL, Cain JM, Garcia FA, Moriarty AT, Waxman AG, Wilbur DC, Wentzensen N, Downs LS Jr, Spitzer M, Moscicki AB, Franco EL, Stoler MH, Schiffman M, Castle PE, Myers ER, Chelmow D, Herzig A, Kim JJ, Kinney W, Herschel WL, Waldman J. American Cancer Society, American Society for Colposcopy and cervical Patholgy and American Society for Clinical Pathology screening guidelines for the prevention and early detection of cervical cancer. American society. J Low Genit Tract Dis. 2012 Jul; 16(3):175–204.

17. Tatti S, Bornstein J, Prendiville W. Colposcopy: a global perspective: introduction to the new IFCPC colposcopy terminology. Obstet Gynecol Clin North Am. 2013 Jun; 40(2):235–50.

18. Waxman AG. Colposcopy, Cervical Screening, and HPV. In: Obstetrics and Gynecology Clinics of North America. 2008, vol 35/No 4.

19. Wright TC Jr, Massad LS, Dunton CJ, Spitzer M, Wilkinson EJ, Solomon D. 2006 consensus guidelines for the management of women with abnormal cervical screening tests. J Low Genit Tract Dis 2007; 11:201-22. Erratum in: J Low Genit Tract Dis. 2008 Jul; 12(3):255.

20. Wright TC Jr, Massad LS, Dunton CJ, Spitzer M, Wilkinson EJ, Solomon D; 2006 American Society for Colposcopy and Cervical Pathology-sponsored Consensus Conference. 2006 consensus guidelines for the management of women with cervical intraepithelial neoplasia or adenocarcinoma in situ. J Low Genit Tract Dis. 2007 Oct; 11(4):223-39. Erratum in: J Low Genit Tract Dis. 2008 Jan;12(1):63.

Useful Links

1. http://www.asccp.org American society of colposcopy and cytopathology

2. http://www.cdc.gov/vaccines/vpd-vac/hpv/default Centres for disease control and prevention: HPV vaccination

3. http://www.cytopathnet.org/ Online Resource for cytopathology

4. http://screening.iarc.fr International agency for research on cancer

5. http://www.ifcpc.org International federation of cervical pathology and colposcopy

6. http://www.ifcpc.org/Healthcare_Professionals/Practice_Improvement/index.asp IFCPC's web based Colposcopy Practice Improvement Program

7. http://www.issvd.org The International Society for the Study of Vulvovaginal Disease

Index